A Textbook of Psychiatric and Mental Health Nursing

2004

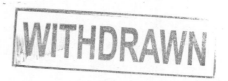

For Churchill Livingstone
Publisher: Mary Law
Project editor: Dinah Thom
Production controller: Nancy Henry
Design: Design Resources Unit
Sales promotion executive: Hilary Brown

A Textbook of Psychiatric and Mental Health Nursing

Edited by

Julia I. Brooking PhD BSc RMN SRN DipN CertEd

Professor and Head of the Department of Nursing Studies, The Medical School, University of Birmingham

Susan A. H. Ritter MA RGN RMN

Lecturer in Psychiatric Nursing, Institute of Psychiatry, University of London;
Honorary Clinical Nurse Specialist, Bethlem Royal and Maudsley Hospital, London

Ben L. Thomas MSc BSc RGN RMN DipN RNT

Chief Nurse Advisor, Director of Quality, Honorary Lecturer, Institute of Psychiatry,
University of London and Bethlem Royal and Maudsley Hospital, London

Foreword by

Jack C. Hayward CBE PhD BSc SRN RMN DipN RNT

Emeritus Professor and Head of the Nursing Research Unit, King's College, University of London

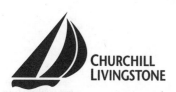

CHURCHILL
LIVINGSTONE

EDINBURGH LONDON MADRID MELBOURNE NEW YORK AND TOKYO 1992

CHURCHILL LIVINGSTONE
Medical Division of Pearson Professional Ltd

Distributed in the United States of America
by Churchill Livingstone Inc.,
650 Avenue of the Americas, New York, 10011,
and by associated companies, branches and
representatives throughout the world.

First published 1992
    Reprinted 1992
    Reprinted 1994
    Reprinted 1996

ISBN 0-443-03461-3

British Library Cataloguing in Publication Data
A catalogue record for this book is available from
the British Library.

Library of Congress Cataloging in Publication Data
A textbook of psychiatric and mental health nursing/edited
    by Julia Irene Brookling, Susan A. H. Ritter,
    Ben L. Thomas;
        foreword by Jack C. Hayward.
            p.   cm.
    Includes index.
    ISBN 0-443-03461-3
    1. Psychiatric nursing. 2. Psychiatric nursing—
    Great Britain.
    I. Brooking, Julia. II. Ritter, Susan. III. Thomas, Ben L.
    [DNLM: 1. Psychiatric Nursing. WY 160 T355]
RC440.T49   1992
610.73′68—dc20
DNLM/DLC
for Library of Congress   91-35319
                                                      CIP

The
publisher's
policy is to use
**paper manufactured
from sustainable forests**

Produced by Longman Singapore Publishers Pte Ltd
Printed in Singapore

Foreword

It is a great pleasure to welcome a new British textbook on psychiatric nursing, especially one which ranges so widely and deeply into the subject. A glance at the contents page shows just how comprehensive is the coverage and suggests that this book will be a valuable addition to the fast-growing body of literature on this oft-neglected area of nursing.

Many of those working in the mental health services are impatient at what they see as a very slow rate of change in prevailing attitudes, customs and practices. Yet changes there have been, and if we single out the area of books and journals written for and by psychiatric nurses they demonstrate that the changes during my own professional lifetime have been dramatic. When training for my RMN in the 1950s there was available one main textbook — the famous 'Red Handbook' — plus a scattering of other texts written largely by non-nurses. Often a nurse was judged on his or her expertise in general nursing or knowledge of psychiatry rather than in what is now recognised as the distinctive body of knowledge underpinning good psychiatric nursing. Although the past 30 years have seen a number of encouraging developments there are, of course, no grounds for complacency and the fight goes on for more resources, greater public awareness and higher levels of professionalism in the mental health services. It is appropriate and timely that this book is aimed fairly and squarely at informing the psychiatric nurse of today and tomorrow.

Only those who have edited a volume of this size and scale will know the personal and practical demands involved before such work reaches publication. Our present authors are to be congratulated on this important addition to the literature which I warmly commend to the reader.

London, 1992   J. C. H.

Preface

This book represents the culmination of several years of work in attempting to bring together in one volume much of the knowledge base from which psychiatric nursing is derived. There are many excellent texts available which help nurses to develop their clinical skills, but this book differs in that it focuses on the research and theory which underlie practice, education and management in psychiatric nursing.

It is our view that psychiatric nursing is now a highly complex and wide-ranging activity and that no single author or small group of authors can reasonably be expected to have expertise across the whole range of the subject. For this reason, we have brought together a large number of contributions from nurses and other mental health professionals, all of whom have specialist expertise in the topics about which they have written.

Almost all of the contributors are working in Britain, so this book to a large extent reflects British thinking and practice, although drawing from research literature published internationally. We recognize that the manifestations of psychiatric disorders and methods of care vary in different cultures and that some chapters (e.g. on mental health legislation) reflect an entirely British perspective. However, we have attempted as far as possible to avoid parochialism and we believe that much in this book will be valuable to nurses in other countries.

Unlike many of the currently available textbooks, this book is not confined to a single model or theory of psychiatric nursing. Our approach is deliberately eclectic, drawing on as many relevant theories as possible. The underlying value system could be described as scientific; each chapter attempts to review and evaluate relevant empirical research. This approach does not result in comfortable certainties for the reader, but we hope it accurately reflects the knowledge base of the discipline, which is characterized by controversy and uncertainty.

Omissions are unavoidable in a single volume, and we make no claim to comprehensiveness. For example, space did not permit the inclusion of important topics such as forensic psychiatric nursing, care of the mentally ill mother and her child, care of people with mental handicap and associated psychiatric problems, and the role of the family in patient management. No doubt the length of this book could easily have doubled and many subjects would still have been omitted.

In an edited textbook, it is inevitable that each chapter will have stylistic differences, reflecting the different interests and approaches of each author. We hope that all provide a useful overview of their subjects, referring the reader to important material in the area, and that all demonstrate a critical, intellectually rigorous and research-based examination of their topics. In short, this book is intended to be a scholarly introduction to psychiatric nursing.

This book has not been written for one particular segment of the nursing market. It should be equally useful for students who need a broad overview and for qualified nurses who need updating on advances in relation to particular topics. We hope that students and practitioners in other mental health professions will also find the material helpful.

J. I. B.
S. A. H. R.
Birmingham and London, 1992   B. L. T.

Acknowledgements

We are grateful to all our contributors for their willingness to participate in this complex and time-consuming project. Our publishers' staff have given us constant encouragement and support and must be thanked for their endless patience in what has been a long and sometimes painful process.

We have been fortunate to work in settings where debate and argument with well-informed colleagues is part of everyday academic and clinical life. Our thinking has been considerably sharpened by contact with nursing and psychiatric colleagues at the Institute of Psychiatry and King's College, University of London, the Bethlem Royal and Maudsley Hospital, London, and the University of Birmingham. We thank our colleagues and friends for their advice, ideas and criticism, particularly Professor Ian Brockington, Mr Eric Byers, Mr Harry Field, Dr Kevin Gournay, Professor Jack Hayward, Professor Isaac Marks, Dr Matthijs Muijen, Professor Robin Murray, Dr Peter Nolan, Ms Lynette Rentoul, Mr David Russell, Professor Gerald Russell, Mrs Pamela Tibbles, Mr Robert Tunmore, Mr Simon Vearnals and Professor Jenifer Wilson-Barnett. As editors, we are of course solely responsible for errors and omissions.

J. I. B.
S. A. H. R.
Birmingham and London, 1992   B. L. T.

Contributors

Ros Alstead BSc SRN RMN
Director of Mental Health Services,
The Royal London Hospital
(St Clements), London

Maura Appleby BSc RGN RHV
Health Visitor, Tameside and Glossop
Health Authority

Christine A. Barnes BA SRN RMN
Genetic Counsellor, South East Thames Genetic
Centre, Guy's Hospital, London;
Formerly Research Associate,
Nursing Research Unit,
King's College, University of London

Alison Bond RGN RMN RCNT CertEd RNT
Tutor, In-Service Education and Training,
Bethlem Royal and Maudsley Hospital
Special Health Authority

Charles Brooker MSc BA DipNEd RNT RMN
Senior Research Fellow, Department of Nursing,
University of Manchester, Manchester

Julia I. Brooking PhD BSc RMN SRN DipN
CertEd
Professor and Head of Department of Nursing
Studies, The Medical School,
University of Birmingham, Birmingham

Gillian E. Chapman PhD MSc BSc RGN RSCN
Nursing Officer, Department of Health;
Formerly Lecturer in Nursing Studies,
King's College, University of London

Michael J. Connolly BSc RGN
Staff Nurse, St Ann's Hospice, Manchester

John K. Davies MSc
Lecturer in Pharmacology, King's College,
University of London

Katherine E. Ferguson MSc BSc RGN RMN
Lecturer, Department of Nursing,
University of Manchester

David Field PhD MA BA AM
Senior Lecturer in Medical Sociology,
Department of Epidemiology and Public Health,
University of Leicester

E. Morva Fordham PhD MSc BSc RGN RNT
Formerly Lecturer in Nursing Studies,
King's College, University of London

Richard James Frisby MSc
Senior Lecturer, Normanby College of
Health Care Studies, London

Kevin Gournay PhD MPhil CPsychol AFBPsS
RMN RNMH CertBehPsychotherapy
Principal Lecturer, Joint Appointment
Schools of Psychology and Health Care Studies,
Middlesex Polytechnic, Middlesex

Sandra Lask MSc BA PGCE RGN RNT
Lecturer in Psychology, Roehampton Institute,
London

Helen Macdonald BSc RGN
Research Associate, Nursing Research Unit,
King's College, University of London

Edana Minghella BSc RMN PGCEA
Lecturer in Interpersonal Skills,
Normanby College of Health Care Studies,
London

Matthijs F. Muijen PhD MD MSc MRCPsych
Director, Research and Development
for Psychiatry, London

Marion Talmadge Reed RN MN CS RMN
Psychiatric Clinical Nurse Specialist,
Emergency Room Psychiatric Crisis Team,
Newton Wellesley Hospital,
Newton, Massachusetts, USA

Lynette Rentoul MSc BSc ChartClinPsychol
Lecturer in Psychology,
Department of Nursing Studies,
King's College, University of London

Robert Rentoul BA
Lecturer in Psychology, Goldsmith's College,
University of London;
Formerly Lecturer in Physiology,
University of Edinburgh

Susan A. H. Ritter MA RGN RMN
Lecturer in Psychiatric Nursing,
Institute of Psychiatry,
University of London;
Honorary Clinical Nurse Specialist,
Bethlem Royal and Maudsley Hospital,
London

David Skidmore PhD MSc RMN RCNT CertEd
DipPE MBISC
Principal Lecturer, Department of Health Care
Studies, Manchester Polytechnic

Steve Taylor PhD MPhil BA LLB
Lecturer in Medical Sociology and Medical Law,
University of London

Ben L. Thomas MSc BSc RGN RMN DipN RNT
Chief Nurse Advisor, Director of Quality,
Honorary Lecturer, Institute of Psychiatry and
the Bethlem Royal and Maudsley Hospital,
London

Robert G. D. Tunmore BSc RGN RMN
Tutor, School of Nursing,
Bethlem Royal and Maudsley Hospital,
London

Stuart W. Turner, MA MD MRCP MRCPsych
Senior Clinical Lecturer and Honorary
Consultant Psychiatrist,
Middlesex Hospital, London

Christine Webb PhD MSc BA SRN RSCN RNT
Professor of Nursing, University of Manchester

Alison E. While PhD MSc BSc RGN RHV
Senior Lecturer, Department of Nursing,
King's College, University of London

Jenifer Wilson-Barnett PhD MSc BA SRN DipN
RNT FRCN
Professor and Head of the Department of
Nursing Studies, King's College,
University of London

Contents

1

Introduction

J. I. Brooking

Psychiatric nursing as a practice discipline uses knowledge from a variety of sources. These include the social and behavioural sciences of psychology, sociology, social policy, politics, economics, management, education and anthropology; the biological sciences of physiology, anatomy, genetics, pharmacology, therapeutics and neurochemistry; the medical sciences including, of course, psychiatry; and the humanities such as ethics, philosophy, law and history. In addition, nursing is rapidly developing as an academic discipline in its own right, as exemplified by the massively increasing volume of research on nursing in recent years, by the development of academic departments of nursing in universities and polytechnics, and by the rapid expansion of undergraduate and postgraduate degrees in nursing.

Another value which underpins this work is the belief that nursing is rarely an activity which can be carried out in isolation from other health professionals. In the past, our largely separate educational systems created barriers between members of the various mental health professions, reducing the effectiveness of teamwork as patients found themselves caught between factions with different ideologies and treatment approaches. This situation is fortunately beginning to change, with a greater emphasis on genuine multidisciplinary teamwork, with shared education, increased recognition of others, skills, greater mutual respect and understanding, and deliberate blurring of roles. The expansion of the case management approach in community psychiatry is a clear example of this welcome trend.

It has in the past been claimed that the fundamental difference between the two major health professions of medicine and nursing lay in the distinction between curing and caring. It was argued that doctors had a primary responsibility for diagnosis and treatment, whereas nurses helped patients to deal with the problems of daily living resulting from the disease process, and cared for the patients' basic physical and psychosocial needs during the period of illness. It was this belief that produced the hostility among some senior nurses to the introduction of nurse behavioural psychotherapists, a group of nurses who undoubtedly have responsibility both for diagnosis and the prescription and implementation of treatment.

It is our view that psychiatrists do not have exclusive expertise in diagnosis and treatment, any more than nurses have the prerogative to caring. Professional role boundaries exist largely to serve the interests of the professions rather than patients, and we consider that the responsibility of nursing as a profession is to identify and respond to the health-related needs of the population. We welcome the blurring of role boundaries in so far as it results in the provision of more effective and efficient services for patients. We therefore hope that this book may be read and found useful by mental health professionals other than nurses.

The book begins with a section on some of the current issues which impact on the development of psychiatric nursing as a profession. Part 2 introduces some of the foundation disciplines which contribute to the knowledge base of psychiatric nursing. Part 3 addresses the principles of practice in a variety of settings. Part 4 deals with nursing interventions for patients with particular types of problems. The final section considers the types of therapeutic approaches which are most commonly used in nursing practice.

The use of the terminology 'psychiatric' nursing rather than the currently more fashionable 'mental health' nursing is deliberate. There is little evidence that many nurses are engaged in much mental health promotion work or, indeed, that primary prevention of mental illness is possible in many circumstances. While we acknowledge that health promotion is important, we are concerned that this trend is resulting in neglect of the most seriously mentally ill. For example, there are already indications that with the move to primary care attachments, some community psychiatric nurses are giving priority to the so-called 'worried well' (those people with minor neurotic disorders) at the expense of those with greatest need, such as the patients suffering from major psychoses. Given that resources will always be limited, we believe that nursing services should be directed at those with the most serious problems, particularly in view of the high rates of spontaneous remission in mild disorders. Hence our preference for the term 'psychiatric' nursing is a reflection of our view that the psychiatrically ill are and should remain the main focus of nursing attention.

Part 1

Issues and developments in psychiatric nursing

2

History

M. J. Connolly

THE VALUE OF HISTORICAL INVESTIGATION

Is psychiatric nursing progressing towards better patient care? Why has psychiatric nursing failed to emerge totally from the shadow of general nursing? Why is the role of the psychiatric nurse so ill-defined and so poorly understood? Why is there a discrepancy between the work described in the literature and the reality of ward-based work?

These and other contemporary questions relating to psychiatric nursing cannot be fully answered by looking into the history of the profession, but such research can shed some light on possible explanations. A study of historical trends and developments enables us to identify some of the factors which have led to the development of psychiatric nursing as we know it today.

For example, historical research has shown that Victorian asylums were completely self-contained communities, in which the nurses and attendants worked in the wards, the infirmary, the laundry and the farms, assisting the patients to maintain that community (Scull 1981). Such information reveals the extent to which the closure of the farms and the infirmaries, coupled with the employment of a separate staff of cleaning, laundry and kitchen workers, and the introduction of occupational therapists has removed many of the previous roles of the nurse. It may also explain the reluctance of psychiatric nurses to give up the institution-based role for a community-based role (Mallinson Report 1983).

Historical studies reveal, too, that in the past psychiatric nurses have tended to be very active over issues such as pay and living standards rather than professional status and the improvement of the profession. This may explain why they are inclined to join the more traditional trade unions, why the general nursing body has tended to look down on them (Maggs 1983), and why research into psychiatric nursing has been neglected compared with other branches of nursing (Wilson-Barnett 1988).

This chapter examines some of these issues, and provides an introduction to methods of inquiry appropriate to the study of nursing history.

METHODS OF HISTORICAL INVESTIGATION

Three methods of inquiry are commonly used:

1. The earliest records are restricted to what are known as secondary sources, such as historical texts specifically related to nursing (e.g. Abel-Smith 1960)
2. Archival sources — that is, documents such as records and reports kept by individuals or institutions — are available for later periods (Nolan 1986)
3. Oral history — that is, information obtained through personal interviews — can be used for the most recent past.

Other useful sources of information are texts concerned with the general social and political conditions (Thompson 1968).

Primary sources, such as archives and oral history, are obviously the most reliable, since they are less likely to be coloured by a second interpretation of the facts (Carr 1981). Secondary literature on psychiatric nursing often reveals what Davies (1980) refers to as the 'self-congratulatory' style, which tends to assume that change necessarily means progress. For example, Goddard (1953) in *The History of Mental Nursing* asserts:

And so gradually the improvements have come. From monks to the trained and efficient nurses; from

doctors who were nonentities to specialists in nerve diseases and psychologists. All go to make the mental hospitals as we know them today (p. 77).

These conventional historical accounts, which present psychiatric nursing as a simple chronology of events or as the outcome of progressive enlightenment, tend to ignore the complex historical, social and cultural centre in which the profession has developed. Fortunately, more objective secondary accounts are also available (notably Walk 1961).

EIGHTEENTH AND NINETEENTH CENTURIES

Walk (1961) describes the changes of attitude towards the care of the insane brought about by Phillipe Pinel (c. 1790) in France, and by William Tuke (c. 1800) in England; almost simultaneously, though independently of each other, these men initiated the first major breakthrough in the case of the insane by unchaining the lunatics in the asylums.

Before Pinel and Tuke, and in some areas even after their work, procedures now seen as cruel were used as forms of treatment. According to Tuke (1820) the routine treatments included blood-letting, starvation, purging, blistering, surprise baths and whipping, and any method of inducing fear or terror was approved. A book published in 1804, entitled *Practical Observations on Insanity*, describes a machine into which four patients were strapped, and which, when worked by a windlass, formed a sort of horizontal swing revolving a hundred times a minute (Cox 1804).

The Earl of Shaftesbury, a 19th century philanthropist and reformer, reported that:

At the present time, when people go into an asylum, they see everything clean, orderly, decent and quiet, and a great number of persons in this later generation cannot believe there was anything terrible in the management of insanity; and many say 'After all, a lunatic asylum is not so terrible as I believed'. When we began our visitations, one of the first rooms we went into contained nearly a hundred and fifty patients, in every form of madness, a large proportion of them chained to the walls, some melancholy, some furious, but the noise and din and roar were such that we positively could not hear each other; every form of disease and every form of madness was there; I never beheld anything so horrible and so miserable (Tuke 1820).

The first change from this state was the 'moral treatment' pioneered in England at the York Retreat set up by Tuke in 1796. This system presumed that the patient was generally 'capable of influence through the kindly affection of the heart and the medium of understanding' (Walk 1961). Jones (1960) suggests that such changes in the public attitude towards the insane in the first half of the 19th century were part of a 'new social conscience' that developed in society generally at this time. There was a desire to tackle poverty, sickness and ignorance, and the country came to share a common ethical principle — a belief that the community had a responsibility to the weak.

The 1845 Lunatics Act was the government's response to public feeling, and was the culmination of the work of the Earl of Shaftesbury.

The growing acceptance of moral treatment of the insane as desirable affected the role of the attendant. John Conolly, the Medical Superintendent of the Middlesex Asylum at Hanwell (the largest asylum at the time) saw the need for a new class of attendant who could understand something of patients' mental conditions and behaviour. Conolly was ahead of his time in suggesting that asylum nursing should be a skilled profession, depending more upon intellectual and personal gifts than a strong nerve and powerful muscles (Jones 1960, p. 14).

The Earl of Shaftesbury, having accomplished the building of a number of Victorian asylums (many of which are still in use today) and helped to bring about significant changes in the law, now turned his attention to the urgent need to recruit male and female nurses of the right type (Jones 1960). He considered that the wages were too low (comparable only to those of a house-maid), and that 'the hours were extremely long and the work exacting'. Significantly, the women tended to be referred to as 'nurses', and the men as 'attendants'. There was no great shortage of nurses, because 'the tendency of a woman's nature is to nurse', but good male attendants were far more difficult to recruit. All who offered

their services were 'of too low a class . . . an uneducated class'. The attendants or 'keepers' were described in 1837 by a Dr Browne as 'the unemployed of other professions . . . if they possess physical strength and a tolerable reputation for sobriety, it is enough; and the latter is frequently dispensed with. They enter upon their duties altogether ignorant of what insanity is' (Browne 1837).

In the middle of the 19th century, many improvements were made, at least in terms of attitudes towards the insane. Attendants were expected to play an example-setting and guiding role with patients, rather than the traditional custodial function. Discussions concerning the need for the education and training of attendants did take place, but their results were not put into practice, owing to expected costs.

Many of the asylums built at this time still function as psychiatric hospitals today, with their archives intact; modern historians are thus able to carry out detailed research, rather than gleaning only a general impression from the work of historians of the period. Archives of particular interest are pay-rolls, rules of the institution, course syllabuses, students' note-books and attendants' reports. Such primary sources not only reveal relevant factual data, but also describe conditions of work in these institutions.

For example, records still available in Springfield Hospital, London, reveal that students at what was then the Surrey Lunatic Asylum received a course of lectures (probably the first in the country) in 1843, from Alexander Morrison, the Asylum's Medical Superintendent. He reports that:

To give the attendants just views of the importance of the duties they have to perform towards the afflicted objects of their care, I have lectured on the principles which ought to regulate their conduct, and I have pleasure in stating that my lecturing has been received with attention, and that the behaviour of both male and female attendants is humane and judicious (Report of the Visiting Justices of the Surrey Lunatic Asylum. Epiphany Quarter 1843).

In 1842, at the Surrey Asylum, the attendants worked from 6.00 am until 9.00 pm, and slept in rooms adjacent to the wards. There were nine male and nine female attendants for 350 patients. The Visiting Justices heard in that year that the attendants were:

The instruments for carrying into effect every remedial measure, and it requires, on their part, firmness and self-control blended with humanity and forbearance; at the same time, they are called upon to perform many menial offices. Their remuneration has therefore been fixed on a very liberal scale, increasing annually during the first five years of service.

This 'liberal remuneration' of between £25 and £30 per year for male attendants was quite generous compared with salaries in other asylums; in 1850, the average pay of male attendants was £26 per year. However, attendants remained amongst the lowest paid workers in the country, and the female attendants earned considerably less; their pay averaged between £12 and £16 per year.

By mid-century, although life for an attendant was far from comfortable, 'there was a spirit of humanity in the treatment. . . Asylums in the real sense of the word, in that they provided refuge from the old bad institutions' (Jones 1960). Unfortunately, the improvement was to be short-lived. The transfer of large numbers of chronically mentally ill people from the workhouses to the asylums, and the admission of mentally ill people who were homeless, unemployed and impoverished, led to overcrowding in the asylums. This, coupled with a period of public complacency, caused standards to fall again. At Surrey, a visiting physician reported, 'everywhere, attendants, we are convinced, maltreat, abuse and terrify patients when the backs of medical officers are turned' (Jones 1960, p. 24). The same physician also noted with dismay that 'the old system of providing incontinent patients with straw palliasses instead of mattresses has been revived'.

Jones (1960) suggests that worries as to the apparent rise in the numbers of insane people in the country led to feelings that the general public needed to be protected, both from the insane, and from being wrongfully declared insane. Public attitudes towards the mentally ill became generally negative, and this was reflected in the Lunacy Act of 1890 which was more concerned with protection of the sane than the insane. The Act viewed insanity merely as a condition which necessitated

depriving a person of his liberty, and as such one that must be clearly defined so that every possible device to limit these circumstances could be used. Since only the Justices of the Peace (a lay authority) had the power to certify a person as insane, and since asylums could only take certified patients, early diagnosis and treatment of both the most mild and the most acute conditions could not take place in the asylums.

This was not only disastrous for patients in need of care and unable to pay privately, but also meant that the work of the asylum attendants became once again largely custodial. The mid-century spirit of humanity in treatment had now, fifty years later, been lost, to be replaced by a situation in which 'large, soulless institutions were being built for thousands at a time, with little sense of community and where attendants were relied upon for strength and intimidation, rather than friendliness and common sense' (Jones 1960).

By 1909, the number of patients in the Surrey Asylum, built for 350 inpatients, had risen to 1235.

At the turn of the century, the morale of attendants was particularly low — 'bad food, broken sleep from the close proximity of noisy patients, and the irksomeness of the many regulations, was responsible for the high staff turnover' (Mercier 1894). The working day commonly began at 6.00 am and ended at 8.00 pm, with an extension to 10.00 pm once a week; this meant an average of 89 hours per week. In 1912, things were no better, if this poem written by an anonymous attendant and printed in a union magazine is to be believed:

It is the wretched victims of this poison in life's cup
who in increasing numbers fill these vast Asylums up;
And with this human wreckage we are herded
All day long.
For all the hours heav'n sends must we
Mix with this mad throng
Repulsive work we have to do and bear
obscene abuse,
And undergo a mental strain from which
there is no truce;
Our tempers through the live long day
are tried full many a time;
But if we make the slightest slip 'tis
counted as a crime.

Small are our wages and our food oft
times unfit to eat
While soul-degrading tyranny our mis'ry
doth complete

                    (quoted in Carpenter 1980, p. 141).

THE UNIONS

The role of organised labour within the asylums has tended not to reflect that of general hospitals, though they do have common starting points. The National Asylum Workers Union (eventually to join other unions to become the Confederation of Health Service Employees) and the College (eventually to become the Royal College) of Nursing, were both preceded by associations set up to provide state registration through examination.

The British Nursing Association (founded in 1887) for general nurses, refused entry to the register to graduates of an examination for 'good attendants' set by the Medico-Psychological Association, which was the association of psychiatrists. Grounds for exclusion were explained in 1895 by Mrs Bedford-Fenwick, the President of the (by then) Royal British Nursing Association:

No person can be considered trained who has only worked in hospitals and asylums for the insane . . . considering the present class of persons known as male attendants, one can hardly believe that their admission will tend to raise the status of the Association (Adams 1969, p. 13).

The fact that the asylum attendants had to work in the asylum's infirmary, caring for physically ill inmates, as well as in their normal wards, suggests that they should have been eligible for inclusion in the register, but it was not to be.

However, it seems likely that a snub from the Royal British Nursing Association would not have troubled asylum attendants very much. It was the Medical Superintendents and the senior attendants who were attempting to achieve status parity with general nursing; the attendants themselves had more pressing worries.

The Asylum Workers Association, set up in 1897, was again dominated by Medical Superintendents and senior attendants, and the 1909 Asylum Officers Superannuation Act (at the request of the Asylum Workers Association) became a vehicle for new contributory pensions. This led to strikes and the formation of the more radical National Asylum Workers Union. This union considered the conditions of service and pay for asylum workers so bad that it did not concern itself with status or professionalism for many years. Professionalism was considered to be pretentious; as is made clear in a letter to the union's journal in 1912, which displayed bitter feelings about the notion that asylum workers were of a higher status than tradesmen:

Why should you grumble because a tradesman works 50 a week and you 80 or 90 or more? Have you not your dignity? Cling to that precious position; feed the wife and children with it when pay day is approaching; when the coal man comes for his bill, try paying him with a dignified look

                    (quoted in Carpenter 1980, p. 142).

The objectives of the National Asylum Workers Union, when it was set up in 1910, were:

— to improve generally the conditions of asylum workers
— to reduce the hours of labour by Act of Parliament
— to provide allowances for the protection of victimised members of the union
— generally to regulate relations between employers and employed

                    (quoted in Adams 1969, p. 18).

The Union presented a Parliamentary Committee with expositions of conditions for attendants; the Committee, however, also heard from spokesmen such as a Dr Cassidy of Lancaster Asylum, who was of the opinion that:

too much freedom would be distinctly demoralizing for the nurse . . . it is in the interest of morality that they should be confined indoors on their off-duty hours

                    (quoted in Carpenter 1980, p. 6).

The first twenty years of the 20th century were times of preoccupation with training and education in nursing, but not until 1920 did the National Asylum Workers Union contribute towards this.

The College of Nursing, set up in 1916, refused further pleas by the Medico-Psychological Association to allow attendants to join, even though attendants were taking the Association's course and examinations in increasing numbers. In fact, the new General Nursing Council started its own course and examination for attendants; hence, there were two qualifications open to attendants. However, neither qualification appears to have carried much weight, because the mental nursing qualification was not essential to gain senior positions in an asylum, and many of the matrons had general training only and no experience of asylums whatsoever.

TWENTIETH CENTURY: 1900–1959

In psychiatry generally, the 20th century brought renewed optimism and interest from the public. The 1930 Mental Treatment Act introduced 'voluntary' and 'temporary' patients, which did away with some of the pessimism associated with the certification process. During both world wars, many staff members were enlisted or redeployed, and many asylums were taken over by the military so that patients had to be redistributed. Asylums thus became very overcrowded in wartime, and once again the work of the attendants was that of containment of large numbers. Allegations of malpractice rose sharply:

The result (of men leaving asylum work for the Services and women leaving for better paid munitions work) was a massive rise in the number of patients dying from diseases such as dysentery and tuberculosis. Years later, scandal broke with the publication of Montagu Lomaz's *The Experiences of an Asylum Doctor* which detailed conditions inside an unidentified asylum during wartime. There was an alleged tendency towards over liberal use of sedatives and laxatives by nursing staff.

Other 'scandals' also came to light, with nursing staff again the main target of criticism
(Carpenter 1980, p. 9).

These allegations led to pressure from the National Asylum Workers Union and the National Council for Lunacy Reform for a Royal Commission into the Lunacy Laws. In 1926 a Royal Commission was set up and it in turn led to the 1930 Mental Treatment Act.

Between the wars there was a change, if only in nomenclature. Asylums eventually became mental hospitals, and both male and female attendants became nurses. The National Asylum Workers Union became the Mental Health and Institutional Workers Union in 1931, and, together with the Hospital and Welfare Services Union, it eventually became the Confederation of Health Service Employees (COHSE) in 1946, with a membership of 40 000.

During the 1930s there was a considerable influx of men into mental nursing from the depressed areas of the country. Attempts to improve standards of nursing between the wars was hampered to some extent by the double examination, but also by the type of people recruited. According to Jones (1960), the entry requirements in the 1930s involved candidates being 'physically fit, able to take part in organized games or play a musical instrument'.

The Regulations and Orders of the Springfield Mental Hospital (1926), a booklet given to all employees, instructs the nurses to show 'kindness and forbearance', and suggests that 'example is better than precept'. However, the strictness of the rules provides a regimental impression of hospital life: patients had to be counted in and out of the wards and gardens:

During the period of night duty, five rounds are to be made in the Female Division. In the Male Division, six rounds are to be made. No dormitory or single room must be left unvisited on each round, unless by special direction of a Medical Officer (p. 21).

Any attendant or servant, through whose negligence a patient escapes, shall pay such proportion of the expense incurred in recovering the patient, as the visiting Justices shall direct (p. 25).

The charge nurse must always be present during the bathing of patients
(quoted from *The Regulations and Orders of the Springfield Mental Hospital* 1926, p. 26).

That such specific rules were thought necessary may be a reflection of the type of nurse/attendant employed, who could not be relied upon to exhibit any responsibility or common sense, or of the concern of the visiting committees wishing to cover themselves from any charges of neglect or maladministration. In any case, they can hardly have been conducive to the moral treatment of patients with forbearance and understanding advocated by Pinel and Tuke, and introduced by Conolly seventy years before.

The variety of duties described in the Regulations and in other archival evidence suggests that around the 1930s the attendants would recruit the labour of their patients for the cleaning and feeding of patients, the cleaning and maintenance of the wards, and the operation of the laundry, the farm and the cricket pitch.

After World War II, plans were made for a National Health Service (NHS) and a new 'Welfare State'. The incorporation of the management of mental health into the NHS at its inception in 1948 changed little, although the category 'rate-aided patient' was abolished and free care became the right of all citizens.

The category of 'voluntary patient' had been extended since its introduction in 1930, and by 1957, 75% of all admissions were on a voluntary basis (Brooking 1984). However, the system of admission and the legal rights of patients had not changed since the 19th century Lunacy Laws. These were only dismantled with the 1959 Mental Health Act, when mental health professionals finally regained control from the magistrates.

Interviews with retired psychiatric nurses employed during the post-war years have provided us with descriptions of mental hospitals during this time. Such interviews reveal that, shortly after World War II, all the wards at Springfield Hospital (formerly Surrey Asylum) were locked, apart from a few geriatric wards. The gardens were also locked and the hospital as a whole was surrounded by fences. The main block was strictly segregated — male staff and male patients on one side; female staff and female patients on the other. Only maintenance staff and doctors regularly saw both sides. The wards themselves were furnished with hard wooden chairs and long workhouse tables, and there were no curtains between the beds.

One nurse reported that the preoccupation with cleanliness and orderliness was almost obsessional, especially on the female side; the beds would sometimes be lined up with pieces of string to ensure perfect regularity. Particular time periods were allocated for each task — so much for bed-making, so much for meal-times, when staff and patients would eat together around the long tables on the wards.

The role of the nurses was varied, and included organising patients in their work: on the wards or on the farm, rolling the cricket pitch or making brooms or furniture. There was also a tailor's workshop where patients would make and maintain clothing and bedding. However, there seems to have been little effort to equip patients for a possible return to the community at large. Yet, in defence of the old system, one nurse reported that by contributing towards the maintenance of the hospital, patients derived a feeling of worth. Today, the employment of ancillary staff in mental hospitals gives the patients — especially long-stay patients — very little sense of contributing to their own environment.

From these accounts of Springfield Hospital (a typical mental hospital of the 1950s), it thus seems that, while there was strict regulation, with rather impersonal procedures for patients, tight discipline and a much-feared hierarchy for nurses, there was nevertheless a sense of common purpose in a community which was self-contained and virtually self-maintaining.

1959 ONWARDS: CONTEMPORARY ISSUES

There have been many changes since the 1950s, not least in the role of the nurse and the opportunities open to the patient. However, not all changes over time constitute progress, and, since Pinel and Tuke's unchaining of 'lunatics', it would be wrong to assume a steady improvement in conditions for patients and their carers in mental hospitals.

During the 1960s, the way forward for psychiatry was planned as a move away from the Victorian institutions towards care for the mentally ill within the community. It was a time of national prosperity, and mental health planners assumed, perhaps naively, that the necessary funds would be allocated for this purpose. Predictions for the mid 1970s and early 1980s were that the care of the mentally ill would be shared equally between community agencies and psychiatric units in general hospitals. However, due to a variety of factors, mainly economic ones, these predictions have not been borne out. While institutional care was run down over this period, community care was not sufficiently built up, and as a result some mentally ill patients have been left homeless and destitute. This problem is central to mental health service planning at the present time.

The Mallinson Report (1983) by the Confederation of Health Service Employees expressed 'serious concern that government cutbacks in the National Health Service will be implemented under the guise of a movement towards community care' (p. 45). The idea that community care would be cheaper was disputed by the Mallinson Report, which implied that more staff rather than less would be required as a result of the closure of hospital wards. There was, however, also concern that hospitals would be completely closed; the Department of Health and Social Security stated that 'reduction in the number of in-patients does not bring matching cost savings unless a hospital is "closed"'.

According to MIND (National Association for Mental Health) (1983) the reason that mental hospital staff opposed the move towards community care and a change in their jobs, was that the underfunding of psychiatry was reflected in low wages. Consequently, the staff felt isolated and sceptical. Furthermore, since there has been little evidence that care in the community is of benefit, they mistrusted the changes, suspecting them of being an excuse for the running down of existing services. The Mallinson Report (1983), while supporting the idea of community care, blamed the low staff morale on the lack of common purpose.

From the interviews and from other descriptive works discussed by Cormack (1983), it would seem that the contemporary role of the psychiatric nurse is unclear, and there exists a discrepancy between the nursing literature and the actual experiences of ward-based nurses. The introduction of occupational therapists may have led to a patient-orientated therapy, but it has also deprived nurses of a clear aspect of their role. In the past, nurses accompanied patients to the hospital workshops, laundry and farm, and taught and encouraged patients to clean the wards and work with them towards the upkeep of the hospital. Today many

of these practices would be frowned upon, as more patient-orientated work is encouraged. A distinction has been made between mental hospital staff and patients existing to keep the hospital running as cheaply as possible, and the hospital and its staff existing to provide care and guardianship of the patients with the aim of alleviating their problems and preparing them for return to the community.

The notion of the 'therapeutic community', an approach to psychiatry pioneered after World War II (Jones 1960), is based on the principle of the patients contributing to the establishment by working in it. It is, however, reminiscent of the old-style approach, the difference being a move towards democratisation and patient involvement in the decision-making. There now exist numerous therapeutic communities where cleaning, cooking and gardening are performed by patients, with nurses facilitating activities, rather than directing them.

Many problems still remain. Cormack (1983) suggested that psychiatric nurses are still largely playing a formal therapeutic role, supporting and monitoring the treatment prescribed by the medical staff. There is some evidence to suggest that this results from a wider multi-disciplinary shift towards one or other of the therapeutic ideologies, rather than a unilateral decision on the part of nurses to fill a personal therapeutic role. Psychiatric nursing, it seems, needs to formulate specific functions, even if these functions are confined to coordinating and integrating the contributions of the various team members. Cormack identified the gap between education and practice in psychiatric nursing as a contributory factor in the problem of role definition. Improvements in nursing training may hold at least some of the answers to the problems facing psychiatric nursing today (see Ch. 5).

CONCLUSION

The purpose of this chapter has been to set some contemporary issues in psychiatric nursing within a historical context. Psychiatric nursing must not be viewed as existing or evolving in isolation from a variety of other forces: developments in psychiatry; changes in the political and socio-economic climate; public opinion; and, most importantly, the aspirations and morale of psychiatric nurses themselves.

REFERENCES

Abel-Smith B 1960 A history of the nursing profession. Heinemann, London

Adams F 1969 From Association to union: professional organisation of asylum attendants 1869–1919. British Journal of Sociology 20: 13, 18

Brooking J 1984 The art of applying the act. Nursing Mirror 159 (10) Sept 19

Browne W 1837 What asylums were, are and ought to be. London

Carpenter R 1980 'All for one' campaigns and pioneers in the making of COHSE. H T Cook, London

Carr E H 1981 What is history? Penguin, Harmondsworth

Cormack D 1983 Psychiatric nursing described. Churchill Livingstone, Edinburgh

Cox 1804 Practical observations on insanity. Quoted in Tuke S 1920 Addresses to mental nurses. London, pp 4, 5

Davies C 1980 Rewriting nursing history. Croom Helm, London

Goddard L 1953 The history of mental nursing. British Journal of Nursing. June: 77

Jones L 1960 Mental health and social policy 1945–59. London

Jones M 1953 The therapeutic community: a new treatment method in psychiatry. Basic Books, New York

Lunacy Act 1890 HMSO, London

Maggs C J 1983 The origins of general nursing. Croom Helm, London

The Mallinson Report 1983 The future of psychiatric services. COHSE, London

Mental Health Act 1959 HMSO, London

Mercier L 1894 Organization and management of asylums

MIND (National Association for Mental Health) 1983 Common concern. Mind Publications, London

Nolan P 1986 Mental Nurse training in the 1920s. The Nursing History Group, Bulletin 10. Royal College of Nursing, London

The Regulations and Orders of Springfield Mental Hospital, nr Tooting, London 1926

Report of the Visiting Justices of the Surrey Lunatic Asylum, Epiphany Quarter 1843

Scull A 1981 Madhouses, mad-doctors and madmen. Athlone, London

Thompson E P 1968 The making of the English working class. Penguin, Harmondsworth

Tuke S 1820 Addresses to mental nurses. London, pp 6, 7

Walk A 1961 The history of mental nursing. Journal of Mental Science 107 (446)

Wilson-Barnett J 1988 Lend me your ear. Nursing Times 84, 17 August: 51–53

3

Theory development

B. L. Thomas

Nursing as a profession has become very conscious of the need for theory development (Walker & Avant 1983). Theories for psychiatric nursing help to stimulate research and extend psychiatric nursing knowledge, the major purpose of which is the improvement of patient care. Unfortunately psychiatric nursing has not progressed very far in this area (Altschul 1986). Numerous reasons have been offered for this shortcoming, including the diversity of psychiatric nursing's subject matter. The intractable nature of the problems which nurses tackle do not lend themselves readily to the discovery of unifying theories, models and concepts (Reed 1987). The complexity of the nurse–patient relationship, which is central to psychiatric nursing, offers many intangibles which do not lend themselves to theory development (Verhonick & Werley 1967). Many psychiatric nurses do not have the preparation or motivation to carry out research and develop theories (Brooking 1986).

This chapter examines the present state of theories for psychiatric nursing. It begins by defining the terms theory, concept and model. A description of the range and various levels of theory is given, and an examination is made of how theories are developed. An argument is made for the development of specific theories which will be of practical use for psychiatric nurses in their day-to-day work with patients. Finally, the problems of developing theories for psychiatric nursing are addressed.

DEFINITIONS OF TERMS

Theory

The meaning of the word theory varies both among professional disciplines and within disciplines themselves (Torres 1986). Psychiatric nurses have already been exposed to many theories, for example, biochemical theories about neurotransmitters, psychological theories about human development, sociological theories about deviant behaviour and psychoanalytic theories about defence mechanisms. In this chapter theory is defined as a proposed explanation of an event or a series of happenings, which demonstrates the relationship of one concept to another.

On the basis of a theory psychiatric nurses formulate hypotheses about what will occur in specific nursing situations. The hypotheses are then subjected to empirical (observation or experimentation) testing in research studies. The outcome of the study may lend support to the theory or may suggest the need for modifications.

Concepts

Chapman (1985) describes a concept as an abstract notion or idea, often conveyed by a single word, although the features of the concept may be extremely complex. Examples of concepts frequently used in psychiatric nursing include communication, behaviour, observation and emotion. Many of the words are used by nurses in everyday language to convey meaning. However, each of these words consists of a body of assumptions, research and conceptual analysis which has accumulated from its use in previous research from other disciplines (Skevington 1984).

Models

In order to give meaning to the relationships between the concepts, models are developed. This enables diagrammatic representation of how one concept influences and logically or causally connects with another. For example, using the concepts, hospital admission, anxiety and information, a linear-directional model is shown in Figure 3.1.

There is much confusion and debate in the nursing literature regarding the status of nursing models, their usefulness and their relationship to theory development (Johnson 1983). The usefulness of nursing models is not contested in the present chapter. On the contrary they have a significant part to play in organizing practice, directing nursing research and in the construction and development of various levels of theory (Harré 1986).

A distinction needs to be made between a model and a theory. Aggleton & Chalmers (1986) suggest that a model is an abstract representation of concepts and linking statements. A theory, in contrast, is more specific and deals with a more limited number of concepts and propositions. A proposition is a statement of the relationships that are possible among the concepts. For example, using the concepts *hospital admission, anxiety* and *information* the following proposition can made.

Anxiety produced by hospital admission can be reduced by giving patients information.

Although some nurses may agree with this statement, as the concepts have not been clearly defined the proposition has different meanings to different people. For example, what is anxiety? Is the level of anxiety the same for all patients admitted to hospital? What information needs to be given? Is it to be given verbally or in writing? It is only when there is a clear definition of the concepts that the proposition can be stated with clarity and the theory tested by research.

Hospital admission ⟶ Anxiety ⟶ Information ⟶ Reduction in anxiety

Fig. 3.1 A linear-directional model.

McFarlane (1986) suggests that nursing models are pre-theoretical. That is, a model identifies and defines the concepts of a nursing situation and describes their relationship. In this way models can generate theories which can then be tested by empirical research. For example, in Orem's model of self-care, the following proposition is made:

The individual's abilities to engage in self-care or dependent care are conditioned by age, developmental state, life experience, sociocultural orientation, health and available resources.

(Orem 1980, p. 27).

The concepts contained in this proposition are self-care or dependent care, age, developmental state, life experience, sociocultural orientation, health and available resources. Each of these concepts must be clearly defined and measurement tools identified. Then the proposition may be stated as a hypothesis and tested by empirical research. Silva (1986) suggests little progress has been made in the testing of theories devised from nursing models. In her own analysis of 62 studies in which the models of Roy, Orem, Rogers and/or Newman were used as a framework for research only nine studies met specified evaluation criteria for the explicit testing of nursing theory.

RANGE OF THEORIES

Nursing models have also been criticized as either being too wide-ranging or too all encompassing for application, or too esoteric for practising nurses (Meleis & Price 1988). Hardy (1974) points out that the pursuit of a 'grand theory of nursing' has deflected the focus from the development of more simple theories which may have more significance to practitioners and may guide their practice safely and creatively.

Not only has there been much confusion in the nursing literature regarding the terms theories and models, but also much confusion regarding the terms, range and levels of theories. Walker & Avant (1983) discuss four levels of theory development in nursing and then describe the range of each of these levels of theory. The first level they name 'meta-theory level'. This level focuses on a broad range of issues related to theory development in nursing, including analysing the purpose and type of theory needed in nursing. Meta-theory examines the meaning of nursing as a practice discipline, that is as a science and a practical discipline.

The next level they identify is the 'grand-theory level'. It is these 'grand theories' which are now commonly referred to as nursing models. While these nursing models have identified the concepts of nursing practice and marked off general boundaries for nursing's professional focus, by virtue of their generality and wide range they are limited for theory development in their present form.

A more workable level of theory development has been proposed by Jacox (1974). Theories at this level are named 'middle-range theories'. They are more limited in their range and contain limited numbers of variables. Middle-range theories share some of the conceptual economy of nursing models, and also provide the specificity needed for usefulness in research and practice. For example, a nursing model of stress and adaptation might not result in any interpretable hypothesis. Refocusing the theory at the level of suspicion as a stressor on the nurse–patient relationship would, however, make the stress theory more operational for both research and practice purposes.

The final level of theory development is the 'practice-theory level'. The range of this type of theory is much more focused. Walker & Avant (1983) suggest that the essence of practice theory is a desired goal and prescriptions for action to achieve the goal. For example, a nursing goal may be to prevent a suicidal patient from harming himself*. Nursing practice theory states that, to prevent self-harm, a particular set of actions must be taken. These could include removal of objects that could be used in a suicide attempt and the nurses' continuous observation of the patient.

These levels of theory have been identified as such on the basis of the range of phenomena that they cover. Each type of theory is used for different purposes. Walker & Avant (1983) propose a

---

* In some chapters 'he' has been used to refer to the patient/client and 'she' to the psychiatric nurse.

model to demonstrate the relationship between the different levels of theory, as shown in Figure 3.2.

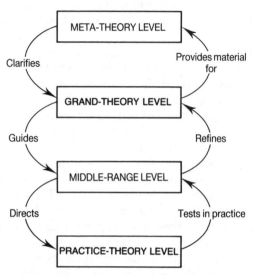

Fig. 3.2 Linkages among levels of theory development (from Walker & Avant 1983).

LEVELS OF THEORY

In a practice discipline like psychiatric nursing it is not enough to describe what is happening. Psychiatric nurses must also prescribe actions (Dickoff et al 1968). In order to do this psychiatric nurses must be able to identify the patient's needs/problems and prescribe nursing interventions that will result in expected outcomes of such interventions. For example, consider the case of a patient who has a low self-esteem and lacks confidence in himself. Having identified the problem the psychiatric nurse will prescribe a nursing intervention which will result in an expected outcome. There are a number of interventions from which the psychiatric nurse may choose. For example the nurse could explore with the patient activities that the patient is good at and engage him in those activities, thereby providing him with an opportunity to be successful. If such a nursing intervention succeeds in promoting the patient's self-esteem, it could be proposed that self-esteem is promoted by engaging patients in activities in which they are successful. Such a proposition can

then be tested with other patients who have a low self-esteem.

Dickoff et al (1968) have identified four levels of theory. They suggest that a practice discipline like psychiatric nursing progresses through four stages of theorizing which eventually lead to a theory base for that discipline.

1. Factor-isolating theories

These theories identify and describe what concepts are used in psychiatric nursing. Anxiety, anger, empathy, isolation, motivation and therapeutic milieu are a few examples. All further development of a theory will expand or refine those concepts and relationships determined in the descriptive phase.

2. Factor-relating theories

These theories attempt to explain how or why the given concepts of a theory relate to and with each other. For example the concepts of patient involvement and care planning may be explained by the concept of psychiatric nurses' attitudes. That is, nurses with positive attitudes to mental illness are more likely to include patients in care planning than those nurses with negative attitudes to mental illness. O'Toole (1981) gives the example of violent behaviour in an inpatient ward. Second-level theory in its simplest form might assert that increased spatial proximity in a ward (defined by numbers of persons per square feet) leads to increased violence.

3. Situation-relating theories

These predict future interactions of the same concepts. In this way they are a test of second-level theory. Hypotheses generated at level two could be tested by empirical research. For example, introducing a teaching package on self-medication for patients may reduce the length of hospitalization. Ideally, an experimental research design which allowed a comparison between a group of patients taught self-medication and a group of patients not taught how to self-medicate would result in a statement of relationships, which could be predictive and be at the third level. For example, patients taught how to self-medicate will need shorter hospitalization than patients who have not been taught how to self-medicate.

4. Situation-producing theories

These may be used to control outcomes. For example if the hypothesis about self-medication was found to be correct on testing it would be possible to reduce length of hospitalization by introducing a self-medication teaching package. Since self-medication may not be possible for all patients, alternative interventions could be proposed and tested. O'Toole (1981) provides a list of 19 studies from the United States which are classified as situation-producing theories. For the most part these studies focused on group therapy and behaviour modification programmes. Other interventions included the use of music, relaxation training and activity therapy. Systematic comparison of such programmes with 'routine' care would lead to decisions about which approach worked best. The intervention itself and the theoretical explanation for why it works becomes the practice theory.

According to Dickoff et al (1968) situation-producing theories are the highest level of theory. They argue that unless nursing functions at this level it cannot be called a profession. This is not to deny the importance of the other levels of theory, since each higher level of theory presupposes the existence of theories at the lower levels.

Skidmore (1975) argues that the strength of a theory is not whether a theory has descriptive, explanatory or predictive powers but rather it is the theory's ability to bring a great deal of thought and information to bear on a specific problem or set of problems, and therefore go far beyond unsystematic thought.

McFarlane (1976) suggests that little theory has been developed at the prescriptive level, not to mention the situation-producing level. For the present McFarlane recommends factor-isolating research and the testing of hypotheses against nursing practice. In exploring recent advances in psychiatric nursing during the past five years Hall (1988) identifies over a hundred concepts in the psychiatric nursing literature. Such an extensive list would suggest that it is time that psychiatric nurses began developing theories at the higher levels, that is at the levels of prescribing, predicting and controlling.

HOW IS THEORY DEVELOPED?

Theories are developed through the use of several strategies that employ inductive and deductive reasoning (Burr 1973). Inductive strategies use concrete observations in the real world to build theories. Data may include direct observations of individuals, groups, situations or events, or they may be case studies of such phenemona reported in the literature. In either instance, the data are examined for regularities, which are then stated as propositions. For example, a nurse may observe that a number of patients on the ward are reported as having very little sleep; they may be going to bed late, having difficulty getting off to sleep and rising early. The nurse may also notice that the patients with sleep difficulties may also drink a large volume of coffee during the day. From such observations the nurse may make a proposition that large caffeine consumption adversely affects psychiatric patients' sleep patterns. If such a hypothesis was confirmed, a health education programme may be introduced regarding the effects of excessive caffeine intake and the introduction of alternative drinks such as decaffinated coffee or herbal teas.

Bunch's (1985) description of how in their daily work on a psychiatric ward nurses are affected by the abnormal communication used by schizophrenic patients illustrates the use of the inductive method. Bunch used participant observation to collect the data. These direct observations of psychiatric nurses and schizophrenic patients were then categorized according to behavioural patterns, and relationships between the categories analysed. Bunch's data led her to propose that nurses had great difficulty operationalizing their professional role, knowledge and understanding of psychopathology and balancing these satisfactorily with the institutional demands. The observed difficulty encountered by the nurses of balancing the structural requirements and establishing therapeutic and meaningful relationships with patients illustrates how bureaucratic organizations may stifle nurses' endeavours to communicate therapeutically.

Deductive methods of theory development start with propositions that are then tested in a variety of specific situations. Field & Morse (1985) suggest that in deductive theory the starting point is identification of a set of concepts and generating hypotheses from previous knowledge. For example, the positive effects of information-giving on stress reduction (Wilson-Barnett & Carrigy 1978), recovery rates (Boore 1979), pain reduction and decreased medication requirements (Hayward 1975), have been widely researched in various aspects of general nursing. Similar theory development could occur in psychiatric nursing. Two examples are providing patients with information prior to hospital admission and also before the administration of electroconvulsive therapy.

McFarlane (1976) points out that in an applied science like nursing, concepts and theories are 'borrowed' from other disciplines or sciences for its practice, education and research. Nursing, however, is no different from other practice disciplines such as medicine and education. McFarlane suggests that by its very nature a practice discipline draws on the pure sciences. In the process of application, however, the pure science is transmuted and McFarlane believes becomes part of the body of knowledge associated with the practice discipline. For example the theory of stress may belong primarily to physiologists. However, the relief of stress in patients by psychiatric nurses using relaxation techniques may be part of the psychiatric nurse's role, and the application of theory to the nursing situation becomes part of nursing theory.

In psychiatric nursing the majority of studies which illustrate this type of theory development have occurred mainly in the specialist area of behavioural therapy. For example a study by Roach & Farley (1986) investigated the effects of behavioural techniques employed by a psychiatric nurse therapist on 300 neurotic patients with behavioural problems. Overall, the results from their data analysis show that the behavioural management of neurosis by the psychiatric nurse is effective only in certain conditions such as social maladjustment, and less effective in others such as phobias and social anxiety.

The relationship of practice and theory development

The relationship of practice and theory requires two simultaneous and complementary processes. The first is practice itself, that is a clear explication of psychiatric nursing by those who practise it. The second is research about practice. Diers (1979) has criticized the tendency of nurses to separate the process of research from practice and the researcher from the practitioner. O'Toole (1981) suggests that the most logical way to advance theory development in nursing is for those who practise psychiatric nursing to raise questions to be researched, and then to conduct the research to find the answers. She argues that if prescriptive or situation-producing theory is the ultimate goal for a practice discipline like psychiatric nursing, then it would logically follow that nurses who prescribe and carry out interventions with patients are in the best position to conduct research to validate their prescriptive interventions. O'Toole has produced the following diagram (Fig. 3.3) to demonstrate this relationship.

The diagram shows how the causal non-systematic observation of a problem in practice leads to more systematic observation and a definition of terms, including the nature of the problem and influencing factors. O'Toole suggests that descriptive, observational and exploratory research designs are useful at this time in more precisely defining a problem or observation. Following this, hypotheses may be developed concerning relationships between identified variables. They may be tested in correlational or survey research designs. Causal relationships between the variables may then be proposed and predictions tested in experimental or quasi-experimental designs in natural or controlled settings, with a specification of the predicted relationship. Only if a causal relationship has been established can one proceed to a prescriptive theoretical level and the testing of specific interventions aimed at changing the problem. In this way prescriptive studies feed back into prac-

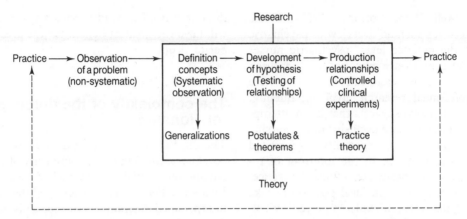

Fig. 3.3   Relationship between practice, theory and research (from O'Toole 1981).

tice to improve the quality of psychiatric nursing care.

O'Toole emphasizes that this progressive process of observing practice, theorizing, testing in research and subsequently modifying practice, must become an essential part of psychiatric nursing if it is to survive as a practice discipline.

Stuart & Sundeen (1983) suggest that in the USA research about the practice of psychiatric nursing has increased in the past decade, and it is obvious that nurses have the ability to construct sophisticated designs, with both theoretical and practical importance. Davis (1986) reports that in the UK, while there is a considerable amount of research available, only a few studies are involved with the experimental manipulation of variables to test hypotheses.

Is it possible to develop theories for psychiatric nursing?

It has been suggested throughout this chapter that psychiatric nurses need to assess their professional role through research into the nature of their work with patients and its effectiveness. Kasch (1986) suggests that the major obstacle to developing nursing theory is the inability to account adequately for the processes by which positive changes in health status are affected.

Four major arguments have been proposed against the development of psychiatric nursing theories. These are described and discussed in the following section.

Developing a theory of psychiatric nursing

The first argument suggests that it is not possible to develop an all-encompassing, unified theory of psychiatric nursing. The fruitlessness of such pursuit has already been mentioned. An examination of other disciplines clearly shows that there is not one unifying theory which accounts for all the various aspects of concern to that discipline. In psychology, for example, there are numerous theories which make up the discipline that studies human behaviour and mental processes. For example, there are developmental theories, learning theories, neurophysiological theories, psychosocial theories, personality theories and humanistic theories. Psychiatric nursing, like psychology, is concerned with the complex issues of human beings, and needs a variety of theories on which to base its practice. Mennell (1974) points out that although some theories are broader in scope than others, no theory can explain everything. Since each theory deals only with specific problems, many theories are needed to deal with all the phenomena of interest in psychiatric nursing.

The work of psychiatric nurses

The intractable nature of the problems with which psychiatric nurses deal seems to have resulted in two major approaches to present theory development. The first approach has been to try to establish what is distinctive about psychiatric nursing (Towell 1975, Cormack 1983). While there is a need for such an overview of psychiatric nursing, at the practice level, psychiatric nurses participate in a multi-disciplinary team approach to care, which in many cases calls for collaborative or inter-professional research involving nursing. Wilson-Barnett (1988) suggests that in an attempt to create a knowledge base exclusive to the nursing care of the mentally ill, the speciality has forfeited many opportunities to be in the forefront of research progress and positively influence practice. Psychiatric nurses are in an ideal position to take advantage of the research skills employed by colleagues in other disciplines which have a longer tradition of researching the effectiveness of their work with patients. For example, there now exists a variety of mental health measurement scales (McDowell & Newell 1987) which could be used by nurses to evaluate therapeutic outcomes.

The second approach has been for nurses to adopt a specific therapeutic role under an identified treatment modality, for example behaviour therapy, cognitive therapy and psychotherapy. While such a shift has resulted in psychiatric nurses being regarded as independent practitioners such emphasis has deflected attention away from basic psychiatric nursing care and from the patient population where these treatments have little or no success, that is the chronically mentally ill. Brooking (1985) has demonstrated that for the most part psychiatric nursing research in this country has concentrated on specialist aspects which are largely irrelevant to the work of most psychiatric nurses. For example, Barker (1987) in a review of two British nursing journals 1970–1985 (inclusive) suggests that descriptions of the use of behavioural approaches with psychiatric patients, or descriptions of the techniques themselves, dominate the literature. Behavioural change following treatment for a specific behavioural problem can be observed directly, which may be the reason for the popularity of research in this area. While not denying the importance of research into specific behavioural problems, there is also a need for research in those areas which demonstrate how the nursing action engaged in by the majority of psychiatric nurses in their day-to-day work can be of benefit to patients. Henderson (1972) suggests

there is a need to study problems whose solution will have the greatest benefit for the greatest number of people.

The complexity of the nurse–patient relationship

The third argument against theory development in psychiatric nursing is the complexity of the nurse–patient relationship (Verhonick & Werley 1967). Ever since Peplau (1952) suggested that theories of interpersonal relations were especially relevant to the work of nurses, there has been a gradual interest in the therapeutic function of the nurse–patient relationship (Altschul 1972). The present emphasis on the nurse–patient relationship and the very nature of psychiatric nursing in dealing with individuals and their needs does mean that research and theory development in this area can be problematic. O'Toole (1981) draws the analogy of comparing psychotherapy with surgical interventions or other medical treatments where the method is clear and easily replicated. O'Toole suggests that in the treatment of the mentally ill, so much of practice resides within the practitioner that to separate them for analysis seems artificial.

McBride (1986) disagrees with this type of argument and suggests that just because there may be methodological problems or many variables that cannot be controlled, there is no reason to shy away from this kind of research. While research into the therapeutic effects of the nurse–patient relationship is scarce, there is a considerable amount of literature which has examined the concepts central to the formation of the nurse–patient relationship (Schmidt 1972, Finkleman 1975, Campiello 1980).

Lego (1980) in an extensive review of the literature on one-to-one nurse–patient relationships concluded that many questions remain to be addressed. Lego suggests that it is necessary to identify what does or what should take place in the one-to-one relationship. Once nurses have identified the concepts which make up the relationship, then hypotheses can be formulated and research undertaken to establish whether such relationships are of value to the patients.

More recently Sundeen et al (1985) have argued that the importance of the interpersonal relationship for psychiatric nurses has led to identification of the essential features of such a relationship. For the most part the essential features are characteristic of all helping relationships and were originally identified by Rogers (1951). These include the concepts of trust, empathy, understanding, respect, genuineness and warm positive regard. There have been some nursing research studies which have explored the link between some of these essential features and the emergence of helping behaviour in nurses.

In order to illustrate the argument the following section examines the concept of empathy and the research conducted to establish its effectiveness as a helping strategy within the nurse–patient relationship.

Kingston (1987) defines empathy as the quality of understanding another person in his own terms. It means being able to see things from the other's point of view, from within his frame of reference. Rogers (1951) argues that empathy is one of the most potent factors in bringing about change and learning. Empathy helps the patient realize that someone understands, cares and values him as a person—the effect of which is that as the patient perceives these new aspects about himself he begins to think of himself as worthwhile and changes his behaviour accordingly.

Hoeffer & Murphy (1982) provide a comprehensive review of the North American psychiatric nursing literature relating to empathy. They demonstrate how the concept of empathy developed in other disciplines has been refined and adapted for use in psychiatric nursing. Ehmann (1971) developed a model for the application of the process of empathy. An adaptation of this model is represented in Figure 3.4.

Kalisch (1973) developed a 'Nurse–patient emphathetic functioning scale' (Table 3.1). Category 0 represents the lowest level of empathy. At this level the nurse may be totally out of touch with the feelings of the patient. As the nurse progresses through the scale, responses demonstrate that the nurse is becoming more attuned to the patient's feelings, firstly to those feelings openly expressed and, by category 4, to deeply hidden indirectly expressed feelings. Sundeen et al (1985) point out the importance of not automatically attaching a higher value to a higher-level response, as a lower response category may be more appropriate to the setting and stage of the relationship. Kalisch's empathetic scale represents the development of an objective measurement tool which can be used to enhance nurses' therapeutic effectiveness.

Forsyth (1980a), in developing psychiatric nursing theory related to empathy, used both inductive and deductive methods of theory development. The deductive approach involved borrowing the

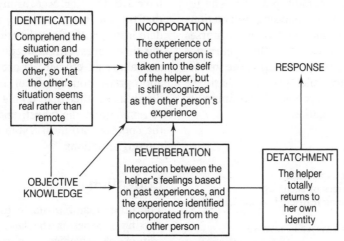

Fig. 3.4 Model of the application of the process of empathy (adapted from Ehmann 1971).

Table 3.1 The nurse–patient empathetic functioning scale: a schematic presentation (from Kalisch 1973)

Categories of nurse empathetic function	Level of patient's feelings	
	Conspicuous current feelings	Hidden current feelings
0	Ignores	Ignores
1	Communicates an awareness that is accurate at times and inaccurate at other times	Ignores
2	Communicates a complete and accurate awareness of the essence and strength of feeling	Communicates an awareness of the presence of hidden feelings but is not accurate in defining their essence or strength; an effort is being made to understand
3	Same as category 2	Communicates an accurate awareness of the hidden feelings slightly beyond what the patient expresses himself
4	Same as category 2	Communicates without uncertainty an accurate awareness of the deepest feelings

concept of empathy from another discipline and applying the concept in nursing practice. The inductive approach involved analysing interactions between nurses and patients and between nurses and patients' families to establish the occurrence of empathy. Forsyth (1980b) developed the following criteria for empathy which provide a basis for operationalizing the concept and determining its occurrence in nursing situations.

Empathy . . . .
1. occurs in consciousness
2. implies relationship
3. involves validation of experience
4. exists in variable degrees of accuracy
5. has temporal dimensions restricted to the here and now
6. involves energy, which varies in intensity
7. requires objectivity
8. requires freedom from judgment or evaluation.

Other research into the use of empathy by psychiatric nurses includes a study by Stotland et al (1978) who investigated the behaviour of nursing students relative to empathy and helping. Students who had been tested regarding their ability to empathize were observed during their clinical experience. Stotland and colleagues (1978) hypothesized that highly empathetic students would spend more time with patients, presumably being more helpful to them. The results did not entirely bear out the hypothesis. In the early part of the clinical placement, highly empathetic students spent less time with clients than the low empathizers. However by the end of the placement this tendency had been reversed, and the highly empathetic students spent more time with patients. The investigators suggested that it was very uncomfortable for the highly empathetic students to be with clients when they were insecure in their own abilities to meet the patients' needs. Later in the placement, they felt more secure in their own nursing abilities and were able to spend more time helping patients.

Mansfield (1973) investigated the verbal and non-verbal behaviours of psychiatric nurses that facilitated empathetic communication with patients during initial interviews. William's (1979) study found that high and low levels of empathetic communication were factors in changing the self-concept of institutionalized patients.

The results of nursing research into empathy have led Hoeffer & Murphy (1982) to conclude that the concept of empathy is one example which demonstrates that psychiatric nurses are concerning themselves with concepts relevant to practice; are taking an efficient approach by borrowing an appropriate concept from related mental health disciplines rather than taking on the laborious task of reinventing the wheel; and are operationalizing the concept into measurable research variables for nursing situations.

Education

The other major obstacle to the development of nursing theories is the lack of educational preparation of psychiatric nurses in research and theory development (Brooking 1985). The successful development and application of psychiatric nursing theories are dependent upon the intellectual capacity and capabilities of psychiatric nurses. Considerable progress has been made in the United States where research and theory have become an established part of basic preparation at the baccalaureate level. Wilson (1985) points out that the question 'Should nursing research be taught at all levels of nursing education?' has been replaced with the contemporary question, 'What should be taught about nursing research, at what level and how?' A number of strategies for incorporating theoretical nursing in undergraduate and graduate programmes have been suggested by Meleis & Price (1988). Advances are also being made in this country, albeit slowly, with the establishment of degree courses for psychiatric nurses. Education of psychiatric nurses has a major role to play in developing and improving the skills required to conduct research and in strengthening the belief that research and theory development can and must be incorporated into psychiatric nurses' routine work.

CONCLUSION

This chapter has examined the state of theory development in psychiatric nursing. The terms concept, model and theory were defined and the distinction drawn between models and theories. The range and levels of theory development were discussed and methods of theory development described. While not denying the importance of existing psychiatric nursing research, much of this research has been of a descriptive nature, concerning either the role of the psychiatric nurse or how psychiatric nurses are prepared for their role. There is a need for the further development of this type of descriptive research, which needs to be used with appropriate rigour and demonstrations of reliability and validity of findings. The argument has been made that if psychiatric nurses are to develop theories which are pertinent to practice, a shift of emphasis is needed in the type of research undertaken. Psychiatric nurses need to research the effect and effectiveness of the various nursing interventions used. Such research will result in the development of the theories required for responsible psychiatric nursing practice.

It has been suggested that psychiatric nursing has not progressed very far in the area of theory development. A number of reasons have been offered for this shortcoming, including the complexity of the nurse–patient relationship. These arguments have been addressed and the concept of empathy has been used as an example to demonstrate the possibility of developing theories for psychiatric nursing.

REFERENCES

Aggleton P, Chalmers H 1986 Nursing models and the nursing process. Macmillan, London

Altschul A T 1972 Nurse–patient interaction: a study of interaction patterns in acute psychiatric wards. Churchill Livingstone, Edinburgh

Altschul A T 1986 Foreword. In: Brooking J I (ed) Psychiatric nursing research. Wiley, Chichester

Barker P 1987 Evaluation in nursing: the nurse as behaviour therapist. In: Milne D (ed) Evaluating mental health practice: methods and applications. Croom Helm, London

Boore J, 1979 Prescription for recovery. RCN, London

Botha M E 1989 Theory development in perspective: the role of conceptual frameworks and models in theory development. Journal of Advanced Nursing 14: 49–55

Brooking J I 1985 Advanced psychiatric nursing education in Britain. Journal of Advanced Nursing 10: 455–468

Brooking J I 1986 Introduction. In: Brooking J I (ed) Psychiatric nursing research. Wiley, Chichester

Bunch E H 1985 Therapeutic communication: is it possible for psychiatric nurses to engage in this on an acute psychiatric ward? In: Altschul A T (ed) Recent advances in nursing: psychiatric nursing. Churchill Livingstone, Edinburgh

Burr W R 1973 Theory, construction and the sociology of the family. Wiley, New York

Campiello J 1980 The process of termination. Journal of Psychiatric Nursing 18: 29

Chapman C M 1985 Theory of nursing: practical application. Harper & Row, London

Coles C R, Gale Grant J 1985 Curriculum evaluation in medical health care education. ASME Medical Education Research Booklet no. 1. ASME, Dundee

Cormack D 1983 Psychiatric nursing described. Churchill Livingstone, Edinburgh

Davis B 1986 A review of recent research in psychiatric nursing. In: Brooking J I (ed) Psychiatric nursing research. Wiley, Chichester

Dickoff J, James P 1968 A theory of theories: a position paper. Nursing Research 17: 197–203

Dickoff J, James P, Wiedenbach E 1968 Theory in a practice discipline. Nursing Research 17: 415–435

Diers D 1979 Faculty research development at Yale. Nursing Research 19(1): 64–71

Duffey M, Muhlenkamp A F 1974 A framework for theory analysis. Nursing Outlook 22: 570–574

Ehmann V 1971 Empathy: its origins, characteristics and process. Perspectives in Psychiatric Care 8(2): 72–80

Field P A, Morse J M 1985 Nursing research: the application of qualitative approaches. Croom Helm, London

Finkleman A 1975 Commitment and responsibility in the therapeutic relationship. Journal of Psychiatric Nursing 13: 10

Forsyth G 1980a Analysis of the concept of empathy: illustration of one approach. Advances in Nursing Sciences 3: 1–7

Forsyth G 1980b Analysis of the concept of empathy: illustration of one approach. Advances in Nursing Sciences 2(2): 33–42

Hall B A 1988 Speciality knowledge in psychiatric nursing: where are we now? Archives of Psychiatric Nursing 4: 191–199

Hardy M E 1974 Theories, components, developments, evaluation. Nursing Research 23: 100–107

Harré R 1986 The principles of scientific thinking. Macmillan, London

Hayward J C 1975 Information — a prescription against pain. Royal College of Nursing, London

Henderson V 1972 Basic principles of nursing care. International Council of Nurses, Geneva

Hoeffer B, Murphy S 1982 The unfinished task: development of nursing theory for psychiatric and mental health nursing practice. Journal of Psychosocial Nursing and Mental Health Services 20: 8–14

Jacox A 1974 Theory construction in nursing. Nursing Research 23: 4–13

Johnson J 1983 Some aspects of the relation between theory and research in nursing. Journal of Advanced Nursing 8: 21–28

Kalisch B 1973 What is empathy? American Journal of Nursing 73: 1548

Kasch C R, 1986 Toward a theory of nursing action: skills and competency in nurse–patient interaction. Nursing Research 35: 226–230

Kingston B 1987 Psychological approaches in psychiatric nursing. Croom Helm, London

Lego S 1980 The one-to-one nurse relationship. Perspectives in Psychiatric Care 18: 67–89

Mansfield E 1973 Empathy: concept and identified psychiatric nursing behaviour. Nursing Research 22: 525

Mathews B P 1962 Measurement of psychological aspects of the nurse–patient relationship. Nursing Research 11: 154–162

McBride A B 1986 Theory and research: present issues and future perspectives of psychosocial nursing. Journal of Psychosocial Nursing 24: (9)27–33

McDowell I, and Newell C 1987 Measuring health: a guide to rating scales and questionnaires. Oxford University Press, New York

McFarlane J K 1976 The role of research and the development of nursing theory. Journal of Advanced Nursing 1: 443–451

McFarlane J K 1986 The value of models for care. In: Kershaw B, Salvage J (eds) Models for nursing. Wiley, Chichester

Meleis A I, Price M J 1988 Strategies and conditions for teaching theoretical nursing: an international perspective. Journal of Advanced Nursing 13(5): 592–604

Mennell S 1974 Sociological theory. Nelson, London

Orem D 1980 Nursing: concepts of practice. McGraw-Hill, New York

O'Toole A W 1981 When the practical becomes theoretical. Journal of Psychiatric Nursing and Mental Health Services 19: 13

Peplau H 1952 Interpersonal relations in nursing. Putnam's New York

Reed P G 1987 Constructing a conceptual framework for psychosocial nursing. Journal of Psychosocial Nursing and Mental Health Services 25(2): 24–28

Roach F, Farley N 1986 The behavioural management of neurosis by practising nurse therapists. In: Brooking J L (ed) Psychiatric nursing research, Wiley. Chichester

Rogers C 1951 Client-centred therapy. Constable, London

Rogers M E 1970 An introduction to the theoretical basis of nursing. Davis, Philadelphia

Roy C 1984 Introduction to nursing: an adaption model. Prentice-Hall, Englewood Cliffs, New Jersey

Schmidt J 1972 Availability: a concept of nursing practice. American Journal of Nursing 72: 1087

Silva M C 1986 Research testing nursing theory: state of the art. Advances in Nursing Science 9(1): 1–11

Skevington S. 1984 Understanding nurses: the social psychology of nursing. Wiley, Chichester

Skidmore W 1975 Theoretical thinking in sociology. Cambridge University Press, New York

Stotland E, Mathews K E, Sherman S E, Hansson R O, Richardson B Z 1978 Empathy, fantasy and helping. Sage Publications, Beverly Hills, Calif

Stuart G W, Sundeen S J 1983 Principles and practice of psychiatric nursing. Mosby, St Louis

Sundeen S J, Stuart G W, Rankin E D, Cohen S A 1985 Nurse–client interaction: implementing the nursing process. Mosby, St Louis

Torres G 1986 Theoretical foundations in nursing. Appleton-Century-Crofts, New York

Towell D 1975 Understanding psychiatric nursing. Royal College of Nursing, London

Verhonick P J, Werley M H 1967 Experimentation in nursing practice in the army. In: Fox D J, Kelly R L (eds) The research process in nursing. Appleton-Century Crofts, New York

Walker L O, Avant K C 1983 Strategies for theory construction in nursing. Appleton-Century-Crofts, New York

Williams C 1979 Empathetic communication and its effect on client outcome. Issues in Mental Health Nursing 2: 16

Wilson H S 1985 Research in nursing. Addison-Wesley, California

Wilson-Barnett J 1988 Lend me your ear. Nursing Times 84(33): 51–53.

Wilson-Barnett J, Carrigy A 1978 Factors affecting patients' responses to hospitalization. Journal of Advanced Nursing 3: 221–228

4

The multi-disciplinary clinical team

S. A. H. Ritter

This chapter follows the Royal Commission on the National Health Service (1979) by defining a multi-disciplinary clinical team (MDCT) as a 'group of colleagues acknowledging a common involvement in the care and treatment of a particular patient' (p. 171).

HISTORICAL BACKGROUND

In 1946 it was hoped that the National Health Service would provide the means necessary by which health care services could both cooperate with each other and maximize their individual contributions to the new service (Ministry of Health 1952). However, by the mid-1950s many management problems that are familiar now had emerged, and indeed appeared intractable. Symptomatic were the scandals which emerged in the 1970s concerning psychiatric and mental handicap hospitals (Martin 1984).

In the 1970s a number of studies of the work of psychiatric nurses found that most direct patient care was carried out by unqualified nurses, and that, despite the qualified nurses' preoccupation with administrative tasks, working relationships with other health care professionals did not appear to be planned around individualized treatment responsibilities and did not reflect the 'common involvement' described by the Royal Commission

(Altschul 1972, Towell 1975, Cormack 1976, Royal Commission 1979).

In 1980 a working party chaired by Nodder was commissioned by the Department of Health and Social Security in order to examine the 'organizational and management problems of mental illness hospitals', where working practices seemed to foster neglect and ill-treatment of patients (DHSS 1980). However, the push towards de-institutionalizing mental health services appears to have overtaken attempts to implement and evaluate the recommendations of the Nodder Report.

There have been many attempts to specify the nature of the relationships within teams, and explanations of why health care teams have so much difficulty in working together are based on a variety of assumptions derived from sociological, psychological and organizational or interdisciplinary theories. Many examinations of teamwork are a blend of different perspectives, sometimes made explicit, sometimes not. A few studies will be reviewed briefly in order to identify some themes.

COLLABORATION WITHIN TEAMS

Collegiality and consensus management are two main ways of defining the nature of collaboration within teams. Campbell-Heider & Pollock (1987) define collegiality as 'interdependent practice between physicians and nurses' (p. 421), while McKeganey and Bloor (1987) define consensus management as a 'quasi-collegiate decision-making system' (p. 154). However, a number of studies have explored collaboration in other terms.

Koerner et al (1986) link collaborative practice both to planning and to quality assurance. Keddy et al (1986) use a grounded theory approach to suggest that nurse–doctor relationships are strongly influenced by the fact that, historically, nurses were often educated and employed by doctors. Guy (1986) concludes that the degree of conflict within a team is a function of the complexity of the unit or environment within which it works: that is, the greater the complexity the greater the conflict. Temkin-Greener's work (1983) implicitly supports this view, and cautions against accepting prescriptions for teamwork

when individual working contexts may differ radically from norms thought to be acceptable by nurses on the one hand and by other disciplines on the other hand. Wolfe & Bushardt (1985) identify a variety of factors which constrain conflict resolution by teams. These include individuals' concern about the outcome of the conflict and concern about relationships with the other people involved. They suggest that to resolve conflict constructively team members need well-developed interpersonal skills and self-awareness, especially as confrontation may be necessary to deal with issues.

THE THERAPEUTIC MILIEU

The therapeutic community emerged in the late 1940s within an anti-authoritarian movement whose rationale was set out in 'a democratic, egalitarian rhetoric' (Cooper 1967, Baron 1987). The most influential views were expressed in publications in the early to mid-1950s. However, there have been many difficulties in realizing the ideals of therapeutic communities in conventional hospital settings. It is suggested that these difficulties stem from the conflicts of ideology and practice among staff with different backgrounds (Bell & Ryan 1985).

Although the evidence for the efficacy of therapeutic communities is contentious, there are aspects of their organization which have been applicable in the settings of 'ordinary' psychiatric hospitals (Islam & Turner 1982). For example, Levine & Wilson (1985) emphasize that a hospital, like a therapeutic community, requires a conceptual framework which identifies both its primary function and the means by which this is carried out. They provide an operation of such a framework, using object relations and systems theories to explain how staff interact with each other and with patients, in order to create a 'holding environment' within which severely disabled patients can be helped by the different disciplines. In another study, Lehman et al (1982) argue that it is essential that patients are carefully monitored to ensure that ward programmes, administrative structures and philosophy actually improve outcomes as well as determine processes of care.

Alanen and colleagues in Finland have taken a different approach to using the components of the therapeutic community by making what they call needs- or case-specific multi-disciplinary treatment plans. Some of the benefits of these plans appear to be associated with long-term contact between patients and a member of the team, irrespective of discipline, but who is intensively supervised (Alanen et al 1985). However, in a large investigation into the effectiveness of treatment programmes in Veterans Administration hospitals, Collins et al (1985) were unable to attribute differences in patient outcome specifically to multi-disciplinary team practices.

Guirguis et al (1983) describe a project to improve staff morale and patient care in a long-stay ward, evaluating it in terms of variables which include clarity of ward aims and goals, well-defined treatment methods, support and direction from outside the ward, and individualization of work. They report that 'sympathetic but firm leadership, which preserved and respected roles whilst appreciating the inevitability of overlap, was essential to keep peace in the team' (p. 592). It is not entirely clear which variables were responsible for the amelioration which took place.

SOCIOLOGICAL PERSPECTIVES

Mechanic & Aiken (1982) examine the perspectives of physicians, nurses and patients in the USA from a sociological point of view, emphasizing the roles of gender, class, economics and technology in the inefficiency of collaborative practice. While they argue that nurses and doctors need to understand the kinds of problems faced by each profession, they suggest quite different strategies to promote positive teamwork, including closer academic ties, greater specialization and higher qualifications for nurses, and greater differentiation within the nursing structure, in order that individuals can negotiate with physicians for a clearly defined and visible position.

In contrast, from a British perspective, Stacey (1988) argues that the relative power of organizations and professions in health care has become a question of bureaucratic rather than professional control, and that the report which introduced

general management to the National Health Service signalled the end of the period of consensus management which characterized hospitals from the 1970s on (Griffiths 1983). General management, encouraged by central government, has challenged the professions and curtailed their freedom to decide how to divide or share the tasks involved in health care work. As a result, the power of nurses, already affected by factors such as gender, race and economic status, has apparently diminished. However, at ward level the effect of general management on the internal functioning of psychiatric clinical teams has been less profound than on their wider organizational contexts.

STRUCTURE, NORMS AND GOALS
Structure

Structure may be thought of as the solution adopted by teams to the problem of operating their ideology or philosophy (Carter et al 1984). The analysis by Strauss et al (1964) of psychiatric ideologies and institutions has remained one of the most influential interpretations of what goes on in teams. According to Strauss et al (1964), the social structure of a psychiatric hospital consists of three elements: first, the number and kinds of professionals who work there; second, the treatment ideologies and professional identities of these professionals; third, the relationships of the institution and its professionals to outside communities. In addition, hospitals develop 'institutional maps' which both shape and are shaped by the activities of their workers.

In order to confirm its shape and place in the institutional map, a team develops its own map. Strauss et al (1964) define the institutional map or structure in terms of a 'negotiated order' in which the total of a hospital's 'rules, agreements and understandings' are maintained by processes of politicking, persuading, bargaining and negotiating (p. 16). A team which does not fit into the institutional map, or a person who does not fit into a team's map, comes under great pressure to conform.

Many of the difficulties encountered by teams can be seen in terms of the conflict involved for individuals in deciding whether to aim for a defined and protected place within the medical divisions of labour, or for a total separateness of knowledge and therapy systems. In the former case, nurses would aim for an acknowledged role in a team, practising something like consensus management. In the latter case, nurses would aim for joint practice within a team: separate and equal (Stacey 1988). It could be argued that the response of the professions to the introduction of general management has been to attempt to maximize their own power at the expense of each other. If this is the case, then it is likely to have had the effect of reinforcing some of the hazards from which teams are at risk.

Norms

The explicit rules of traditional institutions rely on an acceptance by the different professions of the distribution of power. If norms and rules are not made explicit, adaptation and adjustment in an organization occur either through negotiation or through the development of routines (Ashforth & Fried 1988). Morgan et al (1985) examine the notion that nurses in hospital are subject to two kinds of power. The first is bureaucratic power, and the second is charismatic power, usually exercised by doctors. Rosenhan's (1973) observation of the powerlessness of patients suggests that jockeying for power among the professions in psychiatric hospitals is done at the expense of patients.

Strauss et al (1964) discuss norms in terms of ideologies as well as rules. The ideology of a team creates its shape on the institutional map, but is also shaped by the institution's response: whether it endorses or is in conflict with the team's norms. A team's ideology also tends to be determined by the professionals within it who have the most firmly organized ideology. In their 1964 study, Strauss et al found that nurses were characterized by an absence of a 'strong, professionally accepted ideological position' (p. 362). Although they view psychiatric hospitals as places where each profession negotiates its autonomy with the other professions, so that a 'negotiated order' emerges in which authority appears participative and decisions are negotiated, the link between ideology

and power suggests that the participants do not start from equal positions.

One of the most important conclusions reached by Strauss et al (1964) is that the ways in which teams operate their ideologies or philosophies vary widely within and between institutions, so that it is not possible to generalize about nurses' relationships with other professionals. The processes of politicking, persuading, bargaining and negotiating affect, and are affected by, the ideologies of the different professionals (which may not be the same as wider professional ideologies), so that the outcomes in different teams will constitute a unique constellation of factors. If the turnover and replacement of staff is considered, it will be seen that outcomes in the same team will differ according to its membership, and that these processes are likely to be continual.

A development which is related to this view is that of McKeganey & Bloor (1987), who argue that multi-disciplinary clinical teams establish 'therapeutic paradigms', which are used to define the behaviour of both staff and patients. For example, nurses may refuse to answer direct questions from patients in ward groups. The unspoken rationale, or 'therapeutic paradigm', is that learning by experience is a good thing, and patients must learn to take responsibility for themselves. Clearly, such reasoning runs counter to the kind of assumptions usually held outside the institution about answering questions. McKeganey & Bloor (1987) argue that such redefinitions allow staff to select almost any behaviour or event and subject its meaning to a transformation which may not be readily comprehensible.

Goals

Parsons (1951) suggested that the goals of the medical system were to protect the public, protect patients from themselves, protect the vulnerable, provide therapy and to train staff. Of these goals, the nurses were thought to be most concerned with the first three, with subtle control of social relationships being a less welcome by-product. Protecting patients from themselves and protecting the vulnerable may become overt control. The fourth goal, of providing therapy, was largely seen as the area where doctors and psychotherapists exercise control.

PSYCHOLOGICAL PERSPECTIVES

A number of writers have used Tajfel's work on intergroup relations to analyse what happens to relationships between groups of health care professionals (Tajfel 1978, Skevington 1980). Tajfel's theory has three main concepts, involving the perception by group members of their group's status, legitimacy and stability. Eiser (1986) picks out several important aspects of the application of the theory. A group member's self-evaluation depends on processes of social comparison with other groups. Behaviour is the product of specific social situations, and lies on a continuum from interpersonal to intergroup. Finally, group members' perceptions of the legitimacy and stability of intergroup relations determine the likelihood of pressure for group change. The relevance of the theory to multi-disciplinary clinical teams is that it provides an explanation of the behaviour of team members who fail to recognize and tackle problems in their work, while using group meetings to decry other teams' clinical approaches and to congratulate themselves on their own performance.

INTERDISCIPLINARY PERSPECTIVES

Furnham et al (1984) attempt to explore the themes evident in the sociological and psychological literature by analysing the perceptions held of each other by a variety of occupational groups. They conclude that mistaken attributions can be explained by intergroup prejudices triggered by 'the mere separation into groups or professions'. Their remedies include better education about the 'history, role and worth' of another related profession's approach, and clear definition of the purpose and structure of interdisciplinary group meetings.

Values, assumptions and tasks

Understanding differences and negotiating 'shared commitment' are problematic interpersonal ac-

tivities (Carter et al 1984). The values and assumptions which determine organizational practice are therefore often tacitly held. Argyris & Schon (1978) argue that the practices of organizations are continually modified by the fluctuations in their members' understanding of, and adherence to, their values. In the MDCT these fluctuations tend to occur during interaction with colleagues. Carter et al (1984) note that members can choose to agree with their colleagues by accepting the shared rules or by doing as another member tells them. In this way the difficult interpersonal activities of expressing and understanding differences and negotiating 'shared commitment' can be avoided. Similarly, Argyris (1970) notes that in modern organizations, tact and diplomacy are valued at the expense of openness and trust. Difficult interpersonal activities can also be avoided by attending meetings irregularly. A familiar pattern of avoidance is one where an individual will attend a meeting especially to vent a grievance and then not appear for a couple of weeks. Thus he or she expresses a difference without taking responsibility for participating in the understanding and negotiation needed to resolve it.

INTRA-ORGANIZATIONAL PERSPECTIVES

Etzioni (1964) defined organizations as 'planned units, deliberately structured for the purpose of attaining specific goals' (p. 4). Whereas the ward may be described as an organization in Etzioni's terms, it is far more difficult to use the same definition to categorize the MDCT as an organization. Because of the consultation role that some professionals perform within the team, and their multiple attachments to different teams, their commitment to the MDCT is necessarily different from that given to a ward or department. For them, a particular MDCT is characterized by its meetings, which both hold the enterprise together and are the enterprise. Group dynamics necessarily influence the quality of a team's planning and thus its interventions.

Argyris & Schon (1978) initiated a new approach to organizations by suggesting that to speak about learning and behaving is to use a kind of metaphor, since human models which apply to individuals' behaviour cannot be transferred to organizations. Argyris & Schön (1978) state three conditions for considering a collection of people as an organization: procedures for making decisions in the name of the group; procedures for delegating to individuals authority to act for the group; and procedures for defining the boundaries between the group and its environment. Although it is individuals who make decisions and act on them, 'They do these things for the collectivity by virtue of the rules for decision, delegation, and membership' (p. 12). The MDCT is an example of a 'collectivity', or agency. Because it exists, however, mostly in terms of the discrete occasions when members meet together face-to-face, learning and other behaviour may be discontinuous owing to fluctuations in the personnel who actually attend meetings. It is likely that the people who attend regularly will wield most influence, and among these regular attenders the leader(s) will be found.

Ashforth & Fried (1988) attempt to account for the development of 'stagnant mechanistic organization(s)'. They suggest that teams whose members are 'reciprocally interdependent' often develop rigid methods of regulating the behaviour of members in order to reduce unpredictability and to ensure acquiescence to authority, whether exercised by people or by working routines and procedures. Decisions are made as if by reflex, with two adverse consequences. One consequence is that decision-makers are over-confident about the correctness of their actions. The other is that decisions or diagnoses are made on the basis of insufficient or distorted information. For example, in Rosenhan's (1973) study: 'One kindly nurse found a pseudopatient pacing the long hospital corridors. "Nervous, Mr X?" she asked. "No, bored," he said' (p. 253).

Psychodynamics and group dynamics

Intra-organizational perspectives also take into account group dynamics or psychodynamics, or both. The Tavistock Clinic has taken a theoretical and research interest in working groups, of which team meetings are one example. Diamond & Allcorn (1987) provide a four-way classification of such groups of which one category, the autocratic group, is discussed below in the context of leadership. A second category sees individuals and the organization adapting reciprocally to each other, a process which may develop into a symbiotic relationship which prevents the group from learning from and adapting to experience. A third category is the group which attempts consciously to avoid authoritarianism. This can be done by attempting to abolish differences between staff members, said by Hinshelwood (1987) to be an attempt to prevent feelings of guilt and anxiety generated by the perception that other people have different skills. It leads at first to a reluctance to confront shortcomings in colleagues' work, and in an extreme form may be described as a homogenized work group which, according to Diamond & Allcorn (1987), is incapable of work. The fourth category is the integrated team, which recognizes that different members have different skills and is content to leave areas of work to those people who are known to have the relevant expertise.

LEADERSHIP

Where members of teams see organization and teamwork as a system of rational processes, they are primarily interested in how legitimation occurs and where authority is located. In these circumstances, leadership is seen as centrally important, and is treated as a function of role rather than of personal skills, knowledge or experience. Regardless of who acts as leader, this view encourages a style of leadership that is paternalistic and coercive. It is a style which produces special problems when there is a difference between the educational attainments of members of an organization and its leader (Diamond & Allcorn 1987). Such a working group ceases to be able to learn from experience, and Diamond & Allcorn (1987) term it an 'autocratic group', which accomplishes work at the cost of democracy and, implicitly, at the cost of allowing for less rational influences on interpersonal relationships between colleagues.

ROLE OF THE NURSE

In 1968, a report on psychiatric nursing indicated that work with patients and relatives was aimed at the goal of carrying out medical instructions and reporting objectively to the psychiatrist: '. . . Information must be conveyed to other members of the team accurately and precisely and free from subjective bias as far as possible' (Report 1968, p. 17).

The situation as described in 1968 was one where the ward environment was seen as entirely the responsibility of the charge nurse, who co-ordinated the services of other disciplines, supervised all patient care, supervised students, and administered many of the ancillary services provided to a ward. Stacey (1988) suggests that functional management (handing over responsibility for catering, domestic and other services) modified the power of ward nurses. Previously, nursing teams had a good deal of independence, even though their clinical work was carried out under instructions from medical staff. Given nurses' 'clinical subservience' (Stacey 1988), the opportunities to regain power were quite limited, and were, in any case, also being sought by other professionals (DHSS 1973, 1977). Moreover, there is substantial evidence that nurses occupied themselves with administrative and domestic duties at the expense of interaction with patients, so that there has not been a strong base from which to claim rights to specific clinical interventions (Altschul 1972, Towell 1975, Cormack 1976).

Specialization

One way for nurses to achieve parity in a multi-disciplinary team has been by participating in the team's active shaping of its place in its organization's institutional map. In evolving its own systems for managing patient care, a team begins to develop skills in providing certain kinds of treatment. These skills enhance team members' self-appraisal and, it could be argued, their enthusiasm for further definition and modification of clinical management systems.

Thus the role of the psychiatric nurse in the multi-disciplinary clinical team can be seen as comprising the following activities: using accurately recorded observations to structure a bias-free assessment of an individual's mental health; negotiating with individuals the objectives designed to resolve problems defined during assessment; measuring and comparing the cost or outcome, or both, of alternative nursing interventions; collaborating with other health care professionals to implement the interventions required to assist an individual to behave in ways which promote his mental health; collaborating with other health care professionals to define their team's procedures and systems of work. An ability to manage oneself in groups is crucial because, as has been suggested, it is in its meetings that an individual MDCT may be said to exist.

SUMMARY

The functioning of the multi-disciplinary clinical team is reflected in its methods of organizing its work, whether in coordinating case work, managing work-load or designing its procedures. Its strategies for managing change and conflict affect its ability to maintain effective collaborative practices, but it is not clear whether patient outcomes are affected as much as staff outcomes.

Each member of the team is accountable to his or her own professional superior, to the general manager of the service and to the team's authority. How a team constitutes its authority may be more or less negotiable. Traditionally, the consultant psychiatrist has been seen as leader and thus the authority to whom team members defer, but different professions have encouraged their members to see themselves as autonomous practitioners. This has resulted in conflicts of authority within ward-based teams, as nurses, for instance, have come to prefer only nurse-based authority.

The inevitable turnover of staff within teams results in the focusing of authority in the most permanent team members, often the consultant or senior nurse. It can be tempting to try to impose teamworking practices in order thereby to impose stability, but the procedures which suit, say, one occupational therapist are unlikely to suit another. There is necessarily some conflict as new members and the team adjust to one another. This conflict may be both uncomfortable and destructive of effective working relationships, or both uncomfortable and productive of effective collaboration.

The structure of a team affects its communication and decision-making patterns. In a case study, Henry (1954) demonstrates how standard hierarchically organized channels can be used to facilitate or to delay and distort communication in a seemingly paradoxical situation, where key figures in the chain either assert their individual authority (thereby facilitating communication) or attempt to fit in with the multiple demands of the hierarchy (thereby delaying and distorting communication). An organization becomes subject to special stress when its components (in the case of a ward team, the different disciplines) have overlapping functions, similar powers, and low consensus. In these circumstances, because functions of individuals tend not to be clearly defined, a 'guessing game' occurs between staff about who is responsible for what. Interpersonal tensions are the manifestation of stress, under which 'circuit-jumping' occurs (Henry 1954). Circuit-jumping is self-reinforcing. It occurs when 'people take their troubles where they think they will get most satisfaction'; it is characterized by 'suspicion, gossip, rumour, and some truth', as individuals try to establish for themselves a sense of well-being within the organization (p. 148). Since stress affects people in different ways, their behaviour may, according to Henry, be misattributed to personal shortcomings. Personal criticism increases individual stress, and, in providing an explanation for the interpersonal tensions, distracts from the organizational problems which have led to the situation.

Barriers to multi-disciplinary teamwork

At least six barriers can obstruct effective teamwork. Firstly, to hold stereotypical views of each other prevents cooperation between disciplines (Furnham et al 1984). Secondly, collegiality, where professions practise interdependently but autonomously, may degenerate into non-differentiation between disciplines as a way of avoiding conflict (Hinshelwood 1987). Thirdly, a reliance on hierarchy impedes individuals in the deployment of their skills (Margerison & McCann 1986). Fourthly, complete rejection of hierarchy can be just as damaging, especially as the hierarchy usually continues to exist covertly, and power may be exercised insidiously and unaccountably (Baron 1987). Fifthly, the clinical staff at the bottom of a hierarchy have great informal power to influence for good or ill a team's goals; to disregard their goals and aspirations is to jeopardize the team's effective implementation of plans (Carlyn & Stoffelmeyer 1981). (Strauss et al (1964, p. 372) refer to the 'secret work lives of aides'.) Finally, if the team does not specify for each of its tasks who will act as the leader, then time-wasting and potentially damaging conflict can ensue (Belbin 1981).

REFERENCES

Alanen Y O, Räkköläinen V, Rasimus R, Laakso J, Kaljonen J 1985 Psychotherapeutically oriented treatment of schizophrenia: results of 5-year follow-up. Acta Psychiatrica Scandinavica (Supplement) 319: 31–49

Altschul A T 1972 Patient–nurse interaction: a study of interaction patterns in acute psychiatric wards. Churchill Livingstone, Edinburgh

Argyris C 1970 Intervention theory and practice. Addison-Wesley, Reading, Mass

Argyris C, Schön D 1978 What is an organization that it may learn? Addison-Wesley, Reading, Mass

Ashforth B E, Fried Y 1988 The mindlessness of organizational behaviours. Human Relations 41(4): 305–329

Baron C 1987 Asylum to anarchy. Free Association Books, London

Belbin R M 1981 Management teams. Heinemann, London

Bell M D, Ryan E R 1985 Where can therapeutic community ideals be realized? Hospital and Community Psychiatry 36(12): 1286–1291

Campbell-Heider N, Pollock D 1987 Barriers to physician–nurse collegiality: an anthropological perspective. Social Science and Medicine 25(5): 421–425

Carlyn M, Stoffelmeyer B 1981 Diversity of goals in a state mental hospital. Adminstration in Mental Health 9(1): 57–66

Carter et al 1984 Systems management and change. Harper & Row, London

Collins J F et al 1985 Treatment characteristics of psychiatric programmes that correlate with patient community adjustment. Journal of Clinical Psychology 41(3): 299–308

Cooper D 1967 Psychiatry and anti-psychiatry. Tavistock, London

Cormack D 1976 Psychiatric nursing observed. RCN, London

DHSS 1973 The remedial professions. HMSO, London

DHSS 1977 Role of psychologists in the Health Service. HMSO, London

DHSS 1980 Report of the Working Party to examine organizational and management problems of mental illness hospitals (Nodder Report). DHSS, London

Diamond M A, Allcorn S 1987 The psychodynamics of regression in work groups. Human Relations 40(8): 525–543

Eiser J R 1986 Social psychology. Cambridge University Press, London

Etzioni A 1964 Modern organizations. Prentice-Hall, Englewood Cliffs, NJ

Furnham A, Pendieton D, Manicom C 1984 The perception of different occupations within the medical profession. Social Science and Medicine 15(4): 289–300

Griffiths R 1983 NHS Management Inquiry. DHSS, London

Guirguis W R, Rayner R, Hurley M 1983 Evaluation of a planned change on a long-stay rehabilitation ward. British Journal of Psychiatry 143: 591–596

Guy M E 1986 Interdisciplinary conflict and organizational complexity. Hospital and Health Service Administration 31(1): 111–121

Henry J 1954 The formal social structure of a psychiatric hospital. Psychiatry 17: 139–151

Hinshelwood R D 1987 What happens in groups? Free Association Books, London

Islam A, Turner D L 1982 The therapeutic community: a critical reappraisal. Hospital and Community Psychiatry 33(8): 651–653

Keddy B et al 1986 The doctor–nurse relationship: an historical perspective. Journal of Advanced Nursing 11(6): 745–753

Koerner B L, Cohen J T, Armstrong D M 1986 Professional behaviour in collaborative practice. Journal of Nursing Administration 16(10): 39–43

Lehman A F, Strauss J S, Ritzler B A, Kokes R F, Harder D W, Gift T E 1982 First admission psychiatric ward milieu: treatment process and outcome. Archives of General Psyhiatry 39(11): 1293–1298

Levine I, Wilson A 1985 Dynamic interpersonal processes and the inpatient holding environment. Psychiatry 48(4): 341–357

McKeganey N P, Bloor M J 1987 Teamwork, information control and therapeutic effectiveness: a tale of two therapeutic communities. Sociology of Health and Illness 9(2): 154–178

Margerison C, McCann D 1986 High performing management teams. Health Care Management 1(1): 26–31

Martin J P 1984 Hospitals in trouble. Blackwell, Oxford

Mechanic D, Aiken L 1982 A cooperative agenda for medicine and nursing. New England Journal of Medicine 307(12): 747–750

Ministry of Health 1952 Report on Co-operation between Hospitals, Local Authority and General Practitioner Services. HMSO, London

Morgan M, Calnan M, Manning N 1985 Sociological approaches to health and illness. Croom Helm, London

Parsons T 1951 The social system. Routledge & Kegan Paul, London

Report 1968 Psychiatric nursing: today and tomorrow. HMSO, London

Rosenhan D L 1973 On being sane in insane places. Science 179(4070): 250–258

Royal Commission 1979 Report on the National Health Service. HMSO, London

Skevington S 1980 Intergroup relations and social change within a nursing context. British Journal of Social and Clinical Psychology 19: 201–213

Stacey M 1988 The sociology of health and healing. Unwin Hyman, London

Strauss A, Schatzman L, Bucher R et al 1964 Psychiatric ideologies and institutions. Free Press, Glencoe, NJ

Tajfel H (ed) 1978 Differentiation between social groups: studies in the social psychology of intergroup relations. Academic Press, London

Temkin-Greener H 1983 Interprofessional perspectives on teamwork in health care: a case study. Milbank Memorial Fund Quarterly 61(4): 641–658

Towell D 1975 Understanding psychiatric nursing. RCN, London

Wolfe D E, Bushardt S C 1985 Interpersonal conflict: strategies and guidance for resolution. American Medical Record Association Journal 56(2): 18–22

5

Education

B. L. Thomas

There have been considerable changes both in the content and the process of psychiatric nursing education. The content of psychiatric nursing education should be determined by practice. However, the practice of psychiatric nursing has been repeatedly criticized for being ill-defined and psychiatric nurses criticized for lacking identifiable skills (Burnard 1989). This chapter addresses these criticisms by examining some of the changes that have occurred in the content of psychiatric nursing education and some of the influences which brought about these changes. A major change in the process of psychiatric nursing education has been the inclusion of teaching techniques designed to help students to be self-directing, to learn at their own pace and to individualize learning. This move has been influenced by changes in general education. While reference is made to general education, the chapter does not focus on theories of education but rather on their particular application to the education of psychiatric nurses. Where possible the chapter attempts to describe and make recommendations about psychiatric nursing education based on research findings.

RESEARCH PRIORITIES

Psychiatric nursing education has fared reasonably well compared with psychiatric nursing practice in terms of research. Substantial information has been gained regarding career paths and drop out rates (Everest et al 1979, Combes & Rana 1981). Davis (1984a, b, c) has provided insight into the experiences and socialization of student nurses during training. The lack of provision for advanced psychiatric education in the United Kingdom has been demonstrated by Brooking (1985). While not wishing to dispute the importance of previous research, there are, however, many remaining questions which need to be addressed, including the effectivness of psychiatric nurse training in producing competent practitioners. Research in general nursing has found that learners are inadequately prepared in communication and interpersonal skills (Gott 1983, Macleod-Clark 1983). Although similar literature exists in psychiatric nursing (e.g. Altschul 1972, Towell 1975) these finding were derived from research which did not focus specifically on the preparation of nursing students. The dearth of research into the preparation of nurses, especially in the areas of communication and interpersonal skills, is surprising considering the importance accorded to these skills in psychiatric nursing.

Another research priority is to establish whether the skills and knowledge acquired during training have any impact on patient outcomes. The absence of such studies is predictable according to Macilwaine (1983), in view of the complexity of the task and the multiple variables involved. Other research challenges facing nurse educators include the effects of the implementation of Project 2000: A New Preparation for Practice (UKCC 1986) and the implications for nursing of the Government's 'Working for Patients' document (HMSO 1989).

THE INFLUENCE OF PSYCHIATRIC NURSING PRACTICE

Professional education prepares people for practice, therefore it seems pertinent to ask what is the practice of the psychiatric nurse. Cormack (1983) argues that a knowledge of what psychiatric nursing is must precede a discussion of the required educational input. Psychiatric nursing is notoriously difficult to measure, evaluate and define.

However, defining the role of the psychiatric nurse has received considerable attention in research studies (Oppenheim 1955, John 1961, Altschul 1972, Towell 1975, Cormack 1983) and published reports (World Health Organization 1956, 1963, Ministry of Health 1968). These studies have succeeded in making significant advances towards understanding psychiatric nursing. Each study has highlighted deficiencies in the role of the psychiatric nurse and has made recommendations for improvements. Many of these recommendations have slowly been incorporated into the contemporary psychiatric nurse's role. The role continues to evolve over time, adjusting to developments in psychiatry and wider social, economic and political influences.

As well as external pressures there is continuing disagreement within the profession as to the role of the pychiatric nurse and therefore the education and training nurses should receive. Isles (1986) argues that psychiatric nursing has failed to identify a clear role and positive self-image. May & Kelly (1982) also argue that psychiatric nurses possess neither identifiable skills nor unambiguous authority. Peplau (1987), on the other hand, is in no doubt that psychiatric nurses possess skills that 'merit celebration'.

The introduction of Project 2000: A New Preparation for Practice (UKCC 1986) has highlighted the major dichotomy that exists amongst psychiatric nurses. Brooking (1988) commented that one camp consists of those nurses who hold the view that psychiatric nursing is essentially different from general nursing and has its closest affinity with other mental health workers. Proponents of this view identify closely with and advocate more joint education with clinical psychologists, social workers and psychiatrists. Some radical psychiatric nurses would abandon the label nurse altogether, as they claim that their role is more to do with treatment than care. In the other camp are those psychiatric nurses who identify themselves as nurses in the broadest sense, who happen to work in psychiatry. This group believes that nursing has certain essential defining characteristics, irrespective of the area of practice. Their main emphasis is on providing care, not treatment, and providing a 24 hour service.

As Brooking (1988) pointed out each position has a number of implications for psychiatric nurse education. If the psychiatric nurse is viewed primarily as a mental health worker, then there is a need for more multi-disciplinary education and training. While this happens informally in many clinical areas, where staff within a specialty share their expertise, there is also scope for its development in more formal settings. There are numerous topics relevant to all disciplines which could be studied together, including the nature of psychiatric disorders, research methods, ethics, management of violence and communication skills. Such a proposal does not deny that each discipline has its own knowledge base and skills which are most efficiently learned in separate discipline work. Neither does it deny the bureaucratic constraints, such as separate statutory bodies, separate systems of registration and separate funding arrangements.

Those in favour of the opposing position which considers the psychiatric nurse to be first and foremost a nurse must have welcomed the introduction of Project 2000: A New Preparation for Practice (UKCC 1986) and the introduction of a generic preparation before specialization. Their major reservation is the possibility of general nursing being seen as the basic foundation. Concentration on the biological and medical subjects, physical aspects of care and technical procedures may be given precedence with little inclusion of those skills usually associated with the psychiatric nurse's repertoire. It is this concern that has resulted in so many psychiatric nurses protesting against the introduction of a generic nurse training (Butterworth 1986, Briggs 1984).

There is no doubt that psychiatric nurses have considerable skills, particularly in the area of communication, many of which need to be included in a common foundation course. That psychiatric nurses have skills worth teaching general nurses was made explicit in the General Nursing Council Educational Policy Document (1977), which recommended seconding general nursing students to a psychiatric placement for 8 to 12 weeks. However, studies to evaluate the effectiveness of this experience have demonstrated that the use of these skills are quickly relinquished once students return

to work in general wards (Wilkinson 1982, Collister 1983, Thomas 1987).

The dominance of general nursing over psychiatric nursing is not only confined to basic training but is also evident in advanced nursing education. Brooking (1985) found that there were over 20 courses at which it was possible to study full-time for a degree in or with nursing and obtain registration as a general nurse. There were, however, only three courses which were linked with psychiatric nursing registration. The need for graduate nurses has been continually emphasized (Owen 1988). McFarlane (1977) argues that management, research and development, clinical and educational roles all require graduate-level knowledge and skills. If there are few graduate psychiatric nurses and few opportunities for advanced education this will inevitably impede the development of this speciality. Nowhere is this more clearly demonstrated than by the lack of research into psychiatric nursing practice and the paucity of psychiatric nursing theories. Examination of post-basic national board courses reveals a similar picture. Brooking (1985) found that out of a total of 72 certificate courses, 63 were listed as open to general and paediatric nurses whereas only 14 were open to psychiatric nurses.

Concern about the poor status of psychiatric nursing is substantiated by an historical examination of nursing which reveals that psychiatric nursing has long been seen as secondary to general nursing. Evidence of this is provided by Carpenter (1980) who identifies a lack of interest by historians in psychiatric nursing. He argues that nursing history always centres around the history of general hospital nursing. For example, Abel-Smith's *A History of the Nursing Profession* (1960), according to Carpenter 'magnifies the history of general hospital nursing into the history of nursing in general'.

Maggs (1983) pointed out that general nursing came to reign supreme in the occupation, and its representatives decided the structures of nursing until the present day. This point is taken up by Salvage (1985) who argues that general nursing has always been the dominant culture in the profession, as it is now. She suggests that the lack of attention paid to psychiatric nursing reflects the power structures in nursing as well as ignoring the uncomfortable existence of people with 'abnormal' mental conditions. The existence of this power struggle was highlighted by Denny & Denny (1979) in their comparison of mental health nursing education in the United Kingdom and the United States. Denny & Denny were in no doubt that in both countries general nurses did not perceive mental nurses as equal in status and suggested that this may have its origins in the general public's view of mental illness.

Further evidence of psychiatric nurses' secondary significance is supplied by authors who suggest that it was only when psychiatric nurses were able to mimic the role of the general nurse that they became truly identified as nurses. For example Sumner (1981) claims that it was only with the introduction of certain physical forms of treatment for the mentally ill that attendants became known as nurses and their morale improved. Sumner describes how psychiatric nurses scrubbed up to assist with leucotomies, prepared patients for general anaesthetics and cared for unconscious patients. The introduction of somatic treatments, including insulin shock therapy, psychosurgery and electroconvulsive therapy all required medical and surgical nursing skills.

THE CHANGING SYLLABUS OF TRAINING

It is not surprising that psychiatric nursing was so heavily influenced by physical nursing, considering that mental nurse training in the early part of the century was completely controlled by doctors. The Royal Medico-Psychological Association (RMPA), the controlling body, laid down regulations for the training and examination of candidates for the Certificate of Proficiency in Nursing and Attending of the Insane. The emphasis on biological and medical aspects is clearly demonstrated by the mental nurse training curriculum of 1908 (Box 5.1).

The General Nursing Council for England and Wales, set up in 1919, gradually began to assume responsibility for mental nurse training. By 1948 the Royal Medical-Psychological Association had relinquished its function and by 1950 the RMPA

Box 5.1	1908 Curriculum	
1st Year	—	Anatomy
2nd Year	—	Bodily diseases
3rd Year	—	Bodily diseases

examination ceased. The sole responsibility for psychiatric nurse training was then assumed by the General Nursing Council. The content of the mental nursing training syllabus has undergone many changes, as charted by Arton (1981).

In 1952 the General Nursing Council introduced a training syllabus for psychiatric nurses which clearly reflected the belief that psychiatric nursing was similar to general nursing. The first year of training continued to focus on anatomy and physiology, psychiatric topics not being introduced until the final year. In 1957 an experimental syllabus was introduced, based on the educational concept of situation-centred teaching as the most effective method of learning. The content, which included psychology and psychiatry in the first year, was taught on the principle that all subject matter should be capable of being integrated with and applied to the total nursing care of the patient.

In 1964 the experimental syllabus was officially accepted with some minor amendments. It emphasized the importance of relating class teaching as closely as possible with the work undertaken in clinical areas. Essentially the syllabus consisted of three main areas of study — the human individual, the skills needed in dealing with mental disorders, and concepts of mental disorder — which were to be taught at various levels over three years. A substantial amount of the syllabus still concentrated on human biology, psychophysical disturbance, physical illness and first aid. Although skills were mentioned these were concerned with preparation of patients for investigations and procedures, administration of drugs and observation of their effects and side-effects.

The 1974 syllabus continued in a similar vein, but with the introduction of sociological concepts and community care. More attention was given to services provided within hospitals and in the community, such as occupational, recreational and industrial therapy. The syllabus also stated that specialist workers such as doctors, occupational therapists, psychologists, social workers, pharmacists and physiotherapists should give classes where relevant.

The 1982 syllabus showed a considerable change of emphasis from the 1974 syllabus which was essentially a list of topics to be covered by the course. The skills emphasis in the 1982 syllabus was justified as being prompted by several factors. These include a need for the profession to give a clear statement of the skills of the psychiatric nurse. Secondly, the emphasis on skills stamps psychiatric nursing as essentially a 'human activity'. Thirdly, self-awareness skills are vital for all therapeutic interventions. Section two of the syllabus, the knowledge base, is a list of the knowledge to be covered during training, and is similar to the bulk of the 1974 syllabus.

Burnard (1984) argues that the aim of the 1982 syllabus is fairly conventional in that it is said to be providing the skills, attitudes and knowledge to produce a competent practitioner at the end of training. However, the major stated objective is new, that is to cultivate the acquisition of self-directing competence in student nurses which will serve them as a foundation for their professional career. This means that as the course progresses students assess their own competencies and determine their own learning goals and the means of achieving them. A humanistic perspective informs this approach and is based on the work of Rogers (1951) and Maslow (1968). Much psychiatric nurse education had already begun to develop along these lines, concentrating on student-centred as opposed to teacher-centred learning, and placing the personal experience of the student as a starting point of inquiry and reflection (Dietrich 1978).

SELF-DIRECTED LEARNING

Returning to the question of research, one area of investigation required to evaluate the effectiveness of the 1982 syllabus is the determination of the acquistion of self-directing competence in nurses. While professional education is a life-long process, this assumption is not reflected in the majority of

practice. Evidence of this is supplied by the recommendation within Project 2000: A New Preparation for Practice (UKCC 1986) for mandatory periodic refreshment for nurses. Such an idea may be welcomed by many practising nurses, particularly those who have found it difficult in the past to be released from the clinical area because of the usual problems of shortage of staff or lack of funding. However, the proposal implies the old ethos of students being passive recipients of the educational process. As Brooking (1988) explains, education in this instance is regarded as something that is done to nurses on special courses, away from clinical practice.

If during their training nurses had acquired self-directing competence then they would have accepted responsibility for their own professional development and updating. This may not be easy in a bureaucratic organization like the National Health Service and requires a radical shift in thinking, a shift in which learning is valued as part of the 'work ethic' (Treacy 1987) and not separated from it. Regular and frequent updating in teaching sessions, seminars and journal clubs could be built into the daily clinical routine, instead of being unrelated infrequent one-off events.

THE THEORY–PRACTICE DIVIDE

A gap between theory and practice has been highlighted in much research (Fretwell 1982, Melia 1982). One way to lessen the theory–practice divide is for teaching to be seen as a major part of the clinical nurse's role. Teaching skills could be part of the basic education of nurses. Unlike other disciplines nursing has sharply divided the profession into clinical practitioners, teachers, managers and researchers, producing little understanding and credibility between the various fractions. Such artificial divisions have contributed to the lack of professional advancement in nursing.

In most schools of nursing psychiatric nurse tutors are expected to teach most if not the whole of the syllabus (Rodgers 1985). This seems quite unrealistic considering the diversity of knowledge and skills that psychiatric nurses are expected to possess. This system seems to be cultivated early in the nurse teacher's career; Schrock (1975a, b), for example, found that nurse tutor students were expected to teach a wide range of topics including nursing care, drugs, human biology, medical subjects, psychological aspects of nursing and community health.

Reynolds (1984) argues that British psychiatric nurses are unlikely to develop good interpersonal techniques until all nurse educators are clinically based and make fuller use of the learning opportunities to which students are exposed. Reynolds & Cormack (1982) and Reynolds (1982) describe an action research project implementing patient-centred teaching and utilizing clinically based teachers. While potentially beneficial to patients and students, parts of the method appear problematic. For example, the teacher sitting, albeit at a distance, observing the student and patient interacting must be as off-putting as the student recording verbatim notes during the interaction. The method requires refining with further research and testing.

Research has repeatedly shown that nurse tutors lose clinical credibility when they have no clinical involvement, so their teaching is often seen by students as inconsistent and irrelevant to reality (Dalton 1969, Dodd 1973). In 1970 the Department of Health and Social Services produced the Report of the Nurse Tutor Working Party which recommended that nurse tutors should have the opportunity of specializing in their clinical interests. The General Nursing Council's Educational Policy document (1977) makes the point that most nurse teachers should have a close involvement with some part of the practice setting. Gott (1983), Alexander (1982), Reynolds & Cormack (1982) have all recommended that nurse teachers should spend time in the clinical area acting as role models and providing patient-centred learning. Sheahan (1981) in a study of the nurse tutor's role found that while learners perceived a clinical specialization role for nurse tutors, the tutors themselves did not.

For teachers to develop clinical expertise in a particular area also requires rethinking and restructuring of the present system. Time would need to be built into nurse teachers' job descriptions to involve clinical practice and research. This is not to suggest that nurse teachers simply transfer their teaching from the classroom to the clinical area. The arguments for and against the exclusive use of ward-based teaching have been well documented (Bell 1982, Wondrak 1982). The use and advantages of experiential methods in classroom teaching for psychiatric nurse education have also been well documented (Dietrich 1978, Goble 1982). Research has demonstrated that interaction skills can be successfully taught in the classroom (Paxton et al 1988). Simply to transfer all the teaching from the classroom to the ward situation is unhelpful. Rogers (1983) suggests that people need to escape from their surroundings in order to be innovative. Students need to move from the clinical environment to the safety of the classroom and back again to encourage innovation and experimentation. In the classroom they have the opportunity to practise various techniques under expert guidance and without the pressure of the ward environment. In a practice discipline like psychiatric nursing, teaching in both settings is required.

In order to make the best use of both approaches nurse teachers need clinical involvement to maintain their expertise and credibility. Various forms of clinical involvement could be explored. In advanced clinical practice, such as psychotherapy or behaviour therapy, tutors could take on their own case-load. Clinical consultancy, advice and supervision are other areas to be considered. Such involvement could also include relevant clinical research. Clarke (1977) argues that nurse tutors with the right preparation are the ideal people to research into nursing.

One constraint on clinical involvement is the limitation imposed by shortages of qualified tutors. However, Brooking (1988) argues that if nurse tutors did not have to spend so much time teaching pharmacology, clinical psychology, human biology and all the other non-nursing subjects then they would have more time to engage in nursing practice and research and the opportunity to teach practice.

Nurse teachers are in an era where they have to account for the efficiency with which available resources are used, and nurse teachers are themselves a major resource. As an illustration, Fielding & Llewellyn (1987) argue that communication skills training in nursing is expensive, involving a great deal of time, practice and teaching to acquire such skills. However, the effects of such training on patient outcomes have not been evaluated. General managers are therefore likely to give short shrift to training if the benefits to patients and the organization overall have not been demonstrated.

EVALUATING PSYCHIATRIC NURSING EDUCATION

The process of evaluation has become an essential element in the National Health Service (DHSS 1977, DHSS 1980, DHSS 1982, DHSS 1983). Nicklin & Kenworthy (1987) suggest that as nurse education is increasingly scrutinized in a general management climate, carefully planned evaluative processes will be increasingly significant in determining the credibility of nurse education.

Unfortunately, evaluation has by tradition sustained an uneasy relationship with education (Gallego 1985). This is particularly true of nursing education which is clearly under-evaluated, with rare exceptions such as Dodd (1973) and Gallego (1985). The evaluation of psychiatric nurse education is even more impoverished, with the rare exception of an evaluation of a post-basic psychiatric nursing course (Chambers 1988).

Evaluation involves the systematic collection of information for the purpose of decision-making. It involves the collection of quantitative and qualitative data on the structure, process and outcomes of the educational system (Donabedian 1980). In the past, evaluation consisted of figures for recruitment, drop-out rates, teacher/student ratios, examination pass rates and resource and financial allocation. However, it has become recognized that these quantitatively-based measures are insufficient measures of the performance of the training institution.

Recent developments in evaluating and monitoring nurse education have included setting standards against which the quality of education in training institutions can be measured (Table 5.1) referred to as 'performance indicators'. Roques (1988) suggests that an indicator can be defined as a resource which helps to determine whether a service is efficient and effective in comparison with a given standard.

Kershaw & Evans (1986) warn that performance indicators should not replace the process of course evaluation which must remain an integral part of the educational process for an institution or course. Rather, the use of performance indicators should form part of the total evaluative process. Performance indicators will provide substantial amounts of data regarding the structure, process and outcomes of individual schools, and provide a basis from which future developments should be established. In general they do not measure quality as such, but quality identification is needed to give a fuller picture.

Qualitative evaluation using process models is very complex (Wells 1987). Evans (1987), argues that evaluation of the process of education involves observation of the processes by which the varied educational activities undertaken are achieved. Qualitative evaluation can involve collecting

Table 5.1 Examples of perfomance indicators (from Evans 1987)

Standard statement	Structure	Process	Outcome
Research should be incorporated into nurse teaching	Is knowledge expertise of research identified in job description?	Are teachers/students expected to participate in research activities — at what depth?	Is teaching based on recent research findings?
Teachers of nurses should be clinically competent and up to date	Have specialist teaching posts been identified?	How do specialist teachers function?	What do students feel about the use of specialist teachers?

detailed descriptions of the opinions of those who experienced the course, e.g. students, teachers, clinical nurses and others who were involved. Sheahan (1980) suggests that evaluation must take account of the views of the service side of hospitals and the views of any other body entitled to put forward a viewpoint. This is indeed a tall order, but one that must be undertaken. Ideally it should become an aspect of the routine work of all nurse teachers; if not undertaken by them it will become an exclusive role adopted by outside experts.

CONCLUSION

This chapter has examined some of the changes which have occurred in psychiatric nursing education. There has been a definite shift away from the transmission of factual knowledge, particularly biological and medical information, to a more skills-based training. While this movement which has aimed to equip nurses with the practical skills needed in their day-to-day work with patients has been welcomed, areas of concern remain.

At the core of these concerns is the fragmentation of the profession into clinical, teaching, research and management components. The United Kingdom Central Council in its document Project 2000: A new Preparation for Practice (UKCC 1986) recommends that all nurse teachers have an understanding of the care settings to which students are allocated, as well as serving as role models to their students. A further requirement is that all nurse teachers should have an advanced level of knowledge of practice, theory and research in their specialist fields. It has been suggested in this chapter that clinical expertise would enhance the role of the nurse teacher and is an area worth exploring. Lahiff (1984) suggests that the biggest obstacle facing the nursing profession is itself and the ambivalence with which it refuses to allow the exploration of its true potential.

With the current emphasis on effectiveness and efficiency in the health services, evaluation of psychiatric nursing education is increasingly important, but little has been undertaken. This is a deficit which must be made up since without it there is no objective basis on which sensible decisions about the future development of psychiatric nursing education can be made.

REFERENCES

Abel-Smith B 1960 A history of the nursing profession. Heinemann, London

Alexander M F 1982 Integrating theory and practice in nursing. Nursing Times Occasional Papers 78: 65–71

Altschul A T 1972 Patient–nurse interaction: a study of interaction patterns in acute psychiatric wards. Churchill Livingstone, Edinburgh

Altschul A T 1985 Foreword. In: Brooking J (ed) Psychiatric nursing research. Wiley, Chichester

Altschul A T 1986 Branching out. Nursing Times 82: 47–48

Arton M 1981 The development of psychiatric nursing education in England and Wales. Nursing Times 77: 124–127

Bell J 1982 'Strangers in the ward'. Nursing Mirror 155: 14

Briggs K 1984 A very separate training. Nursing Times 80: 41

Brooking I J 1985 Advanced psychiatric nursing education in Britain. Journal of Advanced Nursing 5: 455–456

Brooking I J 1988 Key issues in psychiatric nursing. Paper presented at the Eileen Skellern Memorial Lecture. Institute of Psychiatry, London

Burnard P 1984 The way forward. Senior Nurse 1: 14–18

Burnard P 1989 Fads and fashions. Nursing Times, 85: 69–71

Butterworth T 1986 The future training of psychiatric and general nurses. Nursing Times, July 25: 65–66

Carpenter M 1980 Asylum nursing before 1914: a chapter in the history of labour. In: Davis C (ed) Rewriting nursing history. Croom Helm, London

Central Health Services Council 1968 Psychiatric nursing today and tomorrow. HMSO, London

Chambers M, 1988 Curriculum evaluation: an approach towards appraising a post-basic psychiatric course. Journal of Advanced Nursing 13: 330–340

Clarke M 1977 Research in Nurse Education. Nursing Times 73: 25–28

Collister B 1983 The value of psychiatric experience in general nurse training. Nursing Times Occasional Papers 79: 66–69

Combes R B, Rana S C 1981 An Integrated SRN/RMN course, I and II. Nursing Times 77: 45–52

Cormack D 1983 Psychiatric nursing described. Churchill Livingstone, Edinburgh

Dalton B 1969 Withdrawal from training of RMN student nurses. Nursing Times 65: 129–132

Davis B D 1984a Student nurse wastage and attitudes to treatment. Nurse Education Today 4: 89–91

Davis B D 1984b Student nurse attitudes; their modification and associations. Nurse Education Today 4: 117–120

Davis B D 1984c Interviews with student nurses about their training. Nurse Education Today 4: 136–140

Denny E, Denny J 1979 A comparison of mental health education in the UK and the psychiatric component of a baccalaureate programme in the USA. Journal of Nursing Education 18: 42–49

Department of Health and Social Security 1970 Report of the Nurse Tutor Working Party. DHSS, London

Department of Health and Social Security 1977 Nursing staffing. DHSS, London

Department of Health and Social Security 1980 Recent trends in assessment of nursing workloads and establishment. Maplin Paper 80/11. DHSS, London

Department of Health and Social Security 1982 Nurse manpower: maintaining the balance. DHSS, London

Department of Health and Social Security 1983 Nurse manpower: planning approaches and techniques. DHSS, London

Department of Health and Social Security 1985 Health services management: performance indicators. DHSS, London

Dietrich G C D 1978 Teaching psychiatry in the classroom. Journal of Advanced Nursing 3: 525–534

Dodd A P 1973 Towards an understanding of nursing. PhD thesis, Goldsmiths' College, University of London

Donabedian 1980 The definition of quality and approaches to its assessment. Health Administration Press, Michigan

English and Welsh National Boards for Nursing, Midwifery and Health Visiting 1982 Syllabus of Training Professional Register — Part 3 (Registered Mental Nurse). The English National Board For Nursing, Midwifery and Health Visiting, London

Evans L R 1987 Performance indicators in nurse education. Senior Nurse 7: 7–9

Everest R Richards E, Hanrahan M 1979 What happens to Maudsley Nurses? A follow-up study. International Journal of Nursing Studies 16: 253–266

Fielding R G, Llewellyn S P 1987 Communication training in nursing may damage your health and enthusiasm: some warnings. Journal of Advanced Nursing 12: 281–290

Fretwell J E 1982 Socialization of nurses: teaching and learning in hospital wards. PhD thesis, Warwick University

Gallego A P 1985 Evaluating the school. Royal College of Nursing, London

General Nursing Council for England and Wales 1957 Guide to the training scheme for nurses for mental diseases. The General Nursing Council for England and Wales, London

General Nursing Council for England and Wales 1964 Guide to the Syllabus of Subjects for Examination for the Certificate of Mental Nursing. The General Nursing Council for England and Wales, London

General Nursing Council for England and Wales 1974 Training Syllabus, Register of nurses, Mental Nursing. The General Nursing Council for England and Wales, London

General Nursing Council 1977 Educational policy document 77/19. Enclosures 77/A-D. The General Nursing Council for England and Wales, London

Goble I J 1982 'Ten minutes in an air raid shelter'. Nursing Mirror Education Forum (2) 154: 9

Gott M 1983 The preparation of the student for learning in the clinical setting. In: Davis B D (ed) Research into nurse education. Croom Helm, London

Her Majesty's Stationary Office 1989 Working for patients. HMSO, London

Isles J 1986 An identity crisis perpetuated. Nursing Times 82: 28–32

John A L 1961 A study of the psychiatric nurse. Livingstone, London

Kershaw B J, Evans L R 1986 Testing Skills. Nursing Times 82: 59–60

Lahiff M 1984 Attitudes to continuing education. Nursing Times 80: 27–30

Macilwaine H 1983 The communication patterns of female neurotic patients with nursing staff in psychiatric units of general hospitals. In: Wilson-Barnett J (ed) Nursing research: ten studies in patient care. Wiley. London

Macleod-Clark J 1983 Nurse-patient communication — an analysis of conversations from surgical wards. In: Wilson-Barnett J (ed) Nursing research: ten studies in patient care. Wiley, London

Maggs C J 1983 The origins of general nursing. Croom Helm, London

Maslow A H 1968 Toward a psychology of being. Van Nostrand, New York

May D, Kelly M P 1982 Chancers, pests and poor wee souls: problems of legitimization of psychiatric nursing. Sociology of Health and Illness 4: 279–301

McFarlane 1977 Developing a theory of nursing: the relation of theory to practice, education and research. Journal of Advanced Nursing 2: 261–270

Melia K M 1981 Student nurses' accounts of their work and training: a qualitative analysis. PhD thesis, University of Edinburgh

Melia K M 1982 'Tell it as it is' — Qualitative methodology and nursing research: understanding the student nurse's world. Journal of Advanced Nursing 7: 327–336

Ministry of Health 1968 Psychiatric nursing today and tomorrow. HMSO, London

Nicklin P, Kenworthy N 1987 Educational audit. Senior Nurse 7: 22–24

Oppenheim A N 1955 The function and training of mental health nurses. Chapman and Hall, London

Owen G M 1988 For better, for worse: nursing in higher education. Journal of Advanced Nursing 13: 3–13

Paxton R, Rhodes D, Crooks I 1988 Teaching nurses therapeutic conversations: a pilot study. Journal of Advanced Nursing 13: 401–404

Peplau H E 1987 Tomorrow's world. Nursing Times 83: 29–32

Reynolds W 1982 'Patient centred teaching: A further role for the psychiatric nurse teacher?' Journal of Advanced Nursing 7: 469–476

Reynolds W 1984 Issues arising from teaching interpersonal skills in psychiatric nurse training. In: Kagan C M (ed) Interpersonal skills in nursing: research and application. Croom Helm, London

Reynolds W, Cormack D 1982 Clinical teaching: an evaluation of a problem orientated approach to psychiatric nursing education. Journal of Advanced Nursing 7: 231–237

Rodgers J M 1985 An examination of research priorities in nurse education. Journal of Advanced Nursing 10: 233–236

Rogers C R 1951 Client-centred therapy: its current practice, implications and theory. Houghton Mifflin, Boston

Rogers C R 1983 Freedom to learn for the eighties. Merrill, Columbus

Roques A 1988 Cheers. Nursing Times 84: 35–36

Salvage J 1985 The politics of nursing. Heinemann, London

Schrock R A 1975a Nurse tutor students' experiences in teaching practice 1. Nursing Times Occasional Papers 71: 9–12

Schrock R A 1975b Nurse tutor students' experiences in teaching practice 2. Nursing Times Occasional Papers 71: 13–15

Sheahan J 1981 Some aspects of the teaching and learning of nursing. Journal of Advanced Nursing 5: 491–511

Sumner E C 1981 Psychiatric nursing: the quiet revolution. Nursing 30: 1333–1336

Thomas B L 1987 Are there any benefits? Interviews with general nursing students about their psychiatric secondment. MSc thesis, University of Manchester

Towell D 1975 Understanding psychiatric nursing: a sociological study of modern psychiatric nursing practice.

The Royal College of Nursing, London

Treacy M P 1987 Some aspects of the hidden curriculum. In: Allan P, Jolley M (eds) The curriculum in nursing education. Croom Helm, London

United Kingdom Central Council 1986 Project 2000: a new preparation for practice. UKCC, London

Vousden M 1986 Nobody's fool. Nursing Times 82: 59

Wells J 1987 Curriculum evaluation. In: Allan P, Jolley M (eds) The curriculum in nursing education. Croom Helm, London

Wilkinson D 1982 The effects of a brief psychiatric training on the attitudes of general nursing students to psychiatric patients. Journal of Advanced Nursing 7: 239–253

Wondrak R 1982 Practice without pressure. Nursing Mirror 155: 52–53

World Health Organization 1956 Expert Committee on Psychiatric Nursing: First Report. WHO, Geneva

World Health Organization 1963 The nurse in mental health practice. WHO, Geneva

6

An international perspective

M. T. Reed

The practice of psychiatric nursing is inextricably linked with the mental health practices of a country, as well as that country's history, geography, culture, social climate, politics and economics. In examining the practice of psychiatric nursing world-wide, differences can seem great. The world, however, is an increasingly smaller place: the development of jet age travel and high technology communications means that people and information can travel ever more rapidly around the world. It is important in today's world that we learn more about our international colleagues. Increasing mobility means that more psychiatric nurses will be practising in cultures which are not their own. Psychiatric nurses may also be dealing with client populations from different cultures. Greater understanding of mental health problems and practices globally might aid communications between nurses and clients.

Nurses world-wide also need to learn from each other. Nurses from different continents may be facing similar problems and may be helped by exchanging possible solutions, successes, failures and ideas. Organizations such as the International Council of Nurses are already working to help in the dissemination of information, and events such as the International Congresses of Psychiatric Nursing held in London offer an exciting sharing of ideas. Some of the information in this chapter came from presentations at these Congresses. Friendships formed at such international gatherings are sure to aid in greater understanding of international colleagues and help nurses to feel less insular.

This chapter begins to examine this international perspective. The quality and availability of published literature has influenced the choice of areas covered. In reviewing the literature it is always difficult to find clear descriptions of the practice of psychiatric nursing in particular countries and continents. Descriptions are influenced by the interests and expertise of the contributing authors. Where possible, the background of the author is described for the reader. In some sections the material comes largely from reports of study tours, carried out by Western nurses, and so is influenced by that nurse's own culture. The authors almost always acknowledged their own limitations of time, language and freedom of movement.

Areas which were thought to be of interest to readers, primarily because culture and practice were strikingly different, were intentionally included. Regrettably, large areas of the globe could not be included. This was sometimes due to the lack of available literature, as in the case of South America, and sometimes because their practices seemed to be more similar than dissimilar to those of the West. The text is divided into eight areas and is arranged so that starting from the UK, the focus moves from our nearest neighbours to those most distant. This chapter is intended to broaden the perspective of readers and whet the appetite to learn more.

WESTERN EUROPE

Much has been written about psychiatric nursing in Western Europe. This section will provide an overview of historical trends, discuss current trends in psychiatric nursing, examine nursing education generally and look specifically at the Italian experience.

Historical trends

European countries share a long history of state involvement in the problems of the mentally ill. Throughout Europe, present policies on com-munity care are interwoven with the history of the mental hospital which has dominated psychiatric care for the last one and half centuries. The years following the Napoleonic Wars were a time during which problems of lunacy became a favourite cause of social concern in several European countries. By the middle of the 19th century most insane poor people in Europe were cared for in asylums. Doubts about the effectiveness of asylums were expressed almost from the start, but by the end of the century the network of asylums was complete.

From the turn of the century, Freudian theories began to open up new possibilities, attracting a new and more affluent clientele. Psychoanalytic practice remained rare in Europe in the years before World War II, and was prohibited in Germany from 1933. In England, World War I extended the scope of psychiatry in the treatment of 'shellshock', although the possibility of a 'war neurosis' was officially denied in Germany. This was a time of growing interest in prevention and mental hygiene. The 1920s and 30s saw the beginning of outpatient services which offered screening, early treatment and domiciliary care. Developments were geographically restricted, and the greatest expansions were in Britain, the Netherlands and Denmark. For the majority of patients in Europe the mental hospital, and in some places outpatient practices, were the only services available.

The Second World War years brought new opportunities for psychiatry, with the development of group therapy by the British Army psychiatric service and the beginnings of institutional psychotherapy at St Albans. New physical treatments were introduced in the 1930s and 40s and for a time brought hopes of cure. A common trend in post-war reconstruction was the substantial increase in state involvement in social and economic planning, with each of the countries of Europe developing its own ideas of the welfare state. The introduction of the phenothiazines in the 1950s proved a catalyst to the moves already underway to discharge patients to other forms of care. The mid-50s marked the start of what is now accepted as community care, and such services as day hospitals, outpatient services and hostels were initiated or developed further. The time at which community-based services were formally integrated into official policy varied considerably throughout Europe.

The historical development of mental health services is described more fully in Mangen (1985).

Current trends in psychiatric nursing

Ms Holleran is an Ex-Director of the International Council of Nurses; she discussed her views about trends in psychiatric nursing in an interview for the *Journal of Psychosocial Nursing*. Much of the material that follows is from that interview (Holleran 1984). She suggested that throughout Europe there is now far more emphasis on nursing patients in the community and far more effort being applied to the community preparation of psychiatric nurses. The economic problems which all countries have experienced have produced in some countries a surplus of physicians. Spain, for example, seems to have many more physicians than are needed. This surplus is causing concern among nurses as unemployed doctors try to edge their way into nurses' jobs. There is a move to cut back on procedures which nurses are allowed to perform and to confine these tasks to physicians only. Some governments are also cutting back on the number of nursing positions. Throughout Europe there are great differences in the roles, responsibilities and education of nurses. The formal education of nurses varies widely, from none to several years of hospital training. The Council of Europe (which is larger than the Common Market and contains approximately 20 countries) has a different definition for the Clinical Nurse Specialist (CNS) than the USA. A CNS in the USA is understood to have a master's degree, while a specialist in Europe may be someone 'without a baccalaureate degree'. A grave problem throughout Europe is a lack of well-educated teachers in psychiatric nursing (Holleran 1984).

Nursing education

The variability in nursing education programmes makes it difficult to evaluate similarities and differences among them. The Advisory Committee on Training in Nursing of the European Community (1984) produced a report on the education of psychiatric nurses within the European Community and the feasibility of mutual recognition. This Report highlights the differences between member countries. In only six countries (Luxemburg, Belgium, France, Ireland, The Netherlands and the UK) do nurses require a specific qualification in psychiatric nursing, either basic or post-basic, to practise in this speciality. In Germany, Denmark, Greece and Italy there is no specialist training requirement for nurses working in psychiatric nursing, although all include a psychiatric module in general nurse training. For individual nurses who move country, anomalies arise from this situation. Some host countries, for example, regard general nurses as qualified to work in psychiatric institutions, although they are not considered sufficiently qualified in their country of origin.

After examining the training programmes in the European Community, the Committee concluded that all countries are agreed in principle that psychiatric nurses should have a more or less broad knowledge of general nursing, both theoretical and clinical. It also commented that training in psychiatric nursing includes:

- prevention
- all types of treatment and care for psychiatric patients in all situations
- education and mental health instruction
- rehabilitation and resocialization.

In discussing future trends in training, the Report stated that all countries see the need for the preparation of nurses able to care for psychiatric patients, but this training takes different forms. Of the countries which have no separate basic or post-basic psychiatric nurse training, Greece and Italy have moved towards specialist training at the post-basic level. In countries with a basic psychiatric nurse education, there is a trend towards closer correlation with general nurse training programmes. With the exception of Britain, there appear to be few definite proposals for radical changes in any of the countries. Luxemburg has recently established a 3-year basic psychiatric nurse training. In France the trend is towards separate training for psychiatric and general nurses. Belgium has no plans for changes; Ireland is retaining separate training; Germany is trying to arrive at legal recognition of the additional training; and Denmark has no plans to change the system of general nurse training which makes provisions for psychiatric nursing care.

Italy

The Italian psychiatric reforms have received great attention and much has been written about them, not least because they are different from anything else which has happened in Europe.

The Italian Mental Health Act of 1978 prohibited the building of new psychiatric hospitals and banned new admissions to existing institutions. Institutions were to be replaced by a network of community Mental Health Centres backed up by small psychiatric wards in general hospitals. Medical and social welfare funds were to be reorganized to cope with the new structure in the community with no redundancies. Compulsory admissions were to be scrutinized more closely and all public psychiatric hospitals, it was estimated, would close down within 3 months.

The Community move which had begun in other parts of Europe in the early 60s was at that time still unheard of in Italy. Psychiatric care consisted of long-stay hospitals, owned by local authorities, which were notorious for their use of custodial methods and compulsory admissions (Hicks 1984).

The Italian legal reform came after 15 years of work led by Psychiatrica Democratica (PD), a group of socialists, communist psychiatrists and other mental health professionals, the most famous of whom was the late Franco Basaglia. This movement saw itself as part of a wider Italian political tradition and was influenced by Marxist ideology. One of the first settings for the group's work was Trieste, a northern industrial city. It was in Trieste that the group's adherents gradually opened wards and set up new mental health centres. Over 300 nurses, social workers and psychiatrists now work in teams from the seven mental health centres in Trieste, each of which provides outpatient care and has approximately six beds for short-term use. The general hospital provides an emergency psychiatric service. The teams work according to the PD's collectivist, non-hierarchical principles and seem to have abandoned traditional roles. No staff members have a room or desk of their own; there are no receptionists and no appointments or referrals.

Hicks (1984) interviewed Dr Ramon, Lecturer in Social Work at the London School of Economics and a proponent of the PD model who has paid several visits to Trieste. Dr Ramon's view was that the group's political critiques of traditional approaches have led to some confusion. There is a desire to do away with traditional techniques and methods, but uncertainty as to what to replace them with. Psychiatric nurses in Italy (whom, as previously mentioned, receive no specialist training) form the largest component of the health care work-force, and some of them have strongly resisted the change. In the hospitals at Trieste, the new plans met with a series of strikes by nursing staff who wanted to keep the wards locked. It is psychiatrists and nurses who have had to undergo the most radical modifications of their traditional roles (Ramon 1985). Nurses' roles have expanded to become 'therapists of everyday life'. This change has brought about an identity crisis among nurses. Ms Battaglia, who spoke at a conference on 'Mental Health Care in the European Community', said that the nurses' trade union was not always helpful during this time of great change and that initially the nurses had to fight a battle for a new contract and professional recognition of the new type of work they were doing without the support of the union.

The problems now facing the reformers are enormous. Resources are tight, the service is not adequately funded, and this means that new clients may have to remain with families. The movement is facing a backlash from traditional psychiatry as well as the general public. The law has not been effective throughout Italy; in the South, for example, many institutions remain untouched.

Articles about the Italian experience can at times leave the reader mystified, with evaluations ranging from wild optimism to pessimism and criticism. It is difficult to get a true picture of what really exists. Differences in culture and political ideology between Italy and the UK also contribute to difficulties in our understanding of the experiment. Despite these difficulties, it is worth examining the Italian experience carefully, to learn from both its successes and failures as we move patients out into the community and close down hospitals.

AUSTRALIA

Written reports from the Proceedings of the Australian Congress of Mental Health Nurses, 1985, provided some of the material about the history of psychiatric nursing in Australia as well as the radical changes now occurring.

Historically, psychiatric nursing has developed independently of general nursing. Psychiatric nursing, based on the British model originally, has always offered a 3-year training programme for registration as a psychiatric nurse. This training has provided psychiatric nurses with the knowledge and skills necessary to practise in any psychiatric setting, whether it be based in an institution or the community. There is some course content which is similar to general nursing courses and which provides skills necessary to nurse people with mental health problems and concomitant physical disorders. Apart from this shared area, psychiatric nurse training has claimed to develop skills unique to psychiatric nurses.

Until about 15 years ago psychiatric nurses did not consider it necessary to obtain a certificate in general nursing. The impetus for them to obtain these certificates has come from the development of psychiatric units in or attached to general hospitals. Employers in these units give preference to 'double trained' nurses. In general hospitals, staff with both qualifications can be used in general medical or surgical wards in times of staff absence or emergency. Having this second certificate, the psychiatric nurse has a choice of employment in either the general or psychiatric field. Promotional prospects are also enhanced within the psychiatric setting because higher clinical qualifications are not available in psychiatric nursing.

Mrs Orton, Principal Lecturer at the Department of Health Studies, Sheffield City Polytechnic, completed a 7000 mile study tour within Australia, visiting 20 hospitals. She observed that nursing within Australia presented an exciting drama of change and turmoil (Orton 1985). Australian nurses maintain that the community is increasingly important, with a growing emphasis on the promotion and maintenance of good health. New trends demand a more comprehensive curriculum than that offered in traditional nursing schools.

Australian nurses have for a long time urged the federal government to shift basic nursing education from hospitals to Colleges of Advanced Education. The first report was produced by a nursing leader in 1974 and was the basis for workshop discussions throughout Australia. As a result of these workshops, a policy statement, 'Goals in Nursing Education', was published in 1976. Major areas of concern were:

- the future of nurses trained in conventional settings
- whether educational establishments would be of the right calibre
- whether graduates of the new programmes would be competent practitioners.

An interesting aspect of this policy statement was that it placed responsibility for the preparation of adequately-trained nurses as much on society as on the profession. In 1984, the Federal Government of Australia announced, in principle, its support for the transfer of all nursing education from hospital to college-based programmes by 1993. Since then each state has begun implementing the change, each with a different timetable and different college-based programmes.

These changes have implications for all nurses in Australia, including psychiatric nurses. Another change, affecting psychiatric nurses specifically, has been the proposal to create a single basic course in education, leading to registration in both psychiatric and general nursing. In some states (South Australia and New South Wales, for example) this has already occurred. This has caused concern among psychiatric nurses as there is a fear that the comprehensive training will have an unsatisfactory effect on mental health practices, and that clinical experience in psychiatric settings will be insufficient.

Orton (1985) observed that the increased educational opportunities are associated with a 'new breed' of highly intelligent, well-educated and articulate nurses. High-profile tactics are used by the Royal Australian Nursing Federation to increase the influence of nursing within the public sphere. Quality assurance is a prominent theme, and senior nurses are preoccupied with standards of practice and levels of care. As in Europe, Australian health care budgets are being reduced. A focus of nurses' new found political muscle is the issue of health care funding.

Some nurses have had misgivings and concerns. Some fear that college students will be 'different' and inferior clinically. These concerns are similar to those expressed, in the UK and the USA.

Psychiatric nursing is in the process of much change and development in Australia. The rest of the world will watch with interest the lessons learned and successes achieved as the changes are implemented.

USA

This section is divided into two parts: history, and education and practice. It draws on a number of published sources, as well as the author's own experiences as a psychiatric clinical nurse specialist in the USA.

History

The first American psychiatric nurse graduated in 1873 and helped to prepare the first school for psychiatric nurses. For the next 70 years, the role of the psychiatric nurse was mainly custodial with an emphasis on the use of physical measures. 1947 marked the beginning of a new era for psychiatric nursing in that eight programmes of advanced preparation for nurses to care for psychiatric patients began. It was in these graduate programmes that the first psychiatric nursing leaders were prepared; and in 1952 Dr Hildegard Peplau wrote the first systematic, theoretical framework of psychiatric nursing in her book *Interpersonal Relations in Nursing*.

In 1956, the concept of the Clinical Nurse Specialist (CNS) was formalized under the sponsorship of the National League for Nursing (NLN) and the National Institute of Mental Health. According to a statement made by the NLN, the CNS was to 'bring about advances in the art and science of psychiatric nursing and . . . promote application of new knowledge and methods in the care of patients'.

1960 marked an important year for nursing education with the establishment of the first doctoral programme in nursing. 1960 was also the year of passage of the Comprehensive Community Mental Health Act. Psychiatric nurses were given the go-ahead to 'continue to explore and develop their therapeutic usefulness in individual psychotherapy, group psychotherapy and milieu therapy among others'. By the late 1960s the concept of the psychiatric clinical nurse specialist was widely accepted, and in 1972 the first certifying body for clinical specialists in psychiatric nursing was formed.

Education and practice

Nursing education in the USA differs considerably from most European countries, including the UK. Jane Bruker, director of a nursing programme in an American college, reviewed the American nursing education system and the following comes from her article (Bruker 1985).

In the UK, most nurses are trained in hospital schools of nursing with a few attending nursing degree courses associated with colleges and universities. American nurses have been trained in both settings since the 1950s, and at present there are three methods of preparing students for the nursing profession. (There is specialized education for psychiatric nursing in the USA.)

The first method is the hospital-based diploma programme, quite similar to its British counterpart. These programmes are usually found in general hospitals, and students receive far more clinical experience than in the degree programmes.

The second method, the associated degree in nursing (ADN) programme, is unique to the USA. It began during an acute shortage of trained nurses after World War II and was designed to reduce time spent in training. The community colleges, which are post-secondary educational institutions, were chosen to provide these 2-year programmes. Many of the courses offered by these colleges are vocational in nature and the colleges are supported through taxes from the community they serve. The curriculum content of each ADN programme is determined by the state in which the community college is located; every graduate has to complete theory courses in medical, surgical, maternal/child and psychiatric nursing. Clinical experience must also be gained in the four areas. Nursing students are exposed to students and faculty from other disciplines, and courses are taught by instructors who hold master's and doctoral degrees in their subject.

The third method of education leads to a bachelor of science degree in nursing (BSN) which is awarded after the completion of at least 4 years' study in a college or university. The curriculum for nursing students in the baccalaureate programme must include the same general foundation courses as for non-nursing students in the university. Students therefore receive a well-rounded liberal arts education. The nursing components of the ADN and BSN curricula are the same in the clinical areas that they cover, but the baccalaureate programmes have advanced studies in physical assessment, nursing theory, nursing management, research methods and nursing leadership. The baccalaureate programmes aim to produce analytical people with nursing skills, who are able to identify client needs independent of medical intervention, and to utilize research.

After the completion of any of these three programmes, the graduate then takes an examination which is uniform nationally but given by Boards of Nursing within individual states. Passing this entitles the nurse to use the initials RN (or Registered Nurse) after her name. Nursing licences must be renewed every 2 years and most states now require proof of relevant continuing education before renewing licences.

Thus American RNs could have three very different educational backgrounds and employers can select which type of RN is most suitable for a particular setting. For example, some of the major teaching hospitals prefer to offer work to RNs who are BSN prepared. A nurse who wants to work in psychiatry may find some psychiatric hospitals encouraging or requiring candidates to have 1 to 2 years' general hospital experience. Nursing salaries are good and nursing in general has a higher status in the USA than the UK.

The lack of clinical experience in BSN programmes has been greatly criticized, and employers have developed methods of coping with this problem. Some hospitals offer 'internship' programmes where the new graduate has a year of very close supervision by an experienced nurse, is paid less than other nurses, and spends a considerable amount of time in the classroom.

It is in the graduate programmes that clinical nurse specialists are prepared. Only psychiatric nurses with master's degrees are entitled to call themselves a CNS, and a BSN is a requirement to enter a graduate programme. In the master's programme, the nurse is taught advanced clinical skills, and if the major is psychiatric nursing, the nurse would learn individual, group and family psychotherapy. The master's programme also requires a thesis to be submitted which involves a piece of original research and thus builds on the research knowledge gained at baccalaureate level. Nursing management, education, theory and consultation are also extensively studied. Job markets for the CNS vary over a broad range throughout the country. Doctoral programmes in nursing are widely available, and most teachers in master's programmes are doctoral-prepared or working towards that goal.

There is a strong trend in the USA to make the baccalaureate degree a requirement for entry into the profession. One argument is that nurses should have a comparable educational background to others in the health care team if they are to have equal power. This argument is one which will be closely followed by nurses in other parts of the world as they consider the most appropriate place for nursing education.

Reynolds (1984) conducted a study tour to the USA and found that in American graduate programmes, theory and practice are closely linked. He looked at some of the differences in the UK and USA educational systems and concluded that

USA students are required to implement theory during practice, while UK students are not required to practise psychiatric therapy, and their teachers may not have extensive experience in group, individual or family therapy.

American students always practise theoretical concepts in clinical areas, unlike UK students who are often introduced to theory that they never practise. There is, at all levels of nursing education in the USA, a strong emphasis on nursing diagnosis and much less dependence on a medical model to provide nursing care prescriptions.

Graduate education in the USA seeks to produce researchers. The success of the programmes becomes apparent when the volume and quality of American nursing papers and textbooks are reviewed (Reynolds 1984).

INDIA

Mrs K. Reddemma provided most of the material for the following section on India. She is an Indian psychiatric nurse and in 1982 was one of the very few Indian nurses who had completed the Master of Nursing course with psychiatric nursing as a clinical specialization.

The existing mental health services in India are woefully inadequate. For the current estimated population of 680 000 000, there is one psychiatric bed for 32 500 people, compared with 4.4 beds/1000 in the USA (Doyle 1981). Outpatient services form the main source of mental health care in the urban areas. It can be safely said that there are no significant services for the rural population. It is estimated that the entire health care system provides care for not more than 10% of those requiring urgent mental health treatment (Reddemma 1982).

There is only one training facility for psychiatric nurses in India. The first organized course for psychiatric nursing was begun in 1954, based on the British system, and at present is of 10 months' duration. Although there are only 600 psychiatric nurses in India, the educational system has made great strides forward with the establishment of three MSc programmes and the provision to do a PhD in psychiatric nursing at one university. Due to the limited numbers of psychiatric nurses in

academic work and of teachers, research has a low priority and has yet to become incorporated into the profession (Reddemma 1982).

There are severe problems facing the psychiatric nursing profession in India. Many psychiatric settings are staffed almost entirely with people who have limited training. The role of the professionally prepared nurse in the psychiatric setting is not clearly defined. Educational preparation overall is inadequate. Psychiatric nursing is not well integrated into the basic curriculum due to a lack of teachers and facilities. Trained psychiatric nurses do not have sufficient financial benefits or enough avenues of promotion, and are often left feeling frustrated and inappropriately used (Reddemma 1982).

CARIBBEAN

Rita Frett-Georges RN SCM RMN MA(Psyc) provided much of the factual information about the state of psychiatric nursing in the Caribbean. The information was presented by her at the Second International Congress of Psychiatric Nursing, held in September 1983.

Mental illness in the Caribbean is more often treated by non-medical practitioners than by the few psychiatrists who practise in the country (Frett-Georges 1983). Historically, psychiatric hospitals were built by the British in the late 1800s and British-style mental health care continues, with treatment techniques following British methods rather than American.

The staff and facilities provided for care of mental illness vary greatly from island to island. Barbados has three psychiatrists at its 600-bed hospital, and provides a treatment centre for many neighbouring islands. Antigua has one psychiatrist, two psychiatric nurses and a mental hospital. St Vincent has one trained psychiatric nurse and a mental hospital. There are no mental hospitals on many islands (Frett-Georges 1983).

The socio-political history of the region has left a legacy of beliefs and practices which cannot be ignored. 'Santeria' and 'Esperitismo' or 'Curanismo' in the Spanish-speaking islands, each superimposed by mixtures of Catholicism, Pentecostalism and other beliefs, provide alternative healing systems that are widely used (Frett-Georges 1983).

The diagnosis of mental illness is also influenced by cultural beliefs. For example, personality changes are often seen in the Caribbean as a spiritual phenomenon and not as mental illness. Spiritual possession occurs when a specifically named god enters and 'takes over' the body for a period of time. An individual may become possessed during a religious ceremony or, less frequently, in a variety of secular circumstances (Schwartz 1985).

The practice of obeah is a system of beliefs and practices involving the manipulation of evil spirits. Although most scientific practitioners disregard obeah as superstition, these beliefs are rooted deep in the West Indian culture, and it is perhaps necessary for those involved in mental health to respect the spiritual and cultural beliefs of the people (Frett-Georges 1983).

Psychiatric nursing in the Caribbean is patterned on the mental health model in operation in a particular territory. Numbers of nurses vary, with greater numbers working in Santo Domingo and Puerto Rico. Smaller territories have fewer psychiatric nurses, and where they do exist they may be employed as supervisors or in other areas of the health service. They often work without appropriate psychiatric consultation or support personnel. Salaries are low in the Eastern Caribbean; professionals don't have job variation and career ladders are short or non-existent. Direct care is often given by untrained people, with the better-qualified nurse acting as a supervisor (Frett-Georges 1983).

Obstacles to effective psychiatric nursing practice include lack of appropriate policies, strategies, training and resource management. Inadequately-prepared personnel and the paucity of trained psychiatric nurses, coupled with the absence of psychiatrists and other mental health workers, contribute to the rapid rate of burn-out experienced by psychiatric nurses working in the Carribean (Frett-Georges 1983).

Changes have taken place in the larger territories, with services following the pattern of more developed countries. Nurses who are more capable of a therapist-clinician role with a more broad-based community orientation and with less of the custodial approach are needed, especially in the smaller territories of the Eastern Caribbean.

AFRICA

Most of the material for the following section came from Vincent Wankiiri (1984b), a psychiatric nurse tutor seconded by WHO to the government of Lesotho, Southern Africa. The written material was based on a paper delivered at the International Psychiatric Nursing Congress held in London, 1983.

In many respects, Africa's mental health problems are greater than those in the West. The incidence of such disorders as schizophrenia and affective disorders is much the same as in the West, but conditions relating to infections, malnutrition and childhood brain damage are far more common. Psychosocial changes, such as weakening of the extended family, violent political changes, drought, famine, wars and unemployment, have caused a rising incidence of crime, alcohol and drug abuse and other problems previously unknown in Africa.

Despite these awesome difficulties, psychiatric treatment is largely unavailable. Over 80% of the African population live in remote rural areas where the nearest psychiatric hospital may be hundreds of kilometres away, with few or no roads in between. The few hospitals which do exist are mostly old, overcrowded and understaffed, with a forbidding appearance which contributes to the negative image of psychiatry and psychiatric nurses. This negative image means that most general health workers are unwilling or unable to provide care for mentally ill patients in rural areas (where most patients live). These patients are thus obliged either to travel long distances to urban psychiatric hospitals, or to receive no treatment. A WHO Expert Committee on Mental Health has stated that there are 40 000 000 people in developing countries who suffer from serious neuropsychiatric disorders but who receive no modern treatment at all.

There is a severe shortage of nurses in Africa. The overall ratio of nurses to people is 1.3:10 000, compared with 50:10 000 in New Zealand

(Wankiiri 1984). Over 90% of psychiatric nurses in most African countries live and work in towns where only 15 to 20% of the population lives. The nursing shortage can be attributed partly to lack of adequate training facilities and teachers, and also to the migration of nurses, mainly to the USA, UK and Canada.

One of the main reasons for this migration is inappropriate training. Many nurse-training programmes in Africa are still disease-oriented, hospital-centred and out of line with the mental health needs of African people. Mental health concepts are not well integrated into general nursing education, and often the compulsory psychiatric nursing secondment is not complied with by schools of nursing (Olade 1977). There are inadequate clinical facilities, insufficient teaching personnel trained or interested in psychiatric nursing, and a stigma attached to psychiatric nursing from religious and cultural beliefs (Olade 1977).

The African psychiatric nurse must be able to combine the roles of doctor, social worker, mental health educator, consultant, and tutor to all rural-based primary health workers. Nurses must be community based and most of their work must go beyond traditional psychiatric nursing. They must be able to interview, diagnose, treat, nurse and teach families (Wankiiri 1984).

In Botswana, the role of the nurse is now being expanded. Psychiatric nurses have been given in-service courses in community mental health and have been posted to the community where they are providing excellent services to thousands of families.

In Lesotho, most general health workers are being trained in the community to assist in the treatment of psychiatric patients. Lesotho has also established nine mental health units attached to general hospitals, which are staffed, however, by general nurses who have had only a few weeks' training in psychiatric nursing.

In Zambia, mental health services are being decentralized and integrated into primary health care, and many psychiatric nurses have been posted to district hospitals.

These are all encouraging trends and highlight the important role psychiatric nurses have in developing and implementing programmes to provide mental health services to the majority of African people.

PEOPLE'S REPUBLIC OF CHINA

There is a wealth of information available, mostly from study tours, on Chinese nursing. At times the information found was contradictory, highlighting a problem related to the fact that study tours are of short duration and complicated by a language barrier. The following section is an attempt to consolidate information and provide an overview of psychiatric nursing in China.

The incidence of mental illness in China is difficult to determine. Statistics quoted to a delegation of American nurses visiting China (Tousley 1985) came from cities along the eastern coastline and therefore did not include the vast rural population. Figures on the incidence of major psychoses seem in line with those of the rest of the world.

The Chinese consider mental health a matter of political attitude, and in their controlled society there is little political conflict. Consequently, reported figures on minor mental illness are low compared to other countries (Tousley 1985). Dahl (1983) reported that the diagnosis of depression is rarely given in China. She hypothesizes that the difficulties of identification and measurement of depression, as defined by Western medicine, are due to an entirely different set of cultural beliefs. Emphasis throughout the Chinese belief system of Tao is placed on physical cures to harmony or disharmony with the universe, explained in terms such as Yin and Yang. The emphasis is on physical elements in the definition of all illness. The Tao belief system would therefore seem to preclude defining emotional problems such as depression in any way other than in physical terms (Dahl 1983).

In keeping with these beliefs, psychiatric nurses and doctors interviewed by Dahl had a physiological orientation to psychological treatment. They stated that psychotherapy was considered 'silly', and described patients' problems and progress in behaviouristic terms. There is a strong belief that patients' mental problems are physiologically based and that physical approaches are the most effective. Massage, wax therapy (hot slabs of wax molded around joints), acupuncture, vacuum cupping, exercise and work therapy were all observed to be central to treatment plans (Dahl 1983).

The Cultural Revolution had an enormous impact on nursing in China. In 1966 Mao Tse-tung launched a campaign to 'popularize' medical services. He was severely critical of the education of professionals, and nursing schools were closed. Despite all the setbacks in science and education during the Cultural Revolution, the Chinese have made remarkable strides in health care. It is available at every level of organization at little or no cost to the individual. Since disease is perceived of as a social phenomenon, the Chinese approach to combating disease is to launch a low-level ideological campaign (Tousley 1985). In treating mental illness they have traditionally placed more emphasis on biological causes, with a great emphasis on work therapy in psychiatric treatment. This is related to the political indoctrination which permeates all facets of existence in China and which stresses the social good of the whole rather than the self-actualization of each individual (in contrast to Western philosophy) (Dahl 1983). Political ideology provides the basic support for all activity, and this includes the treatment of mental illness.

During a tour of visiting American nurses, Wilson & Hutchinson (1983) saw patients diagnosed as schizophrenic whom they felt were strikingly different from American schizophrenics. The differences were related to behaviour, affect, sense of motivation and perception of reality. When asked about criteria for diagnosis, they were told that these young people had been involved with the opposite sex or had behaved in ways not beneficial to the Chinese people. Dahl (1983) also reports testimony of a patient hospitalized for a mental condition who attributed her condition to failing to understand the teachings of Mao.

In studying psychiatric treatment, folk beliefs must be considered, as they have a great influence on the Chinese people. Shamanism is the belief in a supernatural power which can descend to a human being, the shaman, to help the client cope with problems. Physiognomy is the belief that there is a close correlation between the structure of a person's face and his entire fate. These devices are not scientifically based, but have been used repeatedly for thousands of years, and may be the first choice of treatment for Chinese people, especially those living in villages (Lee Lo 1976).

As a result of the Cultural Revolution, China has very few nurses (Tousley 1985). Most of a patient's needs are met by the family. If a patient has no family, care is provided by friends from the workplace. Nurses work 48 hours per week, as do all workers in China, and have 2 weeks holiday per year (Chang 1983).

Nursing education programmes take 3 years. After completing the course and passing an examination, graduates are certified as nurses. The government then assigns the nurse to work in a health care setting for the duration of her working life. Nursing schools have shortages of nursing teachers, books and modern equipment. Most nurses in mental health have no formal education in psychiatric nursing (Tousley 1985).

Psychiatric nurses are informally divided into two categories. Recreational nurses work on ward activities and patient management, while therapeutic nurses talk with families about the patient's 'disease' and his readjustment back into the family or production brigade. Psychiatric nurses work in different units representing different levels of nursing care. Patients are discharged when symptoms decrease and their behaviour is no longer disruptive. On return to families and work brigades they resume work gradually through a graded series of jobs (Wilson & Hutchinson 1983).

USSR

The Soviet Union consists of 15 autonomous republics. Although each of the republics has its own health department they are all subordinate to the federal ministry. All major policies thus emanate from Moscow and innovation from any other source is unusual. Decisions on all new developments are made only at the highest level and their implementation is carried out throughout the country. In this way a striking uniformity of practice is achieved (Bloch 1978).

The Soviet health care delivery system was centralized in the 1920s following the Bolshevik

Revolution. During the Revolution and again during World War II, many psychiatric hospitals were destroyed. To cope with so few psychiatric beds, the Soviets developed a system of catchment areas, served by polyclinics for physical ailments and psychiatric dispensaries which are backed up by psychiatric hospitals with inpatient beds.

The Soviet Union presently has made up for its losses and has one of the highest bed/person ratios in the world (Doyle 1981). There are approximately 50 psychiatric hospitals (15 in the highly populated Moscow area). Each hospital has from one to three psychiatric dispensaries associated with it which act as the front lines of defence against inpatient hospitalization.

A patient's initial diagnosis will be made by a doctor. At the first visit, the doctor will also determine treatment goals. On a study tour Doyle (1981) heard contradictory views about the role of the nurse in goal setting. A few speakers said the doctor valued her opinions, but all emphasized that the doctor was in charge, and the nurse only carried out orders. 'Talk therapies' are always conducted by doctors. Medication is prescribed for approximately 90% of all patients seen, as all mental illness is presumed to have a biochemical basis. If the patient doesn't respond at the dispensary level he will be admitted to a psychiatric hospital for from 2 weeks to 2 months. Patients are assured that their jobs will be held for them and receive sick pay while hospitalized. Within 10 days of hospital discharge, the patient is scheduled to see the original dispensary doctor. Should the patient fail to visit, doctor and nurse visit the patient at home.

Inpatient treatment modalities include galvanization, electric stimulation and ultraviolet radiation, carried out by a nurse under doctor's orders. Doyle (1981) was told psychosurgery is no longer done, and that ECT and insulin subcomas continue routinely as a treatment of last choice.

Psychiatric nurses, along with all health care professionals, earn relatively less money than other professionals. The average nurse earns 90 roubles a month, while the average Soviet citizen earns more than double that (a rouble is worth about one pound sterling) (Rogers 1986). The stated rationale is that health care workers are inherently rewarded by the opportunity to serve Socialist comrades and to bring health to the nation (Doyle 1981). Staff shortages are a problem and there is a constant shortage of recruits. The patient load is heavy, and wards are overcrowded. A typical Leningrad ward has 120 patients compared to a UK ward with 20 (Rich 1979).

Nurse training takes 2 years, and is based in a medical training institute. Theory is taught by doctors, with no concept of teaching nursing theory (Rogers 1986). After the initial 2 years the nurse is allocated a place of work where she stays for a further 3 years. Later she can 'specialize' by taking 2 to 4 month courses, also taught by doctors (Rogers 1986). The nurse's responsibility is strictly limited to carrying out the doctor's orders and nurses are very definitely subordinate to doctors.

Soviet psychiatry must be studied within the political system of the Soviet Union. Citizen-provided services are geared towards the growth and productivity of society as a whole, and not towards the individual. The individual is important only in the sense that he fulfils his obligations to the collective. It is the responsibility of everyone to work productively. It is also the right and responsibility of each citizen to be healthy so that he can serve the needs of the state.

Historically, up until the time of the Revolution, Russian and Western psychiatric practices were fairly similar and Freud's theories were accepted by a number of Russian psychiatrists. The virtual obliteration of Freudianism, however, began in the 1930s when Stalin's political controls infiltrated every facet of life and Soviet medicine became isolated from Western influences. Psychoanalysis was officially pronounced as pseudo-scientific and reactionary. The translation of Freud's works ceased and his material became almost inaccessible. The same applied to the work of Jung, Adler and others from the neo-Freudian school. This antipathy to Freud continues to the present, and Freudianism is identified as a bourgeois weapon, related to imperialism (Bloch 1978). In an intensely ideological state like the Soviet Union, the idea that man's behaviour is ruled by irrational, egotistical instincts cannot be tolerated. The psychoanalyst's encouragement to the patient that he adopt an independent and autonomous stance also contradicts the collective thinking of the Soviet Union.

In 1950 a joint session of the Academies of Science and Medical Science, following party dictate, cemented the adoption of the Pavlovian basis of medicine. Pavlov's theories were to be extensively developed and applied to medical practice. The most crucial development arising out of this era has been the immense widening of the criteria for the definition of mental illness, and of schizophrenia in particular. Soviet psychiatrists have introduced a unique scheme for the classification of schizophrenia, which enables dissenting behaviour to be labelled as evidence of the disease. The dissenter is interned in a mental hospital, surrounded by disturbed patients, given drugs for side-effects rather than benefits and loses all rights (Bloch 1978). The Soviet diagnosis of schizophrenia is based upon a set of criteria found unacceptable by WHO standards (Doyle 1981). This broadening of the concept of mental illness has coincided with the widespread misuse of psychiatry for political ends (Bloch 1978).

CONCLUSION

In examining eight different areas of the globe we have seen great differences in the practice of psychiatric nursing with differing climates, policies, economies and social forces all exerting their influence. Despite these vast differences three areas of common concern can be identified.

The first of these is, of course, patient care. Psychiatric nurses everywhere, from the remotest village of Africa to the heart of the world's great cities, are all concerned about the amount, quality and effect of their care. Their patients may bear different diagnoses and be in greatly differing settings, but psychiatric nurses in every country are working to restore mental health and return patients to their homes.

The second common area of concern is education for psychiatric nurses. There seems to be a general feeling, with the exception of the USA, that overall the education of psychiatric nurses is inadequate. In most countries, nursing leaders are calling for more qualified staff, more resources and more research. In many areas, typified by Australia, psychiatric nursing education is being integrated into general nursing courses. Many industrial countries, again typified by Australia, are beginning to move nursing education into institutions of higher and further education. Even in China and the USSR, where information is more limited, education is of concern. The quality of psychiatric nurse education, its most appropriate setting and its relationship to general nurse education are of universal concern to psychiatric nurses.

The third common area of concern is the psychiatric nurse's role in relation to the doctor. In Italy, traditional roles have been altered drastically; in the USSR the psychiatric nurse is clearly subordinate to the doctor; in Africa, psychiatric nurses are often expected to carry out all aspects of the doctor's role; and in the USA, psychiatric nurses are carrying out nursing care plans independently of medical intervention. However varied their roles, psychiatric nurses everywhere are aware and concerned about their relationship with the medical profession.

There are, undoubtedly, additional concerns, as well as ideas and problems, which unite psychiatric nurses globally. The issues raised by the different countries discussed in this chapter will give readers a glimpse of the work of their international colleagues. This glimpse will perhaps inspire readers to learn more and to become increasingly concerned about problem-solving and exchanging ideas on an international level.

REFERENCES

Advisory Committee on Training in Nursing 1984 Report on psychiatric nursing in the European Community. Commission of the European Community, Brussels

Bloch S 1978 Psychiatry as ideology in the USSR. Journal of Medical Ethics 4: 126–131

Bruker J 1985 The American way. Nursing Mirror 160(4): 36–37

Chang M K 1983 Nursing in China. American Journal of Nursing 83: 389–395

Dahl J 1983 Transcultural communication on depression with Chinese nurses and physicians. Journal of Psychosocial Nursing 21(2): 14–18

Dolan J A, Fitzpatrick M L, Hermann E K 1983 Nursing in society. W B Saunders, London

Doyle M C 1981 A nurse's view of Soviet psychiatry. Perspectives in Psychiatric Care 14(1): 21–26

Frett-Georges R 1983 Psychiatric nursing in the Caribbean. Jamaican Nurse 24(2): 21–25

Green N K 1983 Nursing in China. American Journal of Nursing 83: 389–395

Hicks C 1984 The Italian Experience. Nursing Times 80(12): 16–18

Holleran C 1984 The world of psychosocial nursing. Journal of Psychosocial Nursing 22(11): 33–37

Lee Lo M L 1976 Folk beliefs of the Chinese and implications for psychiatric nursing. Journal of Psychosocial Nursing 14(10): 37–42

Mangen S 1985 (ed) Mental health care in the European Community. Croom Helm, London

Olade R 1977 Integration of mental health concepts into general nurse education in Nigeria. International Journal of Nursing Studies 14: 63–68

Orton H 1985 Storming the ark. Nursing Times 82(1): 36–37

Peplau H 1952 Interpersonal relations in nursing.

Proceedings of the Australian Congress of Mental Health Nurses 1985 Implications of the changes in nursing education of mental health nurses and services

Ramon S 1985 The Italian psychiatric reform. In: Mangen S (ed) Mental health care in the European Community. Croom Helm, London

Reddemma K 1982 Psychiatric nursing. The Nursing Journal of India 73(5): 144–146

Reynolds 1984 Psychiatric nursing in the USA. Nursing Mirror 158: 25–27

Rich V 1979 Dr Marina Voikhanskaya. Nursing Times 75(16): 630–633

Rogers R 1986 Health care in the USSR. Senior Nurse 4(2): 29–30

Schwartz D 1985 Caribbean folk beliefs and Western psychiatry. Journal of Psychosocial Nursing 23(11): 26–30

Tousley M M 1985 Psychosocial nursing in the People's Republic. Journal of Psychosocial Nursing 23(5): 28–35

Wankiiri V B 1984a Mental health and psychiatric nursing in Africa. World Health Forum 5: 334

Wankiiri V B 1984b The African dimension. International Nursing Review 31(4): 107—109

Wilson H S, Hutchinson S A 1983 Nursing in China. American Journal of Nursing 83: 389–395

7

Research

D. Skidmore

This chapter provides an examination and, to some extent, critique concerning the current thinking about research in psychiatric nursing.

Research tends to be viewed as one of the mysteries of life by many nurses; in many ways this is the direct result of the various textbooks that try to explain research but instead obscure the issue with jargon and abstruse language. First of all, then, the research process needs to be demystified. It is not a pursuit that lies only within reach of the chosen few, nor is it all mathematics and statistics. Indeed, some of the more useful research projects carried out in psychiatry make little or no use of statistical analysis.

WHY RESEARCH?

In recent years, the sphere of research has attracted a bad press, largely because researchers' motives are not clear. In many ways, research has become synonymous with statistics and it is well known that one can lie (credibly) with these! However, statistics are merely one of the tools that researchers use, and they are not essential, as may be seen, for example, in the works of Davis (1963), Roth (1963) and Goffman (1963, 1964).

Research is a quest, a voyage of discovery. Its motivation lies in questions of the form 'I wonder

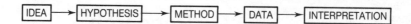

$$\boxed{\text{IDEA}} \rightarrow \boxed{\text{HYPOTHESIS}} \rightarrow \boxed{\text{METHOD}} \rightarrow \boxed{\text{DATA}} \rightarrow \boxed{\text{INTERPRETATION}}$$

why' and 'what of', and its goals are thus to add to knowledge, improve skills, measure cause and effect. The researcher can aim to achieve any or all of these within any one programme.

There are two generally accepted research models: the positivistic, and the non-positivistic stances.

Positivistic stance

In the positivistic research model above, one starts with an idea which is shaped into a hypothesis or statement of intent. This in turn dictates the method chosen, which collects a certain type of data which then gives rise to an interpretation. For example, from the initial idea that dogs are sociable animals, the following hypothesis may be formed:

Dogs, like man, enjoy and need the company of other dogs and seek out social interaction at least once every day.

A method must then be found to test this hypothesis. The hypothesis makes a number of assumptions: it assumes activity on the dog's part; and it assumes social need and intelligence in the fulfilment of that need. Such assumptions will tend to influence the choice of method. In this case, the researcher decides to follow a dog on its daily roam. Suddenly, it starts to bark and growl as it chances upon another dog. Both dogs sniff at each other, give a yip and go their separate ways. Depending upon what one wishes to see, the two dogs can either be old friends who greet each other euphorically, make body contact (sniffing) to advertise their closeness and then offer a short farewell (yip); *or* they are social isolates who hate contact with the same species, react to the meeting with hostility (bark and growl), attempt to intimidate one another (sniffing), and leave with a curse (yip). While both accounts are clearly nonsense, the example illustrates how interpretation depends on how the researcher approaches the evidence. There is so much that the researcher does not

know and — because she cannot ask the dogs concerned — cannot know. The problem here is that she is reading her own values into situations that she knows nothing about.

This is where the positivistic stance falls down in many areas of psychiatric research. This approach is adapted from that used in the 'hard' sciences, where the subject matter is inanimate, there are known constants, and where an experimental design can be used. When it is applied to animal life, however, the data are prone to misinterpretation, because people and animals are not constants. They differ from one another and they change.

For example, one may initially assume the following:

Dog → always attacks → Cat A

However, one has not witnessed every dog–cat relationship. If, say:

Same Dog → is attacked by → Cat A in the home

can one assume that Cat A is tough and intimidates the Dog?
Furthermore:

Cat A attacks → Cat B in the home

Does such a relationship suggest dominance and subservience?

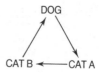

Imagine now a further variable:

Dog → attacks → Cat B outside the home

Is this because the dog is conditioned not to attack in the home?; or perhaps he is short-sighted and does not recognize Cat B outside the home? One simply does not know the dimensions of the relationship; one can only conclude that it is not constant and that it is, perhaps, influenced by many other variables. The positivistic stance, however, leads one to expect to discover reasons and, depending upon one's initial stance, interpret the data accordingly.

Non-positivistic stance

The non-positivistic stance works in reverse, usually commencing with a bland statement, such as:

> 'Find something out about dogs.'

A collection of data-gathering instruments are used with the researcher attempting to make sense of the data at a later stage:

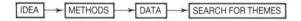

The non-positivistic researcher tends to gather as much data as possible, usually combining several methods (e.g. non-participative and participative observation, interviews and case studies) to check for the influence of her own presence. Used effectively, this approach rarely makes judgemental interpretations, concentrating instead on describing a situation as it occurred in a particular place at a certain time, and allowing the reader to form her own opinion. Rather than attempting to generalize to a total population from a specific population, the non-positivistic researcher tries to adhere to the truism of Dingwall (1976) that any research can only *suggest* (no matter how strongly) what occurs in *certain* situations to *some* persons at a *particular* place and time.

WHAT METHODS ARE APPROPRIATE?

Researchers from both positivistic and non-positivistic camps have a variety of research tools at their disposal, some of which have already been mentioned in passing.

The methods used may be divided into two broad categories:

- *describers*, which provide information about what happens in certain situations
- *explainers*, which attempt to tell us why certain things happen.

The principles of each type of method will now be considered.

Describers

Describers are essentially used to provide descriptive information about what goes on in certain situations; they should never be used as evidence to explain why things happen. Researchers using such methods are very open to the dangers of subjectivity.

Observational methods

Observational methods are of two main types: participative and non-participative.

Participative. The observer becomes a member of the group she is observing (e.g. Goffman 1964, Rosenhan 1973). The danger here is that the researcher can become more participant than observer, and consequently be influenced by the dynamics of interaction, thus losing objectivity (Whyte 1943).

Non-participative. The observer stands outside the group (e.g. Skidmore & Friend 1984), without getting involved in the group activity. There are several problems here:

- seeing what one wishes to see (Roth 1963)
- influencing the actors by your presence (often called the Hawthorne effect)
- being tempted to interpret activities (Argyle et al 1981)
- selective attention, seeing activities out of context.

However, one should remember that all research methods involve some degree of subjectivity on the part of the researcher, and observational methods are very useful when used accurately, since they offer actual accounts concerning the activities of certain groups. As long as one does not then attempt to *explain* these activities, such accounts can provide useful foundations for further research.

Survey methods

Questionnaires — pre-set questions and predetermined answers — are regarded by many as the most used and least useful research tool. However, it is usually the craftsman, rather than the tool, that is at fault. Questionnaires are only information gatherers and even then only offer information about people who fill in questionnaires. However, researchers often fall into the trap of generalizing from their data to the total population. Return rates from questionnaires are always expected to be low, usually about 30%, but in some cases researchers have generalized from a return rate of 0.6%; it is interpretations such as these that give questionnaires a bad name. The national census is perhaps the best example of the effective use of this research tool.

Case studies

The case study can be an excellent means of collecting descriptive data, but tends to be under-used. Davis (1963) provides a good example of use of this method, in which a number of cases are studied and recorded in detail, and then analysed for common points. Such commonality is highlighted, but no attempt is made to draw conclusions, unless to propose some hypothesis for future study. Again, this is a useful method for providing the foundations on which 'explainer' methods can build.

Structured interviews

A structured interview is based on a questionnaire, and is a method much favoured by market researchers. Its advantage is that it allows the subject to explain his actions. For example, consider the question: 'Do you drink beer?' If the subject drinks only one pint per month, he should still answer 'yes', and a large number of such replies in a questionnaire could lead the researcher to conclude (wrongly) that people in a certain area

drink too much. With the questionnaire, the subject's options are limited by the predetermined answers. Questionnaires are widely used and are frequently responsible for inaccurate information because of the limited response they allow. However, if the subject is asked in a structured interview whether or not he drinks beer, he is able to explain how often and thus clarify any misunderstanding.

Describers are neglected by many researchers who tend to overlook their value and prefer to go straight to the explainers. However, they are an integral part of all research and should, when used sensibly, be the first step of any major research project. If one does not know what is happening — and describers do help in forming baselines — how can one seek to explain it?

Explainers

Explainers are methods devised to collect data with the aim of explaining actions or relationships rather than describing them. They rely on two main methods:

Interviews

Interviews are usually of the informal or semi-structured kind, and are often used by the phenomenological school of sociology. Normally, this type of interview is only loosely structured (i.e. the researcher has only a general notion of the areas to be covered in the interview), and the subject is allowed to explain his own responses in his own words. Davis (1984) used a semi-structured technique in order to gather information about students' feelings about their training; whilst Skidmore & Friend (1984) used an unstructured, almost eavesdropping technique, to gather data about community psychiatric nurses' attitudes towards their roles. The value of this method is that one can consider the subject's explanations of events rather than one's own subjective interpretation. However, interviews are still very much open to bias, in that the interviewer can choose to be selective about what she hears, or even 'lead' the interviewee.

Experimental design

Experimental design is a method of measuring cause and effect by having one experimental group matched by a control group. The emphasis is on control so that the effect of the variable under scrutiny can be measured.

Experimental design is very difficult where human subjects are involved, since total control is not feasible. Many researchers have attempted to get around this by way of evaluative research, which attempts to measure the impact of therapeutic intervention (Paykel & Griffith 1983, Freeman & Button 1984, Milne et al 1985). However, interpretation is a major difficulty with this approach, because of the lack of suitable controls. For example, both Ives (1979) and Freeman & Button (1984) examined the impact of intervention for psychosocial disorders which present in general practice, but the two studies draw quite opposite conclusions. Both concur that intervention of a psychotherapeutic nature reduced prescription rates of psychotropic drugs and re-consultation rates. However, Ives concludes from this that there is a case to be made for developing the clinical psychology service within general practice, while Freeman & Button argue that no case can be made for this.

The major problem with 'explainers' is that people are neither the same, nor constant; they differ in their views and a person may change his opinion from day to day. Unfortunately researchers tend to subscribe to the 'collective assumption', i.e. that there exist certain general rules of behaviour, without any real evidence that this is so. Consider, for example, the assumption that people enter crisis because of the lack of social support networks. Now consider the person who enters a crisis (for whatever reason) which causes him to reflect introspectively and only then realize that he never had a support network in the first place. When he reports this to a therapist, it is assumed that this is why he originally entered crisis. In fact, during pre-crisis he had no support network and functioned well; it was only during crisis that the lack of such a support network was recognized, and in post-crisis that this lack is offered as a reason. Similarly, where there is a

professional assumption that de-institutionalization is best for the patient, in the majority of cases the patient has never been consulted. How, then, can the present operational policy be justified?

THE CURRENT STATE

Current research in psychiatric nursing tends to be rather one-sided. It concentrates largely on such staff-oriented questions as what it is like during training, to be a Community Psychiatric Nurse (CPN) or behaviourist; or on staff appraisals of outcome, for example how CPNs have reduced admissions, how more of the elderly are catered for with specialist teams. In short, much current research attempts to justify professional assumptions; it tends to reinforce the created needs of care. Research is frequently short-sighted in its approach, a major reason for the constant changes that take place in psychiatric theory. For example, because various researchers have concluded that community psychiatry 'works', institutional care is now seen as outmoded and, right or wrong, every patient must now receive community care. The patients themselves, however, have not been consulted. It is simply assumed that all hospital inpatients wish to be repatriated into the community; the medical profession — although paying lip-service to the notion of client participation — has decided this for them. Perhaps, had the patients been consulted, rather different conclusions would have been drawn; for example, a dual system of institutional and community care might have been set up which offered the patient a valid choice.

It may be argued, then, that recent research has led to changes in policy, more because it reinforces existing professional and political assumptions than because it demonstrated where the patients' best interests lay.

SOME PROMINENT THEMES

From the reports published, it would appear that the main focus of research is concerned with the nature of services rather than the satisfaction of the consumer of such services. Consider, for example, the well-discussed theme of the CPN base; many papers have argued that there exists a need for primary health care team (PHCT) placement, although there is little evidence to suggest that the CPN can function effectively in that arena. The consumers have not been surveyed, hence we do not have any accurate knowledge of the type of skills needed for any practitioner to be effective, nor do we have any understanding of the resources that will be required.

In the under-researched arena of client satisfaction, the few explorations made there have been interesting and enlightening. Milne et al (1985) suggest that partnership, between client and therapist, in therapy is a viable alternative to the traditional, mechanistic form of intervention. Skidmore & Stoker (1974) suggest that involvement of the client in therapeutic decision-making can potentiate the effects of intervention strategies. Unfortunately, such findings tend to be ignored when it comes to service planning and decisions affecting the clients are made without their consent, or, seemingly, their wishes being considered — a classical example of what Francis Bacon (1561–1626), the father of research, called 'advancement by armchair speculation'.

To summarize, Baconian principles have much to offer research into psychiatric nursing; researchers should rise from those comfortable armchairs and take a look at the real world.

FUTURE DIRECTIONS

De-institutionalization is now inevitable, and in some areas has already taken place. We have not only gone gently into that night but also blindly. This major change in psychiatry will have far-reaching consequences, ranging from the resources needed to the education of future staff, and preparations to cope with these changes should be started now. The American experience suggest that the consequences of de-institutionalization need to be known, and this can surely be gained from examination of the schemes already in operation. Knowledge is required of the clients' needs so that resources and training can be planned accordingly. Similarly, in fairness, the existing population (those in hospital) should be lobbied

to assess their requirements. Suggestions that these patients cannot make a decision since they have no experience of outside life are inane, equivalent to suggestions that all children should have experience of being orphans before they can comment on parent–child bonds. The fact is that such patients are placed in a situation, often not of their own choosing, and should be offered the opportunity of choice prior to professional action being taken on their behalf.

Similarly, the effects of intervention should also be assessed from the consumer point of view. At present, it appears that if an intervention strategy works with one client, everybody receives this same therapy regardless. This is exemplified by the use of ECT some years ago. Poor observation suggested that epileptics never developed schizophrenia; hence, if all schizophrenics were given epilepsy they would be cured. The 'treatment' did not work, but ECT came to be tried on everyone!; because some patients did receive benefit, workers were sufficiently reinforced to continue its indiscriminate use. Unfortunately, many psychiatric interventions are made for similar reasons, for professional rather than client benefit. Professionals can always produce evidence, by selective and subjective data presentation, for continuing chosen methods of practice. Not until a researcher has become truly research-minded in an objective way, can she defend her methods with any justification.

A computer is only as good as its program: contrary to popular belief, computers do make mistakes. Similarly, research is only as good as its interpretation, and the use of a few statistics does not automatically make it good or credible research. For example, consider the following: a thug is placed in the outpatient clinic of a psychiatric unit, and every person that refers himself for consultation is thumped on the nose and prevented from seeing the psychiatrist. After three months, there are no further referrals. This is interpreted as showing that it is psychiatrists who create psychiatric disorder and that 'thump-therapy' is a resounding success: 100% non-re-referral. On paper it looks good, and supports the case for employing professional thumpers, rather than psychiatrists, in every clinic throughout the land; it tells us nothing, however, of consumer outcome.

The example is extreme but mirrors the philosophy of the present research method — the one-sided myopic view. The only honest and fair way to collect data is to gather them from the real world in a 'professional' way. The fact that intervention works on some people does not mean it works on everybody. Hence, the psychiatric nurse should:

- be aware of what is really happening at present, by using describers, and by considering all the parties concerned
- assess the impact of intervention, on both consumers and professional policy, by the use of explainers.

Such an approach would meet the principles of research, namely:

- to improve and add to existing knowledge
- to discover and test new theories
- to develop suitable methods that will enable all involved to cope with existing situations.

If too much knowledge is assumed then the underlying principles of research tend to collapse. How can the what, where, why, when and who be effectively researched if we feel that we already know the what, why and who?

It would seem, then, that a major objective for the prospective psychiatric nurse researcher is to make oneself aware of what one does not know so that one can do something about it. This is the most difficult and yet the most essential step on the road to professional development as it entails that one turns one's back on professional fear and prejudice. The psychiatric nurse is in the front line of psychiatric care, and is consequently well placed for effective and credible research. However, if the ostrich (head in sand) stance continues to be adopted, then others less able and less well positioned will continue to research psychiatric nursing and make policy decisions.

The second essential step is to get into the water. Academics can pontificate for years, one can attend course after course, but the only real way to learn about research is to do it and learn by trial and error. The fear of getting out of one's depth prevents many would-be researchers from becoming involved. However, the fear is unfounded provided that one does not take one's initial steps too seriously, seeing them rather as learning exercises. Remember, small is fun. For example, one may start by developing a small questionnaire, surveying a small population and discovering what the data do and do not tell you. There are many books to help but every researcher has to test the water for herself.

Finally, let us remember that each of us has learned to function in society by gathering data by way of research method, trial and error; we did not get it right all of the time but eventually we got there. Research is quite similar; no one is born a professional researcher, each has had to learn and has done that by getting involved with research. It can be fun, but most of all, when done objectively, it can be of great value to the professional. For psychiatric nurses, research could help them to become leaders rather than followers in the psychiatric arena.

REFERENCES

Argyle M, Furnham A, Graham J 1981 Social situations. Cambridge University Press, Cambridge

Davis F 1963 Passage through crisis. Bobbs Merrill, Indianapolis

Davis B 1984 Interviews with student nurses about their training. Nurse Education Today 4(6): 136–140

Dingwall R 1976 Aspects of illness. Robertson, London

Freeman G K, Button E J 1984 The clinical psychologist in general practice. Journal of the Royal College of General Practitioners 34: 377–380

Goffman E 1963 Stigma. Penguin, Harmondsworth

Goffman E 1964 Asylums. Penguin Harmondsworth

Ives G 1979 Psychological treatment in general practice. Journal of the Royal College of General Practitioners 29: 343–351

Milne D, Walker J, Bentinck V 1985 The value of feedback. Nursing Times 81: 34–36

Paykel E S, Griffith J H 1983 Community psychiatric nursing for neurotic patients. Royal College of Nursing, London

Rosenhan D L 1973 On being sane in insane places. Science 179: 250–258

Roth J 1963 Timetables. Bobbs Merrill, Indianapolis

Skidmore D, Friend W 1984 Muddling through. Community Outlook, 179–181

Skidmore D, Stoker M J 1974 Space age therapy. New Psychiatry 1(4): 15–16

Whyte W F 1943 Street corner society. University of Chicago Press, Chicago

FURTHER READING

Atkinson P 1990 The ethnographic imagination: textual constructions of reality. Routledge and Kegan Paul, London

Herbert M 1990 Planning a research project: a guide for practitioners and trainees in the helping professions. Cassell, London

Mitchell M, Jolley J 1988 Research design explained. Holt, Rinehart & Winston, London

Oyster C K, Hauten W P, Llorens L A 1987 Introduction to research: a guide for the health science professional. Lippincott, Philadelphia.

8

Ethics

M. Fordham

Ethics can be defined as the science of morals, the branch of philosophy which is concerned with human character and conduct. Nursing ethics is primarily concerned with the application of the science of morals to what is considered right or wrong in the conduct of human relationships between nurses and all those people with whom they come into contact in their professional capacity. Much of the time thinking about ethical issues is implicit rather then explicit and behaviour is motivated by an amalgam of ethics, etiquette and pragmatism, tempered by awareness of legal constraints. Harris (1968) said, 'The source of moral obligation is the greater good, and nursing has its origins in this moral obligation.'

Churchill (1977), in his discussion of ethical issues facing nurses, stated that 'ethics is the free, rational assessment of courses of actions in relation to principles, rules, conduct' and that 'critical self-examination is the heart of ethics'. There is no 'God given' code of morality 'writ in heaven' which can be simply taken down and applied impartially. Debate is always possible between those who give greater or lesser weight to competing moral principles. However, there are explicit and generally supported views on the subject. International codes such as the International Council of Nurses (ICN) Code of Nursing Ethics (1973), the Nuremberg Code (1949), the

World Medical Association Declaration of Helsinki (1964, 1975), and national professional codes such as the American Nurses Association (1976) and the British nurses' (UKCC 1984) codes of conduct, and the Royal College of Nursing's 'Ethics Related to Research in Nursing' (RCN 1977) discuss principles and give practical guidelines.

Codes of Ethics do not, however, absolve us from having to think out our own views on issues. Regarding the use of codes of ethics, Kass (1980) stated, 'I increasingly believe that the attempt to replace the often inarticulate yet prudent judgements of discerning physicians with explicit rules and procedures will not lead to better decisions.' Beecher (1966) insisted that 'a more reliable safeguard [than informed consent alone] is provided by the presence of an intelligent, informed, conscientious, compassionate researcher.' However, as Beauchamp & Childress (1983) pointed out, 'persons of good moral character sometimes fail to discern what is right' and are often aware that they do not know what ought to be done in a particular circumstance. Codes of ethics, deliberation of ethics committees, discussion with peers and public debate all influence decisions of society and professions on moral dilemmas.

People generally carry on activities without searching their souls before every word they utter or every move they make. The more unchanging society and the more unchanging and rule-bound the profession the less likely are nurses to meet situations which pose ethical dilemmas. However, society *is* changing — becoming a melting pot for multinational customs of thought and behaviour. The nursing profession is changing and adapting, taking on new roles in therapy and research. Advances in medical science and technology, changes in the law, along with media dissemination of information, have increased both public and professional awareness and debate of ethical issues.

Something — a set of powers, an institution, or a technology — is an ethical problem when its product — an act, a system, or a technique — is capable of good or harm. 'If a human intervention, in some form, can, through its exercise or restraint, result in good or harm, then that inter-vention is by its very nature an ethical problem' (Reich 1981).

There are two main types of situation in which nurses are explicitly forced to face ethical dilemmas. One is when they find themselves in a situation where they are unsure about the right course of action and have an internal moral argument. The other is when they find themselves in dispute with others, be they nurses, other professions, patients or the public. In either circumstance there is a better chance of solving the dilemma if nurses understand and make explicit the theories and principles on which they are attempting to base their thinking and decision taking, and if they have some idea of how to conduct a moral debate.

Beauchamp & Childress (1983) depicted the moral reasoning underlying ethical decision-taking as an hierarchy: ethical theories; principles, e.g. sanctity of life; rules, e.g. wrong to kill innocent humans; particular judgements and actions, e.g. against euthanasia, abortion.

ETHICAL THEORIES

There are two major types of ethical theories, utilitarian and deontological.

Utilitarianism (Hume 1711–76, Bentham 1748–1832, Mills 1806–73) is based on consequentialist or teleological thinking. Teleology is the doctrine of final causes, a view that developments are due to the purpose and design that will be fulfilled by them. Utilitarians argue that morally right action is determined by non-moral values such as pleasure, knowledge, health and freedom from pain. It is not as naive as 'the end justifies the means' but that in all circumstances people ought to promote the greatest possible value over disvalue for all persons affected. Any decision is justified if it produces more good than any alternative would. A basic problem with utilitarianism is that it assumes or requires that people's knowledge of benefits and harm is complete in any given situation and this is patently not true. Whose good or happiness or health are to be considered: the individual's or the total population's? What is the time-scale of future good: now, today, next week, next generation?

What is happiness or good? Nonetheless, ethical decisions about treatment, care and research are often based on utilitarian arguments.

Members of ethics committees and researchers are expected to describe and quantify the harms and benefits for potential patients/clients/subjects before obtaining consent to treatment or participation in research (Beauchamp & Childress 1983). When the benefits to the subject are non-existent (or fortuitous), as in non-therapeutic research, it is argued that the risks should also be negligible (Dworkin 1978). When, however, the benefits are expected to be substantial (life-saving or health improving), as in treatment and therapeutic research, then it can be argued that some risk of harm may be justified. The balancing of risks and benefits is illustrated below. It should be noted that risks have two aspects: their probability of occurrence and their magnitude if they do occur. This reasoning is fraught with possibilities for ethical dispute and raises issues such as the nature of informed consent: who should be taking decisions for whom? The quality versus quantity of life. Are the outcome probabilities for the individual faced with the decision known and can these be conveyed without distortion? The advantages and disadvantages of electroconvulsive therapy largely hinge on a harm/benefit analysis.

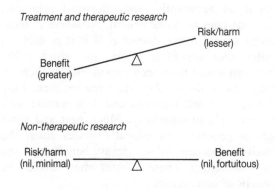

Deontological theorists (Kant 1734–1804, Rawls 1971) hold that some features of acts other than or in addition to their consequences make them right or wrong, i.e. the concept of right or duty is not wholly derivative from the concept of good. (*Deon*

duty.) If a doctor or nurse deceived a patient by giving a placebo, a deontologist would consider both the feature of deception itself (not merely the effects of the deception) and the therapist's motives. For many deontologists deception is wrong, regardless of its consequences. Right-making characteristics in deontological systems include honouring promises, truthfulness and justice.

Some moralists in religious traditions appeal to divine revelation such as the Ten Commandments and Judaeo-Christian absolutes based on the belief that God is good, others to natural law as revealed by human reasoning, others to intuition and common sense. Rawls (1971) appeals to a hypothetical social contract by asking which principles or rational constructs would people adopt if they were placed behind a 'veil of ignorance' and blinded to their talents, abilities and conception of the good life? What moral principles would be espoused if people did not know if they were male or female, rich or poor, black or white, old or young?

PRINCIPLES OF ETHICAL DECISION-MAKING

A number of principles have been mentioned already. Four principles which underpin much decision-taking in biomedical relationships are autonomy, non-maleficence, beneficence and justice (Beauchamp & Childress 1983).

Autonomy

Autonomy is derived from *autos* (self) and *nomes* (rule, governance, or law). Kant — a deontologist — considered that persons should treat one another as autonomous ends and never merely as means to the ends of others. He was concerned with autonomy of will. To be autonomous is to make one's own choices in accordance with universalizable moral principles. Mill — a utilitarian — concentrated on autonomy of action and thought. Autonomy permits all citizens to develop their potential according to their own convictions, so long as they do not interfere with like expression of freedom in others. Veracity, confidentiality and privacy are all based on respect for a person's autonomy. To respect autonomous persons is to recognize their right to self-governance by affirming that they are entitled to autonomous determination free of imposed limitations.⁹ It follows from this that if a person takes a decision without being aware of all relevant information, he or she is only able to exercise limited autonomy. This highlights the difference between consent and informed consent.

Informed consent

Informed consent is largely aimed at protecting the autonomy of patients and subjects of research, but it also serves other functions, listed by Capron (1974) as:

- promotion of individual autonomy
- protection of patients and subjects
- avoidance of fraud and duress
- encouragement of self-scrutiny by medical professionals
- promotion of rational decisions
- involvement of the public (in promoting autonomy as a general social value and in controlling biomedical research).

Informed consent and research. Watson (1982) discussed the informed consent of special subjects for research purposes, including captive groups, acutely ill and dying patients, the mentally ill and legally incompetent. There is a well-accepted trend of giving more information and of more patient/subject involvement in the decision-making process in research. Regarding special subjects including the mentally ill: 'General agreement seems to exist on two points, (a) persons who are unable to give their own informed consent should not be research subjects if other subjects can be used and (b) the less able a person is to protect himself the more vigilant the investigator must be in protecting him' (Hayter 1979). Norton in 1975 expressed concern that 'nurses inexperienced in research are rushing in where the experienced tread warily'.

Non-maleficence

This is the duty of non-infliction of harm, a principle accepted by both rule-deontologists and rule-utilitarians and enshrined in the Hippocratic oath — 'I will use treatment to help the sick according to my ability and judgement, but will never use it to injure or wrong them.' Sometimes stated as '. . . above all or first, do no harm'.

This, like other principles, seems deceptively easy to agree upon in general but can pose enormous problems in specific instances. What is harm? Physicians and nurses have traditionally taken the view that disclosing certain forms of information can be directly harmful to the patient. Thus non-maleficence can come into conflict with autonomy (Simes et al 1986).

Beneficence

This is concerned with the merits of acts of commission rather than omission. It is the duty to confer benefits and actively to prevent or remove harms. It is a principle firmly established in ethics and medicine. Some moral philosophers argue that social and professional duties are violated if one fails to benefit others when in a position to do so; whereas other moral philosophers have argued that although it is virtuous and morally ideal to act beneficently, there is no moral duty to do so. The moral obligation to benefit members of society, including future generations, is often cited as a primary justification for scientific research. Again this is an apparently straightforward principle, until one tries to define benefit. Advances in technology pose a major dilemma. If it is possible to confer some benefit (e.g. save life which a few years ago would have been impossible), is there an obligation to do so? And does the recipient have to accept? Beneficence can and does conflict with the principle of autonomy. Much heat and some light is generated by ethical disputes about the relative importance of autonomy, beneficence and non-maleficence. These debates often invoke the concept of paternalism.

Paternalism

Paternalism is government as by a father. It presupposes that the father is benevolent and that he takes all or some of the decisions relating to his children's welfare rather than letting them make the decisions. Paternalism is likely to be invoked in many situations of inequality of power, state/individual, teacher/pupil, employer/employee. It involves the claim that beneficence should take precedence over autonomy, at least in some cases, although the recipient may argue that he or she does not want good to be done to himself or herself and may regard paternalism as an assault.

The justifications for paternalism are as follows:

1. The harm prevented from occurring or the benefits provided to the person outweigh the loss of independence or the sense of invasion suffered by the interference.
2. The person's condition seriously limits his or her ability to chose autonomously.
3. It is universally justified under relevantly similar circumstances always to treat persons in this way.

(Beauchamp & Childress 1983.)

The danger is that it is easy to justify immoral actions on pseudo-moral grounds when, for example, the true motive for paternalism is expediency, or avoidance of precipitating a situation in which the recipient requires help in coping with knowledge or decision taking.

Justice

The principle of justice is invoked to support arguments about the distribution of social burdens and benefits. Rawls (1971) uses the term 'fairness'. Maxims of distributive justice (or allocation of resources) include:

- to each person an equal share (egalitarian)
- to each person according to individual need (Marxist)
- to each person according to individual effort (libertarian)
- to each person according to societal contribution (libertarian).
- to each person according to merit (libertarian).

(Beauchamp & Childress 1983.)

There is ample scope for ethical dispute about the application of the principle of justice to the mentally ill and handicapped of society as there is for the physically ill. Utilitarians emphasize a mixture of criteria so that public and private utility are maximized. McCormack (1974a) suggested that research on humans is justified because everyone ought to bear certain burdens, usually of a minimal sort, for the common good. Such minimal or negligible burdens are not merely charitable, they are demanded by justice. Beecher (1966) suggested that a prerequisite for experimentation on other people was the willingness of the experimenter to first experiment on himself (although he recognized that self-experimentation might be impracticable and misleading).

Gostin (1986), in a discussion of equity and fairness, said that these concepts are deeply entrenched principles of law and that a government is not obliged to provide health and social services — but once it chooses to provide services it cannot arbitrarily exclude or deprive certain individuals or client groups. He cited the Mental Health Act 1983 as introducing two specific measures which promote an entitlement philosophy: '. . . a mandatory duty of the local authority to provide community aftercare services for detained patients once they are discharged and the right of the patient to publicly financed legal representation, together with public finance for independent psychiatric and social work reports at Mental Health Review tribunals.'

RULES OF ETHICAL DECISION-MAKING

People may recognize that moral reasoning is based on utilitarian or deontological thinking, and espouse certain moral principles. However, even when people agree on basic moral principles there is still room for debate and disagreement about the weight which should be attached to conflicting principles. What rules do their principles lead people to support? If people believe in the sanctity of human life, then the rule that it is wrong to kill follows logically.

Does it follow that one is against abortion in all circumstances or euthanasia in all circumstances or suicide in all circumstances? Do people sometimes take one principle to its logical conclusion and at other times submerge that principle in another? It is quite possible to hold that some behaviour is morally wrong, e.g. suicide, yet also, because of respect for his or her autonomy, that an individual has the right to take his or her own life.

According to Hare (1981) morality has three major characteristics:

1. Prescriptivity — it tells people what to do
2. Universality — universal principles apply in all similar cases
3. Precedence — it overrides convenient or popular behaviour.

It could be argued that before one can be certain what one's principles tell one to do it is essential to be in possession of all the facts of the case. If the application of moral principles was straightforward there would be little need for debate or dispute and few dilemmas. If principles apply to all similar cases it is necessary to be sure what is meant by similar — what aspects of situations make them similar. Does it mean identical? Few situations are identical. The application of principles may indeed be inconvenient, time consuming, result in sanctions against oneself or they may be avoided for expediency. Maybe it is naive to believe or argue as though people's motives for any behaviour are pure. It is so tempting to try to attain and hold the moral high ground, and so easy to see the mote in another's eye whilst ignoring the beam in our own.

Moral argument

This requires that people debate with goodwill and are willing to alter their own views: to argue as though there is an answer, be tolerant to others and sensitive to their own fallibility. A moral stance is likely to consist of a mixture of gut reactions, principles, intuitive responses, value judgements, emotional responses and factual beliefs. Debate requires that people probe and clarify what exactly they are disputing — what are the facts. It is easy for two people to argue at a tangent, only to discover that when they are talking about the same thing they are in agreement. Are they clear about the concepts, e.g. killing or letting die (McCormack 1974b, Glover

1977)? Are they consistent in what they say and what they do? What are the facts? Many a dispute arises because the facts are not known to both parties rather than that the principles are disputed. Nurses need to be cautious in appealing to the argument that they would want to decide in a certain way if they were 'in the patient's shoes' — they could be wrong, especially if they are very different from the patient.

Philosophers can dispute endlessly and agree to differ. Nurses, too, may benefit from discussion of ethical principles and hypothetical circumstances but mostly they are faced with actual circumstances which require action. Steele & Harmon (1983) cited four steps in the decision-making process:

1. identify alternatives
2. evaluate alternatives
3. choose appropriate alternative (decision)
4. convert decision into action (implementation).

Nurses not infrequently complain that they only become involved in step 4, as in medically delegated tasks such as drug administration. If this is so, then a number of possible actions have to be considered. Is the action a nursing action or a legitimately delegated medical action which nurses are competent to perform and contracted to carry out? Are the nurses in possession of facts of which those who took the decision were ignorant, and might the decision-makers have come to a different conclusion if they had been aware of these facts? It is on such grounds that nurses must base their decision to implement the action or attempt to have the decision revised. Is the decision in the province of nursing? The extended role of the nurse has implications for the area of decision taking. Nurses can expend their energies making ethical decisions for other professions, notably doctors, and omit to take ethical decisions about nursing. The debate about electroconvulsive therapy (ECT) has raised this problem and the extent to which professional backing is forthcoming for those who refuse to participate. The proliferation of situations in which nurses may opt out on conscience grounds is not a path that the nursing profession is likely to follow. Assistance in the act of procuring an abortion is the only situation which can be opted from in the UK.

⚭ Murphy & Murphy (1976) discussed the stages of ethical decision-making in more detail:

1. problem identification
2. ethical problem identification
3. identification of persons involved in the decisions
4. identification of the role of the decision-maker
5. consideration of the short- and long-term consequences of each alternative
6. making the decision
7. comparing the decision with the decision-maker's philosophy of patient care ethics
8. follow-up of the results of the decision in order to establish a baseline for making decisions in the future.

Hare (1981) discussed the relationship between the two major methods of settling moral dilemmas — the utilitarian and the absolutist (deontological) views. He suggested that decision taking in situations in which there is little time for reflection before taking action is suited to absolutist thinking and that utilitarian thinking is suited to situations in which there is time to think about general attitudes.

Ascribing 'inalienable rights which there is an absolute duty to respect' (Hare 1981) is a common absolutist stance in arguments about abortion, euthanasia and suicide. Problems arise when a choice has to be made between competing rights. 'A utilitarian is one who thinks that when faced with a moral decision he ought to act in whichever way is best for the interests of those affected' (Hare 1981).

Hare (1981) argues against the views that when faced with conflict of duties people weigh the relative principles and decide for the more weighty or place absolute principles in some order of priority, as the grounds for deciding the weighting or the order are not at all obvious. Instead, he argues for two levels of thinking: firstly, intuitive thinking based on prima facie absolutist duties and inculcated during childhood and the development of conscience; secondly, when dilemmas occur, critical thinking using a utilitarian approach.

The dilemmas which require critical thinking about utility arise 'when the question is asked, what intuitions we ought to have, or what duties we ought to acknowledge, or what would be the content of a sound moral education' (Hare 1981), as intuitive appeal to absolutist principles will not resolve these problems.

Professional codes of conduct make explicit the prima facie principles and duties which apply to its members but do not and cannot absolve nurses from critical thinking. Indeed, 'By doing the best critical thinking of which we are capable when we have the leisure for it, we may be able to get for ourselves a set of fairly simple general prima facie principles for use at the intuitive level. . .' (Hare 1981).

An alternative or parallel way of conceptualizing moral issues is to discuss them in terms of rights and responsibilities instead of in terms of theories and principles.

Patients' rights and nurse advocacy

Patients' rights and nurse advocacy are interrelated issues, in that advocacy is concerned to protect patients' rights. Bandman (1985) discussed the meaning of human rights in the nurse–patient relationship; he noted that rights are complex and many faceted and have been variously defined as permissions, claims, powers and entitlements.

One condition of any right is freedom. To have a right based on freedom is to be accorded a sphere of autonomy or self-determination, to exercise one's rights as one chooses and to be immune to the charge of wrongdoing. . . (p. 16). The right to be free, for patients and health professionals alike, includes the right to be treated rationally, which implies the right not to be coerced, brainwashed, lied to, deceived, unknowingly given drugs, or have one's body entered without the right-holder's consent or permission (p. 17). Secondly, to have rights implies that other relevant persons have corresponding duties to comply with the terms and provisions of one's rights (p. 17).

If the sick have a right to treatment and care, then health professionals have a duty to treat and care. A third condition of any right is that it is consistent with rationally defensible principles of justice, e.g. to each according to their need. There are two kinds of rights — option rights and subsistence rights (Table 8.1). Negative rights are rights to be free from interference and are also

Table 8.1 Characteristics of rights

Conditions	1. Freedom
	2. Corresponding duties
	3. Justice
Types	1. Option rights or negative rights
	2. Subsistence rights or positive rights

called option, or self-determination, rights. They are based on the principle of autonomy, and include the right to give informed consent and to decide what happens in and to one's body. Positive rights are rights to receive social and economic assistance, also called subsistence rights, and include rights to food, clothing, shelter, health care and education at public expense.

The importance of considering human rights is that it is possible to appeal to human rights to justify health care practices. If nurses decide to override a suicidal person's right to freedom from interference, this may be done on the grounds of upholding the patient's right to health care. Many ethical dilemmas are situations in which nurses do not know whether it is right to uphold a person's option or subsistence rights. Bandman (1985) argued that 'in a pinch, subsistence rights are pre-emptive or exclusionary in that such rights exclude and override all other value considerations'. MacCormick (1977) pointed out that freedom to choose is an important patient right but not the only one. Respecting someone's right to freedom makes it possible to die with one's rights preserved (Treffert 1974). Is this preferable to living with one's rights infringed? Are rights automatic? If one demands rights for oneself, one must logically extend these same rights to all other people. Bandman & Bandman (1977) discussed the proposition: 'There is nothing automatic about rights.' Some people regard statements about patients' rights as evidence of new and progressive thinking, whereas others, notably Gaylin (1972), regarded such statements as attempts to 'return to the patients, with an air of largess, some of the rights hospitals have previously stolen from them. It is the thief lecturing the victim on self-protection!'

In general, rights need to be explicitly stated and claimed in situations where there is inequality of power. When debating ethical decisions involv-

ing nurse/patient/client power it may help to recall Kelman's (1972) discussion of the legitimate use of power, including the criteria defining its application, its users, its limits, and the procedures of redress in response to its abuse.

1. 'Those who exercise power and those over whom it is exercised must constitute a community sharing common values and norms.' Is this true of British society? Does the patient/client community share the same values and norms as the health professionals? If not, how do they differ?
2. 'These norms must include some rules that define the limits within which the power holder must operate — the domain of behaviour over which he is entitled to exercise his control, the circumstances under which he may use his power, and the manner in which he may use it; he can be held accountable whenever he violates these rules by going beyond the permissible limits of his power.'
3. 'The person over whom power is exercised may have recourse to mechanisms (such as courts, an ombudsman, public agencies, ethics comittees) through which he can question, challenge, or complain about the way power is exercised over him, and he must have the assurance that these mechanisms have some countervailing power that enables him to protect and defend his own interests in the face of demands from the authorities.' (Kelman 1972).

The ethics of involuntary hospitalization is but a special case of coercive control by some humans over other humans. Libertarians maintain that nothing is more precious than freedom, but how 'free' can a mentally ill person be? (McGarry & Chodoff 1981). 'Internal physiological or psychological processes can contribute to a throttling of the human spirit that is as painful as any applied from the outside' (Chodoff 1976).

It can be argued that society should deprive of liberty only those who can be treated — but some may be better off solely by being 'fed and housed'. Is there a right to asylum? Does compulsory involuntary discharge into the community of long-stay mentally ill differ ethically from compulsory detention?

Two very thorny questions concerning patients' rights are: Does the patient have a right to treatment? Does the patient have the right to refuse treatment?

Is medical and nursing care a right or a privilege? Allocation of finite resources forces health professionals to take pragmatic decisions in which the right to care is regarded as ideal, but care as a privilege is more realistic. Resources include not only national revenue, but also the time and expertise of each individual nurse. Essentially the same issues exist in day-to-day decisions about the allocation of professional resources as in the wider political decisions of society. All people are managers of resources even if the only resource they manage is themselves.

Does the patient/client have the right to refuse treatment? The view that people may refuse the use of heroic or extraordinary measures to prolong life under all conditions is generally accepted, but many decisions, particularly in psychiatry, are about rights to refuse measures which aim to improve the quality of life, or purport to do so more quickly than would the natural course of events.

It seems that many of the ethical disputes in psychiatric nursing are about the rights and/or obligations of the mentally ill to receive or reject treatment or care. Where the nurse advocate tends to intervene is in situations where the hazards of treatment (mainly physical treatments such as psychosurgery, electroconvulsive therapy and drugs) are claimed (by the nurse) to outweigh the benefits, and/or when the attempts by the mentally sick person to refuse treatment are unheard or are unexpressed because the patient does not fully understand the alternatives.

Often the ethical dilemma hinges on the nurse's conception of 'ordinary or extraordinary means' — or, in Beauchamp & Childress' (1983) terminology, 'optional and obligatory' treatment. The dilemma of right to refuse and arguments about what is and what is not obligatory treatment are complex enough in care of physical illness but are even more problematic in care of the mentally ill — particularly as there is the temptation, and in some situations the necessity, to define the recipient of treatment as incompetent and become a 'paternalistic advocate' arguing the case for what nurses think right, or the decision nurses think they would like if they were the patient.

Ordinary and extraordinary measures

The distinction between ordinary and extraordinary treatment is not between low and high technology, simple and elaborate, but between measures which are or are not burdensome to the recipient. The distinction was considered necessary to give patients the freedom to refuse extraordinary treatment without this being regarded as tantamount to suicide by the Roman Catholic Church (Pope Pius XII 1957). Much confusion could be reduced by the use instead of the terms of obligatory and optional treatment (Beauchamp & Childress 1983). Kelly's (1951) criteria for therapy which is obligatory are: that it must offer a reasonable prospect of benefit; and that it must not involve excessive expense, pain or other inconvenience.

The idea that patients have an obligation to accept ordinary treatment is based on the view that the point of human life is to flourish. Although health professionals cannot confer health on anyone, they can aid and abet patients in gaining and maintaining health. When a patient is competent he is in a position to judge for himself what is personally burdensome, and discussions and decisions implicitly or explicitly rely upon views of 'quality of life'. However, some philosophers are opposed to basing decisions or judgements on quality of life as they violate the principle of equality of life. Ramsey (1970) argued that there is an obligation to use the treatment medically indicated when the recipient is an incompetent non-dying patient, or is unconscious. However, McCormack (1978) argued that what is considered medically indicated in itself depends on medical views of the kind of life which will ensue. The moral grounds for regarding some measures as optional or extraordinary are the same for withdrawing as for withholding that treatment (Beauchamp and Childress 1983). Thus optional and obligatory do not refer to the nature of the treatment but to the extent to which it serves the patient's best interests. Parents, guardians and the state have a legal and moral obligation to act in the best interests of children and incompetent people as have nurses and doctors.

The case against rights

In reality no one has absolute option or subsistence rights. Options are curtailed by knowledge, emotions and skills as well as by financial and other environmental limitations. Golding (1978) discussed some of the possible implications of rights, for example: Is there a right to do as one likes with ones own body so long as no one else is harmed? Are there things which a person has no right to do even if others are not harmed? Are there some things which a person has a right to do even if others are likely to be harmed as a result? Is there a right to limit the rights of others? Subsistence rights or welfare rights such as health care can only be logically claimed to the extent that resources exist to satisfy these claims. Another issue concerning welfare rights is whether or not they are mandatory. Is there an obligation to take advantage of such welfare rights as exist?

There seem to be a proliferation of claims to rights. Rights claimed not only impose obligations on others but may curtail the rights of others. Golding (1978), in discussion of the historical development of rights, in particular the emergence of welfare rights, said: 'An uneasy tension, however, exists between the concept of what is right and the concept of (option) rights. But it is because of the partial displacement of the notion of what is right by the concept of rights that we can today ask whether a person can have the right to do what is morally wrong.'

Psychiatric nurses have infinite opportunities to withhold rights, to define rights as privileges and use them for social control and punitive control in the name of expediency and pragmatism in the guise of therapy.

Duty of care

The reciprocal duty which complements patients' rights is the nurse's duty of care. To perform this duty implies that nurses should care in a conscien-

tious and competent fashion. Nurses are accountable to colleagues, other professions and society at large but first and always to patients. If nurses fail in their duty of care they will fail to be nonmaleficent and beneficent.

Patient advocacy

An advocate can be defined as a pleader for the vulnerable. Advocacy involves speaking for and intervening on behalf of another person or group, who for some reason do not have the power to represent themselves. Such people or groups are described as vulnerable by Copp (1986). She described the temporarily vulnerable such as those who are depressed, the episodically vulnerable such as the alcoholic and drug addict, and the permanently or inevitably vulnerable such as the mentally or physically handicapped. The vulnerable person or group is at risk of being dehumanized (Vail 1966). 'Nurses are in a privileged position if they are willing to recognize and accept advocacy opportunities' (Copp 1986).

Curtin (1979) inserted a note of caution into nurses' enthusiasm for the role of advocate: to remember that it is the 'patient's goal, it is their meaning and not ours, their values and not ours and their living and dying not ours' which nurses aim to support. Curtin (1983) pointed out that the nurse as patient advocate tends to be depicted as a supernurse, combining the role of 'lawyer-theologian-psychologist-family counsellor and dragon slayer' in one person. Advocacy is not 'a hobby nor is it to be entered into by the faint-hearted. It requires the advocate to take risks' and to 'be introspective about his or her own motivation, knowledge and skills. It requires self-knowledge of one's value system.' Castledine (1981) discussed the pros and cons of advocacy, including a reminder that 'even if the nurse does act as advocate for the patient, she or he may not be able to do this independently from the constraints of the institution or authority of the employer'. Psychiatric nurses have experienced the personal costs of patient advocacy, the institutional and professional constraints and, perhaps more than other nurses, are aware of both the importance and the pitfalls of this role.

What are nursing values? According to Peplau (1987), 'Nursing is a service for people that enhances healing and health by methods that are humanistic and primarily non-invasive.' She goes on to say, 'This value may once again be put to the test. With the increasing biomedicalization of psychiatry, psychiatric nurses have a remarkable opportunity to use their skills to provide a separate and/or complementary alternative (psychotherapeutic) form of treatment for psychiatric patients.'

If the skills of psychiatric nurses constitute alternative and/or complementary treatments, then it is essential that their efficacy be tested and proven. If advocacy is used *against* a course of action, and not *for* a positive alternative, it can be construed simply as anti-intellectualism or anti-paternalism (Fagin 1975).

What are patient/client values? Do they coincide with nurses' values? There are persons and groups such as the mentally handicapped whose values are difficult to ascertain and who thereby impose 'an unusual burden of ethical responsibility' (de Leon Siantz 1979). How do nurses decide that a person needs an advocate? This depends on judgement of the situation and of the person. Rarely, someone may directly ask for a nurse to be their advocate.

Personhood

Decisions about what is considered right or wrong in the way in which people behave towards one another are sometimes based on the concept of personhood — for example, in determination of the rights of the mentally ill or handicapped, whether or not such people should be treated with respect and dignity. Much of the debate about what it is permissible to do to a fetus, embryo or newborn hinges on this idea (Lockwood 1985). Freedman (1975) argued that the decision to gain consent before surgery 'arises from the right which each of us possesses to be treated as a person, and in the duty which all of us have to respect for persons, to treat a person as such and not as an object'. He goes on to say: 'Perhaps the worst which we may do to a man is to deny him his humanity, for example, by classifying him as mentally incompetent when he is not.'

Personhood is, however, a different type of concept from humanity. It does not merely imply membership of the human species. It is a status which is ascribed on the grounds of certain capacities and potentialities. Thus person is not a biological concept. 'A person is a being that is conscious, in the sense of having the capacity for conscious thought and experiences, but not only that: it must have the capacity for reflective consciousness and self-consciousness. It must have, or at any rate have the ability to acquire, a concept of itself as a being with a past and a future. . . . But a person, in this sense, need not be human' (Lockwood 1985).

Thus the philosophical debate about the definition of the person is invoked in ethical decision taking because of the connection made between personhood and the way in which a person should be treated by others. A person is a being entitled to consideration. A person is not a thing but is free, rational, possessed of dignity and has a right to respect as an end himself, not as a means for others (Kant 1964). Historically, slaves, women and children have been and still are regarded as non-persons in certain circumstances. Debate is possible about the status of embryos, babies, the insane, whales, dolphins and fifth generation computers. What qualities entitle something or someone to consideration — life, consciousness, intelligence related to humans, i.e. the human species?

Defining individuals or groups as non-persons is the standard way of dealing with those who threaten the stability or accepted values of a society. Non-personhood is used to justify treating members of these groups as objects, removing their rights to be respected and thus to be self-determining and limiting their welfare rights. This happens to ethnic minorities at times, to lawbreakers, to the behaviourally unusual, e.g. minority religious sects, non-heterosexuals and so on. One method used to withhold the status of person from some humans is to medicalize and stigmatize the group members with labels of mental illness or mental/moral defect and thus justify control of their lives (Boyers & Orrill 1972, Illich 1976). Often the concepts of 'person' and 'human being' are used interchangeably, although they are different types of concept. The result for the recipient of treatment or care, however, may be the same whether he or she is labelled as a non-person or a subhuman being. There is a long tradition of regarding mental patients as subhuman or animal-like (Deutsch 1938). London (1969) suggested that the ethical issues of behaviour modification revolve around its dehumanizing concept of man, in that it fosters a machine model of man. The therapist is portrayed as a technician or a social reinforcement machine and the patient as a mechanical tool (Krasner 1962).

Consent

One of the major issues in care and treatment of the mentally ill and the mentally handicapped is that of consent.

Arminger (1977) talked of three types of consent:

- informed
- vicarious
- presumed.

Informed consent, according to Arminger (1977), 'means that a person knowingly, voluntarily and intelligently and in a clear and manifest way gives his consent'. There are obvious problems of genuine understanding and shared use of language, of subtle and even unsubtle coercion, and of patients rarely being in an emotional condition to be assertive.

Vicarious consent includes parents' permission for children. This is a particular problem in psychiatric nursing. The Royal College of Nursing (1977) guidelines on research quotes from the Medical Research Council (1963): 'The situation in respect of minor and mentally subnormal or mentally disordered persons is of particular difficulty. In the strict view of the law, parents and guardians of minors cannot give consent on their behalf to any procedures which are of no particular benefit to them and may carry some risk of harm.' When is it necessary to obtain vicarious consent? Mentally disturbed people and children can understand appropriate explanations. Are there certain decisions which should never be allowed by legitimate parents or guardians, such as steriliz-

ation of mentally handicapped people? In clinical practice we presume consent when caring for unconscious patients in emergencies to save life. Informed consent, as it is now understood, is of fairly recent origin. It was not mentioned in the eighteenth century. The legal implications of failure to obtain informed consent are of trespass or assault on the person. Lord Scarman's view (the Sidaway case) is that it is a basic human right to know, i.e. patients have a legal right to know all the risks which may attach to a personal treatment, whereas other Law Lords support the view that patients must prove that circumstances of their right to know take precedence over medical judgement to do what is right for patients. The dilemma of precedence of autonomy over beneficence will not go away, and it is clear that power relationships such as doctor/patient, nurse/patient or client, social worker/client are societal issues in which the values of society as a whole, and not merely the values of the medical, nursing and social work professions, are involved.

Public debate and legal rulings about the nature of informed consent remind nurses that they do not have *carte blanche* to act as they think fit. As members of a profession, nurses are entrusted by society to take certain actions on their behalf — in their case, the care of the sick and maybe the promotion of health — but society retains the right to scrutinize and place limits on how nurses perform these actions. Nurses sometimes need to be reminded that they cannot automatically take on new roles just because they wish to do so. It is also essential to gain the agreement and support of patients/other professions and society in general, because professional relationships are basically contractual. Justification for the right not to be treated without first giving informed consent is based on the view that on the whole patients are the best judges of their own interests, and that their interests are normally much more severely affected than anyone else's. Dworkin (1977) suggested that certain rights can 'trump' other considerations.

Hare (1981) argued that safeguarding patients against treatment against their will will not be achieved by ever more debate about the precise definition of consent but by devising practical rules of conduct. One such rule should be that the people who decide about confinement (lawyers) and the people who decide about release (civil authorities) should not be the people who decide about treatment (psychiatrists).

The issue of informed consent can be circumvented in practice when patient assessment merges imperceptibly into ill-defined treatment with no stated clear objective or plan and consequently no clear opportunity for the patient to agree or disagree to the treatment or care. The argument that cooperation of the patient implies consent is dubious, as subtle and unsubtle duress exists in the relationship and the patient may fear 'loss of face', at least, if he questions the continuation of therapy.

When consent to physical or psychological treatment is refused, this attitude of the patient itself becomes part of the cost–benefit analysis. Merskey (1981) argued that the risk of a high incidence of unfavourable outcomes (serious complications, even death) which follow treatment of the fearful and unwilling general surgical patient also applies to psychotic patients.

Competence

The principle of autonomy of persons under 16 years of age was the basis of legal dispute by Gillick about contraceptive advice Dyer (1985). The judicial ruling was that a child can sometimes give consent if sufficiently mature to understand the consequences. This brings competence into discussions of informed consent. Kilpatrick (1984) discussed the ethical issues and procedural dilemmas in measuring patient competence. She posed the question: 'Is there a line between competence and incompetence or is the difference an arbitrary determination?' She argued that nursing is concerned with ensuring the right of the patient to take decisions, and that uncertainty arises when there are questions about the ability of the patient to make decisions or when the patient makes decisions that will not promote health and have predictable serious sequelae. She went on to discuss the models of competency measurement found in the literature of law, medicine, and philosophy.

Roth et al (1977) described five tests of competence to give consent to treatment (see Table 8.2).

Table 8.2 Summary of tests of competence to give consent

Test	Criteria of incompetence
Roth et al (1977)	
1. Evidencing of choice	No treatment choice manifest
2. Reasonable outcome of choice	Choice not like that of reasonable person
3. Choice based on rational reasons	Cognitive disorder present
4. Ability to understand	Cognitive facts not understood
5. Actual understanding	Treatment situation not completely understood or integrated
Beauchamp & Childress (1983)	
1. Understand the treatment. Weigh risks and benefits of treatment. Make decision in light of such knowledge	Rational reasons not used to meet criteria
Culver and Gert (1982)	
1. Completely incompetent	Infant, severely retarded, senile, comatose
2. Competent to give or refuse SIMPLE consent	Only able to comprehend part of the treatment situation
3. Competent to give or refuse VALID consent,	

Test 1   *Evidencing of choice.* This test for competency requires the patient to show preference for or against treatment. When a patient is verbally silent, behaviour is evaluated, i.e. if the person complies with treatment requirements when given every opportunity to refuse, the patient is considered to be evidencing a choice and therefore competent. Patients who would be judged incompetent by this test are those who are unconscious, delirious or psychiatrically mute.

Test 2   *Reasonable outcome of choice.* This test requires the patient to make the right, or 'reasonable', decision to be considered competent. The reasonable decision is the one that a reasonable person in like circumstances would make. This test is biased to the preservation of health. Thus the patient whose outcome of choice is congruent with this bias is always considered competent, and the patient is considered incompetent when he refuses to acquiesce with treatment. The circular nature of this test reduces its value in clinical use and it has the potential to erode personal autonomy.

Test 3   *Choice based on rational reasons.* The reasons for the patient's decision are evaluated to determine if they are 'rational'. This test equates rational with the absence of mental illness or disordered cognitive function.

Test 4   *Ability to understand.* This is most consistent with current legal and ethical principles of informed consent and requires the patient to answer questions or to show some understanding of risks, benefits and alternatives to treatment. It does not require perfect understanding. Unfortunately, recall is often equated with understanding.

Test 5   *Actual understanding.* This test adds the obligation that the health care provider instructs the patient and then ascertains if the patient really understands the full meaning of the treatment information. This high-level test of competence is considered important in situations when patients agree to treatment that carries high risk or when they refuse beneficial treatment with negligible risk.

Beauchamp and Childress (1983) discussed the concepts of intermittent and limited competence which are arguably particularly important in psychiatry: that 'the same person's ability to make decisions may vary over time', and that an individual 'may at a single time be competent to make certain practical decisions but incompetent to make others'. They cited an example of a man who behaved normally in most areas of living but engaged in self-mutilating behaviour because he believed God was asking him to sacrifice himself for the good of mankind. They argued that to

determine that this individual or a delirious person is totally incompetent to make any treatment decisions limits their self-determination in unnecessary and unjustifiable ways, despite the fact that at times, and/or in some areas, they lack understanding. These authors pointed out that in clinical practice the patient who refuses treatment believed by the health care professional to be necessary and/or beneficial often is deemed incompetent solely because treatment is refused. They stressed that judgement about patient competence should be made independently of the patient's treatment decision. This view would rule out test 2. Culver et al (1980) said the decision should be respected even when the quality is considered irrational, unless there are compelling reasons to override it, such as life-threatening or highly deleterious sequelae. If people are considered incompetent to make a health care decision or to participate in informed consent, then there are further questions to ask. Does someone else have the right to decide on their behalf — parent, daughter/son, guardian, doctor, nurse, court, social worker? Can we wait until the patient is in a better physical or mental state and able to take his own decision? Does the decision have to be made at all?

Culver et al (1980) stated: 'To be competent to give valid consent, the patient must be presented with sufficient information to make an informed decision and must be able to understand and appreciate that information. The aspect of understanding and appreciating the information is crucial.' If, for instance, anxiety results in inability to integrate all of the information, the patient would not give valid consent. Because assessing the understanding requires being with and talking with the patient at some length, Culver & Gert (1982) suggested that, in an inpatient setting, the nurse is often in the best position to determine whether the patient has adequate information and understanding on which to base the decision for treatment. Giving people time to think before making a decision is vital. It is important that decisions about actions which have irreversible and serious consequences should not be made in haste, or they may be regretted at leisure. It has been argued, and with some justification, that some psychiatric treatment itself returns to the mentally ill person their competence to make decisions and that some persons will not be competent unless they receive treatment.

The dilemma for psychiatry and psychiatric nursing is that these practices are dealing with persons who suffer deep emotional and human distress, some of whom may be considered to be a danger to themselves or others and some of whom may be lacking in competence. The risk of, or arguably the necessity for, paternalism is therefore great.

Most voluntary decisions to enter hospital or treatment programmes contain an element of coercion from, for example, family, friends, employers, neighbours, police, and it is argued that institutions are inherently coercive. Voluntary admission and informed consent are ideals towards which to strive but are rarely attained (McGarry & Chodoff 1981).

Quality of life

When discussing ethical decision-making it was noted that when using a utilitarian theory as a basis for decision-making nurses would have to consider the short- and long-term consequences and follow up the results of the decision in order to establish a baseline for making future decisions (Murphy & Murphy 1976). The risk/benefit analysis often requires an assessment of the current versus the expected quality of life. Much of the literature and research on quality of life concerns cancer patients (Pittam 1982, BMJ 1985). However, indices of health similar to those described by Grogono & Woodgate (1971) could be applied or adapted to the mentally ill. They include the following health indices to be judged on a three-point scale:

1. Work: normal, impaired or reduced, prevented?
2. Hobbies and recreation: normal, impaired or reduced, prevented?
3. Is patient free from malaise, pain or suffering?
4. Is patient free from worry or unhappiness?
5. Does patient communicate satisfactorily?
6. Does patient sleep satisfactorily?

7. Is patient independent of others for activities of daily living (washing, feeding, dressing, moving and so on)?
8. Does patient eat and enjoy food?
9. Is micturition and defaecation normal?
10. Has patient's state of health altered his sex life?

Some quality of life assessments have been devised to be completed by patients (Priestman & Baum 1976) and others by health professionals (Spilzer et al 1981).

Confidentiality

Allied to the issue of consent to treatment and care is the issue of consent to the dissemination of personal information obtained in a therapeutic transaction.

When gaining personal private information in psychotherapeutic relationships, 'the sole exception to the rule of confidentiality between therapist and patient is the possibility of "dangerousness" to others' (Karasu 1981). The maxim, 'protective privilege ends where public peril begins' arose from the Tarasoff decision, in which the parents of a murdered girl successfully sued the therapist and psychiatric supervisor for failure to warn them of the confidential disclosure of murder intent by a patient. The balance between healing patients and protecting society which such situations highlight have been much debated, and Roth et al (1977) advocated that the boundaries and limits of confidentiality should be explained to patients, and where possible the patient's permission to warn the potential victim should be obtained.

However, the issue of confidentiality is much broader than this, and concerns information which is less obviously likely to be damaging. Greif (1985) argued: 'Confidentiality is a *sine qua non* in the health professional–patient relationship. It is well rooted in ethics and is governed by law. Revealing information to other parties may lead patients, colleagues or others to personal, social or occupational damages.' He further went on to state that the most common breach of confidentiality by nurses is, 'Naive, well-meant gossiping . . .' Currently, there is much debate and decisions about the patient's potential right of access to his medical records. The worst scenario from the patient's perspective is lack of confidentiality of information between the health professional and other people and at the same time lack of access to his own records, i.e. a lack of confidentiality plus an excess of secrecy.

PSYCHIATRY, PSYCHIATRIC NURSING AND SOCIETY

Psychiatry has been under attack for the past few decades — from some of its own members (e.g. Szasz 1961, 1963, Laing 1965), from consumers (Brown 1985) and from other professions especially the legal profession (Kennedy 1981). Power to enforce hospitalization, the consequences of disease labelling to the individual patient and the flagrant use of psychiatry for social control are some of the major causes of attack — but the whole ethos of psychiatry is under scrutiny, and it is clear that it is the ethical values of society, not solely those of doctors, psychologists, nurses and social workers, which determine what is considered right interpersonal behaviour between the professedly mentally well and the vulnerable mentally ill or handicapped. *Psychiatric ethics* (Bloch & Chodoff 1981) was specifically written to clarify these major ethical issues. As in other branches of medical treatment, the implicit assumption that behaviour — serving the best interests of patients/clients by benevolent paternalism — is being questioned.

Specific psychiatric codes of ethics began to appear in the 1970s. The preamble to The Declaration of Hawaii (1977) states: 'Conflicting loyalties for physicians in contemporary society, the delicate nature of the therapist–patient relationship and the possibility of abuses of psychiatric concepts, knowledge and technology in actions contrary to the laws of humanity all make high ethical standards more necessary than ever for those practising the art and science of psychiatry.' This preamble could equally apply to psychiatric nursing.

The essence of the social control dilemma that psychiatry can be used/abused for sociopolitical ends was stated by Liefer (1970), as follows: 'Because all moral codes are not codified in law, and because the power of the state is limited by a rule of law, the state is unable satisfactorily to control and influence individuals. This requires a new social institution that, under the auspices of an acceptable modern authority, can control and guide conduct without conspicuously violating publicly avowed ideals of freedom and respect for the individual. Psychiatry, in medical disguise, has assumed this historical function.'

Sexism

The systematic bias against women in psychiatry has been extensively discussed. Broverman et al (1981) suggested that therapeutic theories have usually supported rather than questioned stereotypical assumptions about sex roles and different standards of mental health for men and women. Thus therapists have commonly accepted that dependency and passivity are normal qualities in women whereas assertiveness and independence are typical of men, and have designated a woman's dissatisfaction with her traditional role as evidence of psychopathology (Rice & Rice 1973). Other examples of sexism include Freudian antifeminine views; 'blame-the-mother' traditions, e.g. as causes of schizophrenia in their children; and reinforcement of androcentrism by male supervisors (Seiden 1976). 'Ostensibly, therapeutic sexual interaction almost always involves a male therapist and a young female patient and there is little evidence of the therapist providing such help for the fat or ugly who might receive from it more benefit to their self-esteem' (Bancroft 1981).

Mechanic (1981) stated: 'Because psychiatry (and psychiatric nursing) deals with deviance in behaviour, its conceptions run parallel to society's conceptions of social behaviour, personal worth and morality. These conceptions can be viewed from competing vantage points and are therefore amenable to different professional approaches. In the absence of clear evidence about aetiology or treatment, disturbance can be seen as biological in nature, as a failure in development, as a moral crisis, or as a result of socio-economic and other social factors. Remedies may correspondingly be seen in terms of biological restoration, moral realignment, social conditioning or societal change'

(p. 47). Indeed, all of these elements may be present in the same situation — holistic medicine would consider all of them.

CONCLUSION

Ethical controversy surrounds all methods of psychiatric treatment including therapies undertaken by nurses and psychologists. Physical treatments such as psychosurgery, electroconvulsive therapy, drug therapy, behaviour modification techniques and psychoanalysis have all been regarded as forms of 'behaviour control in which the patient has little or no say' (Bloch & Chodoff 1981).

The ethics of psychiatry and psychiatric nursing do not differ from general ethics but are concerned with specific, often puzzling, sometimes unique situations. Some of the particular dilemmas result from imprecision of the boundaries between health and illness, normality and abnormality, conflict between individual and societal good, and seriousness of the outcome of decisions for the consumer. The social consequences of a psychiatric diagnosis such as schizophrenia may be as devastating to the future of the individual as becoming a quadriplegic, even if the symptoms are mild and controlled.

It can be argued that society at large does not behave ethically towards psychiatric nursing or the mentally ill and handicapped in that it 'demands the highest standards whilst providing only the scantiest resources' (Nolan 1985). Some of the ethical dilemmas of psychiatric nursing will not be resolved at individual or local level unless and until political decisions and economic provisions appropriate to the needs of the vulnerable members of society are made.

REFERENCES

American Nurses Association 1976 Code for nurses. ANA, Kansas City

Arminger B 1977 Ethics of nursing research: profile, principles, perspectives. Nursing Research 26 (5): 330–336

Bancroft J 1981 Ethical aspects of sexuality and sex therapy. In: Bloch S, Chodoff P (eds) Psychiatric ethics. Oxford University Press, Ch 9

Bandman E, Bandman B 1977 There is nothing automatic about rights. American Journal of Nursing 77: 867

Bandman B 1985 Human rights in the nurse–patient relationship. In: Carmi A, Schneider S (eds) Nursing law and ethics. Springer Verlag, Berlin, p 14–21

Beauchamp T L, Childress J E 1983 Principles of biomedical ethics, 2nd edn. Oxford University Press

Beecher H K 1966 Ethics and clinical research, New England Journal of Medicine 274: 1354–60

Bentham J 1984 An introduction to the principles of morals and legislation. Hafner, New York

Bloch S, Chodoff P (eds) 1981 Psychiatric ethics. Oxford University Press

Boyers R, Orrill R (eds) 1972 Laing and anti-psychiatry. Penguin, Harmondsworth

British Medical Journal 1985 Leading article. Quality of life in cancer trials. British Medical Journal 291: 685–686

Broverman I K, Broverman D M, Clarkson F E, Rosekrantz P S, Vogel F R 1981 Sex role stereotypes and clinical judgements of mental health. In: Howell E, Bayes M (eds) Women and mental health. Basic Books, New York

Brown P 1985 The Mental Patient's Rights movement and mental health institutional change. In: Brown P (ed) Mental health care and social policy. Routledge & Kegan Paul, Boston, Ch 8

Capron A 1974 Informed consent in catastrophic disease and treatment. University of Pennsylvania Law Review 123: 364–376

Castledine G 1981 The nurse as patient's advocate: pros and cons. Nursing Mirror 11: 138–140

Chodoff P 1976 The case for involuntary hospitalization of the mentally ill. American Journal of Psychiatry 133: 496–501

Churchill L 1977 Ethical issues of a profession in transition. American Journal of Nursing. May: 873

Copp L A 1986 The nurse as advocate for vulnerable persons. Journal of Advanced Nursing. 11: 255–263

Culver C, Fenell R, Green R 1980 ECT and special problems of informed consent. American Journal of Psychiatry 135: 586–591

Culver C, Gert B 1982 Philosophy in medicine. Oxford University Press, New York

Curtin L L 1979 The nurse as advocate: a philosophical foundation for nursing. Nursing Science 1: 1–10

Curtin L L 1983 The nurse as advocate: a cantankerous critique. Nursing Management 14: 9–10

The Declaration of Hawaii 1977 General Assembly of the World Psychiatric Association, Honolulu

de Leon Siantz M L 1979 Human values in determining the fate of persons with mental retardation. Nursing Clinics of North America 14: 57–66

Deutsch A 1938 The mentally ill in America. Columbia University Press, New York

Dworkin R 1977 Taking rights seriously. Harvard University Press, Cambridge, Mass

Dworkin G 1978 Legality of consent to nontherapeutic medical research on infants and young children. Archives of Disease in Childhood 53: 443–446

Dyer C 1985 The Gillick judgement. Contraceptives and the under 16s. House of Lords ruling. British Medical Journal 291(1): 1208–1209

Fagin, C M 1975 Nurses' rights. American Journal of Nursing. 75: 82

Freedman B 1975 A moral theory of informed consent. Hastings Center Report 5: 32

Gaylin W 1972 Genetic screening: the ethics of knowing. New England Journal of Medicine 286: 1361

Glover J 1977 Causing death and saving lives. Penguin, Harmondsworth

Golding M P 1978 The concept of rights: a historical sketch. In: Bandman E L, Bandman B (eds) Bioethics and human rights: a reader for health professionals. Little, Brown, Boston, p 44–50

Gostin L 1986 The ideology of entitlement: the contemporary function of law and its application to psychiatry. In: Carmi A, Schneider S, Hefiz A (eds) Psychiatry, law and ethics. Springer Verlag, Berlin, p 73–79

Greif L C 1985 Issues of confidentiality in health care. In: Carmi A, Schneider S (eds) Nursing law and ethics. Springer Verlag, Berlin, p 70–74

Grogono A W, Woodgate D J 1971 Index for measuring health. Lancet ii: 1024–1026

Hare R M 1981 Moral thinking: its levels, method and point. Clarendon Press, Oxford

Harris E L 1968 Respect for persons. In: de George R T (ed) Ethics and society: original essays on contemporary moral problems. Macmillan, New York

Hayter J 1979 Issues related to human subjects. In: Downs F S, Fleming J W (eds) Issues in nursing research. Appleton-Century-Crofts, New York

Hume D 1888 A treatise on human nature. Selby-Bigge L A (ed). Oxford University Press

Illich I 1976 Limits to medicine. Medical nemesis: the expropriation of Health. Penguin, Harmondsworth

International Council of Nurses 1973 Code for Nurses. Ethical concepts applied to nursing. ICN

Kant I 1964 Groundwork of the metaphysic of morals. Paton H J (trans). Harper & Row, New York

Karasu T 1981 Ethical aspects of psychotherapy. In: Bloch S, Chodoff P (eds) Psychiatric ethics. Oxford University Press, Ch 6

Kass L R 1980 Ethical dilemmas in the case of the ill. Journal of the American Medical Association 244: 1811

Kelman H C 1972 The rights of the subject in social research: an analysis in terms of relative power and legitimacy. American Journal of Psychology 27: 995

Kelly G S J 1951 The duty to preserve life. Theological Studies 12: 550

Kennedy L 1981 The unmasking of medicine. Allen & Unwin, London

Kilpatrick V 1984 Ethical issues and procedural dilemmas in measuring patient competence. Advances in Nursing Science 6: 22–33

Krasner L 1962 The therapist as a social reinforcement machine. In: Strup H, Luborsky L (eds) Research in Psychotherapy. American Psychological Association, Washington DC, Vol 2, p 61–94

Laing R D 1965 The divided self. Penguin, Harmondsworth

Liefer R 1970 The medical model as ideology. International Journal of Psychiatry 9: 13–21

Lockwood M (ed) 1985 Moral dilemmas in modern medicine. Oxford University Press

London P 1969 Behaviour control. Harper & Row, New York

MacCormick D N 1977 Rights in legislation. In: Hacker P, Raz J (eds) Law, morality and society: essays in honour of H L A Hart. Clarendon Press, Oxford, p 188–209

McCormack R 1974a Proxy consent in the experimental situation. Perspectives in Biology and Medicine 18: 2–20

McCormack R 1974b To save or let die: the dilemma of modern medicine. Journal of the American Medical Association 229: 172–96

McCormack R 1978 The quality of life, the sanctity of life. Hastings Center Report 8

McGarry L, Chodoff P 1981 The ethics of involuntary hospitalization. In: Bloch S, Chodoff P (eds) Psychiatric ethics. Oxford University Press, ch II, p 203–219

Mechanic D 1981 The social dimension. In Bloch S, Chodoff P (eds) Psychiatric ethics. Oxford University Press, Ch 4

Medical Research Council 1963 Responsibilities in investigations on human subjects. Report of the Medical Research Council for 1962–63. (Cmnd 2382.) HMSO, London

Merskey H 1981 Ethical aspects of the physical manipulation of the brain. In: Bloch S, Chodoff P (eds) Psychiatric ethics. Oxford University Press

Mills J S 1974 Utilitarianism, On Liberty and Essay on Bentham. Edited with an introduction by Mary Warnock. New American Library, New York

Murphy M A, Murphy J 1976 Making ethical decisions — systematically. Nursing 6 (May): 13–14

Nolan P 1985 Psychiatry under fire. Nursing Mirror 160 (21): 34–38

Norton D 1975 The research ethic. Nursing Times 71: 2048–2049

Nuremberg Code 1949 In: Trials of war criminals before the Nuremberg Military Tribunals under Central Council Law. US Government Printing Office, Washington DC, no 10, Vol 2, p 181–182

Peplau H 1987 Tomorrow's world: Psychiatric skills. Nursing Times 7 (Jan): 29–32

Pittam M R 1982 Does unsuccessful salvage surgery modify the terminal course of patients with squamous carcinomas of head and neck? Clinical Oncology 8: 195–200

Pius XII 1957 Allocution on Ordinary and Extraordinary Means, 24 November, Vatican, Rome

Priestman T J, Baum M 1976 Evaluation of quality of life in patients receiving treatment for advanced breast cancer. Lancet i: 899–901

Ramsey P 1970 The patient as person. Yale University Press, New Haven, Conn.

Rawls J 1971 A theory of justice. Harvard University Press, Cambridge, Mass.

Reich W 1981 Psychiatric diagnosis as an ethical problem. In: Bloch S, Chodoff P (eds) Psychiatric ethics. Oxford University Press, Ch 5

Rice J K, Rice D G 1973 Implications of the Women's Liberation Movement for psychotherapy. American Journal of Psychiatry 130: 191–196

Roth L, Meisel A, Lidz C 1977 Tests of competency to consent to treatment. American Journal of Psychiatry 134: 279–284

Royal College of Nursing 1977 Ethics related to research in nursing. RCN, London

Seiden A M 1976 Overview: research on the psychology of women. II: Women in families, work and psychotherapy. American Journal of Psychiatry 133: 1111–1123

Simes R J, Tattersall M H N, Coates A S, Raghavan D, Solomon H J 1986 Randomized comparison of procedures for obtaining informed consent in clinical trials of treatment for cancer. British Medical Journal 293: 1065–1068

Spitzer W O, Dobson A J, Hall J et al 1981 Measuring the quality of life of cancer patients. Journal of Chronic Diseases 34: 585–587

Steele S M, Harmon V M 1983 Values clarification in nursing, 2nd edn. Appleton-Century-Crofts, New York

Szasz T 1961 The myth of mental illness. Harper & Row, New York

Szasz T 1963 Law, liberty and psychiatry. Macmillan, New York

Treffert D A 1974 Dying with your rights on. 12th Annual Meeting of the American Psychiatric Association, Detroit, Michigan

United Kingdom Central Council 1984 Code of Professional Conduct. UKCC, London

Vail D J 1966 Dehumanization and the institutional career. C C Thomas, Springfield, Ill.

Watson A B 1982 Informed consent of special subjects. Nursing Research 31(1): 43–47

World Medical Association 1964, 1975 Declaration of Helsinki, 18th W M Assembly, Helsinki; 29th W M Assembly, Tokyo

9

Stress

M. Appleby

The nursing profession as a whole has been slow to acknowledge the stressful nature of nursing work. Despite early studies, such as Menzies (1960) and Holsclaw (1965), it is not until recently that nurses have begun to examine the phenomenon of stress in themselves. Patients' suffering and death, frightening tasks and disturbing relationships with patients were seen as potential stresses by Menzies (1960). The emotional high-risk areas identified by Holsclaw (1965) included working with patients with psychiatric problems and being unable to restore patients to well-being.

Stereotypic ideas about the role of the nurse have inhibited the tendency of nurses to seek support. Traditionally, nurses have been told to avoid getting emotionally involved with patients. If this warning was not heeded, the individual nurse received little sympathy from his or her peers (Morton 1984). Jones (1982) has noted how nurses are socialized to believe that it is unacceptable for a good nurse to admit to feelings of stress and frustration. There are many fears which prevent nurses expressing how they feel. Mullins & Barstow (1979) asserted that nurses are afraid of being thought of as unstable, weak or incompetent, and fear being reprimanded for expressing negative emotions such as anger and despair.

During the past decade, there has been much research into the effects of stress in the helping professions (e.g. Cherniss 1980, Freudenberger 1974, Maslach 1979). There is little work specifically studying stress in psychiatric nursing. However, a great deal of the growing body of research into aspects of stress in nursing generally can be applied to this field.

Before attempting to assess the nature of stress in psychiatric nursing and the measures which can be suggested to alleviate it, it is necessary to consider briefly the concept of stress in general terms.

THE NATURE OF STRESS

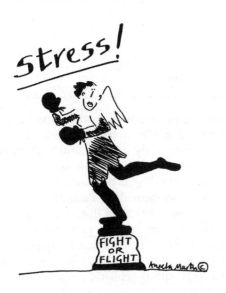

Researchers in physiology, psychology, sociology, medicine and nursing have studied stress using different definitions of the term. No universal definition of stress has been agreed and the way in which it is conceptualized depends largely on the perspective of the individual. Hans Selye undertook pioneering work in the study of stress and his definition is often cited. He defined stress in physiological terms as: 'The non-specific response of the body to the demands made upon it' (Selye 1956). Selye called his model of stress the General Adaptation Syndrome, which is divided into three stages:

1. The alarm reaction, when the individual becomes aware of the situation and the stressor

2. The resistance stage, when the homeostatic mechanisms of the body are mobilized to adjust to the stressor
3. The exhaustion stage, if homeostasis is not restored and stress persists, causing eventual morbidity.

The definition of stress proposed by Lazarus (1971) is also useful when considering the dynamics of stress. Lazarus viewed stress as the environmental or internal demands on an individual that may tax or exceed the resources of the individual's system.

External demands may be, for example, the threat of losing a job. Internal demands may be the desired goals of the individual or the high standards that the individual sets him or herself. Lazarus & Launier (1978) emphasized the importance of psychological stress in enhancing the performance of a person, but if the demands cannot be met, there may be harmful physical and psychological consequences. This can occur when the balance between demands and resources is destroyed, either by increased demands or decreased resources. When an individual cannot meet demands, he or she becomes demoralized, ineffective and has reduced problem-solving skills (Lazarus & Launier 1978). These skills are essential in the helping process, such as in psychiatric nursing; therefore excess stress will have an adverse effect on the performance of nurses and standards of care for patients (Claus 1980).

Both Selye and Lazarus have noted the importance of an individual's perception of a stressor in determining the response. Furthermore, Lazarus (1971) stated that stress reactions are directly related to the cognitive appraisal of the situation by the individual. According to McGrath (1970), the level of stress experienced is a function of the consequence of a failure to meet a demand. Greater stress occurs when the consequence is more important. This has particular relevance to nursing, since nurses are responsible for the well-being and health of patients. McGrath (1970) also suggested that psychological stress can occur when the resources of an individual exceed the demands made and a sense of lack of fulfilment is experienced.

The process of coping with stress begins when the equilibrium between demands and resources is disturbed (see Fig. 9.1). Four modes of coping have been identified by Lazarus & Launier (1978): the search for information, direct action, inhibition of action, and intra-psychic defence. A combination of these methods may be used.

The means of coping depends on the situation: for example, when an individual experiences helplessness, direct action may be inhibited and an intra-psychic method of coping will dominate.

Cherniss (1980) has pointed out that this is common in bureaucracies, such as hospitals, where the individual finds it very difficult to effect change, leading to feelings of helplessness. In a situation of high ambiguity or uncertainty, the coping method may be information seeking, but if this is fruitless, intra-psychic coping will be used. Intra-psychic methods of coping include denial and withdrawal of contact with the stressor; this can be maladaptive and ultimately lead to the phenomenon of burnout.

Job stress and burnout

In order to apply these theoretical ideas to the problem of stress in psychiatric nursing, it is useful to consider a more specific definition of job stress. Job stress occurs when one or more factors at work make demands on the worker, to disrupt psychological or physiological homeostasis (Margolis & Kroes 1974). If homeostasis is not maintained the condition of burnout may result. The term burnout was first coined by Freudenberger in the late 1960s when he recognized the symptoms of exhaustion in his staff of social workers. He described the phenomenon as: 'A syndrome of physical and emotional exhaustion experienced by those in the helping professions when they feel overwhelmed by other people's problems' (Freudenberger 1974).

Maslach (1979) has studied burnout extensively and has noted that the sufferer develops a negative self-concept, negative job attitudes and exhibits loss of concern and feelings for patients or clients. It is this loss of concern which is the most crucial characteristic of burnout, resulting in the tendency to treat clients in a detached manner.

Other theorists have widened the concept to include changes in motivation, including loss of enthusiasm and sense of purpose in work (Cherniss 1980). Storlie (1979) proposed that burnout is typified by disillusionment and what she called 'the collapse of the human spirit'. The process of burnout can be insidious and difficult to identify. She also pointed out that a susceptible host is necessary, this often being a highly idealistic nurse.

There are many physical, behavioural and psychological signs of burnout. McCarthy (1985) following his review of the literature compiled a comprehensive list of burnout indices (see Box 9.1). Three general stages of burnout have been identified (Maslach 1979, Prophit 1983, Spaniol & Caputo 1978).

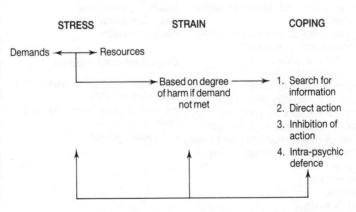

Fig. 9.1 The stress-coping cycle (from Cherniss 1980).

Stage One — Symptoms experienced occasionally but the individual feels emotionally and physically exhausted.

Stage Two — Symptoms become more regular and last longer and cynical, dehumanizing attitudes towards patients develop. The individual may become withdrawn.

Stage Three — Symptoms are chronic, the victim questions the value of his or her work and is unable to control emotions. Often physical symptoms manifest.

There is limited usefulness in identifying the symptoms and stages of burnout because of many individual differences. Nevertheless, identification and awareness of the signs of stress is the first step towards successful coping (Scully 1980).

Box 9.1 Symptoms of burnout among health professionals (after McCarthy 1985)

Emotional indices

Using emotional distancing devices e.g. intellectualization
Feelings of isolation
Feelings of alienation
Feelings of not being appreciated
Feelings of helplessness
Feelings of powerlessness
Feelings of being trapped
Depression
Personal and professional frustration
Poor job satisfaction

Behavioural indices

Irritability and aggression towards patients
Increasing isolation from patients
Inability to perform job as effectively as in past
Narrowing of social and recreational activities
Increased use and abuse of alcohol and drugs
Increased interpersonal difficulties leading to marital and family discord
Increased interpersonal conflict with other staff and students

Attitudinal indices

Development of negative attitudes
Gradual loss of caring about patients
Viewing patients as cases rather than people
Cynical and often dehumanizing perception of patients
Labelling of patients in demeaning terms
Blaming patients for their disorder
Loss of sympathy with patients
Loss of respect for patients
Poor professional self-concept
Distrust of management and peers
Hypercritical of institution and/or peers
Pessimism
Ridicule
Indifference
Boredom

Psychosomatic indices

Fatigue
Muscular aches and pains
Headaches
Menstrual irregularities
Sleep disturbances
Gastrointestinal disorders
Frequent colds

Organizational indices

Deteriorating patient care
Low staff morale
Increased dishonesty and theft
High absenteeism
Increased accidents

SOURCES OF STRESS IN PSYCHIATRIC NURSING

It is essential to identify the factors contributing to stress in psychiatric nursing, in order to see where support, help and change are necessary. The sources of stress can be divided into four broad areas: factors relating to the nature of psychiatric nursing work, individual factors in nurses, organizational factors, and factors relating to change in psychiatric nursing.

The nature of psychiatric nursing work

The nurse in any speciality has a responsibility for the well-being of others and this in itself can be stressful and detrimental to health (Cobb 1974). Menzies (1960) emphasized that it is nurses who bear the major impact of the stresses arising from patient care, because they have the closest and most continual contact with patients. The intense interactions which nurses have with patients and their families is also a source of stress (Bailey 1980). A study by Cronin-Stubbs & Brophy (1985) reported that psychiatric nurses experienced intense interpersonal involvement and frequent conflicts with patients, families and colleagues. Nurses may often experience close contact with very disturbed and distressed individuals. Becoming aware of the frightening world in which some patients live can be quite harrowing and sometimes leads to a nurse questioning many of his or her own values. This can cause anxiety, fear and confusion, and for these reasons Llewelyn (1984) proposed that psychiatric nurses need additional support and guidance.

Students are particularly vulnerable to stress. Inexperience, lack of knowledge and stereotypic notions about psychiatric patients may contribute to this. Burgess (1981) documented some of the fears of general nursing students when beginning psychiatry. These included fear of violence, fear that the patients will demand too much of the nurse and fear about their own mental health. It was noted that students often feel overwhelmed by the initial experience of meeting psychiatric patients. Dealing with depressed patients can greatly impinge on the state of mind of an individual and result in the nurse becoming depressed.

There are certain aspects of psychiatric nursing which are assumed to be more stressful than others, such as working with aggressive or acutely psychotic patients. Hodgkinson et al (1984) in a retrospective survey of assaults on staff in a psychiatric hospital, found that it was the nursing staff who were most frequently assaulted. This is often a source of stress. McCarthy (1985) undertook a small study of burnout in different psychiatric settings, using the Staff Burnout Scale for Health Professionals, developed by Jones (1980). He anticipated that nurses working with acutely distressed, psychotic patients, disturbed psychogeriatric patients and those working night duty would have higher burnout scores. No significant differences were found in the different settings, possibly due to the small size of the sample. Pines & Maslach (1978) did find that the higher the percentage of schizophrenics in the patient population, the less job satisfaction staff members expressed. Further research is necessary to determine which clinical areas in psychiatry are most stressful. However, many stressors are common to all areas of psychiatry.

Psychiatric nursing is still to some extent a low status area of health care. Many patients have chronic, intractable problems which cannot be completely cured or may take years to resolve. This does not fit with the medical model of illness, which nurses are often oriented towards during their training, especially if they have a general nursing background. Nursing interventions are less obvious than in general nursing and potential outcomes less concrete. This may mean that psychiatric nurses get less positive feedback about their work and could experience reduced job satisfaction. Cronin-Stubbs & Brophy (1985) compared the degree of social support received by staff nurses working in psychiatry, intensive care, operating room and medicine. Psychiatric nurses were found to experience less affirmation than other groups. Affirmation was defined as 'feedback about the appropriateness or correctness of thoughts or behaviours, i.e. recognition, acknowledgement or validation by others'. It was noted that social support and affirmation may offset the effects of intense stressors and contribute to the prevention of burnout.

In psychiatry, a diversity of problems are dealt with and there are very few clear-cut answers or forms of therapy. Nolan (1985) went as far as to write: 'Behind therapeutic rhetoric and a professional appearance, psychiatry struggles to contain different and opposing models and theories of illness and treatment.'

Nurses are often at the centre of disagreements about the ethics of certain treatments, and as patient advocates, this can be a source of stress. Inter-disciplinary conflicts exist between psychiatrists, social workers, psychologists, occupational therapists and nurses as to the effectiveness and ethical justification of various treatments. Electroconvulsive therapy (ECT), seclusion, restraint, behaviour modification, psychosurgery, psychotherapy and chemotherapy are all controversial. There is also an increasing public

and media awareness about such practices. These factors may lead to nurses feeling anxious and uncertain and less able to endorse the views of other professionals about particular treatments. Salvage (1985) observed that in 1982 there were at least three hospitals where psychiatric student nurses were sacked for refusing to be involved in ECT. In such circumstances, nurses can be forced to act against their own values and professional judgement, to avoid conflict and loss of their livelihood. These problems are a source of stress to many nurses.

Because of the number of disciplines involved in psychiatry, disagreements about who should undertake certain therapeutic interventions sometimes occur. Many psychiatric nurses feel that their role is being encroached upon by other professionals and that they are being left with more menial or physical aspects of care. It is ironic that this should occur at a time when psychiatric nurse education is improving and nurses are better

---

Box 9.2 Case history of a psychiatric nurse under stress

When Julie Smith got her first job as a staff nurse, she enjoyed the challenge of learning new things. The job was often demanding but she found this rather exhilarating. It was satisfying to prove her competence to herself and others. Julie had many new ideas for the ward. It was a long-stay psychiatric ward but she could see the potential for the rehabilitation of many of the patients. She had high expectations of herself and her patients.

Some of the other staff on the ward were rather cynical about all these new ideas. They felt that Julie was fighting a losing battle. With poor staffing levels, it was difficult to put any new ideas into practice. It all seemed pointless anyway, because rumours suggested that the hospital might soon be closing down.

After working on the ward for a while, these feelings were passed on to Julie. She became disillusioned and felt that without support from her colleagues she could not change anything. Julie's enthusiasm began to wane. She felt very tired, but had difficulty sleeping at night. She was able to get some sleeping tablets from a friend in the nurses home who had the same problem.

Julie eventually began to dread going to work. It was so depressing. She took the occasional day off sick when she could get away with it, but this was only a temporary relief. It all seemed so pointless. Julie felt that the patients themselves were apathetic and did not really want to get better. Finally, she decided to apply for another course and look for other jobs — maybe things would be better on a different type of ward.

equipped than previously to use skills such as counselling and behaviour modification techniques.

The problem of role definition for the psychiatric nurse has been highlighted by Cormack (1983) who stated: 'The new role prescriptions, which supersede those of the nurse custodian and follower of "doctors orders", have undoubtedly confused, rather than clarified, the psychiatric nurse's role' (p. 18). This is relevant, because role conflict and role ambiguity have been identified as major sources of stress (Cherniss 1980). According to Kahn (1974), role conflict causes high job tension and lower levels of job satisfaction. On the basis of research, Cormack (1983) noted that there was a considerable discrepancy between the prescribed role and the actual role of psychiatric charge nurses.

Individual factors

It has already been noted that all individuals perceive potential stressors in different ways. Certain factors within an individual influence his or her reaction to stress and ways of coping.

Cherniss (1980) listed some of the personality traits which influence how susceptible a person is to stress. These traits are: neurotic anxiety, Type A personality, locus of control, flexibility and introversion. High levels of neurotic anxiety, characterized by a strong punitive superego, emotionality, instability and a strong desire for success, conflicting with the individual's fear of competition and need for approval, may increase susceptibility to stress. Often such people rely on psychological defences for coping. It seems that the human services attract individuals who have strong dependency and achievement needs and set unrealistically high goals for themselves (Cherniss 1980). However, a study by Parkes (1980) found that general student nurses were typical, in personality measures, of the female population, except that they tended to be more stable emotionally and more extroverted. Thus it is necessary to be careful when making generalizations.

Type A syndrome is thought to be a common trait in the human services. Friedman & Rosenman (1974) differentiated between two classes of Type A behaviour. Type A1 is when the individual is aggressive, competitive and achievement orientated in any environment. The Type A2 individual must be in a pressurized, hurried environment to exhibit this pattern of behaviour. Tierney & Strom (1980) have emphasized these differences with respect to nurses. They suggested that nurses tend to be Type A2 individuals, who are conscientious and often placed in a setting where there is constant pressure on time. Dillon (1983) cited the work of Sehnert, who proposed that nurses' personalities make them susceptible to stress because they focus on work intensely and allow no time for recreation and spiritual life. Sehnert observed that it is because such behaviour is rewarded during nurse training that so many nurses develop Type A personalities.

The locus of control of an individual is another relevant factor (Rotter 1966). Individuals with an internal locus of control believe that they can influence their own destinies. Conversely, an external locus of control means that the individual feels at the mercy of powers beyond his or her control. Cherniss (1980) has proposed that the latter type of person may be more prone to the feelings of helplessness associated with burnout. Flexible individuals are more susceptible to stress because they find it difficult to refuse requests, and introverts are more likely to withdraw in the face of stress, which can be maladaptive (Cherniss 1980).

Most nurses demand high standards of themselves and aim at effective performance of their work. These internal demands can greatly contribute to stress and burnout. Efficacy is of prime importance when one has responsibility for the well-being and lives of others. Nursing also has a personal significance: it is considered to be a vocation and therefore self-esteem and identity may depend on high standards of performance at work. Cherniss (1980) identified two ways of achieving psychological success: firstly, by the accomplishment of tasks that contribute to the well-being of the patient; and secondly, by having the ability to control the work environment. The latter is not always possible in a hospital organization, and if a nurse feels unable to control and predict events at work, this can lead to the experience of learned helplessness. Seligman (1975) described the effects of learned helplessness, stating that it may result in impaired motivation, cynicism, withdrawal and apathy. This phenomenon appears to be closely related to burnout. Lack of control over one's environment is obviously linked with the organizational factors contributing to stress in nursing.

Organizational factors

Many writers have illustrated the need to explore organizational factors and how they contribute to stress and burnout. Since her classic work in the 1960s, Menzies (1977) has documented how the strategies employed by hospital bureaucracies, that are indirectly aimed at decreasing stress, can actually become sources of stress. There is minimization of nurse–patient contact, protection against developing relationships, minimal decision-making and lack of control over work. Nurses' responsibilities are poorly defined and the bureaucracy is dehumanizing for both staff and patients (Menzies 1977). In recent years, as Coleman (1982) has observed, the link between responsibility and autonomy has been broken down. It is common for nurses to have great practical responsibilities, but no authority at all. The change from consensus management to a system of general management in the National Health Service, as a result of the Griffiths Report (DHSS 1983), may make it even more difficult for nurses to influence decision-making.

Organizational factors also contribute to the problem of role conflict in nursing. The expectations of the hierarchy may not coincide with the professional and personal goals of a nurse. As psychiatric nurses become more professionally oriented, there is an even greater potential for a mismatch of the ideals of the nurse and the organization. Kramer's (1974) work, in the USA, on the problems of nurse graduates when they enter the bureaucracy of the hospital after being in university, is likely to become more relevant to nurses in Britain. Proposals to educate all nurses in the higher education system are currently being examined by the statutory bodies and professional organizations.

The impact of stress caused by shift work, low pay and overtime has been emphasized by Kerr & Poole (1984). High patient–staff ratios have a major influence in reducing self-fulfilment of staff members (Pines & Maslach 1978). Poor career structures and lack of administrative recognition and sensitivity have also been recognized as being instrumental in causing stress in nurses (McCarthy 1985).

The fact that nursing is a female-dominated profession is often cited as being influential in the experience of stress among its members (e.g. Mullins & Barstow 1979, Sanders 1980). Even in psychiatry there is a larger proportion of women than men. Pollock & West (1984) quoted Scottish health statistics showing that only one in four psychiatric nurses is male. In the same paper, they discussed the issues of sexism in psychiatric nursing and observed that men occupy most of the senior positions. Many women attempt to combine family life with a career, but this can cause a great burden on the individual. Lack of nursery provision, shift work and lack of flexibility contribute to the difficulties that women experience (Pollock & West 1984).

Changes in psychiatric nursing

These are closely linked with organizational factors, but in view of the momentous changes occurring in psychiatric nursing, more specific consideration is necessary. Changes in education, administration and the structure of the service are being implemented (see Fig. 9.2). The relationship between stress and change has been examined by Owen (1983). Change can have a positive effect by challenging and stimulating the individual, but negative effects are also common. A major problem with any change is fear of the unknown, which can cause great anxiety. This often stems from poor communication by managers. Staff may feel that they are subjected to change without consultation. Significantly, Coleman (1982) stated that the greatest sufferers in any reorganization tend to be those who have little influence but have most responsibility for facilitating the smooth running of the service. The National Health Service has undergone successive reorganizations in the past

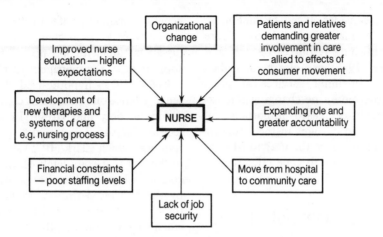

Fig. 9.2 Changes in psychiatric nursing: potential stresses.

decade and the impact of this on nursing staff cannot be ignored.

The move from institutional care to community care of the mentally ill is currently underway. Many psychiatric nurses accept the benefits of this for the patients, but feel that inadequate provision is being made in the community, due to lack of resources. The transition is also occurring very rapidly, giving little time for staff or patients to prepare themselves. Nurses are being moved into the community without always receiving adequate training, and those left in hospitals feel insecure about their jobs. Many large institutions are under threat of closure. To some extent, working in an institution gives a feeling of security, power and is a source of social contacts (Horwitz 1982). Thus, moving out of this environment can be very stressful. Munro (1980) commented that the patients who remain in institutions following these changes are likely to be the most severely disturbed. Consequently, staff will have little relief from dealing with highly dependent patients and stress might be excessive.

Changes in psychiatric nursing practice are also being implemented. The use of the nursing process, individualized patient care and new therapeutic regimens have all been heralded as great improvements. However, without adequate in-service training and support, such new ideas may only serve to create stress and dissatisfaction.

Individualized patient care may remove many of the defences, mentioned by Menzies (1960), that nurses have used to protect themselves from stress in the past.

The education of psychiatric nurses is greatly improving and attempts are being made to provide nurses with wider, more relevant skills. However, the development of a more therapeutic role for the nurse is not welcomed by all (Hocking et al 1976). Psychiatric nurses who were trained many years ago may feel inadequate and under pressure, unless provision for in-service training is made. Hocking et al (1976), in the USA, found that nurses who were willing to extend their role tended to be young, more recently qualified, with few years of nursing experience. With more graduates opting for a career in psychiatric nursing, it is useful to refer to a study by Pines & Maslach (1978). They found that staff members with a higher education tended to enter mental health work for self-fulfilment and had high expectations of themselves and their patients when they began the job. Over a period of time, they became more pessimistic about the potential and usefulness of their work. The experience of stress and risk of burnout may be great for such people.

Finally, it is necessary to be aware of changes in society that influence psychiatric nursing. Economic recession, high unemployment and increased demands on the health services are important factors to consider. It has become more difficult for nurses to maintain standards of care in the face of diminishing resources of staff and equipment. Salvage (1985) has clearly described how nurses are maintaining services at great personal cost. Furthermore, the changing role expectations of women, decreased importance of religious institutions and changes in the structure of family life may all influence the individual's experience of stress and ability to cope effectively.

HOW DO NURSES COPE WITH STRESS?

There are few formal sources of help and support for nurses under stress. This is partly due to the reluctance to admit to the problem and lack of recognition of the widespread needs of nurses. The Briggs Report (DHSS 1972) recommended that a comprehensive nurse counselling service should be established in an attempt to reduce the high drop-out rate of nurse learners. By 1983, there were only 13 nurse counsellors in Britain, and only three of these were full time (Shearer 1983). The Royal College of Nursing runs a counselling service for all nurses, not just members, but the availability of this service is limited because the counsellors have to travel to regional offices to see clients. Most nurses rely on informal support from colleagues, peers and tutors, and the adequacy of such help varies greatly.

Statistics for attrition, absenteeism and suicide in nursing suggest that a proportion of nurses have difficulty coping. Darby (1978) asserted that student nurses leave the profession because they cannot cope with the stress involved. In a study by Birch (1979), it was noted that of the learners in his sample who left nursing, 65% did so because of the stress inherent in the job. More recent work by Murray (1983) showed that 13% of the learners in the sample had considered leaving for the same reasons. This figure did not include those who had actually left. These findings suggest that more effective stress management is necessary to help learners to cope. Help is also needed for qualified staff; there is a high rate of attrition in certain specialities such as intensive care. In

general nursing, Redfern (1981) found that ward sisters were keen to change their jobs because of dissatisfaction with job prospects and insufficient support from the management hierarchy.

Clark (1975) hypothesized that short-term absence from work is often a coping mechanism to reduce anxiety and stress. In her study, absenteeism increased over the period of student training, which Clark (1975) suggested was related to the fact that completely leaving nursing was becoming a less feasible alternative. A recent survey by the *Nursing Mirror* (Campbell 1985) indicated that 55% of respondents had taken time off sick when they were not really ill. Of the qualified staff in the survey, 46.5% said they often felt too tired or stressed to work but carried on, and 48.5% said they occasionally felt this way.

Research into smoking among nurses could also be considered indicative of high levels of unrelieved stress. Hawkins et al (1982) cited an Office of Population Censuses and Surveys (OPCS) study which showed that 48% of female nurses smoked, as compared with 39% of their age/sex counterparts in the general population. These findings were confirmed in a study by Hawkins et al (1982), but it was also noted that psychiatric nurses smoked more heavily than other groups. They proposed that a third of nurses smoke to relieve stress and that stress is influential in acquiring the habit.

Suicide statistics for nurses also make solemn reading. The *Nursing Mirror* (1978) reported that female nurses were three times more likely to commit suicide than any other similar group of working women. On the basis of the indirect evidence quoted, it seems reasonable to suggest that there is a problem of unrelieved and sometimes unrecognized stress or burnout in nursing. In addition to the suffering caused to the nurse, the effects of burnout on patient care can be extensive.

The impact of burnout on patient care

Maslach (1979) has proposed that burnout plays a central role in poor standards of care. By examining the indices of burnout illustrated in Box 9.1 it can be seen that this phenomenon must have far-reaching effects on patient care. It could be argued that the impact of burnout in psychiatry is even greater than in other areas of nursing, because meaningful interaction and communication with patients is even more crucial to the helping process.

Defensive coping strategies can be adopted by an individual or by an entire group within an institution (Cherniss 1980). The custodial norms and dehumanizing practices that are evident in some large institutions may have developed as a collective response to stress and lack of power. This can help to explain the problem of neglect and abuse of patients in some psychiatric hospitals. Nolan (1985) examined this problem in a historical context and concluded that psychiatric nurses themselves have been the victims of abuse. He stated that submissive, compliant individuals were recruited for psychiatric hospitals, and nurse training resulted in them becoming reliant on medical and bureaucratic control. Ultimately, these staff became institutionalized.

Recently, in all areas of nursing there has been an increase in the number of cases to come before the nursing disciplinary body. This increase has been related to the unreasonable pressures of work that many nurses are under (Morton 1984). Thus, for the well-being of both nurses and patients, concerted action needs to be taken to reduce stress levels and prevent burnout.

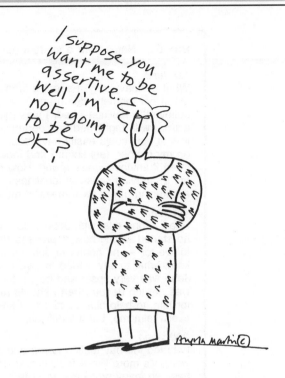

METHODS OF PREVENTION AND REDUCTION OF STRESS AND BURNOUT

Interventions to reduce stress can be divided into four groups: educational, work setting, individual and organizational.

Educational interventions

Widespread education is necessary to promote a change of attitudes in the nursing profession in order to make the seeking of support more acceptable. In-service training for qualified staff is also beneficial, because it increases knowledge and im-

proves problem-solving skills, thereby increasing the resources of a nurse to meet the demands of the work.

The importance of assertiveness training is gradually being acknowleged by nurse educationalists. Many nurses lack assertiveness, because, as women, they have learnt to put the needs of others before their own. Salvage (1985) has described how assertiveness skills can help nurses to cope more positively with the demands made upon them, by being able to refuse requests without feeling guilty. This is preferable to nurses using maladaptive passive or aggressive coping mechanisms.

Gay (1985) suggested that all nurses would benefit from a programme of health education, including advice on diet, exercise, relaxation and stress management techniques. More specifically, schools of nursing could include the teaching of self-awareness and stress recognition and management in their curriculum. Burnard (1984) emphasized the importance of self-awareness training in psychiatric nurse education, in terms of its contribution to producing sensitive, caring

---

Box 9.3 Notes from a student nurse's clinical diary

1st June
What a 'heavy' day. I spent a long time talking to one of the patients about her mother's death and how she coped with it. I could not believe the feelings I had, I was dying to cry, to escape, leave the ward. I was frightened and depressed. Those experiences and feelings in that lady could easily have been mine if my mother died. I depend on my mother, feel secure and independent because I know she is there if anything goes wrong. How could I cope if she suddenly died? I felt a terrifying sense of loneliness; I suppose my reaction was an awakening of my awareness of my own potential for aloneness.

4th June
I had a long chat with John today. I asked him how he was feeling and he started saying how depressed he was. He felt that there was nothing to live for — no home, no job, no friends. I found it very difficult to know what to say. I tried to give him as much hope as possible, but John was very upset and began to cry. I had an awful feeling that I was delving deeper than I should have been. I wanted to do something for him, to help him practically. I knew that I must not let his problems overwhelm me, but it's difficult.

20th June
I started the day feeling bored and apathetic. Maybe bored is the wrong word, it's more like a feeling of disillusionment. The people on the ward have so many problems and I feel overwhelmed by them: inadequate because I don't seem able to do anything. I suppose I'm expecting miracle cures.

25th June First day on the secure unit
We arrived feeling nervous and uncertain. Memories of seeing films about psychopathic killers were at the back of my mind. The environment was surprisingly pleasant, but the atmosphere was strange, very tense. I felt tense and anxious for most of the day; the staff must never be able to relax because they have to be on the alert for potential problems or violence all the time. I was emotionally exhausted after one day, I don't think I could ever work on such a ward for any length of time. Maybe it's just my inexperience that makes me feel this way.

---

nurses. Self-awareness can also help individuals to see their particular weaknesses and help them to understand their reactions to stressors. Maladaptive coping mechanisms can be discussed and an individual can be helped to develop more positive ways of coping. Burnard (1984) documented many of the numerous techniques for developing self-awareness.

One method, which seems to have great potential for stress management in psychiatric nursing, is the technique of reflection. Unconsciously, most people reflect on experiences and clarify thoughts in this way. Recently, authors such as Bond et al (1985) have recognized the importance of reflective activity as a way of turning experience into learning. Writing about personal experiences can aid the exploration of emotions and anxieties and help the nurse to recognize particular stressors. Keeping a diary whilst in the clinical area can help students to be aware of the self-development process, as well as providing a record of significant learning experiences (Walker 1985). Such a diary can be shared and discussed with tutors and peers, or it can be kept as a personal document. This can help an individual to face up to uncomfortable issues or, if shared, can be a basis for co-counselling. Some tutors of psychiatric nursing have adopted the use of student diaries as a tool for learning and these can also have a valuable cathartic effect.

Education about stress and its management is essential to help nurses to understand their own problems, vulnerabilities and resources for coping. The more nurses are aware of their own emotional reactions, the better they can protect themselves. There are stress management workbooks available with practical exercises and suggestions (e.g. Aronson & Mascia 1981, Bond 1986).

Work setting interventions

The need for peer support at work, as a means of preventing and reducing stress, has been noted by Bond (1982) and Maslach (1978). Whether this should take the form of informal support, which stems from colleagues being sensitive to each other's needs, or formal support groups meeting on a regular basis, depends on the situation. When difficulties in interpersonal relationships within the group cause stress, it may be difficult to form and sustain groups as a means of help. However, when staff are well motivated and attempt to begin these groups before there is widespread burnout in a unit, they can be a useful method of prevention (Maslach 1979). Albrecht (1982) has asserted that burnout is a function of the quality of the relationships between a person and his or her colleagues. A framework for informal peer support was suggested by Bond (1982). This provides practical advice about how nurses can help each other. The use of appropriate humour in the work setting is often a beneficial way of easing tension and stress.

A preventative approach to staff stress has been documented by McDermott (1983). This approach begins with 'selective hiring' so that only nurses who are really suited to the work are taken on. At the interview, nurses were told about the advantages and disadvantages of working in the particular unit and nurses were asked to describe personal strengths, weaknesses, their support systems and the way they coped with stress. McDermott (1983) also emphasized the importance of giving nurses a choice of work assignments, so that a nurse is not constantly in a high stress area. Maslach (1978) claimed that in psychiatric settings, sharing the load of more difficult patients by rotation of staff between wards and by work-sharing is an excellent way of reducing pressure on certain members of staff and making work more varied and stimulating. It has also been proposed that work rotas should be organized so that no nurse has to work more than 5 consecutive days (Gaudinski 1982).

It is possible that the structuring of patient care in a nursing process framework can help to reduce stress by giving nurses responsibility for the total care of a smaller number of patients. However, with a high patient–staff ratio and no support for nurses taking this responsibility, stress levels may increase. Realistic goal-setting and care planning for/with patients is very important in psychiatric nursing. Lamb (1979) noted high levels of frustration and burnout in staff working with long-term psychiatric patients. He suggested that this was partly related to unrealistic expectations of the potential of patients for rehabilitation. Staff may need to be satisfied with improving the quality of a patient's life rather than increasing his or her level of functioning.

Individual interventions

There are many ways that an individual can increase personal resources for coping with stress. Gaudinski (1982) recommended that nurses should always separate work and home life. This point was echoed by Maslach (1978), who also commented on the need for mental health workers to focus some attention on themselves and their own needs, not just on the needs of the patients. By having interests outside work, coping outlets are increased and stress may become more manageable.

Various methods of relaxation can be used by individuals to cope with stress, such as yoga and meditation. Exercise is also a useful outlet for ten-

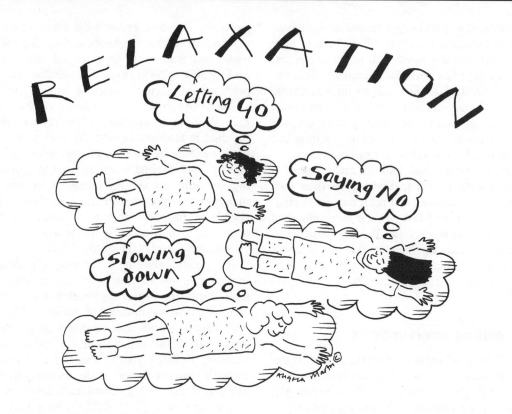

sion and aggression. Townsend & Linsley (1980) discussed co-counselling as a self-help method of increasing a person's ability to deal with stress. It can be learnt relatively quickly and easily. Many other methods of individual therapy have been identified and obviously the individual needs to decide what suits him or her best. However, the most important principles of coping with stress are to be aware of personal needs and to maintain good standards of physical health (Maslach 1979).

Organizational interventions

According to Charles-Edwards (1983), the ability of staff to care for each other and for their patients correlates with the degree that they feel cared for by the organization. He stated that formal support is necessary to prevent staff becoming alienated from the organization and work. Some hospitals have successfully employed nurse counsellors (Annandale-Steiner 1979), but these workers need to be seen as independent of management and the training school. Thus, Salaman (1983) and Cang (1983) have questioned the value of formal counselling services.

These services may be viewed with suspicion by junior members of staff and therefore under-used. Furthermore, Salaman (1983) argued that: 'Counselling *personalizes* organizational problems and inefficiencies. It defines structural, organizational problems as individual problems, possibly even individual *illness*, which thus require individual treatment — that is counselling.'

A more beneficial approach to reducing stress due to organizational factors would be to introduce regular meetings between managers and ward staff, so that difficulties, anxieties and aspirations could be discussed (Salaman 1983). The provision of such a forum could help nurses to feel more involved in decision-making and reduce feelings of powerlessness. Nurses' annual appraisal interviews could also be orientated towards mutual problem-solving and goal-setting.

Reducing patient–staff ratios, shortening working hours and adopting a flexible approach to provision of breaks or 'time outs' for staff have all been identified as necessary changes in many institutions (Maslach 1978). Breaks from direct patient contact should be possible without detriment to patient care because of poor staffing levels. An increase in the provision of child care facilities and a greater willingness to promote job-sharing could also reduce the stress experienced by many nurses.

CONCLUSION

The problem of stress in psychiatric nursing should not be underestimated. The profession is facing a period of great change and the need for support and help for nurses will be substantial.

More research is needed to examine particular areas of stress in psychiatric nursing and to evaluate the effectiveness of systems of support. The impetus for such research must come from within the profession itself. It is essential for nurses to form a cohesive body which can exert pressure and make realistic suggestions for change.

Nurses need to become more sensitive and aware of the needs of their colleagues. It must be made acceptable for individuals to express their feelings or seek help. There are certain stresses inherent in nursing work, but there are also many unnecessary sources of stress which can be prevented or changed. If the problem of stress in nursing is addressed in a coordinated way, the benefits to both nurses and patients are potentially great.

REFERENCES

Albrecht T L 1982 What job stress means for the staff nurse. Nursing Administration Quarterly 7(1): 1–11

Annandale-Steiner D 1979 The nurse counsellor's role at Guy's. Nursing Times, August 9: 1345

Aronson S, Mascia M F 1981 The stress management workbook: an action plan for taking control of your life and health. Appleton-Century-Crofts, New York

Bailey J T 1980 Job stress and other related problems. In: Claus K E, Bailey J T (eds) Living with stress and promoting well-being. C V Mosby, St Louis

Birch J 1979 The anxious learners. Nursing Mirror 148: 17–22

Bond D, Keogh R, Walker D 1985 Reflection: turning experience into learning. Kegan Page, London

Bond M 1982 Do you care about your colleagues? Nursing Mirror 155, October 20: 42–44

Bond M 1986 Stress and self awareness: a guide for nurses. Heinemann, London

Burgess A W 1981 Psychiatric Nursing in the hospital and the community; 3rd edn. Prentice-Hall, New Jersey

Burnard P 1984 Training to be aware. Senior Nurse 1(23) September 5: 25–27

Campbell C 1985 Disturbing findings, Nursing Mirror 160(26) June 26: 17–19

Cang S 1983 Nursing organization and the question of counselling. Nursing Times 79, January 19: 37–38

Charles-Edwards D 1983 Carry on caring for the staff. Health and Social Services Journal 93 April 21: 472–473

Cherniss C 1980 Staff burnout: job stress in the human services. Sage, London

Clark J 1975 Time out: a survey of absenteeism among nurses. RCN, London

Claus K E 1980 The nature of stress. In: Claus K E, Bailey J T (eds) Living with stress and promoting well-being. C V Mosby, St Louis

Cobb S 1974 Role responsibility: the differentiation of a concept. In: Maclean A (ed) Occupational stress. Charles C Thomas, Springfield, Illinois

Coleman V 1982 Warning: hospitals can damage your health. Nursing Mirror 154, June 16: 20–21

Cormack D F S 1983 Psychiatric nursing described. Studies in nursing series. Churchill Livingstone, Edinburgh

Cronin-Stubbs D, Brophy E B 1985 Burnout: can social support save the psych nurse? Journal of Psychosocial Nursing 23(7): 8–13

Darby C 1978 News item. Nursing Mirror 147, December 14: 2

DHSS 1972 Report of the Committee on Nursing (Briggs Report). HMSO, London

DHSS 1983 NHS Management Inquiry Report (Griffiths Report). HMSO, London

Dillon A 1983 Reducing your stress: six experts tell you how. Nursing Life 3(3) May/June: 17–24

Freudenberger H J 1974 Staff burnout. Journal of Social Issues 30(i): 159–166

Friedman M, Rosenman R H 1974 Type A behaviour and your heart. Alfred A Knopf, New York

Gaudinski M A 1982 Coping with and expanding nursing practice, knowledge and technology. In: McConnell E A (ed) Burnout in the nursing profession. C V Mosby, St Louis

Gay J E 1985 Nursing under stress. Occupational Health, May: 225–228

Hawkins L, White M, Morris L 1982 Smoking, stress and nurses. Nursing Mirror, October 13: 18–22

Hocking I L, Hassenein S, Bahr R T 1976 Willingness of psychiatric nurses to assume the extended role. Nursing Research 25(1): 44–48

Hodgkinson P, Hillis T, Russell D 1984 Assaults on staff in a psychiatric hospital. Nursing Times 80(16) April 18: 44–46

Holsclaw P A 1965 Nursing in high emotional risk areas. Nursing Forum 4(4): 36–45

Horwitz A V 1982 The social control of mental illness. Academic Press, London

Jones E M 1982 Who supports the nurse? In: McConnell E A (ed) Burnout in the nursing profession. C V Mosby, St Louis

Jones W J 1980 Preliminary test manual: the staff burnout scale for health professionals (SBS-HP). London House Press, Park Ridge

Kahn R L 1974 Conflict, ambiguity and overload — three elements in job stress. In: Maclean A (ed) Occupational stress. Charles C Thomas, Springfield, Illinois

Kerr A, Poole R 1984 Prescription for survival: health and safety in the Health Service. Macmillan, London

Kramer M 1974 Reality shock. C V Mosby, St Louis

Lamb H R 1979 Staff burnout in work with long-term patients. Hospital and Community Psychiatry 30(6): 396–398

Lazarus R 1971 The concept of stress and disease. In: Levi L (ed) Society, stress and disease, vol 1, The psychosocial environment and psychosomatic disease. Oxford University Press, London

Lazarus R, Launier R 1978 Stress related transactions between person and environment. In: Pervin L A, Lewis M (eds) Perspectives in interactional psychology. Plenum Press, New York

Llewelyn S P 1984 The cost of giving: emotional growth and emotional stress. In: Skevington S (ed) Understanding nurses; the social psychology of nursing. J Wiley & Sons Ltd, Chichester

Margolis B, Kroes W 1974 Occupational stress and strain. In: Maclean A (ed) Occupational stress. Charles C Thomas, Springfield, Illinois

Maslach C 1978 Job burnout: how people cope. Public Welfare 36: 56–58

Maslach C 1979 The burnout syndrome and patient care. In: Garfield C A (ed) Stress and survival — the emotional realities of life-threatening illness. C V Mosby, St Louis

McCarthy P 1985 Burnout in psychiatric nursing. Journal of Advanced Nursing 10: 305–310

McDermott B 1983 A preventative approach to staff stress. Canadian Nurse 79(2): 27–29

McGrath J E (ed) 1970 Social and psychological factors in stress. Holt, Rinehart and Winston, New York

Menzies I E P 1960 Nurses under stress. International Nursing Review 7(6): 9–16

Menzies I E P 1977 The functioning of social systems as a defence against anxiety. Tavistock Institute, London

Morton A 1984 The nurse addict — a state of emotional bankruptcy? Nursing Mirror 159(6) August 22: 16–20

Mullins A C, Barstow R E 1979 Care for the caretakers. American Journal of Nursing, August: 1425–1427

Munro J D 1980 Preventing front-line collapse in institutional settings. Hospital and Community Psychiatry 31(3): 179–182

Murray M 1983 Role conflict and intention to leave nursing. Journal of Advanced Nursing 8: 29–31

Nolan P 1985 Psychiatry under fire. Nursing Mirror 160(21) May 22: 34–38

Nursing Mirror 1978 News item: RCN orders high suicide rate probe. Nursing Mirror 146, February 23: 2

Owen G M 1983 The stress of change. Nursing Times, Occasional Papers 79(4): 44–46

Parkes K 1980 Occupational stress among student nurses. Nursing Times 76, October 30: 113–116

Pines A, Maslach C 1978 Characteristics of staff burnout in mental health settings. Hospital and Community Psychiatry 29(4): 233–237

Pollock L, West E 1984 On being a woman and a psychiatric nurse. Senior Nurse 1(17): 10–13

Prophit P 1983 Burnout. Personal Communication

Redfern S J 1981 Hospital sisters. RCN, London

Rotter J B, Mulry R C 1966 Internal versus external control of reinforcement and decision time. Journal of Personality and Social Psychology 2: 598–604

Salaman G 1983 Counselling organizations: trust or conspiracy? Nursing Times 79, January 19: 38–39

Salvage J 1985 The politics of nursing. Heinemann, London

Sanders M M 1980 Stressed? or burnout? The Canadian Nurse 76(9): 30–33

Scully R 1980 Stress in the nurse. American Journal of Nursing 80(5): 912–915

Seligman E 1975 Helplessness: on depression, development and death. Freeman, Oxford

Selye H 1956 The stress of life. McGraw-Hill, New York

Shearer A 1983 The minders: angels in hell. The Guardian, June 29: 11

Spaniol L, Caputo J J 1978 Professional burnout: A personal survival kit. Human Service Association, Lexington, Mass.

Storlie F J 1979 Burnout: the elaboration of a concept. American Journal of Nursing, December: 2108–2111

Tierney M J G, Strom L M 1980 Stress: type A behaviour in the nurse. American Journal of Nursing, May: 915–917

Townsend I, Linsley W 1980 Creating a climate for carers. Nursing Times, July 3: 1188–1190

Walker D 1985 Writing and reflection. In: Bond D, Keogh R, Walker D (eds) Reflection: turning experience into learning. Kegan Page, London

10

Politics, power and psychiatric nursing*

G. E. Chapman

There is a paradox associated with politics and power about which writers in political science have commented (Dunsire 1984, Held & Leftwich 1984, Leftwich 1984). On the one hand individuals involved in political decision-making are accorded the formal symbols of social prestige, while on the other it is commonly believed, in everyday life, that politics is concerned with cynical manipulation, deceit and artful manoeuvring. Many nurses may view themselves as apolitical and share this common perception of political life, both admiring political activity and distrusting the politicians who engage in it. Dunsire (1984) states that two propositions which inform the paradox are true:

Politics is at once important and trivial, and . . . . politicians are both worthy of respect and contempt.

To resolve the paradox it is necessary to distinguish between the activity of politics and the practice of politicians, and to understand the structures in which particular political action occurs. Similarly, the processes through and around which political power is manifest need to be identified.

---

* The contents of this and Chapters 26 and 41 represent the views of the author alone and in no way commit the Department of Health. The chapters were written before the author joined the Department.

These issues as they relate to psychiatric nursing and the health services in which they work, will be the subject of this chapter. First, definitions of politics and power will be outlined. Second, British National Health Service (NHS) politics and policy decisions about mental health services will be explored as a means of identifying the political structures in which psychiatric nurses work. Third, inter-disciplinary politics and the impact of professional associations and trade unions will be discussed as they relate to the power and autonomy of psychiatric nurses. Finally, guidelines on interpersonal assertiveness and political skills will be provided.

POLITICS AND POWER

What is politics and how is political power gained and maintained? The traditional academic view (Moodie 1984) divides politics into two broad sections: first, theory related to classical works like Plato's *The Republic* (427–347 BC) and Hobbes' *Leviathan* (1588–1679) which reflected on the proper relations between rulers and ruled; and second, the study of institutions and empirical examination of organizations of central and local government. Later, definitions of politics expanded to include Marx's theory of class subordination and antagonism and the economic determinants of social action (Gilbert 1981). American studies of the behaviour of political leaders and the electorate followed (Dahl 1963).

Contemporary political analysts seem to adopt one of two main approaches which draw on those traditions. The first represents the view that politics is about government and the second that politics refers to all social activity. Moodie (1984) believes, for example, that politics is about governing: the process of making rules by which social, economic and cultural conduct can be regulated. The mechanisms through which governing occurs are rule-making and application, policy-making and implementation, and making use of legal and other sanctions to ensure rules and policies are observed.

Rule breaking and conflict usually occur around the production and distribution of valued, scarce economic and social resources, for example,

finance, housing, material goods, social prestige and health care. Nicholson (1984) appears generally to agree that politics is about government but stresses the role of power. He argues that what distinguishes the politics of government from political interactions between individuals and groups is that the government claims a 'monopoly of the legitimate use of force' (Gerth & Wright Mills 1970). Governments use force to ensure obedience when goodwill, persuasion and deceit fail. The miners' strike of 1984 and the print union dispute of 1985/86 provide an example of the resources of physical coercion available to government (in this case the police) when disputes are not resolved by negotiation.

Leftwich (1984), however, adopts a much broader definition of politics as being concerned with all collective social activity. In formal and informal settings, on private or public occasions, and within all human groups (the family, clubs, institutions such as hospitals, nations and states) politics arise. He argues that politics is fundamental to human activity and not the preserve of government:

Politics comprises all activities of cooperation and conflict, within and between societies, whereby the human species goes about organizing the use, production and distribution of human, natural and other resources in the course of the production and reproduction of its biological and social life.

This view of politics stresses the negotiations and interactions which occur at all levels of society around the control and use of resources: it acknowledges, and to some extent was influenced by, feminist politics. Feminism, after an analysis of the subordinate relationship between women and men, produced the phrase 'the personal is political' (Oakley 1981).

Writers in nursing politics also stress the impact of the division of labour by gender, and the subsequent doctor/nurse, male/female relationships on health service politics (Salvage 1985, Leeson & Gray 1978, Ehrenreich & English 1979).

A definition of politics which encompasses social activity makes it possible to understand power, not as a thing owned by some and not others (Lukes 1979, Johnson 1977), but as a process occurring in and between the relations between people

(Foucault 1982). As such it suggests that as politics is to be found everywhere, in small and large social groups, each individual has an opportunity to affect or be involved in political decisions. An example is easily provided from a scenario familiar to psychiatric nurses. Humans are a creative and productive species actively involved in organizing and communicating in a variety of productive social activities, the provision of consistent nursing care for the mentally ill not being the least of these activities. Cooperation is required if this care is to be continuous over a 24-hour period; disputes and political activity are likely to arise if one group or another is unhappy with the way, for example, decisions are made about the distribution of valued resources such as extra duty payments, overtime, weekends off and allocation of prime season annual leave. Negotiations and decisions relating to the sharing of resources amongst staff may not only occur at ward level, but also at hospital and national level with the involvement of government institutions and trade unions and professional associations.

Leftwich (1984) identifies four main elements in all such political activity:

1. The principles and processes which govern the ownership, control and use of major productive sources in any given culture (in health care — capital, revenue, knowledge, technology, manpower)
2. The structure of power and decision-making, that is the people/groups which regularly have more access to power and influence on decision-making. These groups may be linked by virtue of gender, class, wealth (in health care — occupational groups, hierarchies)
3. The social organization and patterns of relations between people and groups (in health care — the division of labour of nursing, medical, ancillary staff, paramedics and so on)
4. The network of ideas, values and sets of beliefs which govern action (in health care — that doctors are more skilled than nurses, males are better managers than females, staff know better than their clients).

These elements can be used to study the politics of any organization. It is a similar model to that which Klein (1983) used in his general analysis of politics in the British National Health Service.

THE BRITISH NATIONAL HEALTH SERVICE

For the purposes of this discussion it should be noted that while a small private sector exists in Britain, the state, through the Department of Health (DOH), provides the major proportion of health care. Decision-making about distribution of resources and policy occurs at three levels: regional health authorities (RHAs), district health authorities (DHAs) and hospital or service units.

Earlier it was stated that in order to understand the political processes and structures which impinge on psychiatric nurses, a knowledge of the politics of the organization in which they work is necessary. Most psychiatric nurses work within the National Health Service — 50 804 in 1982 (Gray 1986) — and all are effected by the policy-making and political structures which surround it. From wages policy to catering policy, bricks and mortar to therapeutic philosophy, nurses' personal and professional lives are affected by the decisions which are made at national level in the DOH and at local level by the RHAs and DHAs. Fuller understanding of how and why these bodies were set up in the way they were can only be gained via an historical analysis of the political decisions surrounding the setting up of the National Health Service. Klein (1983) charts the different socio-economic and political circumstances which have influenced its development. The creation of the NHS, he argues, grew out of all-party recognition in the 1930s that the hospital and general practitioner services were inadequate, patchy, inefficient and irrational in their management. Some 1000 hospitals were run by bodies as varied as local authorities and a mixture of charitable associations. The distribution of resources, then as now (DHSS 1976b), was unevenly distributed, favouring the richer well-populated south. Charitable incomes had decreased and municipal hospitals refused entry to patients outside their area. The Second World War pointed to the need for centrally-organized facilities. Both major political parties were committed to a nationally organized scheme, partly as a result of anxieties about the electorate's disaffection with government following years of recession and unemployment, and partly in recognition of years of suffering in the war (Forsythe 1975). The Beveridge Report of 1942 included an assumption that a social welfare programme should embrace a comprehensive national health service, and was generally popular. The medical profession, however, mostly opposed such schemes (Fraser 1978, Forsythe 1975, Klein 1983). Their resistance and campaign against the NHS was based on their wish to retain private practice, pay beds and independent status. The British Medical Association, largely representing general practitioners, was particularly vehement in its opposition. Bevan, Minister of Health in the Labour government which followed the war, negotiated a settlement with the medical profession which made it possible to inaugurate the NHS. Klein argues that Bevan first 'bought off' the hospital specialists by agreeing to retain pay beds and private practice, by introducing a system of merit awards, and by ensuring that doctors would have places on governing bodies. The general practitioners' continuing opposition was resolved by agreeing a payment per capitation fee, and the provision of local health centres and maintenance of independent status.

Klein states that the irony of the NHS is that these compromises set up a system in which the gatekeepers and spenders of NHS resources, the medical profession, were effectively outwith managerial and political control.

No other occupational group in health care was involved in the negotiations. While the NHS exploited its position as monopoly employer to hold down the income of doctors, at the same time the medical profession permeated the decision-making machinery of the NHS and obtained an effective right of veto over the policy agenda (Klein 1983). In 1948 medical membership of regional health boards averaged 32%, and in hospital management committees 20–27%. The institutionalized medical voice in the NHS, according to Klein, enabled

doctors to medicalize management. More importantly, once defined as a medical problem a subject became taboo for lay discussion.

The political implications of this for other occupations including nursing were profound. Initially the views and interests of nurses and others in the NHS were not considered and their voice has always been muted. By the late 1960s and 1970s, however, technological and managerial changes in health care as well as changes in social values saw the erosion of differentials and perceptions between and within health care occupations. Trade unions and professional associations became more militant and the NHS dispute-prone on issues concerning pay, conditions of service and the policy related to pay beds. A central political problem became how to restrain the demands of the consumers and producers of health care. Attempts at rational planning were introduced by the 1960s as it became clear that scarce resources required rationing. The managerial and administrative imperative associated with rational planning led to four reorganizations of the NHS, the first in 1974 (DHSS 1972), the second in 1982 (DHSS 1979), the third in 1984 (DHSS 1984) and finally, the NHS Review culminating in its White Paper, 'Working for Patients', in 1989 (DOH 1989a), which is being implemented at the time of going to press. In 1974 the administrative management structure echoed that of the 1969 Salmon reorganization of nursing management (Ministry of Health 1966). Nurses in the 1974 and 1982 restructuring were to be involved at all levels of decision-making: regional, area, and district health authorities and the Department of Health and Social Security. Some writers believe that nurse managers failed to grasp the opportunities 1974 and 1982 provided in terms of influencing decision-making. Dimmock (1986), for example, argues that a clash of values between the service orientation of nursing and self-interest elements of politics ensured that nurse managers failed to gain more power and control, because they lacked an instinct for machiavellian machinations. Unlike doctors in the NHS, 80% of whom are men, it is also possible that nurse managers failed to make an impact on the broader aspects of NHS politics (as opposed to nurse politics) on the basis of their gender and educational backgrounds. Approximately 90% of nurses are women and like many women may not have been encouraged to value their intellectual and academic achievements. The phenomenon of lack of female assertiveness together with a systematic discrimination and lack of opportunity for women in the larger political and educational arena has been well charted in the feminist literature (Oakley 1981).

In 1982 a fresh opportunity was provided with a reorganization which saw the end of area health authorities and introduced units co-managed by a unit administrator, director of nursing services and medical representative. The directors of nursing services became involved in unit budgetary control and policy-making and they have demonstrated their skills in this area. In 1983, the Griffiths' proposals introduced the concept of general management into the NHS, and a range of organizational arrangements were also introduced. Some nurse managers had general management function added to their job descriptions, or became general managers, while others retained a professional advisory role.

Views about the Griffiths' proposals were mixed during the period (Dunn 1986, Vousden 1986a, McIntegart 1986, Killen 1986, PNA 1986, Young 1986, Pownall 1986). However, a new set of opportunities yet to unfold face nurse managers in the 1990s as a result of the NHS Review White Paper 'Working for Patients', which reconsidered the nature of the relationship between health authorities as purchasers and providers of health care (DOH 1989a).

THE MENTAL HEALTH SERVICE

It is a truism to state that the psychiatric services within the British National Health Service are under-resourced. Historically, as a low status speciality in medicine and nursing this has always been so, and the experience in other countries is similar. Various government reports and commissions have made recommendations to redress the balance. Policy statements regarding the development of new patterns of service include

'Better Services for the Mentally Ill' (DHSS 1975), 'Priorities for Health and Social Services' DHSS 1976a), and 'Care in Action' (DHSS 1981). The Nodder Report (DHSS 1977) looked also at the organizational and management problems in mental hospitals. These and other policy statements are discussed in other chapters. Briefly, the main thrust of the DHSS guidelines were that:

1. Mental health and community health services should have a priority in the distribution of funds.
2. Patients should be able to receive treatment from the family doctor and outpatient departments at local district general hospitals.
3. Service initiatives in the community, including community psychiatric nurses, social workers and members of the primary health care team, should be developed to care for the long-term mentally ill.
4. Hospital-based care should no longer be based in large institutions miles away in the countryside.
5. These policies should result in closure of old large asylums in inaccessible parts of the country.

In 1989 the White Paper 'Caring for People' outlined a new approach to caring for the mentally ill in the community which will be implemented in the 1990s (DOH 1989a).

All these decisions affect psychiatric nurses. For some, the new initiatives have been welcomed and enabled expansion of the nurse's role in rehabilitation and community programmes (Dick 1986, Jenkins & Spencer 1986). The development of community psychiatric nursing services over the last decade provides an example of this. For other nurses, despite evidence of poor standards of care and neglect of patients in large mental hospitals (Martin 1984), the policies have been resisted.

This is not always a function of reactionary beliefs, but due to strongly-held views that the 'glamorous' areas of psychiatric nursing will draw away committed nurses from the 'bread and butter' areas of long-term care (Vousden 1986b). Similarly, there is the idea that skills learnt in the large mental hospitals, like containment of violence, might also be lost (Gostin 1985). Lack of agreement about such ideas and their implications for clinical practice is the material out of which political conflict grows. Salvage (1985) reports, for example, that trade unions have sometimes been placed in the awkward position of having to defend reactionary attitudes, because members feared their jobs were threatened and new jobs in the community would not materialize (Vousden 1986c, Gaze 1985). An irony of the debate is that by 1986 only one large mental illness hospital had been closed (Vousden 1986d).

Some attention will be paid to trade union politics in the next section; here it is noted that for psychiatric nurses to be politically credible in their policy initiatives related to matters of patient care, their arguments should be cogent, relevant and backed up by valid knowledge/evidence. The issue of psychiatric nurses' knowledge base is at the heart of their struggle for clinical and professional autonomy, and recognition in society at large and in relation to other occupations. It will be discussed more fully below.

PROFESSIONAL ORGANIZATIONS AND TRADE UNIONS

Much has been written in the sociological literature about the power of any given occupation to define its own area of work and achieve status and recognition in society as a whole. Power is said to be linked to the notion of professionalism. While there has been criticism of the approach (Friedson 1983), most sociologists agree that the core components of a profession are that:

1. It is based on a body of theoretical knowledge and research
2. Members command special skills and competence in the application of that knowledge
3. Professional conduct is guided by a code of ethics which focuses on the protection of the client (Toren 1969).

Occupations which lack one or more of these characteristics are usually defined as semi-professions, and nursing (which lacks (1)) is usually classified in this way (Etzioni, 1969). Semi-professions are usually well adapted to the organizations in which they are situated, have shorter training, and individual practioners have less independence and personal autonomy than their colleagues in the medical profession. As Klein's (1983) analysis of the NHS demonstrated, they have less power as a group as well. Similarly their work is more closely bounded by organizational procedures and regulations.

Occupations aspiring to full professional status, and the power and autonomy this brings, are said to engage in a range of professionalizing activities. The key activities, as far as psychiatric nurses are concerned, include:

- Boundary maintenance and disputes with other neighbouring occupations (e.g. social workers, occupational therapists, psychologists)
- Developing the power to define and control their own work and that of others
- Developing a body of research-based knowledge which they own and control
- Placing training in colleges of further education and universities.

All of these professionalizing activities are in effect political activities aimed at enhancing the interests of the occupation in relation to others. Claims that such activity improves the quality of care for patients (which it well may do) are also political claims which justify and legitimate the aspirations of the interested parties. However, the professionalizing route to political power is not the only one. Trade unions, who base their claims on the needs and aspirations of the collectivity of the members, offer a different route. Salvage (1985) argues that nursing (including psychiatric nursing) is divided in its approach to its own development between professionalists and unionists. First, professionalists are said to be drawn from the ranks of managers, teachers, trained staff and students aspiring to the status and rewards of professionalism noted above. The strategies taken, she argues, are elitist (they seek to control entry into the profession), and fail to recognize the needs and aspirations of untrained nurses and those not keen to take the educationally-based route to status and power. As such, the political strategy is said to be divisive and contains certain risks, not least of which is an active acceptance of the establishment's moral and behavioural codes, for example, that professionals should not strike. Professionalists, it is argued, seek to impose a uniform view of nurses and are largely represented by the Royal College of Nursing.

The second approach, that of trade unionists, is historically more prevalent in psychiatric nursing. Trade unions, traditionally linked to the working class socialist movements, tend to be concerned with the protection of members and the improvement of their well-being via better pay and conditions. They have not in the past been involved in debates about the nature of nursing or with 'professional' issues such as standards of care or education. Their concern has been directed towards labour relations and management/trade union negotiations. Furthermore they do not rule out the possibility of strike action in the battle for better pay and conditions. White (1985) provides a more rigorous analysis of the same phenomenon. She categorizes nurses as being either generalists, specialists or managers. Table 10.1 outlines the main characteristics of these groups. Articles in the psychiatric nursing press seem to reflect the tensions which exist between these groups about the proper identity of psychiatric nursing: that is,

whether they adopt a specialist approach, concerned with the acquisition of specific nursing skills, or a more common-sense pragmatic approach to care (Isles 1986, Fox 1986, Cormack 1986).

Of the four main health service unions (National Union of Public Employees, Confederation of Health Service Employees and National Association of Local Government Officers), COHSE has traditionally been strongest in psychiatric nursing. This can be explained in part by the fact that the Royal College of Nursing (RCN) initially only admitted female trained nurses. Male nurses and attendants in mental hospitals historically were drawn from working class backgrounds and had more sympathy with the ideals of socialist trade unions than professional associations (Carpenter 1980). The political conflict between trade unions has been expressed in their competition for members by offering better services. The RCN has become more militant (Nursing Standard 1986) and the unions have been increasingly concerned with professional issues (Howie 1986). In 1982 RCN membership stood at 250 000 and included students and trained staff. Of 230 000 COHSE members, half were nurses in 1986 (Vousden 1986e), and NUPE had 60 000 nurse members across all categories of nursing (Howie 1986). Conflict between the above organizations is understandable given that they tend to represent different constituencies, yet they have demonstrated a capacity to work together in the face of common threats. For example, the 1982 pay campaign was fought jointly (Vousden 1986e).

Each organization has its own particular difficulties. While the RCN seeks to retain the loyalty of students, the unions have to address the problem of lack of women representatives at senior level. Each must find the appropriate balance with respect to the conflicting needs of its members. The RCN, for example, was felt not to adequately reflect the interests of psychiatric nurses despite the creation of special interests groups. This led to the creation of the Psychiatric Nurses Association and the Community Psychiatric Nurses Association: neither of which are full professional organizations or trade unions but both of which focus on the professional interests of the nurses concerned.

Table 10.1 Interest groups in nursing. (The table is the author's but the concepts are drawn from White 1985)

	Generalists	Specialists	Managers
Type of work	Unskilled Semi-skilled Supervised	Skilled Personally accountable Unsupervised	Planner Policy maker Supervisor
Type of training	Minimum	Post- registration University	Management Budgetary systems
Primary interest	Material rewards	Professional status	Resources/ control
Attitude to skills	Practical Anti- academic	Conceptual Intellectual valued	Ambivalent
Politics	Hierarchical Activism	Personal autonomy Independence	Equality with peers
Promotion	Experience	Qualification	Lateral movement

LEVELS OF POLITICAL ACTION

So far, a broad picture of NHS politics and the politics of representation has been outlined. However, while this might describe the context in which nurses work, the issues may not be experienced as immediately relevant to the nurse working in direct patient care. More readily experienced by psychiatric nurses might be the day-to-day impact of political decisions on their patients' recovery; the possible threats to jobs caused by hospital and ward closures; and the day-to-day inter-professional politics of the multi-disciplinary team. Each will be discussed in turn.

Patients' lives

Recent research outlined in this volume and elsewhere (e.g. Brown & Harris 1978) has demonstrated that stressful life events are linked in complex ways to mental illness. Similarly, it has been argued that unemployment, poverty and social class are statistically associated with the prevalence of psychiatric disorder (see Chapter 16). At the same time lack of resources in the NHS makes funding of progressive care units like group homes, community care etc. problematic. The phenomenon of poverty and the distribution of wealth in society, together with the provisions made for mental health care, are a function of political and economic policies of governments. While, as a professional involved in a therapeutic programme with an individual patient, such knowledge may help provide insight into a patient's plight, direct political action is not appropriate at this level. Careful consideration of research evidence, and party political manifestos regarding the economy and health care provision, should rather inform nurses as voters in general elections. A *Nursing Times* poll in 1986 demonstrated that nurses were thinking politically about the NHS in Britain (Cole 1986). Furthermore, a psychiatric nurse may make a contribution to political debate about causes and provision for mental health care through informed interest in consumer groups like MIND, and contributions within representative bodies such as trade unions and professional associations. These pressure groups can have an impact. Certainly the RCN adopted a high profile in 1986 with its 'Manifesto for Nursing and Health' (RCN 1986) aimed at influencing political parties in the run up to a general election.

Policies about the provision of mental health services are made at national, regional and district level. If nurses as individuals or as a group do have an interest in influencing such decisions they should be aware of the consultation machinery available to them at these levels. First, they may have an opportunity to comment through their own line manager about local policy decisions concerning the organization of patient care in their speciality. Second, most districts have a professional advisory committee in which nurse representatives may put forward their view. Knowledge of how this works should be of concern to all psychiatric nurses. Third, most districts also have a joint staff committee in which representatives of trade unions and professional associations meet with management. This too, via the representatives, may prove a useful channel for directing comment. Fourth, most health authorities have a nurse advisor and it would be helpful to nurses to discover what means she has set up to take account of nurses' views. Fifth, some of the new unit general managers have set up a mechanism for consultation at unit level, and this should be used effectively.

Multi-disciplinary politics

Nurses have shown a mixed reaction to being assertive with respect to their ideas and plans as members of a clinical multi-disciplinary team. Some authors believe that social workers, occupational therapists and nurses are happy to leave decision-making and leadership to the medical profession (Goldie 1977). Many doctors argue that as they are ultimately responsible for the clinical decisions related to patient welfare they should retain their leadership role. They believe this because they are legally accountable for clinical decisions (Batchelor & Mcfarlane 1980).

It is possible that there is considerable misunderstanding about the legal aspects of accountability. In general terms doctors are legally accountable for medical decisions, but nurses remain legally accountable for provision of adequate standards of nursing care. For example, while doctors may be accountable for the pharmacological and physiological consequences of drugs they have prescribed for patients, nurses are accountable for the actual administration of the drugs. In order for the health authority to accept vicarious responsibility for the nurse's actions she should be able to demonstrate that she has followed its procedures and guidelines (Young 1981). Similarly, in cases where patients have been neglected or abused in mental hospitals by nurses it is the nurse, not the doctor, who has often been found negligent. The United Kingdom Central Council Code of Professional Conduct for the Nurse, Midwife and Health Visitor (UKCC 1984) explicitly recognizes that nurses are accountable for certain aspects of patient care. It is therefore pertinent to consider how effective nurses are in multi-disciplinary settings at presenting their ideas about appropriate delivery and organization of patient care. This is an empirical question as yet unanswered by research. It is certainly pertinent to consider the skills required to ensure that individual psychiatric nurses negotiate and present their arguments cogently, and it is this which will provide the focus of the last section.

POLITICAL SKILLS

Political skills amount to skills in interpersonal relationships, an area in which most psychiatric nurses have considerable experience. At a personal level a key area of skill, which nurses are not always encouraged to adopt, is that of assertiveness (Briggs 1986). At a professional level some understanding of negotiating skills between interest groups is of use. Each will be discussed in detail.

Assertiveness

Briggs (1986) notes that nurse training and clinical practice fosters a submissive attitude to authority figures and members of other professions (particularly doctors). In a training exercise with psychiatric nurses he identified eight personal rights which if internalized and upheld might result in nurses being professionally more effec-

tive. These are listed in Box 10.1. He acknowledges that for nurses the exercise of these rights is problematic, in that they may often be perceived as aggressive if they do. It is important therefore to distinguish between assertive behaviour guided by principles of human rights, and non-assertive behaviour characterized by aggressiveness, manipulation and submission. The main elements of the latter behaviour are listed in Table 10.2. A cautionary note should perhaps be made about the exercise of these rights in work settings. It is important to recognize that the parameters of the right to say 'no' or 'yes' with respect to certain tasks, to decide what to do with one's own time, and to do anything, are defined to some extent by the contract of work within a particular health authority. Work contracts, signed by all employees

---

Box 10.1 Identification of personal rights (adopted from Briggs 1986)

1. The right to opinions and to state them
2. The right to say yes or no without guilt
3. The right to decide what to do with one's time, body or property
4. The right to make mistakes and to be responsible for them
5. The right to ask for wants
6. The right to be treated with respect and dignity
7. The right to be listened to
8. The right to do anything which does not violate others' rights

---

Table 10.2 Characteristics of assertive and non-assertive behaviour (adapted from Briggs 1986)

Aggressive	Manipulative	Submissive	Assertive
Forcing	Conning	Self-denigration	Honesty
Attacking	Guilt inducing	Not expressing wants	Self-respect
Blaming	Undermining	Abrogating responsibility	Respecting others
Ordering	Insincerity		Praising others
Dominating		Violating own rights	Accepting criticism
Violating			Owning decisions

of the National Health Service, contain job descriptions which usually include an agreement to follow district procedures within the constraints of professional responsibility. It is therefore vital for nurses to be informed and understand, before signing a contract, the implications of these requirements, and to base their assertion of rights on a foundation of firm professional knowledge.

Dainow (1986) discusses the way assertiveness techniques can be used in work situations. She notes that 'assertion means sharing thoughts and feelings in such a way that the other person does not feel put down or discounted'. A formula she suggests using is characterized by the words report, relate, request and result. Reporting means describing what is happening, and being specific about the behaviour of the other person which is of concern. Relating means explaining the effect of the behaviour or its emotional impact. Requesting means asking for change in concrete terms. Result refers to the positive or negative consequences if the change is or is not made. An example of this formula is provided in Box 10.2. Dainow claims that it is important not to criticize people for what they are but for what they have done. In the example provided, a statement like 'You are thoughtless and don't care about other staff's training and development' would be less effective. Dainow further outlines the principles which should govern assertive negotiations. These are:

1. Identify and deal with problems separately.
2. Discover the interests of all involved and establish shared interests.
3. Identify and explore as many options to resolve conflicts as possible, and think through the consequences of each option. Further, be prepared to compromise by suggesting time-limited solutions, partial changes, pilot studies and so on.
4. Turn alternative options into firm proposals with a recommended option, requesting others' views and reasoning rather than adopting political positions.
5. Be prepared to fail if the opposition is all powerful or unprincipled.

An additional item might be to explore the possibilities informally before making formal

---

Box 10.2	An example of an assertive exchange
Report:	'I can see that you have changed my off-duty in my absence.'
Relate:	'I am unhappy about that because I have a long-term arrangement to go to a conference on that day.'
Request:	'I would like you to alter the off-duty back to the original.'
Result:	'This would mean that the conference fee is not forfeited and I would be available for duty at the weekend as previously agreed.'

proposals, which should usually be presented in written form.

The principles of assertiveness described above, interestingly, echo the ideas of political theorists outlined earlier. It is the political theorists who provide an account of political strategies described in the last section.

Political strategy

Dunsire's (1984) insight that political activity is paradoxically perceived as worthy of both contempt and esteem can be explained by acknowledging that politics is about principles and policies, and people and personalities. He cites March & Simons' (1958) analysis of what people actually do to support this. The political process seems to be as follows:

1. Problem solving

When all members of the negotiating group have the same objective, information is pooled about the subject of discussion and ingenuity is used to find a solution satisfactory to all.

> *Example*: Team meetings deciding a therapeutic programme for a schizophrenic patient.

2. Persuasion

If the above fails, persuasion is attempted. One member induces the view in others that if they relax their own goals it would be possible to achieve a shared objective.

> *Example*: A psychiatrist may relax his 'right' to admit patients to a therapeutic community without prior consultation with the nurses, in the interests of developing a therapeutic milieu.

3. Bargaining

If the objectives are not shared, neither problem-solving nor persuasion will work. In this situation a trade-off occurs where no one surrenders their goals unilaterally, and no one goes away empty handed.

> *Example*: The nursing service agrees to staff a weekly Modecate clinic which has a pharmacological research-based orientation, while the psychiatrist agrees to support and refer patients to a weekly relatives' support group run by nurses.

In situations of bargaining, interested parties should know and understand the principles and priorities upon which they are basing their arguments, and make clear which principles they are not prepared to relinquish.

4. Politics

In situations where the above activities fail, politics proper occurs. One of three things can happen.

First, the definition of the group is altered — either the people are changed or the decision is referred to a higher authority.

> *Example*: Psychiatric nurses may not be invited as members of key meetings, or if they are, the unit general manager arbitrates when professionals disagree.

Second, the definition of the problem may be altered and be related to wider issues.

> *Example*: Disputes about staffing ratios on a specific ward may be decided on the basis of national guidelines, thus changing the definition of the problem of staff shortage into the problem of meeting nationally agreed standards.

Third, the solution of the problem may be changed. In these circumstances it is accepted that the solution may not be satisfactory to all, but satisfactory to the majority (or more powerful) of interested parties. In the NHS, decisions of this kind usually flow in favour of medicine or general management.

> *Example*: Closure of a small, popular but under-utilized local clinic in favour of closure of acute admission beds when rationalizing services.

Decisions like this are rarely achieved in formal settings, but arise out of backroom coalition building and bargaining outside the formal arena. As such, majority decisions are rarely valued by those whose interests have been ignored. In this case the next political strategy may be adopted.

Resistance violence

While in British politics violence is only rarely resorted to (Northern Ireland and the inner city riots of the 1980s being the recent exceptions), strategies of resistance do occur. They may take the form of passive non-compliance, industrial disputes, work to rule or strike action. This form of resistance was used by psychiatric nurses in the pay and conditions disputes of the 1970s and 1980s.

CONCLUSION

It has been argued that nurses should understand the historical and contemporary political context of the health services in which they work if they are to be involved in policy decisions about mental health care, and if they are to understand their own experiences at work. The power of medicine in relation to nursing and other occupations has been traced in the historical developments associated with the inaugauration of the British National Health Service. The maintenance of the disparities of power between medicine and psychiatric nursing has been explored in terms of sociologists' accounts of the role of knowledge in enhancing professional status and prestige. Some conflicts within nursing and between professional associations and trade unions have been identified. While these conflicts may be difficult to resolve, it is suggested that debates about a strategy for psychiatric nursing should rest on an informed analysis of the political environment surrounding it. In keeping with this suggestion, political theory and techniques associated with personal assertiveness and political strategic skills have been outlined. The overall message is that none of us exists outside politics; we all, by virtue of our involvement in everyday social life, become involved in political processes. The challenge for psychiatric nurses is to develop the practical political skills, not only to advance the development of the profession, but also to improve the delivery of patient care.

REFERENCES

Batchelor I, McFarlane J 1980 Multidisciplinary clinical teams. Kings Fund Centre, London
Beveridge Report 1942 The report on social insurance and allied services (CMD. 6404). HMSO, London
Briggs K 1986 Speak your mind. Nursing Times June 25: 24–26
Brown G, Harris T 1978 The social origins of depression. Tavistock Publications, London
Carpenter M 1980 Asylum nursing before 1914: a chapter in the history of nursing. In: Davies C (ed) Rewriting nursing history. Croom Helm, London
Cole A 1986 Who will win your vote? Nursing Times Oct 8: 24–27
Cormack D 1986 Psychogeriatric nursing in 2005. Nursing Times Sept 10: 39–41
Dahl R A 1963 Modern political analysis. Prentice-Hall, Englewood Cliffs, New Jersey
Dainow S 1986 Believe in yourself. Nursing Times July 2: 49–51
Department of Health and Social Security 1972 NHS reorganization in England. HMSO, London
Department of Health and Social Security 1975 Better services for the mentally ill. HMSO, London
Department of Health and Social Security 1976a Priorities for health and personal social services. HMSO, London
Department of Health and Social Security 1976b Report for the resource allocation working party: sharing resources for health in England. HMSO, London
Department of Health and Social Security 1977 Organizational and management problems of mental illness hospitals (Nodder Report). HMSO, London
Department of Health and Social Security 1979 Patients first. HMSO, London
Department of Health and Social Security 1981 Care in action. HMSO, London
Department of Health and Social Security 1984 Circular DS (84)20. HMSO, London
Department of Health 1989a Working for patients. HMSO, London
Department of Health 1989b Caring for people. HMSO, London
Dick D 1986 Why change ? Mental Health Nursing: Nursing Times Jan 15: 55–56
Dimmock S 1986 Machiavellian machinations. Nursing Times April 9: 35–36
Dunn A 1986 Action stations. Lampada No 6 Winter 86. Royal College of Nursing, London
Dunsire A 1984 The levels of politics. In: Leftwich A (ed) What is politics? Blackwell, Oxford, p 85–106
Ehrenreich B, English D 1979 For her own good. Pluto Press, London
Etzioni E 1969 (ed) The semi-professions and their organization. Collier Macmillan Co, London
Foucault M 1982 The subject and power. Critical Enquiry 8, University of Chicago Press, pp 778–795
Forsythe G 1975 Doctors state medicine. Pitman Medical, London
Fox J C 1986 Participating in change. Nursing Times June 18: 33–34
Fraser D 1978 The evolution of the British Welfare State. Macmillan Press, London
Friedson E 1983 The theory of professions: state of the art. In: Dingwall R, Lewis P (eds) The sociology of the professions: lawyers, doctors and others. Macmillan Press, London
Gaze H 1985 When to blow the whistle. Nursing Times Dec 11: 18–19
Gerth H M, Wright Mills C (eds) 1970 From Max Weber essays in sociology. Routledge, London
Gilbert A 1981 Marx's politics. Oxford University Press, Oxford
Goldie N 1977 The division of labour amongst mental health professions. A negotiated or an imposed order? In: Stacey M (ed) Health and the division of labour. Croom Helm, London
Gostin L (ed) 1985 Secure provision: a review of special services for the mentally ill and mentally handicapped in England & Wales. Tavistock Publications, London
Gray A 1986 Anatomy of a profession. Nursing Times March 26: 24–26
Held D, Leftwich A 1984 A discipline of politics. In: Leftwich A (ed) What is politics? Blackwell, Oxford, pp 139–160
Howie C 1986 Running for cover. Nursing Times Dec 4: 18–19
Isles J 1986 An identity crisis perpetuated. Nursing Times

June 18: 28–30

Jenkins J, Spencer F 1986 Home benefits. Mental health nursing. Nursing Times Jan 15: 57

Johnson T 1977 Professions and power. Macmillan, London

Killen S 1986 Not waving but drowning. Nursing Times July 16: 56–57

Klein R 1983 The politics of the National Health Service. Longman, London

Leeson J, Gray J 1978 Women and medicine. Tavistock, London

Leftwich A 1984 Politics, people, resources & power. In: Leftwich A (ed) What is politics? The activity and its study. Blackwell, Oxford, pp 62–85

Lukes S 1979 Power: a radical view. Macmillan, London

March J G, Simon H A 1958 Organizations. Wiley, Chichester

Martin J P 1984 Hospitals in trouble. Basil Blackwell, Oxford

McIntegart J 1986 Turning a blind eye to Griffiths' Mental Health Nursing. Nursing Times July 16: 55–56

Ministry of Health 1966 Report on the committee on senior nursing staff structure. HMSO, London

Moodie G C 1984 Politics is about government. In: Leftwich A (ed) What is Politics? Blackwell, Oxford, pp 19–33

Nicholson P P 1984 Politics and force. In: Leftwich A (ed) What is Politics? Basil Blackwell, Oxford

Nursing Standard 1986 Spelling out the harsh realities of health care. Nursing Standard No 467 Oct 9: 1

Oakley A 1981 Subject women. Fontana, Glasgow

PNA Editorial 1986 On trial. Mental health nursing. Nursing Times Jan 15: 54

Pownall M 1986 No place to die. News focus. Nursing Times Sept 10: 16–17

Royal College of Nursing 1986 A manifesto for nursing and health. Royal College of Nursing, London

Salvage J 1985 The politics of nursing. Heinemann, London

Toren N 1969 Semi-professionals and social work: a theoretical perspective. In: Etzioni E (ed) The semi-professions and their organization. Collier Macmillan, London, pp 141–196

UKCC 1984 Code of professional conduct for the nurse, midwife and health visitor, 2nd ed. United Kingdom Central Council for Nursing Midwifery and Health Visiting, London

Vousden M 1986a Sheila's hat trick. Nursing Times July 16: 59

Vousden M 1986b Agents of change or caregivers? Nursing Times June 25: 51–52

Vousden M 1986c Trouble at Tooting. Nursing Times July 30: 18–19

Vousden M 1986d Closing time. Nursing Times March 19: 16–17

Vousden M 1986e The voice of pragmatism. Nursing Times June 18: 20–21

White R 1985 Political regulation in British nursing. In: White R (ed) Political issues in Nursing, vol 1. Wiley, Chichester

Young A P 1981 Legal problems in nursing practice. Harper and Row, London

Young D 1986 Is there life after Griffiths? Nursing Times Feb 12: 33–35

Klein R 1983 The politics of the National Health Service. Longman, London

Leftwich A (ed) 1984 What is politics? The activity and its study. Basil Blackwell, Oxford

White R (ed) 1985 Political issues in nursing, vol 1. Wiley, Chichester

White R (ed) 1986 Political issues in nursing, vol 2. Wiley, London

Salvage J 1985 The politics of nursing. Heinemann, London

Part 2

The knowledge base: an introduction to relevant disciplines

11

Mental health legislation

S. A. H. Ritter

This chapter is intended to provide an overview of the development of contemporary mental health legislation. For detailed explication of the Mental Health Act 1983 itself there are several excellent expositions of what are called 'mental health services', and readers are referred to these (Hoggett 1984, Jones 1985, Gostin 1986a).

SUMMARY

The complicated history of modern mental health legislation in the UK begins toward the end of the eighteenth century. The large number of Acts of Parliament concerning lunacy and idiocy reflects the initially piecemeal and subsequently consolidated legislation which was eventually to constitute a state approach to poverty, disease and crime, beginning in the Regency and continuing through the reign of Queen Victoria, as social problems which had reasonably been seen as the concern of individuals and families before the mid-eighteenth century gradually became the concern of communities and the organizations which were responsible for their government (Midwinter 1968).

The legislature was for a long time only concerned with the land and other estates of well-off lunatics and idiots, while the judiciary was engaged in the practical matters of determining whether individuals were insane or idiots. Once the legislature became interested in vagrants and beggars, the role of the judiciary included determining the disposal of the whole spectrum of poor, unemployed and homeless lunatics and idiots as well as of landed lunatics and idiots.

The shift from a feudal economy which characterized the Tudor period meant that fluctuations in trade superimposed upon a different pattern of land ownership and management and of fluctuating harvests caused, for the first time, an unemployed and sometimes unemployable population without material support. The attempts since Tudor times to control the social effects of poverty form the background to modern mental health legislation. Plague, oscillations in trade, crop and harvest failure led to poverty and unemployment, which in their turn led to vagrancy and crime. Vagabonds and criminals were identified in Tudor legislation, which attempted more or less savagely to restrict vagrancy.

In the sixteenth century, for the first time there appeared organized attempts to provide for the poor, however their poverty was caused. The dissolution of the monasteries during the reign of Henry VIII meant that the sick became the responsibility of secular organizations. The Tudor poor laws, combined with the common law, provided a framework within which local justices of the peace could order detention of lunatics in the workhouse or house of correction, and could order the allocation of parish funds towards the support of a lunatic. A series of acts starting with The Beggars Act 1531 attempted to deal with the unemployed who wandered the countryside and towns, begging and committing crimes.

From the sixteenth century, idle unemployed people began to threaten social order, because if they were able to make a living without working there was not much point in labouring for a living. If there was no labour, wealth would collapse. The system of poor relief was used to keep wages low, ensuring the profitability of manufacturing (Hill 1969). The mentally disordered could not be exempted from this system, otherwise it would be to the advantage of the poor to pretend to be mad (Scull 1989).

'The interplay of lunacy and poor laws' (Mellet 1981 p. 246) which characterized nineteenth century developments in psychiatry progressed inevitably from earlier concerns about the ability of the insane to support themselves. Porter (1987) suggests that the netting of lunatics in the poor law provisions affected the development of psychiatry as a respectable branch of medicine. The fate of pauper lunatics was closely linked with the development of the large public asylums in the nineteenth century. One effect of the legislation of the twentieth century, which finally brought together the mentally impaired with the mentally ill and which created a health service that no longer discriminated between those who could or could not pay, was to draw into psychiatry's net the necessary social range of clients for ensuring pressure to effect and validate beneficial results. Mental health and poor relief legislation always ran ahead of medical involvement and of doctors' capacities to intervene productively in mental disorder. Custodial provision as it developed from 1808 provided the setting in which psychiatry developed and established itself as a branch of clinical science (Mellet 1981).

Hard evidence, such as from examination of parish records for accounts of the disposal of lunatics under the poor laws, is still not available in large enough quantities to draw conclusive inferences about mental disorder and its management before the mid-eighteenth century. Partly because of the lack of evidence for earlier times, historians of mental disorder and its management have concentrated on the eighteenth and nineteenth centuries. Allderidge (1978) emphasizes that limited conclusions must be drawn from limited evidence. Parry-Jones, in his authoritative history of the 'trade in lunacy', could not find 'officially documented information' dating from before 1774, the year of the Act for Regulating Madhouses, although 'houses for lunatics' can be traced from the early seventeenth century (Parry-Jones 1972).

DEFINITIONS

Coke's (1626) definitions of idiot and lunatic are quoted by Ray (1838).

Lord Coke says there are four kinds of men who may be said to be *non compos mentis*: 1. An idiot, who from his nativity is *non compos*; 2. He that by sickness, grief, or other accident, wholly loses his memory and understanding; 3. A lunatic that hath sometimes his understanding, and sometimes not, *aliquando gaudet lucidis intervallis*; and therefore he is called *non compos mentis*, so long as he hath not understanding; 4. He that by his own vicious act for a time deprivith himself of his memory and understanding, as he that is drunken (Coke 1626 in Ray 1838 p. 14).

Pitt-Lewis et al (1895) points out that the legal term was lunacy and the medical term insanity; idiocy was the legal term, amentia the medical one. He clarified the issues for the mentally disordered person and the law as follows: treatment; civil rights; criminal liability; capacity to be a witness or to make or revoke a will (p. 136). The importance of legal definitions of idiocy and lunacy lay in the need to determine rights over the property of the idiot or lunatic, and to determine responsibility for their financial support. It is these aspects of property and land which, according to some historians, took control of the disposal of idiots and lunatics along with other classes of the poor and dispossessed who were seen as a threat to social stability and prosperity.

LEGAL PROVISIONS IN PRE-MEDIEVAL IRELAND, WALES, ENGLAND AND SCOTLAND

Ireland

Early Irish law codes contain accounts of medical psychology which are related to contemporary religious beliefs and practices. There are certain provisions for maintaining mad women who had no landed estate, and for regulating the marriage and divorce of 'insane persons'. Clarke (1975) cites two Irish legal documents dating from the eighth century which refer to 'fools', 'half-wits', 'idiots' and 'lunatics', although the exact nature of society's responsibility is not clear, nor is the question of whether any sort of nosology is implied by the terms. However, what is clear is that in

Ireland, 'normally the deranged and the defective were wholly in the custodial care of relatives' (p. 32).

Wales

The earliest readily available Welsh legal codes date from the tenth century and contain little reference to insanity. Where it is mentioned it is not related to medical practice. One reference is to the qualifications required to become a judge. A second is to 'persons, of whom no one is to stand in judgement: one of them is, a person deranged by insanity, and who is required to be bound or watched at times. . .' (Record Commission 1841).

England

A number of different Anglo-Saxon legal codes developed in pre-Norman times, in which mental disorder as a concept does not appear except in relation to liability for crimes, and then in a variety of terms whose distinctions are now difficult to disentangle. Relatives were liable for compensating damage by mentally disturbed people. After the Conquest, a practice gradually developed of referring to the Crown judgements of serious crimes by the mentally disturbed. Medical practice was not a feature of assessing or managing the mentally disturbed (Clarke 1975).

Scotland

References to lunacy in Scottish legal documents, written in Latin, are of uncertain dates. The problems of lunacy appear to be seen in terms of management of property. By the sixteenth century the concept of *curator bonis* had appeared (Regiam Maiestam Lib IV 1585c 15 III 396).

MEDIEVAL LEGAL PROVISIONS IN ENGLAND

Apart from being able to assert that in the Middle Ages families took responsibility for mentally disturbed members, it is not possible to say confidently what the categories and supposed aetiology of such disturbance were. Except in relation to property and to criminal offences the law was not used to regulate social provision for the mentally disordered. Up to the seventeenth century, where the judiciary did become involved, there appears to have been a 'relative consistency of assessment' despite the heterogeneous explanations of causality and the varieties of disorder, perhaps because of the relatively small number of cases involved (Clarke 1975).

Two statutes from the reign of Edward II make it clear that, probably for mixed economic and political reasons, the Crown assumed custody of the land belonging to the mentally disordered. In 1810 these statutes, 'Prerogativa Regis', were termed 'The Custody of Lands of Idiots', 'idiot' being a gloss from the literal translation from the Latin, 'natural fools', and 'Of Lands of Lunaticks', 'lunatick being a gloss of the Latin 'non . . . compos mentis' (Statutes of the Realm 1810 p. 226).

Allderidge (1978) notes scattered references in medieval year books to common law restraint and confinement of madmen, including a fifteenth century case which provided a precedent for legally imprisoning a potentially dangerous lunatic. To be a furious lunatic — *demens and furiosus non per feloniam* — was not necessarily a defence against conviction for criminal actions, and there is evidence from the medieval period that lunatics who committed serious crimes were imprisoned in places such as castles or bishop's palaces (Hibbert 1963, Clarke 1975). Another fourteenth century case indicated that it was lawful to beat a mad person with rods, as long as he or she was a relative of the flogger (Allderidge 1978). Clarke (1975) cites evidence that beggars in the sixteenth century traded on the popular image of ex-inmates of Bedlam (Tom O'Bedlam or the Abram-man) by displaying bruises as from floggings and by threats of violence. Later, whipping was specifically prohibited at Bethlem and in private madhouses (Porter 1987 p. 285).

DEVELOPMENTS IN TUDOR AND STUART LEGISLATION

It was not until the reign of Henry VIII that the second and third strands appeared of the four which were to dominate later mental health legislation. The first had concerned the management of the affairs of idiots and lunatics. The second concerned the question of how lunacy affected the trial and conviction of people accused of crimes. The third was the question of how to deal with the unemployed and unemployable, and by extension the unemployed mentally disturbed.

Before this period, Clarke (1975) argues, 'There was no great social pressure to go much further than [a very limited provision for broad classes of mental disability] while custody was a family matter and only a community matter when family provision was unavailable or broke down' (p. 56). Additionally, the state of medical knowledge and the variety of classifications of not necessarily accurately observed and described phenomena meant that the influence of doctors on family management of disturbed members was completely peripheral. Beliefs which arose from the prevailing culture, such as anti-Semitism or demonology, witchcraft or heresy, were more likely to influence treatment of the mentally disturbed.

Management of the affairs of the mentally disturbed

Court of Wards and Liveries

In 1540 the question of the management of the affairs of 'Ideottes and fooles naturall' was again addressed by a statute which gave the Crown authority over their estates, administered by the Court of the King's Wards. Further legislation concerning the Court of Wards and Liveries was enacted in 1618, and referred to lunatics as well as idiots (Hunter & MacAlpine 1963). The Court's functions did not survive the Civil War, and during the Protectorate legislation was passed to recompense those who had suffered as a result (Firth & Rait 1911).

Lunacy and trial of criminals

In 1541 a statute of Henry VIII dealt with the 'Real or pretended Lunacy of Persons having committed Treason, while sane. . .' Once convicted, such people were to be executed even if they became mad subsequently. If they committed treason while sane and became mad before trial, they were to be tried and convicted as necessary whether they were present in court and did or did not plead.

For the same period Hunter & MacAlpine (1963) reprint a late sixteenth century account of different 'degrees' of 'wants of understanding and reason'. In a discussion of whether three defendants on trial for treason were mad or not, Richard Cosin, Master in Chancery, offered a sevenfold categorization: *'Furor sive Rabies: Dementia sive Amentia: Insania sive Phrenesis: Fatuitas, Stultitia, Lethargia, & Delirium'*, and considered whether any of the three accused men fitted the classification. Since he based his judgement as much on their utterances as on their behaviour, and they had been tortured as part of the investigation, it is difficult to evaluate what meaning these categories had for Elizabethans (Hunter & MacAlpine 1963 p. 43).

Poverty, vagrancy and unemployment

From 1547–52 at least four Acts attempted during the reign of Edward VI to deal with the wandering unemployed. Penalties at one stage included slavery, branding, flogging and chaining. Gradually, certain provisions emerged which were to remain stable until the nineteenth century: raising money from parishes for poor relief, and removal of sick and aged poor to their own parishes. The reign of Philip and Mary continued the attempts to tackle poor relief, but it was Elizabethan legislation which remained the basis for subsequent poor laws.

From 1562, under 'An Act for the Releife of the Poore', a bureaucracy developed which was designed to raise and distribute relief. In 1576 an 'Acte for the setting of the Poore on Worke, and for the avoyding of Ydleness' provided for houses of correction on the model of Bridewell in each county for 'punishing and employing Rogues and unsettled Poor'; with further provision for whipping. Nineteen years later an 'Acte for the Releife of the Poore' consolidated all previous Tudor legislation for the poor, providing for collection of

rates, penalties for non-payment and declaring all Beggars to be Rogues. Although JPs were responsible for erecting and maintaining houses of correction in which vagabonds could be confined and whipped, the legislation was not effective, and in that year, another 'Acte for erecting of Hospitalls or abiding and working Howses for the Poore' designed for 'pore needy maymed or ympotent people' was passed.

Finally, in 1601 an 'Acte for the Releife of the Poore' re-enacted previous legislation, providing for taxation of parish inhabitants to provide materials for setting the poor to work, and for removal to the house of correction or to gaol for paupers who refused to work. This statute remained in force until the mid-nineteenth century (Pound 1986). James I added legislation to punish rogues, vagabonds and sturdy beggars with branding, and for confining violent patients in a house of correction (Statutes of the Realm 1810).

1601–1714

Political upheaval was to characterize the rest of the seventeenth century. By 1714, the substratum of the unemployed, the poor, those without property or land and thus without rights which had emerged during the reign of Henry VIII was beginning to be identified with urbanization. Parry-Jones (1972) notes that provisions for parishes to raise money to be used for the support of paupers led to the practice of 'boarding-out' of pauper lunatics who would be placed, at the expense of the parish, in houses belonging to individuals prepared to offer a degree of supervision. Better-off lunatics from respectable families were boarded with doctors and clergymen. Hunter & MacAlpine (1972) tell the story of the Reverend John Ashbourne who was murdered by a patient in about 1661.

The Restoration in 1660 restored the Anglican Church as well as the monarchy. The transition from Restoration culture to the neo-classical Age of Reason was accompanied by a rejection of the religious turmoil which had characterized the Civil War. Secularization of the ruling culture ensured that religious enthusiasm became identified with unreason and, by a short further step, with insanity (MacDonald 1981). Medicine was still irrelevant to the management of insanity. The reality for lunatics was confinement in a madhouse if they had means, and poor relief in one form or other if they had not (Hunter & MacAlpine 1963).

Developments in scientific methods gradually drew medicine away from its arts-based background towards reasoned observation and speculation about causes and classifications. Clarke (1975) suggests that the development of printing had been responsible for disseminating many ideas such as humoral explanations which hindered development of medical science. In the seventeenth century distinctions between psychological and physiological phenomena began to be more sharply defined and used as the basis for nosologies, theories of aetiology and for rationales of treatment. Eighteenth century developments in medicine meant that diverse descriptions of mental disorder began to lead towards classifications of mental illness which are recognizable today (Leigh 1961). Along with such developments came restrictions on the activities of lay therapists of physical and mental disorder (Allderidge 1978). However, Scull (1989) quotes from a 1684 textbook of medicine which provides a summary conveniently close to the end of the seventeenth century of one view of madness: 'Furious Madmen are sooner or more certainly cured by punishment and hard usage in a strait room, than by *Physick* or medicines' (p. 62).

1714–74

In 1714 lunatics were specifically mentioned for the first time in legislation designed to control vagrancy, begging and poverty: this was an 'Act for reducing the laws relating to Rogues Vagabonds Sturdy Beggars & Vagrants into one Act of Parliament & for the more effectual punishing of such Rogues Vagabonds Sturdy Beggars and Vagrants & sending them whither they ought to be sent.' The Act applied to 'Persons of little or no Estates, who, by Lunacy, or otherwise, are furiously Mad, and dangerous to be permitted to go Abroad'; and provided that 'two Justices may make order for apprehending and securing pauper lunatics, and sending them to their Place of Settlement' (Statutes of the Realm 1810 vol. 29 p. 981, Hunter & MacAlpine 1963 p. 299).

The Justices Commitment Act 1744, also known as the Vagrant Act, reinforced the powers of justices to authorize the capture of dangerous lunatics, to send them to their parish of settlement, and if they were paupers, to be supported there (Greig & Gattie 1915).

This period was marked by urbanization, further dislocation of the poor and landless, emigration, colonization, transportation, and a particular savagery of the criminal law as well as restrictiveness of the poor law. It culminated in the long drawn out mental illness of George III which began in 1765 and ended in 1820 (Jones 1955, Leigh 1979). The repeated public examination of the King's physicians, and the political problems of establishing a regency during his illnesses ensured that madness as a phenomenon became a question of social policy. The three broad headings which emerged during the sixteenth century now become four: management of the affairs of lunatics and idiots; criminal lunacy; the Poor Law and other social and welfare provisions; and custody of lunatics. It is possible to trace the progress of each issue through to contemporary legislation. Towards the end of the nineteenth century idiocy was distinguished from lunacy in separate legislation, the Idiots Act 1886 and subsequently the Mental Deficiency Act 1913. Eventually, in the Mental Health Act 1959 the term 'mental disorder' was adopted in order to integrate provisions for care, treatment and management of patients irrespective of the supposed aetiology of their mental disturbance.

Management of the affairs of lunatics

As described in relation to the Court of Wards and Liveries, legislation concerning lunacy originally centred round the management of estates and other property. After the abolition of the Court of Wards and Liveries in the mid-seventeenth century, the Lord Chancellor's office was responsible for issuing writs '*de idiota*' or '*de lunatico inquirendo*' in order that the mental state of people thought to be lunatics or idiots could be tried by jury. The aim was to prevent the dissipation of estates and income and to protect the interests of relatives of lunatics and idiots. If the person in question was found by the jury to be '*non compos mentis*' the Masters in Chancery became responsible for supervision of his estates. Such persons were known as Chancery lunatics. Subsequently, the Lord Chancellor appointed three commissioners who would issue the writs (Tuke 1882).

In 1833, legislation was passed to appoint three Chancery Visitors who provided reports annually on Chancery lunatics (Jones 1955). In 1842 a new Act enabled the Lord Chancellor to appoint two 'Commissioners in Lunacy' to deal with the writs of '*de lunatico inquirendo*' (Tuke 1882). In 1845 the term 'Masters in Lunacy' replaced that of Commissioners, and the responsibility of the Masters in Chancery for supervising the estates of idiots and lunatics was passed to the Masters in Lunacy. The Masters in Lunacy were thus part of the Chancery Division of the High Court (Tuke 1882, Mellet 1981). Tuke (1882) recorded that in 1881 in England and Wales there were 992 Chancery lunatics.

The process of *de lunatico inquirendo* continued through nineteenth and twentieth century changes in procedures for administering the property of idiots and lunatics. The Percy Commission (Report 1957) recommended that what had become known as the Court of Protection (the Judge and Master in Lunacy) within the Chancery Division of the High Court should restrict its activities to the 'protection and control of patients' property' (p. 267), abolishing the procedure of inquisition. The Mental Health Act 1959 established the procedure whereby the Court of Protection acted after receiving appropriate medical evidence about a person's capacity to manage his affairs. Under the Mental Health Act 1983 the nearest relative or any interested person can apply on behalf of a person to the Court of Protection (Gostin 1983, Carson 1987).

A Commission in Lunacy originally meant an enquiry into the circumstances of a lunatic or idiot in order to ascertain the rights of interested parties in the estate of the lunatic or idiot, a process described in detail by Tuke (1882) (Pitt-Lewis et al 1895). The term Commission was also used from 1774 in quite another sense, and confusingly referred to the process of supervising custodial provisions for lunatics.

During the nineteenth century, the development of state intervention through parliamentary legislation was accompanied by the growth of central control through the statutory bodies set up to implement the provisions of the various reforming Acts. Such bodies included the Poor Law Commission, afterwards the Poor Law Board and the Local Government Board (Midwinter 1968). The 1774 Act for Regulating Madhouses appointed five commissioners who were Fellows of the Royal College of Physicians, to be responsible for inspecting madhouses in London, but their responsibilities existed only on paper. The Madhouse Act 1828 appointed 15 Metropolitan Commissioners, including five physicians and five magistrates, who were to be responsible for inspecting madhouses. Their reports managed to be both cursory and verbose, deliberately avoiding detailed examination of issues (Mellet 1981).

Nevertheless, under the Lunatic Asylums Act 1843 the Metropolitan Commissioners were empowered to visit all metropolitan and provincial public and private asylums in England and Wales, expect Bethlem. The Metropolitan Commissioners included the reformers Somerset and Ashley (Lord Shaftesbury), and in 1844 they published their survey of all provision for lunatics in England and Wales, which became the basis of legislation in the following year. In 1845 the Metropolitan Commissioners were replaced by the Board of Commissioners in Lunacy, which consisted of up to 11 members and which later became known as the Board of Control. They were responsible for all lunatics except Chancery lunatics. That is, the Board existed to protect the civil liberties of people confined under various types of legislation, and to regulate institutional provision under the same legislation (Mellet 1981). Six were salaried professional commissioners, three of whom had to be physicians, three lawyers. Up to five were honorary commissioners. The Board employed a number of secretarial and clerical staff (Parry-Jones 1972, Mellet 1981).

In 1890 the Commissioners' role incorporated that of the Masters in Lunacy and of the Chancery Visitors. The 1911 Act increased the number of Lunacy Commissioners to 13. The Mental Deficiency Act 1913 increased the number to 15, four of whom were medical practitioners, four lawyers and two women; 12 of them were paid. The chairman of the Board of Control was appointed by the Secretary of State. They produced annual reports (Greig & Gattie 1915).

The Commissioners in Lunacy were responsible for ensuring that the Lunacy Acts were properly complied with, and were in fact inspectors as well as administrators. They were part of a general Victorian trend of establishing inspectorates to invigilate the implementation of reforming legislation, much as the factory inspectors did with the Factory Act 1833. As a major reform of the 1845 Lunacy Act, along with other inspectors, 'They eventually taught their countrymen to accept the value of itinerant overlookers in all aspects of social administration' (Midwinter 1968 p. 65).

The 1926 Royal Commission found that the powers of the Board of Control were in fact inadequate to carry out effectively its duties. Its visiting staff was too small, while the Board itself was unwieldy in size. The Commission recommended that the Board should consist of up to six members, with a visiting staff of at least 15 assistant commissioners, and that the administrative staff should be increased (Report 1926). The Mental Treatment Act 1930 implemented these recommendations. The Board of Control consisted of five senior commissioners, of whom one was a lawyer, two were medical practitioners and one a woman. The Minister of Health provided at his discretion a number of paid commissioners responsible for visiting and inspecting institutions under the Lunacy and Mental Deficiency Acts. The Board of Control was empowered to make rules approved by Parliament for the conduct of mental health services.

The National Health Service Act 1946 removed from the Board of Control its administrative functions of generally supervising and approving the provision of mental health services: approving medical practitioners, managing state institutions such as Rampton and Moss Side, supervising standards of and licensing accommodation for the mentally disordered, and supervising local authorities. The Board of Control retained its quasi-judicial responsibilities for supervising patients' civil liberties, visiting and inspecting institutions, and visiting voluntary as well as detained patients in all kinds of institutions. The provision of administrative staff to the Board of Control became the responsibility of the Minister of Health (Ministry of Health 1948).

The Percy Commission recommended the abolition of the Board of Control, believing that its other recommendations would make the Board's functions superfluous, by ensuring the availability of treatment without compulsion, by centralizing administrative responsibilities in the Ministry of Health, and by creating Mental Health Review Tribunals (Report 1957). Accordingly, the Mental Health Act 1959 dissolved the Board of Control, constituted Mental Health Review Tribunals in each regional hospital board, and, as described, laid down the functions and powers of the judiciary in relation to the Court of Protection.

However, under the Mental Health (Amendment) Act 1982 a new Mental Health Act Commission was established. According to Gostin (1986) the main reason for the reappearance of a commission resulted from the 'intractable problems concerning consent to treatment (p. 22). It is a special health authority established under the National Health Service Reorganization Act 1977. Under the Mental Health Act 1933 the Secretary of State was empowered to delegate to the Mental Health Act Commission responsibility for preparing a code of practice, monitoring procedures for obtaining consent to treatment from detained patients, visiting and inspecting hospitals, and preparing biannual reports.

THE MENTAL WELFARE COMMISSION

Under part II of the Mental Health (Scotland) Act 1984 a body of at least 10 commissioners is responsible for exercising 'protective functions in respect of persons who may, by reason of mental disorder, be incapable of adequately protecting their persons or their interests'. The Commission publishes a yearly report, and provides a small information booklet for 'all patients detained in a psychiatric ward under the Mental Health Act'. However, its responsibilities include all patients, 'whether they are in hospital or not, and whether they are informal or detained patients' (Mental Welfare Commission 1986 p. 11). Patients who are detained under the Act can appeal against their detention to a sheriff or to the Mental Welfare Commission. Another person can appeal on the patient's behalf. The Mental Welfare Commission will also investigate and report on complaints by patients.

CRIMINAL LUNACY

Criminal Lunatics Act 1800

The first modern legislation to deal with mentally disordered people who committed crimes was rushed through in 1800 after James Hadfield shot at George III at the Theatre Royal, Drury Lane. Under existing legislation there had been no provision for someone like Hadfield who was found at trial to be insane, and subsequently not guilty of the offence of high treason. Because he was thought to be still in need of safe custody, the common law was used to detain him in hospital. He was kept at the Bethlem Hospital where his reputation ensured his notoriety until, it was said, he was displaced by Jonathan Martin who was admitted a few years later after nearly succeeding in razing York Minster by arson.

The 1800 Act provided that any offender who was guilty of an offence but insane should be kept in custody during His Majesty's Pleasure: in effect, indefinitely. The courts were empowered to empanel a jury to 'try the sanity' of accused persons who, if they were found to be insane, could also be kept during His Majesty's Pleasure (Lushington 1895).

Further evidence that the Act was a response to the attack on George III was in Section 4 which provided for the detention of apparently insane persons who attempted to intrude upon the King.

The 1800 Act only applied to accused persons who were found guilty but insane. It did not apply to prisoners who became insane subsequent to their conviction.

Criminal Lunatics Acts 1838–84

The 1838 Act repealed parts of the 1800 Act and extended the powers over apparently insane and dangerous people who could now be detained in an institution if they appeared to be intent on committing an indictable offence. Discharge depended on cure or the agreement of two Justices of the Peace.

The 1884 Act was designed to 'consolidate and amend the law relating to Criminal Lunatics' (Greig & Gattie 1915 p. 720). It repealed the 1864, 1867 and 1869 Acts which had amended the provisions for confining and maintaining mentally disordered prisoners. In 1843 the trial of Daniel McNaughton for the attempted murder of the secretary of Sir Robert Peel had resulted in the formulation of the McNaughton Rules. These rules had the effect of establishing that 'every man is to be presumed sane until the contrary is proved' (Hibbert 1963). They can be summarized as the 'right and wrong' principle, which has ever since been extensively criticized in legal practice in the UK and USA. This principle involves a jury's deciding whether an accused person knew at the time of the offence that 'he was acting contrary to law', and if they decide that this is so, finding the person guilty. The rules themselves can be found in Hunter & MacAlpine (1963 pp. 919–922).

The 1884 Act defined a criminal lunatic as: (a) 'Any person for whose safe custody during Her Majesty's Pleasure Her Majesty or the Admiralty is pleased to give order; and (b) 'Any prisoner whom a Secretary of State or the Admiralty has in pursuance of any Act of Parliament directed to be removed to an asylum or other place for the reception of insane persons' (Greig & Gattie 1915 p. 733). Included in the general notion of criminal lunatic were people who had committed no offence but who were thought to be in danger of doing so. A criminal lunatic could be directed by the Secretary of State to be removed to and detained in a named asylum 'until he ceases to be a criminal lunatic' (Greig & Gattie 1915 p. 720).

Certification as a criminal lunatic was initiated by two medical practitioners. If the prisoner was under sentence of death two or more registered medical practitioners were appointed to assess him. Once detained, the criminal lunatic was subject to yearly reports to the Secretary of State who, once every three years, had to consider continued detention or discharge. The criminal lunatic could be absolutely or conditionally discharged by the Secretary of State or became classified as a lunatic or pauper lunatic on the expiry of the prison sentence to which he was subject. He could be further detained by a justice of the peace in a named asylum and supported by the union or parish in which he resided at the time of the offence.

A number of conditions were imposed on the transfer of patients from criminal lunatic asylums to ordinary asylums, including certification by a registered medical practitioner and agreement by the receiving asylum.

The 1884 Act effectively brought idiots for the first time into the scope of criminal lunatic legislation (Greig & Gattie 1915). This was despite attempts in the Criminal Lunatic Asylums Act 1860 and the Criminal Lunatics Act 1867 to deal with idiots or imbeciles who also appeared to be lunatics. The 1884 Act repealed the 1867 Act and the section of the 1860 Act dealing with imbeciles.

The costs of continued detention of the criminal lunatic who recovered before the expiry of his prison sentence were supported, if necessary, by the Treasury. Meanwhile the affairs and property of a criminal lunatic could be taken over and managed by the authority of the Lord Chancellor.

Assisting the escape of a criminal lunatic was punishable by penal servitude or imprisonment with or without hard labour. Carelessly allowing a criminal lunatic to escape was punishable by a fine (Greig & Gattie 1915).

The term 'lunatic' persisted in the legislation for criminal lunatics. The Criminal Lunatics Act 1884 ran alongside the Lunacy and Mental Treatment Acts 1890–1930. It was amended under the National Health Service Act 1946 when the term 'Broadmoor patients' was introduced, but substantial changes did not occur until the Mental Health Act 1959.

Criminal Lunatic Asylums Act ('Broadmoor Act') 1860

In 1807 a Select Committee Report recommended that a central asylum for criminal lunatics be established. In 1816 Bethlem Hospital incorporated 60 beds for criminal lunatics. The 1860 Act finally provided the legislation for the establishing of asylums for criminal lunatics. The Broadmoor Asylum was established under this Act and opened in 1863. Offenders or accused persons who would otherwise be transferred to a county lunatic asylum could be removed to the appointed asylum for criminal lunatics, although such people could still be detained in a county asylum. Under the 1860 Act rules for the administration of Broadmoor were drawn up on behalf of the Secretary of State along with a 'council of supervision'. The Act also provided for the capture of criminal lunatics who escaped, whether from Broadmoor or another asylum, and for the punishment of those who helped them to escape. The Commissioners in Lunacy were required to visit Broadmoor at least once a year and to report to the Secretary of State every March.

Trial of Lunatics Act 1883

The 1883 Act repealed Section 1 of the 1800 Act, dealing with treason, murder or felony, so that the new Act applied to a person accused of any offence. According to a contemporary commentary, the 'Act accordingly abolishes the verdict of acquittal on the grounds of insanity, and substitutes a special verdict of guilty, but insane at the time of the commission of the offence' (Lushington 1895). The aim was to avoid the need to determine whether an accused person was sane, and to ensure that the trial was of the offence as it was committed. The court was not given the power to detain people who were found innocent, even though they might appear insane. Where the verdict of guilty but insane was found, the prisoners could be detained in an asylum for criminal lunatics during Her Majesty's Pleasure.

Criminal Justice Act 1948

This Act designated criminal lunatic asylums as 'Broadmoor institutions', vested in the Minister of Health and managed by the Board of Control; and termed criminal lunatics as 'Broadmoor patients'. Responsibility for Broadmoor was transferred from the Home Office to the Ministry of Health, under the Board of Control.

Homicide Act 1957

The Homicide Act 1957 introduced the concept of diminished responsibility, whereby a person would not be convicted of murder 'if he was suffering from such abnormality of mind . . . as substantially impaired his mental responsibility for his acts and omissions in doing or being a party to the killing'.

Mental Health Act 1959

The Mental Health Act 1959 replaced much of the existing legislation for criminal lunacy. The term psychopath was introduced as part of the wider concept of mental disorder defined at the beginning of the Act. A number of provisions opened the possibility of hospital treatment for offenders, as well as of transfer from other hospitals to Broadmoor of non-offenders. A system of hospital orders under the Mental Health Act 1959 provided compulsory hospitalization for mentally disordered offenders, but as Hoggett (1984) notes, the offender need not consent to the substitution of a hospital order for a prison sentence. A hospital order could be made with or without a restriction order, which among other conditions, meant that only the Home Secretary could authorize the discharge of the patient.

Patients who were subject to a restriction order could not apply directly to a Mental Health Review Tribunal, but had to make a request in writing to the Secretary of State, who then referred the patient's case to the Tribunal for advice. As a result of these provisions and of the vagueness of those relating to compulsory treatment, increasing numbers of patients were treated against their will and without recourse to appeal.

Criminal Procedure (Insanity) Act 1964

This Act returned to the question of the verdict referred to in the Trial of Lunatics Act 1883: 'Not guilty by reason of insanity.' The Act lays down the procedures for accused persons who are thought to be unfit to be tried (to be determined by a jury), and for returning a 'special verdict that the accused is not guilty by reason of insanity'. The Act empowers the court to order admission to hospital. If an accused person later becomes fit to be tried he can later be transferred to prison or remand centre.

NATIONAL HEALTH REORGANIZATION 1973

Under this reorganization, Broadmoor, Rampton and Moss Side Hospitals became known as the 'special hospitals', for the treatment of patients requiring special security but who otherwise fell into the same categories of mental disorder as patients treated in ordinary hospitals (Report 1975).

Report of the Committee on Mentally Abnormal Offenders (Butler Report) 1975

The Butler Report drew attention to the many problems besetting the arrangements for mentally disordered offenders, despite the success of the underlying principles of the Mental Health Act 1959 (Report 1975). Difficulties included the lack of coordination of services, the difficulties and delays in getting some offenders admitted or transferred to ordinary psychiatric units, the tension between custodial and 'open-door' policies of treatment, overcrowding and isolation of the special hospitals, shortcomings of social services and aftercare facilities, use of the prison service for the mentally ill, questions of definition of mental abnormality in relation to sex offenders, and neglect of patients' rights, for example, to consent to treatment. Among the Committee's recommendations were provision of secure units for patients who require secure conditions, increased development of multi-disciplinary forensic psychiatric services, better medical and psychiatric services in prisons, easing of transfer of patients to local hospitals, more effective use of hospital orders, and a widening of access to Mental Health Review Tribunals, together with attention to the need for consent to treatment.

Mental Health Act 1983

Some of the Butler Committee's recommendations were implemented in the Mental Health Act 1983. Whereas under the Mental Health Act 1959 provisions for patients concerned in criminal proceedings and for prisoners were lumped together in two broad groupings, under the Mental Health Act 1983 provisions were divided under five headings. New provisions included the remand of accused persons to hospital for reports or treatment or both; the transfer of unsentenced prisoners to hospital; and interim hospital orders, whereby a convicted prisoner could be admitted to hospital before sentencing. Under Section 70, patients who were subject to a restriction order could now apply to a Mental Health Review Tribunal. Under Section 73, the Mental Health Review Tribunal was empowered to order the discharge of restricted patients.

THE POOR LAW

For many years the Poor Law represented the only form of social and welfare services available. Hobsbawm's (1968) view of the Poor Law was that it was designed to provide the minimum necessary to enable paupers to survive, this being below the lowest wage available. 'The Poor Law was not so much intended to help the unfortunate as to stigmatize the self-confessed failures of society' (p. 69). Medical services for the unemployed, that is, the money-less, just did not exist. The redistribution of public funds, such as it was, under the Poor Law meant that medical services to poor law institutions were of the same bare minimum as that urged by the legislation as the level

of expenditure on maintaining pauper inmates of workhouses (Hobsbawm 1968).

In England and Wales, the population was 5.5 million in 1700, 13 million in 1831, and 29 million in 1900, gradually becoming concentrated in urban areas. In 1832 10% of the population were registered as paupers. 'In 1846 there were 1 331 000 paupers, of whom only 199 000 were "in" paupers, leaving 1 132 000 "out" paupers' (Midwinter 1968 p. 31, 32). 'To the central poor law authority, throughout the century, pauper lunatics were first and foremost paupers. . . . By January 1847, 8986 lunatics were known to be confined in workhouses in England and Wales' (Mellet 1981 p. 237). In 1836 the Committee of Vestry of the Parish of St George, Hanover Square, reported on the 'immense expenditure on the [County] Pauper Lunatic Asylum at Hanwell', referring to the excessive outlay of public monies on the maintenance of pauper lunatics (p. 1).

In 1834, the Poor Law Amendment Act was the prelude to more than 70 years of legislation which attempted to tackle public health problems manifested in successive epidemics of cholera, typhus, smallpox and other forms of enteric and respiratory disorders. There were no reliable freshwater supplies, or sewage systems. All utilities were privately owned. The police system was inadequate, and the penal system (including transportation, convict hulks and flogging) was both savage and inadequate. There was overcrowding of graveyards as well as of living accommodation, which was sometimes shared with unburied bodies.

The dramatic effects of nineteenth century improvements in public health contrast with a lack of effect either of prevention or cure in lunacy. Lunacy law regulated institutional provision for the insane, but interlocked awkwardly with welfare provision that was governed by a collection of overlapping laws whose complexity effectively prevented any kind of integrated approach. By the early years of the twentieth century, institutions for the mentally disordered ranged from county and borough asylums to licensed private houses to the workhouse. Poor law infirmaries were administered by the poor law authorities, providing a number of hospital services. Via the vagrancy laws, workhouses rather than the infirmaries were used for custody of pauper lunatics. The development of public lunatic asylums was distinct from the development of other hospital services such as the voluntary hospitals. Mental health services remained separate from other health and social services, although some voluntary hospitals did become registered for the purpose of treating mentally disordered patients. The study of mental disorder largely developed in institutions staffed by isolated communities centred round them. The location of an institution on the continuum of custody and therapy was a matter of chance aggregation of local circumstances, largely out of contact with other institutions.

Justices of the peace, as well as being judicial authorities, were, until the Local Government Act 1888, responsible for much of the administration of central government legislation as it affected local communities. The growth of conurbations and other heavily populated areas meant that the existing resources of local justices and parishes became inadequate to carry out their administrative functions. The various commissions and boards were central government's attempt to oversee local implementation of legislation. Inevitably, tension between local and central government grew in proportion to the relative power of each to control allocation of resources to services (Report 1957).

The Poor Law and the workhouse haunted any person without financial support. The possibility of emergency detention in a workhouse was seen as a procedure which 'pauperized' — at least temporarily — 'persons who are in fact in good circumstances' (Report 1926 p. 32). The stigma of mental illness was integral to the stigma of poverty. To be a rate-aided case as opposed to a private case could mean the difference between personal catastrophe and temporary inconvenience. Certification became associated in the public's mind with the loss of all civil rights and liberties.

In 1926 the Royal Commission recognized the need to extricate mental health from Poor Law legislation (Report 1926) but it was not until the

introduction of the National Health Service and the subsequent reforms of mental health law that the separation could take place.

NATIONAL HEALTH SERVICE ACT 1946

When the National Health Service Act 1946 was introduced, it was acknowledged that the complexity of detention procedures under existing mental health legislation made substantial change impossible. Changes were confined to administrative and financial provision (Ministry of Health 1948). Part V of the Act laid down the 'special provisions for mental health services'. A document published by the Ministry of Health in 1948 summarized and explained the changes to what was acknowledged to be the 'already complicated provision of the Lunacy and Mental Treatment Acts and the Mental Deficiency Acts' (Ministry of Health 1948). As part of the 'comprehensive health service for England and Wales', the Minister of Health took over responsibility for providing 'hospital and institutional accommodation for mentally ill or mentally defective patients', along with the 'supervisory functions of the Board of Control' (Ministry of Health 1948 p. 1). That is, the Ministry of Health took over the duty of providing mental hospitals. The running of these institutions and services was delegated to the 14 regional hospital boards, with the exception of designated teaching hospitals. The regional boards delegated the supervision of mental health services to a standing Mental Health Committee advised by the Regional Officer of Mental Health (Ministry of Health 1948).

In accordance with the tripartite division of the NHS into hospital, general practitioner and local government health services, certain responsibilities were delegated to local health authorities. These included the 'initial care and removal to hospital of persons who were dealt with under the Lunacy and Mental Treatment Acts; the ascertainment and (where necessary) removal to institutions of mental defectives; and the supervision, guardianship, training, and occupation of those in the community; the preventive care and after-care of all types of patient' (Ministry of Health 1948 p. 12).

The National Health Service Act 1946 abolished the term rate-aided and repealed part X of the Lunacy Act 1890, which was entitled 'Expenses of Pauper Lunatics'. The Act also repealed the provisions for emergency detention of mentally ill people in workhouses. As has subsequently become clear, the stigma of pauperization and certification could not be abolished with the legislation, not least because many of the workhouse buildings were retained under different nomenclature for the accommodation of the mentally ill (Ministry of Health 1948).

NATIONAL HEALTH SERVICE REORGANIZATION

Reorganization of the National Health Service began in 1974 and continues to date. Since 1974 there have been further attempts to constrain the demands of the NHS upon national resources, by redistributing management and administrative responsibilities, with many direct and indirect effects on mental health services.

In 1974, the Regional Hospital Boards, except in Wales, became Regional Health Authorities, defined by new geographical boundaries, conforming to local authority boundaries. Responsibility for community health services was transferred from local authorities, which retained responsibility for social services and took over hospital social work provision. The first Health Service Commissioner (ombudsman) was appointed, and Community Health Service Councils were set up to 'represent the interests in the health service of the public in its district'. The term 'special hospitals' was introduced as part of the definition of the service provided by the Secretary of State for patients detained under the Mental Health Act 1959 who 'require treatment under conditions of special security on account of their dangerous, violent or criminal propensities'.

In 1977 a consolidating Act to tidy up existing legislation was passed (National Health Service Reorganization Act 1977). In 1976, a Royal Commission on the National Health Service had been set up. It did not report until 1979, in the same

year that a change of government from Labour to Conservative took place. As a result, although some of the Commission's conclusions formed the basis of government planning, the report as a whole was overtaken by other pressures for further reform.

It drew attention to the way in which reformed hospital services had not materialized to replace the large mental illness hospitals which were beginning to close as a result of the Hospital Plan (1962) and of the White Paper 'Better Services for the Mentally Ill' (DHSS 1975). It recommended that the closure programme be modified to ensure the future existence of 'most of the mental illness hospitals' (Report 1979 p. 138). The Commission's report also highlighted the problem of low morale of staff in such hospitals, a problem which received further attention the following year in the report of the working party on the 'Organizational and Management Problems of Mental Illness Hospitals' (DHSS 1980). However, the impetus towards community care was now too strong, despite the lack of genuine alternatives to hospital services for the mentally ill, and a series of measures designed to promote deinstitutionalization have proceeded to date. Ostensibly, these can be justified by reference to the Percy recommendations as to community care (Report 1957) and to the Mental Health Act 1959, but they have been based on fluctuating assumptions and constrained by lack of resources (Malin 1987).

In 1982 another National Health Service reorganization took place. Its results included the arrangement of services into units of management, and withdrawal from involvement with local authorities by abolishing area health authorities. It was followed closely by another report, of the NHS Management Inquiry, which resulted in the implementation of general management at all levels of the NHS (Griffiths 1983). The long-term effect on mental health services is as yet difficult to assess.

A report of the House of Commons Social Services Committee concluded that 'the stage has now been reached where the rhetoric of community care has to be matched by action' (House of Commons 1985 p. cxiii). Among many other recommendations the Committee proposed that health and social services for the mentally disabled should be brought together. The Government responded by saying that 'the way ahead lies in better coordination and cooperation rather than in amalgamation' (DHSS 1985 p. 5).

In 1986, the Government commissioned a report on community care policy from the writer of the NHS Management Inquiry (Griffiths 1983). Griffiths (1988) defined health authorities' responsibilities in terms of health promotion and the prevention of ill-health. They 'should not provide services which fall outside this definition' (Griffiths 1983 p. 15). He recommended that social services authorities lead and direct the assessment of community care needs, as well as the resulting action to be taken. It is not at the time of writing clear how mental health services will be organized in the future.

CUSTODY OF LUNATICS

Foucault (1967) argued that the Age of Reason (c.1650–c.1800) could not tolerate unreason in the form of madness because it subverted the values and foundations of social stability. Madmen were therefore to be confined, at first in the houses of correction and workhouses, along with the other indigent poor, and finally in purpose-built asylums. Foucault's history of ideas offered an attractive explanation of why what he calls the 'great confinement' took place from the mid-seventeenth century, but it has been one that has been more difficult to sustain as empirical evidence emerges of institutional provisions before 1650. It is difficult to know, for example, how to fit Foucault's thesis with the decline of foundling hospitals during this period, which, from pre-medieval times to the Renaissance had housed enormous numbers of abandoned children (Boswell 1988). Why there should have been a shift, if shift there was, from incarcerating foundlings to incarcerating lunatics is not at all clear. Moreover, Parry-Jones cites the considerable evidence that 'the confinement of the insane in private madhouses was a well-established practice by the beginning of the eighteenth century' (Parry-Jones 1972 p. 9).

In Britain, early industrialization further affected provision for the insane. Scull (1989) argues that one effect of the Industrial Revolution was to mechanize further the violent restraint already applied to mad people and which was powerfully symbolized by the sight and sound of clanking chains, swinging chairs, mechanical showers and ducking apparatus.

Attempts had already been made throughout the century to introduce legislation to control the practices of madhouse proprietors. Daniel Defoe had argued in 1697 for the establishing of asylums for idiots, and in 1728 for the licensing and inspecting of private madhouses (Hunter & MacAlpine 1963). The first Act for Regulating Madhouses was passed in 1774 following a select committee report on the confinement of patients in London madhouses (Jones 1955, Parry-Jones 1972). This Act, although it was never effectively implemented, marked the beginning of the nineteenth century developments of legislation for the insane.

Public lunatic asylums

In 1808 the County Asylums Act was the first legislation which provided for the setting up of public lunatic asylums. Whereas before a select committee report of 1807 only a few thousand lunatics were housed in institutions, in the next 100 years this number was to increase twentyfold, so that the 1808 Act was one of the main landmarks of nineteenth century legislation (Porter 1987). The Act was designed to tackle the injustices, neglect and ill-treatment which followed the incarceration of lunatics in workhouses and houses of correction. It was to provide 'asylums for paupers and criminal lunatics', funded by county authorities (Hoggett 1984). However, it was the Overseers of the Poor who were responsible for applying to justices of the peace for the 'conveyance' of lunatics to an asylum, thus maintaining the link between poor law and lunacy legislation (Hoggett 1984). The few asylums built under the 1808 Act rapidly became overcrowded and institutional abuses developed.

Problems arose with the procedures for admitting, certifying and discharging patients (Jones 1955).

Following the 1808 Act a number of amendments were passed which were eventually consolidated in the County Lunatic Asylums Act 1828, also known as the Madhouse Act (Gostin 1986a). An unsuccessful attempt made in 1814 to repeal the 1774 Act for regulating madhouses and to remedy its defects was followed by the establishing of another select committee which reported four times in 1815. Three further attempts at reforming legislation failed in 1816, 1817 and 1819 (Parry-Jones 1972). Although the Madhouse Acts provided for the construction of public asylums, the building of county asylums was not made mandatory until 1845.

Until 1845 pauper lunatics continued to be mainly boarded out by parishes in private madhouses. With the compulsory building of county lunatic asylums under the Lunatic Asylums and Pauper Lunatics Act, pauper lunatics began to be warehoused in huge institutions. Between 1807 and 1890 the percentage per 10 000 of the population who appeared in official statistics as lunatics grew from 2.26% to 29.26%. Of these, 90% were paupers (Parry-Jones 1972, Hoggett 1984).

Other legislation in 1845 included the Lunacy Act 1845, for the 'Regulation of the Care and Treatment of Lunatics'. It was passed as a result of the Metropolitan Commissioners' Report made in 1844, and known as the 'Domesday Book of the Insane' (Hunter & MacAlpine 1963). According to Mellet (1981) this report contained 'dichotomies which were to haunt the inspectorate for the rest of the century' (p. 224). Examples were the Commissioners' concern for the civil liberties of patients versus their concern that patients should be hospitalized and treated as quickly as possible; and their recognition that pauper lunatics were improperly kept in workhouses versus their inability to do anything about the overcrowding of public asylums (Mellet 1981).

All subsequent legislation has oscillated between legalism (protecting patients' liberties by a hedge of provisions and conditions) and a more laissez-faire (reducing the restrictions on practice) reliance on the good faith of medical practitioners and others responsible for caring for the insane.

Accordingly, the Lunacy Act 1845 was subsequently amended by a series of Acts beginning with the Lunacy Amendment Act 1862. One of the provisions of this Act required relieving officers to bring an alleged lunatic in front of a magistrate, in order that he could be admitted to an asylum rather than the workhouse, but the legislation proved ineffective (Mellet 1981). The amending Acts, which followed a select committee report in 1860, failed to assuage public concern about wrongful confinement which began to dominate concern about the conditions under which lunatics were treated. It had taken until 1845 to achieve the legislative reforms demanded by Ashley, Lord Shaftsbury, and practices in the asylums had begun to improve with the development of moral treatment, but another select committee reported in 1877. As a result, the Lunacy Act 1890 was eventually passed after being withdrawn twice (Jones 1960).

Lunacy Act 1890

The sheer amount of legislation which was enacted in the last half of the nineteenth century is overwhelming, but additionally the complexity of procedures, provisions, regulations and amendments led to undoubted inadvertent abuses as well as to intentional abuse of mentally disordered people. The centre-piece was the Lunacy Act 1890, most of which remained in force until 1959. This Act represented, above all, the legalistic approach to lunacy. Upon its detention procedures hinge its other provisions. In particular, the procedure of certification symbolized the status of lunatics in society.

Certification

One of the main provisions of the County Lunatic Asylums Act 1828 was the refining of the procedure for ordering the confinement of people. An order for confinement was given on the production of a certificate signed by two medical practitioners, unless the person was a pauper lunatic, when only one medical certificate was necessary. The 1828 Act was designed to protect the interests of well-off patients, and made no provision for regulating admission to poor law institutions (Hoggett 1984).

Thus the term certification was derived from the medical certificate which a magistrate used to help decide whether to order admission. Private patients had the right to demand to be seen by the magistrate who had to furnish a report to the Lunacy Commissioners (London County Council 1947). The medical certificate became the method used to 'establish the patient's eligibility for . . . care at public expense' (Report 1957 p. 46). If someone applied to a 'judicial authority' (usually a magistrate) for a relative to be detained as a lunatic, the Justice was required to consider the evidence of one or two doctors and possibly to interview the 'alleged lunatic' before making a reception order (ordering an institution to receive the lunatic). If the alleged lunatic was thought to be unable to pay for treatment, then he or she was admitted to the local county or borough asylum.

These procedures meant that unless a person could pay for psychiatric treatment he could not be a voluntary patient. Pauper status was automatically achieved because many people could not afford treatment for mental disturbance. A magistrate examined the alleged lunatic, acting on information received from the relieving officer of the poor law institution of the area, and on one medical recommendation. A judicial order was required under the Poor Law to classify and admit a pauper to the workhouse for rate-aided treatment, in order to exclude people who had or were capable of earning the means to support themselves. Both a judicial order and a medical certificate were required to admit paupers to a poor law hospital, again in order to exclude people who could pay for their treatment. Since the poor law authorities funded the maintenance of patients in the public asylums as well as the other poor law institutions, they preferred to maintain harmless lunatics in the cheaper workhouses. Only patients who were subject to detention (that is, people who were paupers or dangerous or both) were admitted to an asylum (Report 1926, London County Council 1947). By 1958 'this certificate, originally intended as a safeguard against improper deten-

tion, [had] become the evil genius, so to speak, of the whole system' (Rolph 1958).

Report of the Royal Commission on Lunacy and Mental Disorder 1926

The Royal Commission was set up to investigate the 'existing law and administrative machinery in connection with the certification, detention, and care of persons who are or are alleged to be of unsound mind' (Report 1926 p. ii). It criticized the complexity of the detention procedures of the 1890 Act and their association with the Poor Law, but the distinction between private and rate-aided patients remained until the National Health Service Act 1946. Under existing legislation the complexity and number of procedures constituted an administrative maze which reflected the economics of the financial provision for health and welfare services generally and mentally disordered people in particular.

The Commission recommended two classes of admission to care: voluntary and involuntary. The involuntary patient would be dealt with by a provisional treatment order, a reception order, or an emergency procedure. The magistrate was still to be involved in making the orders. The Commission also recommended that the scope and size of the Board of Control should be increased, along with the documentation of involuntary admissions and reports. They recommended changes in the procedure for discharging involuntary patients.

To ease the financial burden imposed on local authorities by the Commission's recommendations of transfer of maintenance costs to the county or borough rate, it also recommended a block grant system from central government funds. It recognized the potential conflicts in running private institutions for profit, but did not find that the private houses wrongfully detained patients.

Mental Treatment Act 1930

The Mental Treatment Act 1930 amended the existing lunacy legislation, which, as a result, became known and was cited as the Lunacy and Mental Treatment Acts 1890–1930.

Lunacy and Mental Treatment Acts 1890–1930

Under the Lunacy and Mental Treatment Acts 1890–1930, patients were classified into four types of status: 'voluntary', 'temporary', 'certified', and an 'inquisition case' (after *de lunatico inquirendo*). 'Lunatics not so found by inquisition' were dealt with differently depending on whether they were private or rate-aided. The distinction between those who were self-supporting (private) and those (paupers) who were maintained in hospital by public funds (rate-aided) was integral to their status in relation to admission and discharge. Voluntary patients entered hospital of their own volition, but had to give 72 hours notice if they wished to be discharged. Temporary patients were detained in hospital, but were not subject to a reception order. They were admitted on application from the nearest relative and with two medical recommendations. Detention was for six months initially, and could be extended for up to a further six months by the Board of Control. Certified patients were those for whom a reception order to an 'institution for lunatics' was made by a magistrate following an application and one or two medical recommendations (Lunacy Act 1890). 'Lunatics so found by inquisition' were the responsibility of the Master in Lunacy and the Chancery Visitors (Mills & Poyser 1934).

Before the National Health Service Act 1946 an institution could be either 'designated', 'registered', or 'licensed'. This did not stop other hospitals from taking mentally disordered patients, but they were not empowered under the Lunacy and Mental Treatment Acts 1890–1930 to detain patients. Conversely, the classification of voluntary and other patients did not apply to them either. Designated hospitals were those designated by the Ministry of Health as 'mental hospitals' (Lunacy and Mental Treatment Acts 1890–1930). Another form of designation was of institutions which could accept and detain patients in an emergency under Section 20 of the Lunacy Act 1890. Section 20 refers specifically to the workhouse, sometimes known for this purpose as an observation ward.

Private patients were admitted to registered hospitals (also known as voluntary hospitals), to 'licensed houses' (private nursing homes), and to 'single-care' in nursing homes. There were two classes of private patient. One class (the 'private list') paid the rate-aided maintenance rate. The other class paid a higher rate for special accommodation. Rate-aided patients were admitted to public mental hospitals (designated hospitals), workhouses, voluntary and public health hospitals (London County Council 1947).

The National Health Service Act 1946 used the term 'mental hospital' to cover the range of asylums, hospitals and other institutions which existed under previous legislation, including workhouses, where pauper lunatics were accommodated, and which had been taken over by local authorities under the Local Government Act 1929 (Report 1957). Because of the separate administration of mental health services, subject as it was to the Board of Control, they took longer to integrate with other health services.

MENTAL HEALTH ACT 1959

The Mental Health Act 1959 was introduced following the Report of the Royal Commission on the Law Relating to Mental Illness and Mental Deficiency (Percy Commission) (Report 1957). The key proposal of the Percy Commission was that patients should be assumed to be willing to enter hospital. The role of the magistrate was to be removed from detention procedures, and that of the doctor made central. The safeguard against improper detention represented by the magistrate was to be taken over by Mental Health Review Tribunals, appointed by the Lord Chancellor.

The Mental Health Act 1959 states: '*Nothing in this Act shall be construed as preventing a patient* who requires treatment for mental disorder *from being admitted to any* hospital or mental nursing home in pursuance of arrangements made in that behalf and without any application, order or direction rendering him liable to be detained under this Act, *or from remaining in any hospital or mental nursing home* in pursuance of such arrangements after he has ceased to be so liable to be detained' (Section 5). Emphases have been added to indicate the two reforms which occurred as a result of this Act.

Mental Health Review Tribunals

The Mental Health Act 1959 introduced a Mental Health Review Tribunal for each regional hospital board. The rights of patients to appeal against detention in hospital remained fairly circumscribed. Despite the safeguards intended by the introduction of tribunals, gradually abuses grew, particularly of treatment without the patient's consent. The Mental Health Act 1959 was deliberately vague about compulsory treatment, shifting far from the legalistic approach of the Lunacy and Mental Treatment Acts 1890–1930, and placing reliance on the judgement and good faith of hospital staff to provide appropriate treatment. As a result of what was felt to be a too sweeping removal of statutory control, a movement began in the 1970s for reform of the Mental Health Act 1959. The need for reform became further evident with a succession of scandals of mistreatment of patients in mental handicap and mental illness hospitals (Martin 1984).

White Paper 1981

The aims of mental health reform were set out in the White Paper (DHSS et al 1981) as follows: to improve safeguards for detained patients, clarify the position of staff looking after them, and to remove legal uncertainties. The principal changes were: reduction in the period of detention allowed before review, permission for detention only for certain groups people thought to be treatable, increased access to Mental Health Review Tribunals, clarification of consent to treatment provisions, establishment of the Mental Health Act Commission, improved guardianship provisions, and the introduction of interim hospital orders for assessment of accused persons appearing in court.

MENTAL HEALTH ACT 1983

The Mental Health Act 1983 was preceded by the Mental Health (Amendment) Act 1982. It was designed to 'consolidate the law relating to mentally disordered persons'. As outlined in the White Paper (DHSS et al 1981) the principal changes in the Mental Health Act 1983, which represented a return to a more legalistic approach, concerned patients who were detained in hospital (Gostin 1986a). The restoration of the Mental Health Act Commission is described elsewhere in this chapter.

Among other changes in terminology was the replacement of the term 'subnormality' with that of 'mental impairment'. The 1983 Act removed age limits for treatment of psychopathy, and instead referred to the need to establish that 'such treatment is likely to alleviate or prevent a deterioration of . . . condition'. Whereas under the Mental Health Act 1959 patients who were admitted for observation were not entitled to appeal to a Mental Health Review Tribunal, under the Mental Health Act 1983 patients detained under section 2 (admission for observation) could apply within 14 days of their detention. The Act also strengthened the rights of the nearest relative to be informed about changes in status and treatment of patients, along with the rights of detained patients themselves to be kept informed by staff (Gostin 1986a).

Guardianship

To a general statement about guardianship made in the Mental Health Act 1959, the Mental Health Act 1983 added three specific clauses defining the powers of a guardian. These were 'the power to require the patient to reside at a place specified by the authority or person named as guardian'; to 'require the patient to attend' specific therapy, education or training; to 'require access to the patient to be given' to anyone specified by the guardian.

Consent to treatment

For the first time, the Mental Health Act 1983 explicitly stated the circumstances in which people, whether detained in hospital or not, could be treated against their will. As Gostin (1986b) points out, the Mental Health Act 1983 refers to medical treatment, so that interventions designed merely to control behaviour are not covered by the Act's provisions for setting aside the requirement to obtain consent.

Power of registered mental nurses to detain patient in hospital

The nurses' six hour holding power was another major innovation of the Mental Health Act 1983. The power to detain a patient in hospital for up to six hours is one which the nurse exercises as part of his or her professional judgement as to the need to restrain a person from leaving hospital. Although the detention period lasts only until a doctor can assess the patient, or for six hours, whichever is shorter, no doctor or other member of staff can order the nurse to exercise the holding power. In this way the Mental Health Act 1983 recognizes the professional autonomy of psychiatric nurses and registered mental handicap nurses.

The implementation of the Mental Health Act 1983 did not go entirely smoothly, especially in relation to the Mental Health Act Commission and its code of practice. At the time of writing, two drafts of the code had been rejected and a third was being written. However, the Commission, together with the Health Advisory Service, monitors practice in hospitals for the mentally disordered, in particular the use of compulsory treatment. A major gap in the mental health legislation which continues to provoke much debate is the question of compulsory treatment in the community. Section 17 of the Mental Health Act 1983 (concerning leave of absence of detained patients) has on occasion been used to enforce long-term treatment in the community, but High Court judgements have shown that this is unlawful (Mental Health Act Commission 1986). The purpose, it is said, of a community treatment power is to maintain people in the community who might otherwise be admitted to hospital. However, this statement is misleadingly simple because of the many possible circumstances in which people are determined to be in need for care and treatment. In 1986 the opinion of the Mental Health Act Commission was that the guardianship provisions of the Mental Health Act 1983 should be thoroughly tested and then possibly extended (Mental Health Act Commission 1986). However, the uncertainty about the future relationship of social and mental health services has delayed any decision about introducing new provisions.

MENTAL IMPAIRMENT

The Idiots Act 1886

The mid-nineteenth century saw greater attention to the need for provision of services for mentally impaired people. The Idiots Act 1886 arose from 'consideration of the Lunacy Acts Amendment Bill in the House of Lords in the session of 1886 [when] it was thought desirable to cut out from the Bill certain new provisions for the regulation of hospitals, institutions and licensed houses for the training and education of idiots and imbeciles, and for simplifying the forms of admission of the inmates and to incorporate these provisions in a separate Bill' (Lushington 1895 p. 811).

The Idiots Act 1886 specified that '"idiots" or "imbeciles" do not include lunatics', and that '"lunatic" does not mean or include idiot or imbecile'. There is no further definition of idiot or imbecile. '"Hospital" and "institution" mean any hospital or institution or part of a hospital or institution (not being an asylum for lunatics) wherein idiots and imbeciles are received . . .'

It should be noted that Section 341 of the Lunacy Act 1890 included idiot in its definition of lunatic, thus ensuring that confusion remained.

Mental Deficiency Acts 1913–38

Following the report of a Royal Commission (Report 1908) a new Act was passed in 1913. Among other provisions, the Mental Deficiency Act 1913 repealed the Idiots Act 1886, classified mentally impaired people, established 'State institutions' for 'defectives of dangerous or violent propensities', detailed the 'regulations for management of institutions for defectives', provided for removal to a place of safety, and for detention of defectives, and replaced the Lunacy Commissioners with a Board of Control.

Mental Health Act 1959

The Mental Health Act 1959 finally amalgamated the two types of legislation for the mentally impaired and mentally ill. However, health services for the mentally impaired remain distinct from those for the mentally ill. Once again it appears that mental health legislation ran ahead of social awareness and provision for the needs of the

people whose disorder is thought to require them to be protected by the law.

SELECTED LIST OF ACTS OF PARLIAMENT

Date	Reference	Title	Date	Reference	Title
1531	22 H VIII c 12	AN ACTE concerning punysshement of Beggers and Vacabundes	1808	48 Geo III c 96	Lunatic Papers or Criminals Act
			1828	9 Geo 4 c 41	County Lunatic Asylums Act
1540	32 H VIII c 46	Court of Wards	1833	3 & 4 Will IV c 36	Commissioners of Lunacy Act
1541	33 H VIII c 20	AN ACTE for due Pces to be had in Highe Treason in Cases of Lunacye or Madnes	1834	4 & 5 Will IV c 76	Poor Law Amendment Act
			1838	Act 1 & 2 Vict c 14	Criminal Lunatics Act
			1842	5 & 6 Vict c 84	Lunacy Act
			1843	5 & 6 Vict c 87	Lunatics Asylums Act
1541	33 H VIII c 22	AN ACTE Concerninge the Order of Wardes and Lyveries	1845	8 & 9 Vict c 100	Lunatics Act
			1845	8 & 9 Vict c 126	Lunatics Act (Asylums)
			1860	23 & 24 Vict c 75	Criminal Lunatic Asylums Act
1562	5 Eliz I c 3	Act for the Releife of the Poore	1862	25 & 26 Vict c 111	Lunacy Acts Amendments
1576	18 Eliz I c 3	Act for the Setting of the Poore on Worke and for the avoyding of Ydleness	1867	30 & 31 Vict c 12	Criminal Lunatics Act
			1883	46 & 47 Vict c 38	Trial of Lunatics Act
			1884	47 & 48 Vict c 64	Criminal Lunatics Act
			1886	49 & 50 Vict c 25	Idiots Act
1595	39 Eliz I c 3	Act for the Releife of the Poore	1888	51 & 52 Vict c 4	Local Government Act
			1890	53 & 54 Vict c 5	Lunacy Act
1595	39 Eliz I c 5	Act for erecting of Hospitalls or a biding working Howses for the Poore	1911	1 & 2 Geo V c 40	Lunacy Act
			1913	3 & 4 Geo V c 28	Mental Deficiency Act
			1930	20 & 21 Geo V c 23	Mental Treatment Act
			1946	9 & 10 Geo VI c 81	National Health Service Act
1601	43 Eliz 1 c 2	Act for the Releife of the Poore	1948	11 & 12 Geo VI c 58	Criminal Justice Act
1714	13 Ann c 26	Act for Reducing the Laws relating to Rogues, Vagabonds, Sturdy Beggars and Vagrants	1957	5 & 6 Eliz 2 c 11	Homicide Act
			1959	7 & 8 Eliz 2 c 72	Mental Health Act
			1964	Eliz 2 c 84	Criminal Procedure (Insanity) Act
1744	17 Geo 2 c 5	Justices Commitment Act	1977	c 49	National Health Service Reorganization Act
1774	14 Geo III c 49	Act for Regulating Madhouses	1982	c 51	Mental Health (Amendment) Act
1800	39 & 40 Geo III c 94	Criminal Lunatics Act	1983	c 20	Mental Health Act
			1984	31 Eliz II c 36	Mental Health (Scotland) Act

REFERENCES

Allderidge P 1979 Hospitals, madhouses and asylums: cycles in the care of the insane. British Journal of Psychiatry 134: 321–334

Boswell J 1988 The Kindness of strangers. Pantheon, London

Carson D (ed) 1987 Making the most of the Court of Protection. King Edward's Hospital Fund, London

Clarke B 1975 Mental disorder in early Britain. University of Wales Press, Cardiff

DHSS 1975 Better services for the mentally ill. HMSO, London

DHSS 1980 Organizational and management problems of mental illness hospitals. Department of Health and Social Security, London

DHSS et al 1981 Reform of mental health legislation. HMSO, London

DHSS 1985 Government response to the Second Report from the Social Services Committee. 1984–1985 session: community care. HMSO, London

Firth C H, Rait R S (eds) 1911 Acts and ordinances of the Interregnum 1642–60, Vol 2. HMSO, London

Foucault M 1967 Madness and civilization. Tavistock, London

Gostin L 1983 The Court of Protection. National Association for Mental Health, London

Gostin L 1986a Mental health services: law and practice. Shaw, London

Gostin L 1986b Institutions observed. King Edward's Hospital Fund, London

Greig J W, Gattie W H 1915 Archbold's lunacy and mental deficiency, 5th edn. Butterworth, London

Griffiths R 1983 NHS management inquiry. HMSO, London

Griffiths R 1988 Community care: agenda for action. HMSO, London

Hibbert C 1963 Roots of evil. Penguin, Harmondsworth

Hill C 1969 Reformation to industrial revolution. Penguin, Harmondsworth

House of Commons 1985 Second Report from the Social Services Committee. Session 1984–1985. HMSO, London

Hobsbawm E J 1968 Industry and empire. Weidenfeld & Nicholson, London

Hoggett B M 1984 Mental health law. Sweet & Maxwell, London

Hunter R, MacAlpine I (eds) 1963 300 years of psychiatry: 1535–1860. Oxford University Press, Oxford

Hunter R, MacAlpine I 1972 The Reverend John Ashbourne (ca 1611–1661) and the origins of the private madhouse system. British Medical Journal 2 (5813): 513–515

Jones K 1955 Lunacy law and conscience: 1744–1845. Routledge & Kegan Paul, London

Jones K 1960 Mental health and social policy 1845–1959. Routledge & Kegan Paul, London

Jones K 1972 History of the mental health services. Routledge & Kegan Paul, London

Jones R (ed) 1985 Mental Health Act manual. Sweet & Maxwell, London

Leigh D 1961 The historical development of British Psychiatry Vol 1: 18th and 19th centuries. Pergamon, Oxford

Leigh D 1979 Historical perspectives on depression. Roche, Nutley, N.J.

London County Council 1947 Handbook on mental health social work. London County Council, London

Lushington S G 1895 Archbold's lunacy, 4th edn. Shaw, London

MacDonald M 1981 Insanity and the realities of history in early modern England. Psychological Medicine 11: 11–25

Malin M 1987 Community care: principles, policy and practice. In: Malin N (ed) Reassessing community care. Croom Helm, Beckenham

Martin J P 1984 Hospitals in trouble. Blackwell, Oxford

Matthews F B 1948 Mental health services. Shaw, London

Mellet D J 1981 Bureaucracy and mental illness: the Commissioners in Lunacy 1845–1890. Medical History 25: 221–250

Mental Health Act Commission 1986 Compulsory treatment in the community. MHAC, London

Mental Welfare Commission 1986 Information for patients. Mental Welfare Commission, Edinburgh

Midwinter E C 1968 Victorian social reform. Longman, London

Mills G E, Poyser A H R W 1934 Lunacy practice. Butterworth & Shaw, London

Ministry of Health 1948 The National Health Service Act 1946: provisions relating to the mental health services. HMSO, London

Parry-Jones W 1972 The trade in lunacy. Routledge & Kegan Paul, London

Pitt-Lewis G, Smith R P, Hawke J A 1895 The insane and the law: a plain guide for medical men, solicitors, and others. Churchill, London

Porter R 1987 Mind forg'd manacles. Athlone, London

Pound J 1986 Poverty and vagrancy in Tudor England, 2nd edn. Longman, Harlow

Ray I 1838 The medical jurisprudence of insanity. Little Brown, Boston

Record Commission 1841 Ancient laws and institutes of Wales. Commissioners on Public Records, London

Report 1860 Select Committee of the House of Commons

Report 1877 Select Committee of the House of Commons

Report 1908 Royal Commission on the Care and Control of the Feeble-Minded, Cmnd 4202. HMSO, London

Report 1926 Royal Commission on Lunacy and Mental Disorder. HMSO, London

Report 1957 Royal Commission on the Law Relating to Mental Illness and Mental Deficiency 1954–1957 (Percy Commission). HMSO, London

Report 1975 Committee on Mentally Abnormal Offenders (Butler Report). HMSO, London

Report 1979 Royal Commission on the National Health Service. HMSO, London

Rolph C H 1958 Mental disorder. National Association for Mental Health, London

Scull A 1979 Museums of madness. Allen Lane, London

Scull A 1989 Social order/mental disorder. Routledge, London

Statutes of the Realm 1810 Vol 129

Tuke D H 1882 Chapters in the history of the insane in the British Isles. Kegan Paul, London

Committee of Vestry of the Parish of St George, Hanover Square 1836 Third Report on the Expenditure of the County of Middlesex. Bridgewater, London

1962 Hospital plan. HMSO, London

12

The contribution of sociology

D. Field and S. Taylor

WHAT IS SOCIOLOGY?

The simplest definition of sociology is that it is the study of human societies. The sociologist's problem is trying to explain how societies, or parts of society, work in the way that they do (Berger 1968). However, this definition does not take us far enough. We all know to our cost that there are politicians, moralists and other pundits of one sort or another only too willing to tell us what is wrong with society and what should be done to put it right. Almost everyone, it seems, has an opinion as to why society is as it is. Even if we go further and claim that sociology is the *academic* study of society, then we are still confronted by the problem that there are other academic disciplines — such as history, politics and anthropology — that also have their subject matter in human societies. Therefore, as sociologists have no monopoly over the subject of societies, it is better to outline some of the ways in which sociology offers a distinct interpretation of human societies.

Sociologists argue, and attempt to demonstrate, that the nature of the society into which we are born and in which we live our lives influences, or structures, our behaviour and how we perceive ourselves and the world around us. In our individualistic modern world most people assume that societies are merely aggregates of their component individuals and that it is the study of the individual and his or her basic 'needs' or 'drives' that provides the key to understanding societies. In challenging this assumption sociologists do not reject the study of the 'individual' in favour of the 'group'. Rather, they explore the *relationships* between individuals and societies, and between the various institutions that make up a society. Sociologists see this as a two-way process. Clearly, societies are necessarily the creation of individuals but, as individuals, we are also the *products* of our societies. Implicit in a sociological approach to society is the assumption that social life is not merely a consequence of individual activity, but rather that it exerts an independent and constraining influence over people.

From this position sociologists have shown that the relationships between people and between different parts, or institutions, of society do not occur randomly, but tend to be regular or patterned. For example, birth and death rates remain relatively stable in a given country year after year: some groups within a country have a consistently higher life expectancy than others; some groups regularly commit more crimes than others. Even when sociologists engage in more detailed, first-hand, observation of, for example, doctor–patient, teacher–pupil, police officer–suspect interaction, they still find certain regular and consistent patterns of communication and behaviour. Sociologists conclude that social life is structured and governed by particular sets of rules. Of course, some of the rules are obvious to all. There are laws and moral and ethical values proscribing certain kinds of conduct and sanctions may be applied to transgressors. However, sociologists go further than this and argue that many of the rules of social life are hidden, or latent, such that people are themselves unaware of the extent to which collective social life and the expectations of others are influencing and shaping their behaviour and consciousness. Sociologists see one of their main tasks as documenting and attempting to explain these processes.

In seeking to explain why societies or parts of societies work in the way they do, sociologists attempt to go beyond speculation, subjective opinion and philosophical debate. They try to make their accounts as systematic and objective as possible. First, as with other sciences, a large part of sociological work involves careful observation and description of the subject under consideration. This may involve various sources ranging from official statistics, questionnaires and interviews, historical and documentary sources to direct, or participant, observation. Sociologists try to systematize their accounts by using clearly defined conceptual tools. For example, a sociologist studying patterns of inequality in health would do so in terms of a clearly identified concept of social class — based either on ownership or non-ownership of the means of generating wealth or on categories of occupation — and a concept of health based, for example, on life expectancy and vulnerability to long-standing illnesses. The sociologist might then construct a provisional hypothesis about a particular pattern of relationships. For example, a positive relationship between relatively poor health and manual occupations may suggest links between the stresses and dangers of types of manual work and poor health. This hypothesis will then guide further observations. For example, the sociologist may then want to look much more closely at the illness rates of particular occupational activities. As a result of this further research, the original hypothesis regarding work conditions and illness may be developed and confirmed, or it may need to be modified or even rejected.

Sometimes, the sociologist's research may produce a theory of some aspect, or aspects, of human life. However, a major problem for the social and psychological sciences is that they are usually denied the opportunity to test theories under 'closed', or controlled, conditions. As far as sociology is concerned, it would normally be unethical, if not impossible, to conduct 'social experiments' on large groups of people. However, sometimes the 'real' world resembles a 'quasi-experimental' situation. If, for example, a new form of teaching or policing or health care practice is introduced, then sociologists may learn a great deal about education or crime or health care by observing the changes. Sociologists also make a great deal of use of *comparative* study. For example, one of the present authors, in a research study of how decisions are made about children suspected of having been abused, has recently made a study of two different authorities. One is known to have a 'hard-line' policy over taking children into care, while in the other, every effort is made to keep children out of care. By comparing two very different responses to what is essentially the same problem, the researcher is in a better position to make certain general statements about child care.

The general lack of controlled experimental evidence has led some to doubt whether it makes any sense to talk about social *sciences*. We cannot examine this issue here, but it must be conceded that the social sciences can never achieve the certainty and predictive power of the natural sciences. However, sociologists can still go well beyond opinion, rhetoric and guesswork by using clearly defined conceptual tools, constructing logically consistent theoretical statements, and by showing that their explanations are consistent with the available evidence. Sociologists, like other scientists, must also expect their favourite theories either to be replaced by a more logical and plausible explanation, or to be refuted by contradictory evidence.

SOCIOLOGY APPLIED TO HEALTH AND ILLNESS

Sociological ideas, methods and concepts have been applied to the study of physical and mental health in a number of different ways. Some sociologists examine the way in which society, or social factors, influence the distribution of health and illness. For example, as we implied above, sociological research has revealed links between social inequality and health inequality. In Britain, those who have manual occupations are, on average, two and a half times as likely to die before retirement age than those from managerial or professional backgrounds (Townsend & Davidson 1982).

Sociologists have also established links between physical and mental disease and the nature, or quality, of people's interpersonal relationships. In general, people appear to be more vulnerable to disease when they lack close, socially supporting ties to others (Berkman & Syme 1979). From this kind of evidence, sociologists have argued that many diseases, rather than being *purely* biological in origin, have their roots in society and different forms of social interaction.

Other sociologists have been more concerned with examining how certain physiological states or types of behaviour come to be labelled as 'illnesses', and also with exploring the effects of illness labels on individual patients. It is argued that 'diseases' are not simply facts of nature waiting to be 'recognized' and classified by experts, but, rather, are products of *social definition* (Wright & Treacher 1982). Sociologists have shown that the ideas a society has about what constitutes health and illness, and even medical knowledge itself, do not exist in a 'medical vacuum', but change in response to social changes and development (Jewson 1976, Armstrong 1983). For example, in modern society, child bearing, child rearing, excessive unhappiness, madness, ageing and even dying have all been brought under medical supervision and control (Freidson 1970). The growth of medical power and influence has led sociologists to argue that rather than being 'detached' and value free, medicine is now one of the most important *socializing* agencies in society, that is, it is one of the most important ways in which certain ideas and values are consolidated and transmitted through society. Dr Michael Gossop (1987 p. 54) has put it thus:

One of the striking developments of recent years is the way in which health has been elevated to a supreme value. In the name of health and treatment, the medical bureaucracy is increasingly able to violate such important social values as the individual's freedom of choice and rights of privacy. The distinction between good and bad has been largely replaced by that of healthy and unhealthy (or as it is sometimes expressed — good for you, and bad for you).

Clearly, these observations are particularly relevant to mental illness, where the main criterion for labelling people as 'ill' is that their behaviour and communications contradict others' views of what is normal and rational.

Sociologists also study interaction between health professionals and patients and examine peoples' experiences of illness. Once a person is defined as sick and enters into the 'sick-role', important social changes follow. For example, the person may be given certain rights and privileges and be excused many of his or her social obligations. However, illness labels may also be constricting and stigmatizing, and may have a negative effect on the individual's sense of identity and personal worth. Sociologists have shown that the ideas that a social group holds about a particular illness or disability can have a profound effect on the sufferer's perception and experience of that condition. For example, in his research on blindness, Scott (1969) observes that in the United States — where blindness tends to be perceived in terms of mourning and grieving for lost sight — the blind are characterized by melancholy, dependence and helplessness. Scott argues that this 'blind personality' is not inherent in the condition of blindness, but is transmitted to the blind by professional workers. Thus, it is the health and welfare workers who, as Scott puts it, 'create for blind people the experience of being blind'. In contrast, in Sweden, where blindness is viewed more as a technical handicap, the blind tend to be less dependent, more involved in their own welfare provisions and there is much less evidence of the 'blind personality'.

This section has outlined some of the major characteristics of a sociological approach to the study of society and some of the ways in which this is applicable to the study of health and medicine. In the following sections we develop these ideas in relation to topics of particular relevance to psychiatric nursing. First, we consider patterns of social differentiation and their relationship to the occurrence and treatment of mental illness. Second, we look at the labelling and definition of people as mentally ill. Finally, we discuss the care and treatment of the mentally ill, and examine the argument that mental illness is used as a form of social control.

SOCIAL DIFFERENTIATION AND MENTAL DISORDER

We have already noted that sociologists look at regularities and patterns in social life and the relationship of these to health and illness. Together with other researchers, sociologists have contributed to our understanding of the ways in which patterns of social differentiation relate to the incidence and distribution of mental disorders. Patterns of reported mental disorder vary by age, gender, social class position, and by ethnic group — although the data bearing upon the latter within British society is less well documented or understood.

High rates of psychiatric morbidity are found among the aged, who occupy nearly half of all psychiatric beds, and symptomatology increases sharply with age. These differences are partly attributable to biological processes of maturation and ageing, but are also linked to the social aspects of such processes. For example, there is an obvious organic link between old age and Alzheimer's disease (senile dementia). However, confusion among the elderly may be a product of social isolation, inadequate diet, drug interactions, hospitalization, and other factors related to an old person's *social environment* rather than to senility. Such socially-induced confusion may be mistakenly diagnosed as dementia. Once diagnosed as demented, the reactions of nursing and other staff to the patient may serve to maintain such confusion and to enhance the confusion of the genuinely demented. For example, further drug therapy may reinforce rather than clear up confusion, while the belief that it is futile to try to communicate normally with patients may reinforce their isolation and remove important social orienting cues about time and place (Browne 1984).

Age effects are also evident in earlier years. Among males, hospitalization for mental disorder is highest in the twenties, mainly for schizophrenia, alcoholism and personality disorders. Women are more likely to be treated for neurotic disorders, with hospitalization at its peak in the forties. Another high risk group are women with young children. These patterns of age differentiation interact with gender differences, and seem to be at least partly explicable in terms of gender differentiation in our society.

There are clear differences in the reported rates of mental disorder between the sexes in our society. Females are more likely to be diagnosed as suffering from psychoneurotic, psychosomatic and manic-depressive psychoses than males. Males are more likely to be diagnosed as suffering from personality disorders. Rates of diagnosed schizophrenia are similar. Most psychiatric cases are treated at the primary care level, and here females are twice as likely to be diagnosed by GPs as having psychiatric disorders than males. These gender differences are accentuated by marriage, with married men least likely to show psychiatric disorders, whilst married women are *most* likely to do so — thus supporting Nathanson's (1975) conclusion that 'from the standpoint of health status, the married state is less advantageous to women than to men'.

A number of explanations can be offered for these striking differences. First, they seem to be linked to conceptions of self and gender roles in our society — help-seeking and 'emotionality' are congruent with idealized female roles and attributes, whereas male roles and attributes tend to restrain the expression of emotion, encourage the denial of illness and restrict the use of health services. Thus, it is claimed, women are more likely than men to see their problems as some type of mental disorder and are more willing to seek psychiatric help for them. Both the patterning of mental disorder and the level of reported use of services seem to be affected by gender-related patterns of interpretation and lay referral. It is also likely that the diagnostic practices of psychiatrists are shaped by gender expectations, and that the pattern of females being more likely than males to be diagnosed as mentally ill is at least in part the result of professional patterns of gender-based diagnosis. Unfortunately, despite some evidence that gender influences diagnosis and treatment, there is no systematic picture of how this works (Miles 1987). A final explanation for gender differences is that the differing work, family and leisure experiences of males and females generate different levels and types of mental disorder. For example, alcoholism is more prevalent among males than females, and this seems to be related to patterns of male sociability and leisure. Female alcoholism and depression are similarly linked to patterns of female domestic life.

Ethnic group differences in diagnosed mental illness seem to be largely the product of the low social class position of migrant groups in our society. It is also highly likely that diagnostic and referral patterns will vary by ethnic group and that the perception of GPs and psychiatrists as to the likely relevance or success of referral for psychiatric treatment will vary by ethnic status. Some groups — e.g. inner city migrants from the New Commonwealth — may well be grossly under-represented in the psychiatric patient population due to these factors. It is also probable that the pattern of symptomatology will vary by ethnic status. Despite the many difficulties in arriving at 'true rates' of mental disorder for ethnic groups, Mangen (1982), in his review of the evidence, concludes that 'immigrant groups do not have uniformly higher rates of mental disorder than the host community' (p. 60).

Social class differences associated with mental illness have been well researched by sociologists and others, especially in the USA. The classic study by Hollingshead & Redlich (1958) in New Haven, found that the prevalence of diagnosed psychiatric disorder was inversely related to social class, with the lowest class having by far the highest rates. Types of treatment and types of disorder were also related to social class, with lower social classes most likely to receive institutional 'custodial' care (and to be re-admitted after discharge) and upper classes most likely to be receiving psychotherapy. Schizophrenia and psychotic disorders were more common in the lower classes. Hollingshead & Redlich suggested that there was a causative relationship between social class and mental disorder, and that the adverse life situation of lower (manual) social class members generated stresses which caused high rates of mental disorder. They also showed that psychiatrists used different criteria in defining people from different social classes as mentally ill, and that members of the lower social classes were more likely to be diagnosed in this way than members of other social classes with similar conditions.

Another important study was of Midtown Manhattan (Srole et al 1962). The study generated some controversy at the time because of the very high rates of psychiatric impairment and disorder which it reported, although subsequent studies in other settings also produced similarly high rates. High rates of untreated symptomatology have also been reported from surveys of physical health and illness (e.g. Wadsworth et al 1971). In addition to the link between social class and mental disorder found in New Haven, this study found evidence of downward social mobility or 'drift' as a result of mental disorder. Further studies in the USA, UK and elsewhere have confirmed the findings of these two studies: that there is a clear relationship between social class and mental disorder, that this is mainly due to the adverse social conditions of the lower classes, and that there is also a significant 'downward drift' of the mentally ill into the lower social classes (Dohrenwend & Dohrenwend 1981, Miles 1987).

How might low social class be a causal influence on depressive illness? The Camberwell community study by Brown & Harris (1978) investigated depression among working class and middle class women, and attempted to identify the differing life situations and associated stress factors which led to higher rates of depression among the former. Working class women were doubly disadvantaged. They were more likely to experience either a long-term major life difficulty (e.g. poor housing, financial difficulty) or major stressful life events (e.g. death of a family member, job loss, marital breakdown) which Brown & Harris identify as primary causes of depression. They were also more vulnerable to the effect of such stresses. While only a fifth of the women experiencing such factors developed clinical depression, working class women were much more likely to do so. This greater vulnerability seemed to be directly linked to the past and present social experiences of the women. Brown & Harris identified four 'vulnerability factors', all of which were more common among working class women. Working class women were more likely to have three or more children under the age of 14 in the home, a situation which generates a set of problems and stresses. They were more likely to have experienced the loss of their mother before the age of 11, and thus to lack an important female role model. They were less likely to be in paid employment, which provides an alternative source of stimulation and achievement and independence

from the home. Finally, they were less likely to have social support in the sense of an 'intimate' or confiding relationship with their partner, mainly due to the patterning of role relationships within working class families along more clearly demarcated gender divisions. These factors interacted with each other to increase vulnerability, and all are hypothesized to work through their effect on the women's self-esteem: the pattern of working class life for women being less productive of high levels of self-esteem than the pattern of middle class experiences (Mangen 1982; pp. 110–114).

BECOMING AND BEING 'MENTALLY ILL'

Studies of physical illness have shown that the presence of symptoms is not in itself sufficient to lead people to consult a physician. Indeed, most people exhibit symptoms of disease which they either ignore or treat themselves (Wadsworth et al 1971). As Zola (1973) and others have demonstrated, people must recognize and interpret their symptoms as requiring medical rather than any other type of action to be taken, usually as part of a process of 'lay referral' with close others. Sociologists emphasize that meanings are shared within social groups and transmitted and reinforced within groups. Thus, the nature of social networks and of social definitions of health and illness within groups must be understood if we are to understand people's 'illness behaviour'.

The ways in which social and personal life are viewed may vary markedly by social group. Using Freidson's (1961) distinction between 'parochial' and 'cosmopolitan' attitudes, we can describe two general attitudes towards health and illness in our society which seem class related (Fig. 12.1). Parochial attitudes are found in the lower social classes which emphasize dependence on the social group, and whose definitions of health and illness are often different from current medical views and practice. Familiarity with the range and availability of services may also be lacking. In such groups utilization of services tends to be low. Cosmopolitan attitudes are found among professional and managerial groups which emphasize individual responsibility and which are more knowledgeable and accepting of current medical views. These groups are also likely to be aware of the full range of options available to them, and to be adept at 'working the system' to receive treatment acceptable to them.

LAY CULTURE

		Cosmopolitan	Parochial
SOCIAL NETWORKS	Loose & truncated	Medium/high use Professional & managerial	Medium/low use Working class in new towns
	Cohesive & extended	High use ?	Low use Traditional working class

Fig. 12.1 Lay culture, social networks and utilization of services (based on Freidson E 1961 Patients' views of medical practice).

Similar processes occur with respect to the recognition and definition of 'mental illness', although two additional factors complicate matters. First, the negative attitudes held towards mental

disorders make both lay people and general practitioners less likely to define problems in terms of mental disorder. Second, the difficulty in recognizing and defining mental disorders has a similar effect. As with physical illnesses, there are more cases of unreported mental disorders in the community than are being treated within the health service, and both the affected individuals and their families show similar processes of accommodation and adjustment to sometimes extreme departures from normal behaviour.

In this context, sociologists have been less concerned with the social causes of mental illness than with exploring how social influences structure the meaning and experiences of behaviour that experts *define* as 'mental illness'. For example, Scheff (1966) argues that the most important feature of becoming and being mentally ill is the act of being labelled 'mentally ill' by others (see Fig. 12.2). For Scheff, the meaning and reality of mental illness do not inhere in an objective pathological state, and are not simply properties of the behaviour of the mentally ill. Mental illness is a label

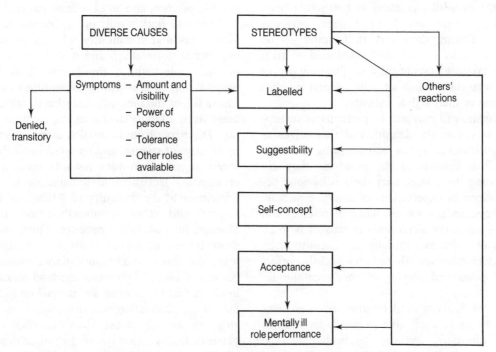

Fig. 12.2 The 'labelling theory' of mental illness (based on Scheff T 1966 Being mentally ill).

applied to people displaying a wide variety of behaviours. Further, similar behaviours are not necessarily defined as mentally ill. The label is applied to make sense of the behaviour of people who consistently violate common and taken-for-granted expectations about behaviour, usually after other explanations have been tried and found wanting. Accounts of how spouses come to define their partners as mentally ill support Scheff's thesis, and also demonstrate their great reluctance to do so, even in the face of extremely disruptive and bizarre behaviour (Miles 1987). However, once a person has been labelled as mentally ill, stereotypes learned in childhood and reinforced in the mass media become influential in shaping the reactions of others to the mentally ill, whose past behaviour is usually reinterpreted in the light of their new social position — what was once seen as an acceptable idiosyncrasy comes to be seen as a sign of mental disorder. Professional health workers, it seems, are not immune from this tendency to reinterpret a person's behaviour in terms of the mental illness label. In one study (Rosenhan 1973), nine pseudopatients faked the symptoms of schizophrenia until admission to hospital, whereupon they were asked to behave perfectly normally. During their stay in hospital — on average 9 weeks — the staff continued to treat them as seriously psychotically ill. The only people to challenge their status as 'real' mental patients were some of their fellow patients.

The mentally ill may also be particularly susceptible to accepting the definition of themselves as mentally ill, and accepting and adopting the mentally ill role because of the problems they are experiencing. In a large part their behaviour becomes shaped by expectations of others, especially those of doctors and nurses. They themselves will also have learnt the stereotypes of what it is to be mentally ill which may initially lead them to resist such a definition, and then, subsequently, affect their adoption and playing of the 'mentally ill' role.

Critics of Scheff's model claim that his ideas seem to be more applicable to psychotic than to neurotic disorders, and that he underplays the extent to which the 'victims' may be willing and grateful collaborators in seeking psychiatric help (Gove 1975). Entry to the sick role often offers a solution to crisis or long-term difficulty for *all* parties concerned. The ill person can legitimately give up the struggle to live a normal life and seek professional help, while family and friends can finally give up the pretence that 'everything is normal' and find some explanation for the person's behaviour. It also seems that the stereotypes of the mentally ill as bizarre, dangerous and unpredictable, are being complemented by more accepting and less stigmatizing ideas of less severe mental disorders. For example, the idea of 'nervous conditions', which are essentially similar to minor physical conditions, and which are amenable to chemotherapy by the general practitioner, seems to be quite widespread. Greater acceptance and less fear and mistrust of the mentally ill are now evident (Miles 1987).

Despite the apparently greater recognition and acceptance of mental disorders as part of everyday life, the mentally ill still suffer from discrimination and stigmatization at work and in the community. The idea that mental disorder is essentially incurable persists, and so ex-mental patients may be avoided and find it difficult to resume their previous work and community roles. They may also experience quite sharp and negative re-definition of their roles within the family. Entering the hospital may thus assume great significance for the future life of the mentally disordered, which treatment from a family doctor in the community may not. Discharge from hospital is often accompanied by feelings of stigma, and by often justifiable fears about negative attitudes towards them and discriminatory treatment in society. Such attitudes contribute to the difficulty of setting up 'halfway houses' and other community-based treatment schemes for ex-hospital patients. Thus, one of the most important set of skills for ex-patients to learn are those concerning 'stigma management' (Goffman 1963). The most common strategy followed is that of 'passing' for normal by hiding the fact of hospitalization and diagnosis from others, although this, of course, does not work with the patient's family, upon whom they often depend for help in re-establishing a normal life. The presence of ex-patients may also have a negative effect upon other family members both directly and in terms of the disruption and strain which they cause, and indirectly through the 'courtesy stigma' which may be applied to other family members because of their relationship with the ex-patient. Family members may try to hide the fact of the ex-patient's hospitalization, and to distance themselves from it in various ways. These negative consequences are most likely when patients with long-lasting conditions, or those with socially embarrassing symptoms, are discharged home with their symptoms controlled by drugs. A fuller account of the ex-patient phase can be found in Miles (1987).

INSTITUTIONAL CARE OF THE MENTALLY ILL

Despite the move away from the treatment of the mentally disordered in hospitals, this is still a major source of treatment for them — nearly a third of hospital beds are still occupied by psychiatric patients. The two main groups caring for the mentally disordered in hospitals are doctors and nurses, even though other therapists and social workers may also play important roles.

Admission to hospital is known to be associated with negative psychological effects for physically ill patients stemming from the problems of adjusting to a new and potentially dangerous environment, loss of independence, restricted communication and lack of information from staff. These aspects of hospital life are partly the result of the organization of hospitals. Hospitals are complex organizations which employ a great range of staff engaged in a variety of activities. To co-ordinate these various activities — running from the mundane but essential provision of cleaning and catering, through the routine nursing care of unproblematic cases, clinical therapy, clinical research and high technology treatment of the critically ill — requires the development of a strict set of bureaucratic rules and routines. The various formal rules and informal routines provide an institutional framework within which nursing work takes place, but within this context there is a con-

tinuous process of negotiation between staff and patients as to the meaning and applicability of rules and arrangements (Strauss et al 1965). Patients are not in a very powerful position to influence their care, and tend to be 'fitted in' to ongoing practices and routines regardless of their individual needs and requirements. Psychiatric patients may be particularly vulnerable to such 'depersonalization' given the nature of their disorders. Research has shown that patients who are perceived as disruptive or demanding too much attention run the risk of being labelled by staff as 'bad patients' (Kelly & May 1982). The typical response to such problematic patients is for nurses to avoid them.

Relationships between carers importantly influence patient care, especially where there is disagreement about treatment. The day-to-day contact and care is the province of the nurses, whose activities are largely under the direction of the doctors. The key feature of nursing as an occupation is its definition in relation to the medical profession as a subordinate and ancillary activity. This largely stems from the concentration of nursing work in the hospital, where the parameters of nursing activity are controlled largely by other groups within the hospital hierarchy. Nurses are recruited predominantly from young females (although psychiatric nursing attracts more males than other types of nursing), and the doctor–nurse relationship of superordination/subordination reflects traditional male–female relationships within Western society. The fact that most nurses are female appears to contribute significantly to the continuation of the subordinate position of the nurse in the hospital hierarchy, despite general changes towards greater equality (Game & Pringle 1983), and may contribute to the reluctance of nurses to go against 'doctor's orders' or to challenge their decisions on the basis of their greater contact with, and knowledge of, patients. This may greatly reduce the therapeutic role of the nurse.

Sociological studies of mental hospitals (e.g. Goffman 1961, Strauss et al 1964) have shown that differing 'psychiatric ideologies' about treatment held by the various professionals, and the consequent disagreements and negotiations about patient care among staff, may adversely affect patient care. They also demonstrate that those who have most frequent contact with patients, i.e. nurses and aides, exert most influence on patient behaviour and recovery prospects both through the way in which they interact with patients and through their definition of patients. Towell's (1975) study of a group of psychiatric student nurses also shows the important impact of treatment philosophies on the way in which the students came to perceive their role and how they should interact with patients. He also found that for most students their training was perceived as inadequate.

There have been a large number of studies of the interaction between nurses and patients (for overviews see Rosenthal et al 1980, Kelly 1982, Bond & Bond 1986). We have already mentioned that nurses tend to categorize patients in various ways and react towards them in different ways as a result of such 'typifications'. For example, children are treated more indulgently than adults, professional males are more likely to be given full information about their case than other patients, alcoholics are treated more roughly and with less respect, and so on. Such typifications, as the examples suggest, are not only confined to clinically relevant aspects of the patient's condition, but also reflect widely-held prejudices and beliefs within society.

Typification of patients is one example of the depersonalization of hospital patients. One of the major problems for patients in hospital is that their individual and social needs are frequently overlooked. Indeed, doctors and nurses frequently do not know of their patient's psychological condition (Duff & Hollingshead 1968). One of the main complaints from patients is that hospital staff do not provide them with sufficient information about what is happening to them while they are in hospital. Nurses and doctors may deliberately control the information they give to patients as one way of maintaining their control over their work with patients. More commonly, information is withheld for a variety of other reasons. There is a general reluctance to break 'bad news' or uncertain prognoses

to patients because of the psychological problems this is thought to entail. Where nursing work is organized along task-specific lines, and/or where there are high levels of patient turnover, nurses may not establish close contacts with patients. Nurses may be reluctant to become involved with patients and try to maintain personal distance from difficult or emotionally demanding nursing work such as that found in acute psychiatric wards — something which may be hard to maintain where the nursing process or primary nursing is in use. Finally, nurses tend to be reluctant to answer patients' questions and may well be forbidden by doctors to reveal information to a patient, even if they themselves want to.

Taken as a whole, these processes may result in what Goffman (1961) has called a 'mortification' of the patient's self-concept. Having movement restricted, fitting into routines organized by the hospital and having to ask permission for, or help with, things previously taken for granted, tend to return the patient to a state of child-like dependency that undermines his or her sense of autonomy and identity. Admission to hospital tends to disrupt, as Goffman puts it, 'precisely those actions that in civil society have the role of attesting to the actor that . . . he is a person with "adult" self-determination, autonomy and freedom of action' (p. 47). In this context, a particular problem for the mental patient is that the child-like behaviour relatively common to all inmates of enclosed, or total, institutions may be interpreted as further evidence of mental illness and deterioration.

Another of the dangers for chronically ill psychiatric patients is that they may become 'institutionalized'. A number of studies of mental hospitals in the 1950s and 1960s described this aspect of patient life, and although it appears to have diminished as a problem, patients in psychogeriatric wards in British hospitals can still commonly be found who have become so adjusted to their long-term stay in the hospital that they are unable to function adequately in the community. In such wards, characterized by low levels of staffing, high levels of organic care, and many confused patients, a vicious circle of neglect, lack of stimulation of patients, and low staff morale can be found. Confusion and apathy among patients in these situations are as much a product of poor institutional care as of mental disorder.

CARE OR CONTROL?

Underlying psychiatric professional expertise, mental health legislation and the organization of the care and treatment of the mentally ill is the assumption that there exist recognizable diseases called mental illnesses. It is believed that it is in the interests of both patients and wider society that these illnesses are diagnosed and treated. These assumptions have not gone unquestioned. We have already seen that some sociologists have argued that the definition of someone as mentally ill owes more to social than clinical considerations. People are labelled as mentally ill because their behaviour and communications appear bizarre and nonsensical to others. Therefore, to define something as a symptom of mental illness involves making the value judgement of comparing the patient's behaviour with what is generally considered normal and acceptable. From this position, it is argued that psychiatry helps to perform an important social control function in modern societies. That is, by defining people who think and behave in 'deviant' ways as 'ill', psychiatry is helping to reinforce more accepted ways of thinking and behaving and legitimizing the treatment, and sometimes detention, of those who violate these norms. Szasz (1961, 1970) has argued that defining what are really moral and ethical problems in living as 'mental illnesses' has given the 'Therapeutic State' an unacceptable power of regulation and control over peoples' lives.

Szasz and other 'anti-psychiatrists' have been criticized both for underestimating the effectiveness of contemporary psychiatry in diagnosing and treating mental illnesses and overestimating its control function (Clare 1976). However, it does seem impossible for psychiatry to avoid the moral and ethical implications of its practices, especially in such contentious areas as compulsory hospitalization, psychosurgery and widespread administration of the major tranquillizers. In this context, Hayes (1979) and Flanagan (1986) argue that psychiatric nurses are also caught up in these moral and ethical dilemmas, and are in a position to act as a powerful voice on behalf of patients' rights and liberties. One of the achievements of sociological and social-psychiatric work in this area is to raise the crucial question of whether the 'medicalization' of human madness and desperation tends to serve the interests of the vulnerable patient or those of wider society in controlling those it finds troublesome.

CONCLUSION

In this chapter we have sketched out some of the ways in which sociological research can contribute towards our understanding of health and illness generally, and mental illness in particular. First, sociologists have shown that many of the conditions which come to be seen as mental illnesses have their origins in distinct patterns of social interaction and forms of social organization. Second, sociologists have drawn attention to the importance of social attitudes and beliefs, especially professional attitudes, in shaping for people the meaning and experiences of mental illness. Third, sociologists have examined the organization of the care of the mentally ill, and contributed to an important process of questioning the concept of mental illness and its application in the treatment and control of those we call mentally ill.

REFERENCES

Armstrong D 1983 The political anatomy of the body: medical knowledge in Britain in the 20th century. Cambridge University Press, Cambridge

Berkman L F, Syme S L 1979 Social networks, host resistance and mortality: a nine year follow-up study of Alameda County Residents. American Journal of Epidemiology 109: 186–204

Bond J, Bond S 1986 Sociology and health care: An introduction for nurses and other health care professionals. Churchill Livingstone, Edinburgh

Brown G W, Harris T 1978 Social origins of depression: a study of psychiatric disorder in women. Tavistock, London

Browne K 1984 Confusion in the elderly. Nursing 2: 698–705

Clare A 1976 Psychiatry in dissent. Tavistock, London

Dohrenwend B P, Dohrenwend B S 1981 (eds) Stressful life events and their contexts. Produst, New York

Duff R S, Hollingshead A B 1968 Sickness and society. Harper & Row, New York

Flanagan L 1986 A question of ethics. Nursing Times, August 27: 39–41

Freidson E 1961 Patients' views of medical practice. Russell Sage, New York

Freidson E 1970 Profession of medicine: a study of the sociology of applied knowledge. Dodd Mead, New York

Game A, Pringle R 1983 Gender at work. Allen & Unwin, London

Goffman E 1961 Asylums: essays on the social situation of mental patients and other inmates. Penguin, Harmondsworth

Goffman E 1963 Stigma: notes on the management of spoiled identity. Prentice Hall, Englewood Cliffs, N J

Gossop M 1987 Living with drugs, 2nd edn. Wildwood House, Aldershot

Gove W R 1975 Labelling and mental illness: a critique. In: Gove W R (ed) The labelling of deviance: evaluating a perspective. Wiley, New York

Hayes E W 1979 Anti-Psychiatric nursing — a personal overview. Canadian Journal of Psychiatric Nursing 20

Hollingshead A B, Redlich R C 1958 Social class and mental illness. Wiley, New York

Jewson N K 1976 The disappearance of the sick-man from medical cosmologies 1770–1870. Sociology 10: 225–244

Kelly M P, May D 1982 Good and bad patients: a review of the literature and a theoretical critique. Journal of Advanced Nursing 7: 147–156

Mangen S P 1982 Sociology and mental health: an introduction for nurses and other care-givers. Churchill Livingstone, Edinburgh

Miles A 1987 The mentally ill in contemporary society, 2nd edn. Blackwell, Oxford

Nathanson C A 1975 Illness and the feminine role: a theoretical review. Social Science and Medicine 9: 57–62

Rosenhan D 1973 On being sane in insane places. Science 179: 250–258

Rosenthal C J, Marshall V W, Macpherson A B, French S E 1980 Nurses, patients and families. Croom Helm, London

Scheff T J 1966 Being mentally ill: a sociological theory. Aldine, Chicago

Scott R A 1969 The making of blind men. Russell Sage, New York

Srole L, Langner T S, Michael S T, Opler M K, Rennie T A C 1962 Mental health in the metropolis: the midtown Manhattan Study. McGraw-Hill, New York

Strauss A L, Schatzman L, Bucher R, Ehrlich D, Sabshin M 1963 Psychiatric ideologies and institutions. Free Press, New York.

Strauss A L, Schatzman L, Bucher R, Ehrlich D, Sabshin M 1963 The hospital and its negotiated order. In: Freidson E (ed) The hospital in modern society. Free Press, New York

Szasz T 1961 The making of mental illness. Harper & Row, New York

Szasz T 1970 The manufacture of madness. Harper & Row, New York

Towell D 1975 Understanding psychiatric nursing: a sociological analysis of modern psychiatric practice. Royal College of Nursing, London.

Townsend P, Davidson N 1982 Inequalities in health. Pelican, Harmondsworth

Wadsworth M, Butterfield W J, Blaney R 1971 Health and sickness: the choice of treatment. Tavistock, London

Wright P, Treacher A (eds) 1982 The problem of medical knowledge: examining the social construction of medicine. Edinburgh University Press, Edinburgh

Zola I K 1973 Pathways to the doctor: from person to patient. Social Science & Medicine 7: 677–689

The contribution of psychology

L. Rentoul and R. Rentoul

The aim of this chapter is to provide the reader with some understanding of psychology: its nature, its scope and what it can and cannot do for the psychiatric nurse. An attempt will be made to confront some of the broad characteristics of psychology as a discipline: for example, the methodological problems of studying man, the extent to which psychology can appropriately be regarded as a science and the different types or levels of explanation it offers. Themes and topics in psychology which are particularly pertinent to psychiatric nursing will be discussed, acknowledging the theoretical conflicts and controversies as well as the growing body of knowledge about which there is broad agreement. Psychology is an important part of the knowledge base of nursing generally and psychiatric nursing in particular. It can be seen as both providing a frame of reference in which questions can be formulated and complex material coherently organized, as well as furnishing the nurse with useful information derived from empirical research. It is clearly a daunting task to embrace the full scope of psychology and emphasize its relevance to psychiatric nursing in one chapter. Although the aim is to do justice to the discipline of psychology, the material included, and by implication excluded, as well as the thrust of the arguments proposed, are likely to reflect the interests and preferences of the authors.

Psychology is the systematic study of human behaviour and mental activity, and concerns itself with both normal and pathological aspects of development. Many areas of human experience have become the focus of psychological enquiry, for example, perception, motivation, memory, cognition, intelligence, personality, psychopathology, learning, human development, attitudes and group behaviour. In some senses all of psychology is relevant to psychiatric nursing in as far as it concerns itself with human nature and development; nevertheless a more fruitful approach is to draw from psychology those areas most clearly related to nursing assessment and practice. There are many different and equally defensible ways of doing this; indeed a review of the related literature reveals a number of approaches (see, for example, Hall 1982, Altschul 1975, Watling & Muller 1984, McGhie 1973). Some texts provide a review of psychology very much along the lines of an introductory psychology textbook; others focus upon nursing practice, and, by drawing on the psychological data, look at topics such as relationships in nursing, the cost of giving, nurses' perceptions of the patient and the psychological impact of the hospital environment. Another strategy is to focus upon the major theoretical approaches in psychology and consider the ways in which they throw light upon patients, nurses and the hospital environment. It is this latter approach which is largely adopted in this chapter.

THE ROOTS OF CONTEMPORARY PSYCHOLOGY

In order to make sense of the schools of thought that exist in psychology today it is important to consider their origins and lines of development. Academic psychology arose first with the setting up of Wundt's laboratory in Leipzig in 1879 as an attempt to develop a stringent science of the mind, and several rigorous lines were developed from this early work. One was physiological psychology, in which it was proposed that the most useful or scientific way to comprehend the mind was to understand the brain and ancillary systems. Another was the development of sophisticated introspective techniques facilitating the examination and exploration of the contents of consciousness. At the same time Freud, in Vienna, was arguing forcefully for the importance of the unconscious as a major determinant of human motivation and development, whilst in America a vigorous reaction to the difficulties of the introspective method (for example, those of replication and validation) arose in the form of behaviourism. Watson, its major proponent, argued that neither the mind nor consciousness were the proper subjects of scientific enquiry; behaviour, on the other hand, was, being public, reproducible and measurable. The limitations of such an approach began to be most forcefully and cogently expressed with the rise of cognitive psychology in the 1960s and 70s. During this time, and subsequently, a range of developments in psychology, such as work emphasizing the analogy between brain and computer, new methods and theories derived from the study of the acquisition and generation of language and insights from developmental psychology, can be seen as psychology returning to the study of the mind. For a fuller discussion of the history of psychology the reader is referred to Wertheimer (1979), Thompson (1968), Miller (1966), and Lloyd et al (1984).

Scientific method

Throughout its history there has been in psychology a commitment to the experimental method, in some instances as a means of testing theoretical propositions, and in other instances as a major defining characteristic of scientific psychology (see, for example, Wright et al 1970). The word 'scientific' itself may generate problems: some see it as a commitment to rigorously defined procedures, whilst others see it as synonymous with 'knowledge'. These differences in definition clearly have consequences for what is accepted as science, and are also sources of great controversy within psychology. The systematic study of the parameters of scientific enquiry is the proper concern of the philosophy of science (see, for example, Popper 1963, Kuhn 1970, Bolton 1979), although it is generally agreed in psychology that whatever is asserted must stand or fall in the light of empirical evidence. Although many areas of human experience do not lend themselves readily to scientific treatment, because of their relatively inaccessible, subjective or even irrational nature, to ignore the canons of scientific methodology would, in the words of Taylor et al (1982), 'condemn psychology to perpetual uncertainty or to the realm of fancy'. Concerns about what do and do not constitute appropriate methods of scientific enquiry, although important, should not be permitted to obscure the true aim of research which is, continuing in the words of Taylor et al, 'to ask interesting and important questions and attempt to answer them as fully and as objectively as circumstances permit'.

In an attempt to meet this aim a wide range of research methods have been devised, including experimentation, surveys, naturalistic observations, correlational studies, case studies and psychological testing. A proliferation of research methods implies some conflict about appropriate research strategies. However, it is also likely that different approaches provide complementary material to what is, after all, an extremely complex focus of enquiry, namely human social life.

Models of man

A brief review of the contentious history of psychology reveals that from its inception there have been fundamental disagreements both about what constitutes appropriate areas of study and also how psychological research should be carried out. This fragmentation of psychology, reflected in the development of competing theoretical perspectives, is in part a function of the particular history of psychology, and in part a function of the complex nature of psychological enquiry. The lack of consensus in psychology at every level of enquiry, including the underlying assumptions about the nature of man and human development, is one aspect of psychology that many students find perplexing and difficult to absorb. The disagreements between the different schools of thought suggest that much of psychology is in what the American philosopher of science Thomas Kuhn (1970) refers to as a state of 'paradigm clash', where additional information does not necessarily

clarify issues and promote consensus, but rather may fuel controversy and increase the distance between the advocates of different points of view.

In attempting to comprehend complex material the concept of the 'model' has proved useful both in the social and natural sciences. Models are theoretical frameworks in which data can be organized and classified, rendering that data more manageable and more meaningful. In psychology a number of models of man have been developed, reflecting different assumptions about the essential nature of human beings and human development. These differing assumptions have repercussions for the way in which data are gathered, organized and interpreted. An important feature of a model in science is that it relies upon analogy, that is, when we are puzzled by complex phenomena we think about them in a way we find easier and more familiar. Thus, for example, a famous nuclear physicist reports thinking about the structure of the atom in terms of billiard balls circling around each other. One danger with this in psychology is that we may forget the 'as if' status of the analogy. For example, it may be useful in the formulation of ideas about certain mental disorders to think of them in terms of illness or disease. One may then move to a point where the initial analogy is lost and one assumes they are in fact physical diseases (they may be, of course, but the important thing is to recognize the shift).

In psychology the use of a model enables one to select relevant material, provides a mode of representation of that material and facilitates the organization of data, especially in the elucidation of causal relationships. However, models should be used with care, since they are an incomplete representation of human nature and potentialities, and should not be used beyond the scope originally intended. This latter criticism has, for example, been levelled against the medical model of mental illness. A number of authors have looked critically at the increasing medicalization of a range of problems and issues (see, for example, Illich 1977, Szasz 1961, Zola 1975, Ingleby 1981, Parton 1985, Conrad & Schneider 1980). They have criticized the appropriateness of a medical framework to comprehend and deal with issues and problems such as alcoholism, child abuse, homosexuality, death and dying and a wide range of personal miseries and anxieties. The main drawback of a model is that in as far as it narrows the range of information considered it may lead essentially complex material to be viewed in a blinkered or oversimplified manner. A frame of reference may become so powerful that vital information, which is not readily incorporated into the model, may be disregarded. It has been argued that medicine, with its focus largely on physiological variables, has failed to incorporate crucial determinants of health and disease, such as environmental, sociological and psychological factors (see for example the work of Powles 1973, McKeown 1979).

MAJOR THEORETICAL MODELS IN PSYCHOLOGY

Any science must be informed by a theory or theories which organize information. In psychology, as has already been emphasized, there are a number of perspectives, some complementary, some in conflict. The perspectives, characterized by different underpinning assumptions about the nature of human development, provide a technical language, an orientation to research, and have implications for therapeutic manoeuvres in a clinical setting. Since there has been in psychology a strong tradition to work within the confines of one theoretical framework, many have argued that there has been, as a consequence, minimal cross-fertilization of ideas between the major schools of thought.

The biological model

This approach has two main tenets: firstly an emphasis on biological continuity between man and animal, and secondly an interest in physiological, biochemical, neurological and hormonal mechanisms that underlie thought, feeling and behaviour. In terms of endocrinological continuity, ethological approaches have long been popular, where the focus is on instinctive or 'wired-in' patterns of behaviour studied under representative conditions. Ethological theory and empirical evidence derived from animal work carried out

within this frame of reference have served as inspiration to a number of researchers looking at human growth and development in areas particularly relevant to psychiatric nursing: in particular, the seminal work of Bowlby (1969, 1973, 1980) on the pathological sequelae of separation and loss in childhood, and the moving accounts provided by Parkes (1972) on normal patterns of bereavement and the effects of unresolved grief on mental health.

A more recent synthesis is provided by sociobiology, which attempts to understand social phenomena in terms of evolutionary adaptiveness. What advantage did it confer, for example, on a species to develop altruism? Sociobiologists give evolutionary theory a particular twist, seeing the gene, rather than the individual or the species, as the target of the adaptive process. However, all biological approaches have in common some commitment to evolutionary explanations as an extension of the notion of biological continuity referred to above.

Clearly, a review of the physiological, biochemical and hormonal mechanisms underlying human conduct cannot be undertaken in this chapter; however, for those interested in a fuller account the following references are suggested (Teyler 1978, Carlson 1981, Kolb & Wishaw 1990). However, certain topics within the biological perspective are likely to be of relevance to psychiatric nursing. Of particular interest is the set of neurotransmitters or substances which convey an impulse from one neuron to another. Current techniques allow for the examination of these mechanisms and how they might be manipulated by drugs. An example illustrates both the approach and the implications for psychopathology, that is, the dopamine hypothesis of the genesis of schizophrenia. Schizophrenia, a particularly debilitating disorder and one of the most prevalent of the psychoses, is characterized by thought disorder, emotional disturbance and social withdrawal.

Dopamine is one of the neurotransmitters found in the basal ganglia, and a series of considerations led to the proposal that schizophrenia was a 'dopamine disorder', that is, that a person with schizophrenia had abnormally high dopamine activity, whether caused by oversensitivity of the receptors, inactivity of the pharmacological inhibitors or superfluity of the substance itself. The considerations leading to this proposal were firstly that drugs (the phenothiazines) which alleviate the symptoms of schizophrenia are found in animal experiments to block the activity of dopamine. Secondly, the more effective the drug is in alleviating the symptoms, the more powerful is its ability to block dopamine activity. Finally, drugs such as the amphetamines, which are known to enhance dopamine activity, exacerbate schizophrenic symptoms. There are, however, difficulties with the argument. In particular, it may take two weeks for the phenothiazines to have a significant effect on schizophrenic symptoms, yet the drug works instantly at the neurotransmitter level. Furthermore, the dopaminergic part of the brain is primarily motoric in function, whereas the defining characteristics of schizophrenia are those associated with the neocortex, for example thought disorder.

These and other considerations (e.g. an increase or decrease in the number of dopamine receptors in the brains of schizophrenic patients which appears to be an artifact of medication) lead the 'dopamine hypothesis' to be no more than suggestive (for a more detailed review of this literature see Hornykiewicz 1982). And a fundamental difficulty relates to the distinction between 'correlation' and 'cause'. Does high dopamine activity, if it reliably accompanies schizophrenia, *cause* the illness or is it a *consequence* of it?

This approach can be seen as illustrative of the medical model of psychopathology. It is usual to differentiate between the organic disorders (those associated with brain damage or metabolic pathology) and functional disorders. Some researchers argue that the latter only await neurological explanation; if techniques were refined enough it would be possible to find the 'machine defect' at the heart of the problem. Two versions of the medical model of mental illness have been discussed (see, for example, Price 1978): firstly that all psychopathology is organically caused and therefore treatable in principle by medicine or surgery. Alternatively, it has been suggested that the term mental illness may also be used within medicine

as a metaphor. Thus, the psychopathologies are modelled upon the disease framework, dominant in medicine. The disorders may not be organically caused; there may not be any physical pathology, but understanding of the disorders is enhanced by a biological frame of reference. Only the second of the two approaches outlined allows any significant role for psychological causality. In both approaches the notions of diagnosis, aetiology, prognosis, treatment, cure, symptom and syndrome are applicable. This model implies that doctors and nurses are best suited to treat the mentally ill, and the hospital is the most appropriate treatment centre. There have been a number of reviews of the medical model of mental illness, for example Clare (1980) and Siegler & Osmond (1966) provide accounts sympathetic to medicine. On the other hand, ferocious critiques of this approach have also been published (for example, Szasz 1961, 1971, Laing 1970, Ingleby 1981).

The psychoanalytic model

This is the creation of Sigmund Freud, although it has been modified and revised more recently by writers working within this tradition. His ambition was to extract from psychopathology that which would be of benefit to normal psychology and ultimately 'to elucidate the human mind'. He sought to develop a model of man which incorporated thought and feeling and which embraced man's essential nature, especially vulnerabilites, anxieties, loneliness and despair, which were consequent upon man's unique capacity to reflect upon his situation. One of the fundamental concepts of psychoanalysis emerged from Freud's struggle to find answers to questions posed by the hysterias, namely the concept of the unconscious. From his early experience with hypnotized patients he found that he was able to have access to material not normally available to patients, and that this appeared to be causally related to the neurosis. Freud did not invent the concept; what was novel was the use he made of the unconscious in constructing a model of human personality. Freud acknowledged the permeability of the unconscious, recognizing that unconscious material can be made conscious. However, individuals are normally reluctant to confront unconscious feelings and conflicts, and Freud introduced the idea of a counteracting force (repression) that is used to ensure that unconscious material remains so. He saw man as dominated by biological drives from birth. These remain largely unconscious and are potentially both constructive and destructive in nature.

Freud laid great emphasis on the significance of early family life experiences. The first five years of life were considered to be of crucial importance because experiences during this time provided a framework within which personality was integrated. The vital components of personality, including defensive manoeuvres, once established tend to become entrenched and resistant to change. In this way the early years are seen to determine adult personality, including adult psychopathology. Hence the famous, and often cited quotation, 'the child is father to the man'. The tradition of making sense of adult personality by referring to childhood experiences has influenced the development of ideas in many spheres (see, for example, the work of Bowlby 1965, 1969, 1973, 1980, Lidz 1976, Bateson et al 1956, Kempe & Kempe 1978, Winnicott 1986, Erikson 1963, Miller 1987, Pincus 1976, Parkes 1972).

The psychoanalytic model highlights the potential for much conflict, both between the competing aspects of personality, and between the individual and society. Such conflict generates anxiety, and in an effort to deal with this and achieve some degree of psychological equilibrium the individual may resort to the use of mechanisms of defence. Often, the individual remains unaware of the nature of the threat and even that defensive strategies have been adopted.

There is a close relationship between normal personality development and psychopathology; the same mechanisms are imputed, but in the neuroses and psychoses the defensive strategies become maladaptive and entrenched and lead to pathological development. This is in many ways similar to the relationship between anatomy (and physiology) and pathology in medicine. Human emotional existence is thus seen in terms of a continuum; at one end is normal, healthy development (which nevertheless includes the possibility of unhappiness, loneliness, distress, guilt and anxiety), moving through a range of neurotic disorders to severe psychotic disorders at the other end of the spectrum. Symptoms of mental disorders are seen as maladaptive coping strategies designed to deal with either intra-psychic conflict or unpalatable realities. However, with the adoption of such strategies, which do bring temporary relief, there comes a new arena of problems.

More recently Freud's ideas have been revised and developed in a number of ways. In the area of psychopathology his work has continued to inspire researchers looking at the aetiology of a range of disorders (see, for example, the work of Bruch (1978) on anorexia nervosa; the work of Lidz (1974), Bateson et al (1956) and Karon & Vanderbos (1981) on schizophrenia; the work of Bowlby (1972) on agoraphobia; the work of Bowlby (1980) on depression and loss; and the work of Kempe & Kempe (1978) on the psychopathological roots of child abuse). There has been a proliferation of therapies derived from psychoanalysis, including different individual therapeutic techniques as well as family and group therapies. His ideas have also influenced work in child development (for example, Kelmer-Pringle 1974, De Mause 1974, Bettleheim 1987), and developmental issues in adulthood, such as crises of mid-life (Jaques 1965, Sheehy 1978, Levinson et al 1974) and of old age (Butler 1963, Erikson 1963). Finally the vast literature on death and dying clearly indicates the influence of psychoanalytic ideas, both implicitly (Kubler-Ross 1972) and explicitly (Parkes 1972, Bowlby 1980).

Psychoanalytic psychology has been the subject of much critical appraisal. The target of much of the criticism has been the methods employed by researchers and clinicians for the gathering of data and the generation of ideas. It has been argued, for example, that psychoanalysis should have no place in a psychological science since it does not lead to refutable hypotheses. Breger (1981) in defence of psychoanalysis suggests that although it does not meet many of the criteria typically associated with scientific endeavour it nevertheless remains a fruitful and valid framework for understanding human experience and behaviour.

Indeed, he goes further and suggests that the problems raised by the relationship between psychoanalysis and science highlight the inadequacies of traditional approaches. Psychoanalytic theory continues to provoke much controversy, but the boldness of Freud's insights have assured his place as a profound thinker, and his doctrines a place in the clinic and as part of our culture. For a review of the scientific status of psychoanalysis, and its relationship to psychology, see, for example, Frosh (1989).

The behavioural model

Attempting to understand human behaviour and experience in a framework which could strictly be referred to as scientific, poses many problems. One attempt to solve these problems, that adopted by the behaviourists, was to limit the field of psychology to 'things that can be observed' (Watson 1931), that is, to behaviour. This was because behaviour was seen as more amenable to the strict application of rigorous scientific method, in particular the tenets of replicability, quantification and objectivity. In this way this model of man sought to formulate laws about behaviour, in particular learning. More recently Skinner (1974) has differentiated between 'methodological behaviourism' (that which is primarily concerned with the scientific study of behaviour) and 'logical or analytical behaviourism' (the philosophical interpretation of that science). During the ascendancy of behaviourism, psychologists were, on the whole, preoccupied with what they considered to be the fundamental problems of human learning.

There are two major paradigms within learning theory, those of classical and operant conditioning. Classical conditioning was originally delineated in an experiment by Pavlov (1955). When a dog salivates in the presence of meat powder this is called an unconditional response since this response is part of the animal's biological endowment. If the presentation of the meat powder is consistently accompanied by, say, a buzzer, the dog will eventually salivate to the sound of the buzzer alone. This is a classically conditioned response, not part of the repertoire the animal was born with, and thought to be a paradigm of much human learning. To this can be added operant conditioning (sometimes called Skinnerian after its discoverer, B. F. Skinner), where the individual has to act or operate upon the environment to produce reinforcement. Reinforcement is a crucial concept in an operant paradigm and is seen as a major determinant of behaviour. The basic and fundamental stance of behaviourism is that behaviour can be understood by relating it to the setting and conditions in which it occurs and to the consequences of the behaviour in those conditions. This approach has provided explanations of both normal and pathological development and has generated a wide range of psychological therapies for the treatment of mental disorders. For a fuller discussion of the theoretical underpinnings of behaviourism and the implications of this perspective for the treatment of mental disorders the reader is referred to the following texts: Hilgard & Bower (1981), Walker (1984), Dickinson (1980), Blackman (1980).

Just as the psychoanalytic model has been the subject of development and revision in the face of new information, so has the behavioural model. In particular there has been increasingly an incorporation of cognitive variables into the model and much greater attention paid to internal mental events, such as the individual's appraisal of situations. The cognitive-behavioural model of development during infancy and early childhood has provided major insights into early styles of learning and the development of early social behaviour and attachment. Much of this work stands as a significant challenge to the work of the psychoanalysts (see, for example, the work of Clarke & Clarke 1976, Schaffer 1977). The development of Bandura's (1977) work on imitation and modelling as an explanation of human learning, has also proved fruitful. In particular, his empirical studies on the development of aggression, on the origins and development of sex roles and on the nature of adolescence have led to a much greater understanding of these issues. Finally, in recent years there has been a vast proliferation of therapies derived from this school of thought, and it is in this area that the relevance to nursing practice is most evident.

The humanistic and existential model

A number of strands contributed to this point of view. One was the philosophical movements of existentialism and phenomenology. In contrast to 'Anglo-Saxon' philosophy which has tended to be concerned with problems of logic and linguistic analysis; existentialism, a more continental development, was concerned with the dilemmas of existence: the choices we face in our everyday lives and the sincerity with which we cope with them. Such writers as Bertrand Russell typify the former approach and Jean-Paul Sartre the latter.

Phenomenology, essentially the product of Edmund Husserl, attempted to concentrate philosophy on the analysis of mental phenomena, rather than, say, the relationship between logic and mathematics. These two strands, then, provided a powerful boost from philosophy to any social science to consider the nature of human existence, rather than to concern itself with elaborate abstract models. In psychology they were to interact with 'self-theory', that is a movement which reacted against what was seen as Freud's exaggeration of the importance of the id instincts to the detriment of the ego. This gave rise to what is sometimes referred to in psychology as the 'third force' (to contrast it with behaviourism and psychoanalysis, the two predominant theoretical frameworks at that time). This movement is a heterogeneous collection of theories and therapies which share a common concern for human suffering, human dilemmas and human experience, which they see as being at the forefront of their endeavour. Their view of academic psychology is that its preoccupation with method and scientific respectability has led it to displace its subject from the centre of the stage.

Humanistic or existential psychology concerns itself with such notions as the importance of the will, of responsibility for one's actions, and 'reciprocal determinism', which is the view that one affects one's environment as much as one is affected by it. Further, the positive aspects of living are stressed in such terms as 'self-actualization', rather than the libido-dominated theories of analysis or the passive conditioned reflexes of behaviourism. This concentration on human experience is accompanied by a revolt against what is seen as the naive determinism of the alternatives.

Because of its heterogeneous nature, humanistic psychology is hard to exemplify. A central concept is the self, which is grounded in values, either acquired from our own experience, or 'introjected' or absorbed from others, in which latter case the danger of mis-labelling our true nature can arise. The emphasis is on experience, feelings and perceptions, which may be deep, vivid and accurate if the self is integrated, and to be contrasted with the 'divided self' as described by Laing (1965) where experience is blunted, perceptions distorted and growth slowed or halted. Theorists such as Maslow (1968, 1971) have argued for a 'hierarchy of needs' holding that deficiency motives such as food, drink, safety, affiliation, affection, acceptance and approval need to be met before growth motives, such as understanding, the appreciation of beauty and, most particularly, self-actualization, can occur. This is not to say that the self-actualized individual may not experience conflicts and problems, anxieties and guilts, but rather that such problems arise from growth, and not deficiency motivation.

Fear of dying, the concept of responsibility and the importance of the will are central to the existential approach. Feeling that we are special is a coping strategy to enable us to deal with the appreciation of our own mortality. For example, 'workaholics' may believe that they have a special contribution to make and that they are irreplaceable. Fusion is another strategy: by joining clubs, groups or marrying we attempt to diffuse our fear of isolation and individual obliteration. More generally, behaving authentically, rather than, for example, behaving merely in order to please others, is advocated. Further, we should accept responsibility for our own actions, feelings and lives, and we should be aware of the ways in which language leads us to deny this. (We typically say, for example, 'It broke' rather than 'I broke it'). And our will comes into play in terms of the goals we set ourselves; we should take risks and suffer the pain of finding out what we really want and then doing it.

The cognitive model

Three different strands have become interwoven in what is loosely referred to as 'cognitive psychology'. Firstly, there is the development of a branch of academic psychology devoted to the understanding of thinking, and using computer programs as its principal metaphor. There is a distinction between the systems analyst/computer programmer on the one hand, who is concerned with the 'software' or programs which computers execute, and the electronics engineer on the other, with an interest in 'hardware', that is, the machinery of the computer which enables it to execute programs. This distinction is paralleled in psychology where the biological approach is concerned with the central nervous and endocrine systems (the 'hardware', the province of the physiological psychologist). The cognitive psychologist is concerned with the mind and how it functions; this may be thought of in terms of 'software'.

From this viewpoint the human being is thought of as an 'information-processing-device': just as computers receive, store, transform and retrieve information, so do humans. This approach is concerned with modelling human behaviour in terms of computer programs or similar well-specified procedures, and as such is of limited interest to the nurse. It should not be confused with the use of computers as diagnostic aids or information storing and retrieving methods, which clearly can aid nurses a great deal.

Secondly is the particular development within behaviour therapy which includes what is now often referred to as 'cognitive-behaviour therapy'. Reacting to the limitations of behaviourism in a clinical setting, some psychologists, notably Beck (1976) and Ellis (1979), elaborated on the idea of changing cognitions by manipulating behaviour, or indeed by directly confronting the defective cognitions themselves. For an expansion of this see the section below on 'therapies'.

Finally there is the cognitive-developmental approach associated with the work of Piaget (1952) and Kohlberg (1968). This approach focused on the way in which man's capacity to reason about the world changed throughout childhood and adolescence, and examined the development of thinking itself. The acquisition of logical categories, the development of morality, and, more recently, and initially associated with Chomsky (1972), the acquisition of language, have been examined. Language is a case in point where the contrast with behaviourism could not be more marked; what is acquired by the child is not a set of discrete responses associated with environmental 'triggers', where no recourse to mental entities is necessary, but rather an organized body of knowledge which is 'rule-bound'; that is, strategies enabling children to generate sentences they have never heard before, are acquired. Indeed, in part they are 'wired-in' (being part of what Chomsky called the 'Language Acquisition Device'), and have a common substrate in all languages. To understand this system one must have recourse to what is inferred to be going on in the mind, and this is a feature of contemporary cognitive psychology. Some of the mystery involved in this has been removed by the information-processing or computer analogy; what is important in the understanding of the functioning of a computer program (surely much simpler than a mind) is manifestly not its component parts, since different hardware can execute the same program, nor its 'responses' as a biological psychologist or a behaviourist respectively might see it, but the logic of its operations. What such an approach seems to leave out of account is what psychoanalysis was concerned to treat, namely, the realm of feeling.

Thus we can see that three psychological approaches concern themselves with broadly defined psychologic processes. Behaviourism is concerned with what we do, psychoanalysis with what we feel, and cognitive psychology with how we think. A more refined examination shows that it is not so simple: cognitive developments of behaviourism deal with how thoughts affect behaviour; psychoanalysis is also concerned with how we think about our feelings (even giving rise to the view in some quarters that it is a theory of thought); and 'hot' cognition is an attempt to introduce affect into information-processing approaches.

PSYCHOLOGICAL ASSESSMENT

Psychological assessment plays an important role in many areas of applied psychology, especially clinical, educational and occupational, as well as being an important research tool. Before carrying out any kind of psychological assessment it should always be clear to those involved the purpose of the tests and the ways in which the test results can be incorporated into planned interventions. Thus, for example, in psychiatry, detailed assessments should normally be carried out in the context of an overall treatment strategy. This can be interpreted as a plea against any attempt at routinization of testing.

The role of the clinical psychologist

In psychiatry, assessment of patients' problems may be undertaken by a range of personnel, but the systematic use of psychological tests, questionnaires and inventories is normally only undertaken within the health services by a clinical psychologist. A clinical psychologist is an individual who has carried out undergraduate studies in psychology and who has subsequently undertaken postgraduate training, both academic and practical, in clinical psychology. In the early days clinical psychologists were appointed to devise objective techniques of clinical assessment and subsequently apply them when psychiatrists encountered problems of differential diagnosis. At the time of the development of the profession there were few clear guidelines with regard to tasks, roles and responsibilities, and this continues to be the case. However, the work nowadays carried out by clinical psychologists is far more wide ranging, with responsibilities for research, assessment, therapy, training and teaching (including an important commitment to the teaching of psychiatric nurses). They have responsibility for a broad client group, including acute psychiatric patients, long-stay psychiatric patients, the care and assessment of disturbed children, mentally handicapped children and adults, and increasingly they are assuming responsibility for a wide range of patients in a general medical setting, dealing with the psychological sequelae of a number of acute and chronic medical conditions. They are generally employed by health authorities to work either in the community or in a hospital, though increasingly local authority social service departments are also employing them. For a fuller description of the role and responsibilities of clinical psychologists, the reader is referred to Liddell (1978).

Psychological tests

There exist a wide range of psychological tests which structure the process of assessment. Statistical norms for these tests were established during their development by the repeated administration of the tests to many people at different times. This process is called standardization, and once it has been carried out responses of individual patients can then be compared to the standardized norms in order to provide diagnostic information that should be both reliable and valid. Several types of psychological tests have been developed reflecting both differences in psychological orientation and differences in the kind of problem under scrutiny. They include: projective tests, personality inventories, tests of organic brain damage, tests of intelligence and behavioural assessment.

Projective tests

This group of tests reflects a psychoanalytic orientation to assessment. The subject is required to respond to vague and ambiguous material which permits wide variation in response. It is assumed, because the stimulus material is unstructured, that the subject's responses are largely determined by unconscious processes and will reveal deep-seated attitudes, motivations, fears and desires. Not only must the subject provide interpretations of the material, but also the assessor must subsequently interpret those responses. The main types of techniques in use include: responding to highly ambiguous stimuli such as the Rorschach Inkblot Test (Rorschach 1921), sentence completion (Holsopple 1955), pictorial techniques, such as the TAT and the CAT (Bellak 1954), where the patient is required to describe fully a vague and ambiguous picture, and a range of play techniques, used with children, such as the Family Relations Test (Bene & Antony 1959).

Personality inventories

These are standardized tests which present a range of statements, typically descriptions of self, to the patient, who is required to indicate whether they do or do not apply. It is rare that these tests lack reliability but problems may exist with regard to their validity, that is, the extent to which they provide an accurate measure of whatever it is they set out to assess. Inventories tend to be used to facilitate diagnosis by providing both further evidence of the extent to which the individual is disturbed and a more precise description of that disturbance. This may be reflected in a score, a profile, or may include descriptive terminology. There are many of these in common use, for example the Eysenck Personality Inventory (Eysenck & Edwards 1964).

Tests of organic brain damage

A wide battery of tests has been designed to facilitate the diagnosis of organic brain dysfunction, and the weight of evidence suggests that they are useful (see, for example, Lezak 1983). The assessment of an individual patient often involves the use of wide range of tests in an attempt to ascertain not only the extent of the damage but also that exact location of the area of the brain affected. Common tests in use at the moment include, for example, the Halstead-Reitan Neuropsychological Test Battery, the Luria-Nebraska Neuropsychological Test Battery and the Michigan Neuropsychological Test Battery. There is debate currently in the field of neuropsychological assessment about whether it is preferable to adopt an individualized approach or whether one should administer a uniform battery for all patients. The obvious advantage of using a standard battery of tests is the comprehensiveness of this approach. However, a serious disadvantage of batteries is that they may be providing redundancy of information in some areas of functioning, whilst achieving insufficiency of information in others. For a fuller description of tests of organic brain damage, and contemporary debates about their use, the reader is referred to the following texts: Golden (1978), Hersen et al (1983), Mittler (1974) and Anastasi (1976).

Intelligence tests

The use of intelligence tests in a clinical rather than an educational setting plays an important role in the diagnosis of mental handicap in providing significant information about the abilities of patients, which is especially important when planning care and rehabilitation, and may be useful as a preliminary tool in the assessment of brain damage and dementia. As with all tests, intelligence tests should be used with humility and should not, is isolation, be regarded as a final statement on the intellectual ability and potential of the patient. The most frequently used intelligence test is the Wechsler Adult Intelligence Scale.

Behavioural assessment

As well as carrying out specific psychological tests, clinical psychologists may also be involved in behavioural assessment. This includes a range of techniques which have been developed within a behaviourist tradition, and thus largely reflects the underlying ideology of that school of thought. These techniques include direct observation of behaviour (in real life as well as in contrived, experimental conditions), role-playing, and self-reports of likely responses in invented or real situations. A range of physiological measurements may also be taken as part of a behavioural assessment; these include heart rate, conductivity of the skin, tension in the muscles and blood flow in various parts of the body.

PSYCHOLOGICAL THERAPIES

Though the contours of psychiatric disorders vary greatly there are nonetheless common themes and features, such as misery, anxiety and anger. The presenting picture may be one of fear, tension, and even panic, of loneliness, isolation, unhappiness and despair, of guilt and self-punishment or contempt for others. Mental disorders vary in extent from a vague expression of general unhappiness and dissatisfaction to the experience of excruciating torment. Sometimes there is a veneer of coping, belying an inner world of psychological turmoil and discontent; or there might be an outward expression of madness. It is likely, with such wide disparities in the clinical picture and aetiological background of mental disorders, that appropriate and useful therapeutic interventions will take a variety of forms. Whatever form psychological therapy takes, it is likely to provide help in the following ways: the provision of an emotional cushion at the time of crisis, clarification of the nature of the problem, and the removal of any external agents which may be aggravating the problem. Essential to all therapies, and irrespective of the type of therapy offered, is the effect of the relationship between patient and therapist. The main parameters of this relationship, trust, safeness and rapport, all combine to play an important role in the outcome of therapy.

In psychiatry, the definition of therapeutic success is fraught with problems. It is usually not possible to talk of 'cure' in the sense that this is often used in other medical fields. Kovel (1978), in discussing this issue, describes the promise of a dramatic breakthrough in the following terms, 'as tedious and old fashioned as the tidings of a new Messiah or the miracle at Lourdes'. If reference to 'cures' or dramatic breakthroughs is not normally a helpful or useful aim of therapy, what then might usefully be regarded as an appropriate expectation of therapeutic success? For most people it implies gradual and positive change, which may mean coming to terms with life's losses and tragedies, increasing self-understanding, forming new relationships, freedom from distorted perceptions or persistent thoughts and more generally assuming greater control in both personal and professional aspects of life.

Different schools of thought within psychology have generated a range of therapies which can be divided into the following categories: analytic therapies, post-analytic therapies, group and family therapies, behaviour therapies and cognitive-behavioural therapies.

Analytic therapies

Freud can be regarded as the progenitor of modern psychotherapy, for not only do all the analytic schools derive directly from his ideas, but also many of the non-analytic schools owe much of their impetus to ideas introduced by him. Psychoanalysis was the therapy developed by Freud and can be seen as a direct application of his principles of human development in a clinical setting. Much emphasis is laid upon infantile sexuality and dynamically repressed unconscious mental processes. In this model, anxiety, generated by unconscious conflict, is seen as at least psychologically debilitating or at worst, highly destructive. The main goal of psychoanalysis is to gain insight into the childhood orgins of distress and the basic rule is to say whatever comes to mind (referred to as free-association). Psychoanalysis takes place through the interpretation of material brought forward in this manner, by attention to resistance, that is, blocks in the path revealing unconscious mental life, and transference, that is, the reliving of significant past conflicts in the safety of the analytic setting. The special circumstances of the analytic situation — of understanding, safety and non-judgement — facilitate both an airing and a reliving of past experiences, a crucial part in the process of freeing oneself from past emotional shackles. The aims of psychoanalysis are not radical in the sense of 'cure', but rather in Freud's terms, 'to succeed in transforming neurotic misery into common unhappiness. With a mental life restored to health you will be better armed against that unhappiness'.

Psychoanalysis has been revised both by Freud's contemporaries (e.g. Jung and Adler) as well as by later followers, for example the Neo-Freudians such as Rank, Horney, Stack-Sullivan and Fromm; and by the 'British School' (e.g. Klein and Winnicott). It can also be seen as a major influence on the more existential work of Rollo May and Laing.

Post-analytic therapies (the Human Potential movement)

Those authors who revised and developed Freud's ideas in their own ways have themselves been the subject of further revisions and developments. For example Gestalt therapy, developed in the 1960s by Fritz Perls (1973), was largely influenced by the earlier work of Reich and Jung. Rogerian therapy, developed in the 1950s and 60s by the American Carl Rogers, was a highly individual approach to therapy, yet as Kovel (1978) suggests, reflects, 'a typical blend of American pragmatism and optimistic faith in the individual'. Rogers' basic contention was that what humans require from birth is to be granted 'unconditional positive regard', that is, they should be valued in and for themselves, and not only conditionally upon behaviour or performance. Such unconditional affection will in turn allow them to develop 'unconditional positive self-regard'. They will develop a robust belief in themselves and this self-esteem will enable them to overcome those situations where their ideal for themselves does not accord with the facts — the diligent student, for example, who fails an examination. Such eventualities, Rogers argues, give rise to 'incongruity' (between the ideal self and experience) and positive unconditional self-regard helps the individual to cope with it.

If there has been a lack of unconditional positive regard from parents, for example, the child is unlikely to develop unconditional positive self-regard, and hence the perceived incongruity will be greater, leading potentially to disorganized behaviour, distorted perceptions and devaluation of self.

The task for the therapist is to supply what was missing, to provide the 'client' with the approval he previously lacked, and so to create 'conditions of worth' in which he can develop self-esteem. Despite the idealistic and utopian sound of much of this, Rogers has to be given credit for trying to codify his practice (by the use of videos and the like) in order to be able to transmit his techniques, and for having carried out extensive outcome evaluations. Neither of these things has in general been done by others of the humanistic persuasion, who tend to feel that their activity is its own justification.

During the 1960s the United States of America, in particular, witnessed the proliferation of group techniques: for example, Encounter Groups (influenced by psychoanalysis, Rogerian and Gestalt therapies); and Transactional Analysis (developed by Eric Berne in 1968). Many of these approaches have been linked together under the umbrella term 'The Human Potential Movement', or the 'Growth Movement'. What they all have in common is that they attempt to provide an altered life experience with peers and a leader or guide who directly affect the individual and render him more psychologically 'open' and more emotionally honest. These group techniques are further addressed in the next section.

Group and family therapies

So far the stress has been on individual therapy, but this can prove expensive, both in terms of money and therapist and patient time. One of the driving forces behind group approaches was the desire to economize; if patients could be treated effectively in groups, then a considerable saving would be achieved. Another idea which led to this approach was that most significant behaviour is social: actions occurring between two or more people. It therefore seemed sensible to try to treat people in a group setting, where processes that might only occur in such a setting could be examined.

Group therapy is characterized by a range of theoretical orientations which have in common the use of group processes to deal with psychological issues. These issues are most likely to be psychological problems, but groups are also concerned with personal growth, support, even companionship. Groups can in theory help with most problems in which individual therapy might be efficacious, provided that the individual accepts the group and an appropriate one is available (see Levine 1979 for an expansion of this argument). And the factors presumed to be curative in a group have been summarized by Yalom (1975) as the following: the imparting of information; instilling hope; universality — learning that others have similar problems; altruism — demoralized individuals learn that they can help others; interpersonal learning; modelling; a chance to work out with a surrogate family conflicts that were not resolved the first time; catharsis — the open expression of feelings; and group cohesiveness. Individuals may also gain greater self-awareness through role-reversal and role-playing in a group setting.

Encounter groups can be seen as an extension of group therapy applied in non-psychopathological settings, although they developed from training-groups ('T-Groups') devised for reducing racial tension. Kurt Lewin was the originator of this project, believing that groups were potent arenas for improving problem-solving skills and interpersonal relationships. More generally, encounter groups are held to facilitate growth and change, the realization of an individual's potential, heightened self-awareness, and richer and more accurate perceptions and feelings (Stoller 1970, Korchin 1976). Encounter groups have as their aim to present people with a degree of emotional intensity that is rarely, if ever, 'encountered' in normal life — we use all sorts of evasions to avoid confronting each other with naked affection or aggression. It is assumed that such confrontation can lead to the sorts of change referred to above, but clearly there are dangers — psychological defences built up over a lifetime are hardly going to disappear after a weekend's haranguing. Also, there can be casualties of this immersion in emotional intensity, so that the leadership of such a group is critical; one of the biggest dangers being 'scapegoating', or picking on one individual on whom the group vents its collective anger, frustration and tension.

Marathon-groups carry this logic further, where 24 or even 30 hours of intensity are tolerated — the rationale being that fatigue may lead to the dropping of defences and the emergence of more spontaneous and authentic behaviour.

In all group settings, the individual must trust the group in order to make the sort of disclosures that are often demanded. Social groups may model the family in more ways than one: they might be a crushing or inhibiting influence to some. All group therapy, however, assumes that change is most usefully brought about in a social setting. For a discussion of marathon groups see Schwartz & Schwartz (1969); and for a more general evaluation of group approaches see Lieberman (1975).

The family is such a social group, and indeed can be seen as the prototype and progenitor of all such groups. For example, it is with its parents initially, and then with siblings, that a child first begins to understand the give and take of social interactions, the overt and covert 'rules' of such exchanges, such as turn-taking in conversation. Therefore some therapists felt that the family, or a significant part of it, rather than the individual, should be treated. It might be possible to produce considerable improvement in an individual's functioning, but if the family 'require' him to behave in a particular way — as a scapegoat, for example — then as soon as the individual is returned to them he is liable to revert to pre-treatment behaviour. The problem of relapse following discharge home has received considerable attention, in particular the undermining effects of high levels of expressed emotion and critical attitudes in the family.

Two approaches to family therapy will be described briefly: conjoint and structured. In conjoint therapy the therapist attempts to understand the communications of the family, ultimately with the aim of ensuring that families can communicate clearly, specifically, directly, and with consensus. The therapist attempts to ensure that each member is seen, heard, and understood, and that each individual can give and accept feedback without it being punitive. Further, it is intended that family decisions provide for the needs and wants of each individual, their uniqueness being valued, and that the differences between individuals is used for growth rather than as a barrier to understanding. For a fuller account see McPeak (1979).

Minuchin (1974) has argued for a more active role in the family than the above. It is not enough, he maintains, to examine the communications in a clinical setting, but preferably to see them in their natural setting. Thus advocates of the structured approach will join in family activities rather than examine or reconstruct them in the clinic. Mealtimes, it is argued, provide a wealth of information as to the interactions and perceptions that are going on.

Another approach to family therapy is represented by the 'Milan' school (it being first founded there), where systems theory is applied to analysis. Each family is seen as a functional system, where every interaction is part of a self-supporting complex of interactions or systems. The therapist's task is to identify the functional components of the system, to enable the protagonists to understand what they are doing for and to each other, and by using techniques like 'paradoxical intervention' (where an insight at odds with the clients' usual view of their relationship is presented), the therapist attempts to produce constructive movement. For a brief but wide-ranging introduction to family therapy see Kovel (1978).

Behaviour therapies

A range of therapies were developed in the 1950s and 60s that derived from a radically different tradition in psychology. Behaviourism and, more specifically, the psychology of learning generated a number of treatments. In contrast to most schools of thought, behaviourists do not regard behavioural abnormalities as symptomatic of underlying pathology, but see them essentially as the problem. This philosophy can be illustrated by the remark made by Eysenck 'if you get rid of the symptom. . . . you have eliminated the neurosis'.

Behaviour therapy was developed initially in the USA, but was readily embraced by psychologists in Britain who were eager to develop a range of therapies that were distinctly psychological and which adhered to scientific rigour, which was stressed in their approach to the discipline. Although there are a number of different techniques, deriving from different paradigms within the psychology of learning, what all behaviour therapies have in common is the emphasis laid upon the role of the environment in maintaining and reinforcing abnormal behaviour. This can be contrasted, for example, with the psychoanalytic model which emphasizes the significance of events occurring in early infancy and childhood as important determinants of adult pathology.

A useful distinction within this approach to therapy, which has been discussed by McKay (1974), is between those who are primarily interested in developing and utilizing a range of behavioural 'packages' (such as, for example, systematic desensitization, flooding, response prevention, token economy or aversion therapy) and those who are more concerned with the assessment of individual pathology, and who use a range of behavioural approaches, cognitive therapies and counselling. This latter approach is referred to as 'behavioural psychotherapy'.

The criticisms of this approach, and the consequent revisions and developments that have taken place, can be seen in terms of the merging of two main lines of argument. Firstly, radical behaviourism, as a school of thought within psychology, became increasingly the subject of critical review and appraisal. New developments and evidence in academic psychology, in particular in developmental psychology, cognitive psychology and information processing, could not be readily accommodated within this model, and raised major doubts about the underlying assumptions of this approach. Many authors increasingly questioned the failure of behaviourists to look beyond the presenting behavioural pathology, either in understanding the nature and development of that pathology or in the treatment of it.

Secondly, a number of criticisms were increasingly voiced in clinical settings as a consequence of the implementation of insensitive behavioural programmes. These doubts reflected both ethical and therapeutic concerns, although were not necessarily attacks upon the basic tenets of behaviour therapy. Blackman (1980), for example, an advocate of academic behaviourism, suggested that, 'the enthusiastic advocacy of the techniques of behaviour modification by some who have an unduly crude and ill-formulated view of contemporary behaviourism is likely to result in insensitive programmes. It is probably inevitable that professions such as nursing and teaching will turn to behaviour modification merely as a set of effective techniques.'

Cognitive-behavioural therapies

The cognitive approach in therapy is an outgrowth from, as well as a reaction to, behaviourism, and hence has given rise to the notion of 'cognitive-behavioural' therapy. Behaviourism tried to exclude mental events from its brief; the lack of a lever on what was mediating the connection between environmental stimuli and responses led behaviour therapists to introduce these 'mediating variables', perceiving them to be false or destructive cognitions which could lead to maladaptive behaviour. The basic assumptions of this point of view are threefold: firstly, that cognitive processes are causal, that is, our thoughts are not merely 'epiphenomena' accompanying neurophysiological activity. The second assumption is that disordered cognitive processes can cause some psychological disorders; while the third is that changing faulty cognitions can alleviate such disorders.

Such cognitive processes may be in the form of expectations, appraisals or attributions, all of which may vary along a number of dimensions. For example, an individual might expect to fail an examination because his view of his own efficacy is low. If he did fail, he might attribute this to his own stupidity, which can be seen as an internal, stable and global attribution; or to the fact that the room was too warm — an external, transient and specific attribution.

More crucial for psychopathology in the view of such psychologists as Beck and Ellis are long-term cognitive processes or beliefs. Ellis (1979) in the development of his particular treatment, rational-emotive therapy, has propounded the notion that such unconscious beliefs can cause maladaptive behaviour; he terms these 'irrational beliefs' as they do not correspond with reality. These might be of the following form: 'Everyone should love me; I must be competent, adequate and achieving at all times; I am worthless and it is a catastrophe if I am not', and the like. This he has referred to as the 'tyranny of the shoulds', and one of the tasks of the cognitive-behavioural therapist is to correct such distorted cognitions, by encouraging reality-testing and by outright confrontation. The therapist will attack such irrational beliefs directly, and at the same time address the second task, of training new and more productive habits, by cajoling or even bullying the patient into behaviour which will invalidate irrational beliefs. An excellent account of rational-emotive therapy is provided by Dryden & Golden (1987).

Arnold Lazarus is one extreme example of an eclectic approach where more or less all of the above are mobilized by the therapist as deemed necessary. Lazarus has advocated 'multimodal therapy' where insight, behaviour modification, modelling, cognitive restructuring and, where appropriate, drug treatments, are all used (Lazarus 1981).

A number of authors have noted the difficulties in attempting to compare and contrast the different approaches to therapy (see, for example, Kovel 1978). Outcome studies and comparisons of success rates of different therapies are fraught with problems. This situation is likely to pose difficulties for the clinician, especially the training clinician who may be seeking to establish a particular therapeutic style and orientation. The repercussions for the psychiatric patient, or prospective psychiatric patient, are likely to be far greater, presenting what may appear to be a bewildering and perplexing picture of treatment strategies.

Since different approaches to therapy derive from different models in psychology, the underlying assumptions are often at cross purposes and the language very different. Even the aims of therapy are not comparable. For some, 'cure' is a most inappropriate concept. Those, on the other hand, who define the pathology in terms of observable behaviours, may find it a useful concept, synonymous with the elimination of maladaptive behaviours. Nor do outcome studies give a clear indication about the relative efficacy of different approaches. Indeed there is evidence to suggest that irrespective of the particular therapy adopted the quality of the therapist is most important. Kovel (1978) suggests that the successful therapist must possess certain characteristics. She must be able to make sense of what is going on psychologically; be attuned to communications; be able to adapt to changing circumstances without losing identity or purpose; and most essential of all, care in a mature manner for the well-being of the patient.

CONCLUSION

With the increasing professionalization of psychiatric nursing there has been a concomitant increase in the demands made on the psychiatric nurse. A review of the literature reveals an emphasis on the broad scope of the work and the wide-ranging expectations inherent in the role (see, for example, Altschul & Simpson 1977, Cormack 1983, Baker 1976, Maddison et al 1975). The psychiatric nurse is expected to have adequate knowledge of psychiatric disorders since identification and assessment of patient behaviour are significant prerequisites to the planning and implementation of nursing care. The psychiatric nurse is also required to possess a range of technical skills for the physical care of patients, and psychotherapeutic skills facilitating interpersonal communication and counselling. The nurse–patient relationship, characterized, according to Maddison et al (1975), by nursing attitudes of acceptance, reliability, responsibility, humility and professionalism, is an important therapeutic tool, but in order to use it effectively the nurse must be well informed. Psychiatric nursing, like a number of other medical and non-medical professions, requires a multi-disciplinary knowledge base. It draws upon a range of theories and empirical data developed in the context of various academic disciplines within the biological and social sciences. Psychology, thus viewed, is one of the major disciplines, contributing to the knowledge base of psychiatric nursing, and can be seen as providing information relevant to each stage of the nursing process. Altschul & Simpson (1977) suggest that psychiatric nursing is concerned with the promotion of mental health, the prevention of mental disorder and the nursing care of patients who suffer from mental disorders. Psychology provides theory and evidence relevant to all these areas. It provides normative data on the nature of human growth and development (both cognitive and emotional aspects), on healthy modes of interaction and on healthy coping strategies in the face of stress (especially the stresses inherent in facing significant separations and losses). It provides theoretical models which facilitate an understanding of the ways in which psychopathology occurs and in which care can be organized. In addition to this it may be seen as providing information which helps nurses to understand themselves and their relationships better, both with colleagues and patients. It may also help them to understand more clearly the constraints of the setting in which they work, including the ideological constraints of the medical model in which much psychiatric care is organized, the physical constraints of the often oppressive atmosphere of the large ward in an old-fashioned hospital, and the organizational and bureaucratic constraints of the profession in which they work.

REFERENCES

Adler G 1948 Studies in analytic psychology. Routledge, London

Altschul A 1975 Psychology for nurses. Ballière Tindall, London

Altschul A, Simpson R 1977 Psychiatric nursing. Balliere Tindall, London

Anastasi A 1976 Psychological testing. Macmillan, Basingstoke

Baker A A 1976 Comprehensive psychiatric care. Blackwell, Oxford

Bandura A 1971 Social learning theory. Prentice-Hall, Englewood Cliffs, NJ

Bateson G, Jackson P, Haley J, Weakland J 1956 Toward a theory of schizophrenia. Behavioural Science 1: 251–264

Beck 1976 Cognitive therapy and the emotional disorders. International University Press, New York

Bellack C 1954 The Thematic Apperception Test and the Children's Apperception Test in clinical use. Grune & Stratton, New York

Bene E, Antony E J 1959 The family relations' test manual. National Foundation for Educational Research, London

Berne E 1968 Games people play: the psychology of human relations. Penguin, Harmondsworth

Bettleheim B 1987 The good enough parent. Thames, London.

Blackman D 1980 Images of man in contemporary behaviourism. In: Chapman A J, Jones D M (eds) Models of man. British Psychological Society, Leicester

Bolton N (ed) 1979 Philosophical problems in psychology. Methuen, London

Bowlby J 1965 Child care and the growth of love, 2nd edn. Penguin, Harmondsworth

Bowlby J 1969 Attachment and loss. Volume 1 Attachment. Hogarth, London

Bowlby J 1973 Attachment and loss. Volume 2 Separation: anxiety and anger. Hogarth, London

Bowlby J 1980 Attachment and loss. Volume 3 Loss: sadness and depression. Hogarth, London

Breger L 1981 Freud's unfinished journey: conventional and critical perspectives in psychoanalytic theory. Routledge, London

Bruch H 1978 The golden cage: the enigma of anorexia nervosa. Fontana, London

Butler R N 1963 The life review: an interpretation of reminiscence in the aged. In: Allman L R, Jaffe D T (eds) Readings in adult psychology: contemporary perspectives. Harper & Row, New York

Carlson N R 1981 The physiology of behaviour, 2nd edn. Allyn & Bacon, Boston

Chomsky N 1972 Language and mind, enlarged edn. Harcourt Brace Jovanovich, New York

Clare A 1980 Psychiatry in dissent, 2nd edn. Tavistock, London

Clerke A M, Clerke A D B 1976 Early experience: myth and evidence. Fontana, London

Conrad P, Schneider J W 1980 Deviance and medicalization. Mosby, London

Cormack D 1983 Psychiatric nursing described. Churchill Livingstone, Edinburgh

De Mause L 1974 The history of childhood. Souvenir Press, London

Dickinson A 1980 Contemporary animal learning theory. Cambridge University Press, Cambridge

Dryden W, Golden W L 1987 Cognitive-behavioural approaches to psychotherapy. Hemisphere, London

Ellis A 1979 The theory of rational-emotive therapy. In: Ellis A, Whitely J M (eds) Theoretical and empirical foundation of rational-emotive therapy. Brooks/Cole, Monterey, California

Erikson E 1963 Childhood and society, 2nd edn. Penguin, Harmondsworth

Eysenck H J, Edwards S 1964 Eysenck personality inventory. National Foundation for Educational Research, Nelson, Windsor

Fromm E 1957 The art of loving. Allen & Unwin, London

Fromm E 1974 The anatomy of human destructiveness. Cape, London

Frosh S 1989 Psychoanalysis and psychology. Macmillan, London

Golden C J 1978 Diagnosis and rehabilitation in clinical neuropsychology. Thomas, Springfield, Illinois

Hall J 1982 Psychology for nurses and health visitors. British Psychological Society, Leicester

Hersen M, Kazdin A E, Bellack A S 1983 The clinical psychology handbook. Pergamon, Oxford

Hilgard E R, Bower G H 1981 Theories of learning, 5th edn. Prentice-Hall, Englewood Cliffs, New Jersey

Holsopple J Q 1955 Sentence completion: a projective method for the study of personality. Thomas, Springfield, Illinois

Horney K 1939 New ways in psychoanalysis. Kegan Paul, London

Hornykiewicz O 1982 Brain catecholamines in schizophrenia — a good case for noradrenaline. Nature 299: 484–486

Husserl E 1980 Ideas pertaining to a pure phenomenology and to a phenomenological philosophy. 3rd book: Phenomenology and the foundations of the sciences. Translated by Klein T E, Pohl W E. Nijhoff, The Hague

Illich I 1977 Limits to medicine. Pelican, Harmondsworth

Ingleby D 1981 Critical psychiatry. Penguin, Harmondsworth

Jaques E 1965 Death and the mid-life crisis. International Journal of Psychoanalysis, October

Jung C G 1968 Analytic psychology: its theory and practice. In: Barker M, Game M (eds) The Tavistock lectures. Routledge & Kegan Paul, London

Karon B P, Vanderbos G R 1981 Psychotherapy of schizophrenia: treatment of choice. Jason Aronson, New York

Kelmer-Pringle M 1974 The needs of children. Hutchinson, London

Kempe R S, Kempe C H 1978 Child abuse. Fontana, London

Klein M 1975 Envy and gratitude and other works 1946–1963 Hogarth. Institute of Psychoanalysis, London

Kolb B, Wishaw I 1990 Fundamentals of human neuropsychology. Freeman, New York

Kohlberg L 1973 The child as moral philosopher. Psychology Today 2(4): 25–30

Korchin S K 1976 Modern clinical psychology. Basic Books, New York

Kovel J 1978 A complete guide to therapy: from psychoanalysis to behaviour modification. Penguin, Harmondsworth

Kubler-Ross E 1972 On death and dying. In: Allman L R, Jaffe D T (eds) Readings in adult psychology: contemporary perspectives. Harper & Row, New York

Kuhn T 1970 The structure of scientific revolutions. University of Chicago Press, Chicago

Laing R D 1970 The divided self. Penguin, Harmondsworth

Lazarus A A 1981 The practice of multi-modal therapy: systematic, comprehensive, and effective psychotherapy. McGraw Hill, New York

Levine B 1976 Group psychotherapy: practice and development. Prentice-Hall, Englewood-Cliffs, New Jersey

Levinson D, Klein E B, Levinson M H, McKee B 1974 The psychosocial development of men in early adulthood and the mid-life transition. In: Ricks D F, Thomas A, Roff M (eds) Life history research in psychopathology. University of Minnesota Press, Minneapolis, MN

Lewin K 1964 Field theory in social science: selected theoretical papers. Harper & Row, London

Lezak D 1983 Neuropsychological assessment. Oxford University Press, Oxford

Liddell A 1978 The practice of clinical psychology in Great Britain. Wiley, London

Lidz T 1974 Family studies and a theory of schizophrenia. In: Cancro R (ed) The Schizophrenic Syndrome 13. Brunner Mazel, New York

Lidz T 1976 The person: his and her development throughout the life cycle. Basic Books, New York

Lieberman M A 1975 Group methods. In: Kanfer F H, Goldstein A P (eds) Helping people change. Pergamon, New York

Lloyd P, Mayes A, Manstead A S R, Mendell P R, Wagner H L 1984 Introduction to psychology: an integrated approach. Fontana, London

McGhie A 1973 Psychology as applied to nursing. Churchill Livingstone, Edinburgh

McKay D 1974 Clinical psychology: theory and therapy. Methuen, London

McKeown T 1979 The role of medicine: dream, mirage or nemisis? Blackwell, Oxford

McPeak W R 1979 Family therapies. In: Goldstein A P, Kanfer F H (eds) Maximizing treatment gains: transfer enhancement in psychotherapy. Academic Press, New York

Maddison D, Day P, Leadbeater B 1975 Psychiatric nursing. Churchill Livingstone, Edinburgh

Maslow A H 1968 Towards a psychology of being. Van Nostrand, New York

Maslow A H 1971 The farther reaches of human nature. Viking, New York

May R 1981 Freedom and destiny. Norton, London

Miller A 1987 For their own good: the roots of violence in child-rearing. Virago, London

Miller G A 1966 Psychology: the science of mental life. Penguin, Harmondsworth

Milner P M 1971 Physiological psychology. Holt, New York

Minuchin S 1974 Families and family therapy. Harvard University Press, Cambridge, Massachusetts

Mittler P 1974 The psychological assessment of mental and physical handicap. Tavistock, London

Parkes C M 1972 Bereavement. Penguin, Harmondsworth

Parton N 1985 The politics of child abuse. Macmillan, Basingstoke

Pavlov I P 1955 Selected works. Foreign Languages Publishing House, Moscow

Piaget J 1959 The language and thought of the child. Routledge & Kegan Paul, London

Perls F 1973 Gestalt therapy: excitement and growth in the human personality. Penguin, Harmondsworth

Pincus L 1976 Death and the family. Faber & Faber, London

Popper K R 1963 Conjectures and refutations. Routledge, London

Powles J 1973 On the limitations of modern medicine. Science, Medicine and Man 1: 1–30

Price R 1978 Abnormal behaviour: perspectives in conflict, 2nd edn. Holt, New York

Rank O 1973 The trauma of birth. Harper & Row, New York

Reich W 1983 The function of the orgasm: sex-economic problems of biological energy. Translated by Carfagno V R. Souvenir, London

Rogers C R 1973 Encounter groups. Penguin, Harmondsworth

Rorschach H 1921 Rorschach psychodiagnostic test. Grune & Stratton, New York

Sartre J P 1969 Being and nothingness: an essay on phenomenological ontology. Methuen, London

Schaffer H R 1977 Mothering. Fontana, London

Schwartz J J, Schwartz R 1969 Growth encounters. Voices 5: 7–16

Sheehy G 1978 Passages. Bantam Books, London

Siegler M, Osmond H 1966 Models of madness. British Journal of Psychiatry 112: 1193–1203

Skinner B F 1974 About behaviourism. Jonathan Cape, London

Stoller F H 1970 A stage for trust. In: Burton A (ed) Encounter. Jossey-Bass, San Francisco

Szasz T 1961 The myth of mental illness. Harper & Row, New York

Szasz T 1971 The manufacture of madness. Routledge, London

Taylor A, Sluckin W, Davies D R, Reason J T, Thompson R, Coleman A M 1982 Introducing psychology, 2nd edn. Penguin, Harmondsworth

Teyler T J 1978 A Primer of psychobiology. Freeman, Oxford

Thompson R 1968 The Pelican history of psychology. Penguin, Harmondsworth

Walker S 1984 Learning theory and behaviour modification. Methuen, London

Watling L A, Muller P J 1984 Investigating psychology: a practical approach for nursing. Harper & Row, London

Watson J B 1931 Behaviourism, 2nd edn. Kegan, Paul, Trench and Traubner, London

Wechsler D 1971 A British supplement to the manual of the Wechsler Adult Intelligence Scale: incorporating decimal currency items and British amendments to the test administration section. Prepared by Saville P, National Foundation for Educational Research, Nelson, Windsor

Wertheimer M 1979 A brief history of psychology, revised edn. Holt, London

Winnicott D W 1986 Home is where we come from. Penguin, Harmondsworth

Wright D S, Taylor A M, Davies D et al 1970 Introducing psychology: an experimental approach. Penguin, Harmondsworth

Yalom I 1975 The theory and practice of group psychotherapy. Basic Books, New York

Zola I K 1975 Healthism and disabling medicalization. In: Illich I (ed) Disabling professions. Marion Boyars, London

14

The contribution of biological sciences

A. Bond

A relationship between the biological sciences and psychiatry has been historically accepted, although at times it has proved to be a delicate one. The purpose of this chapter is to introduce the reader to a new and exciting era within this relationship. This is a time when new discoveries are occurring at a breathtaking pace, many of which will have important clinical implications for psychiatric nursing in the near future.

EPILEPSY

Because of its varied manifestations, ranging from the classical motor convulsions to a more complex selection of abnormal behaviours and subjective experiences, epilepsy stands between the disciplines of neurology and psychiatry.

The Greeks explained epilepsy as a sacred disease. How else could a healthy person suddenly be thrown to the ground, lose their senses, convulse and return eventually to their former self if they were not invaded by a god? Later in history mad people were labelled 'maniacs' as they were believed to be invaded by evil spirits. The New Testament refers to a 'deaf and dumb spirit' of which Jesus relieves a young man with convulsions (St Mark 9: 17–27).

It was not until the nineteenth century that epilepsy began to be separated from madness, when it became linked with the new discipline of neurology. Hughlings Jackson first described epilepsy in 1873: 'Epilepsy is the name for occasional, sudden, excessive, rapid, local discharges of grey matter.' Jackson realized that this description presented certain complications, as he acknowledged by stating that 'a sneeze is a healthy sort of epilepsy'. In 1890 Jackson announced that he would only 'use the term "epilepsy" for that neurosis which is often called genuine or ordinary epilepsy'. It was not until Berger (1929) used electroencephalography (EEG) to record the electrical rhythms of the brain that Jackson's description was fully supported.

Nowadays, an epileptic attack is accepted as the manifestation of abnormal electrical discharges in some part of the brain, although it is still not fully understood.

Towards the end of this century epilepsy was removed from the national and international classifications of psychiatric illness (Hill 1981) and more recent research has begun to concentrate on the possible contribution of complex biological and psychosocial factors which may affect people with epilepsy.

The genetics of epilepsy have been extensively studied. Although large-scale studies have indicated a genetic contribution, a specific pattern has not yet been identified. Alstrom (1950) suggests that this is hardly surprising, considering that the symptoms of epilepsy may occur in numerous forms of cerebral disorder. Providing precipitating factors are present, a large proportion of the population is capable of having an epileptic attack. This suggests that injury or infection may determine a person's susceptibility to epilepsy, or that there may be a genetic factor influencing a person's susceptibility to epilepsy.

Today it is recognized that if one partner has a normal EEG and a negative family history and the second partner has a focal type of epilepsy, then the risk of a child from that relationship being an epileptic will probably not be more that 1 in 40. However, if one or both partners have a strong familial history of epilepsy then the chances of a child being epileptic will be greatly enhanced.

The generalized epilepsies

During a generalized epileptic attack electrical disturbances derive from the reticular formation and the nuclei of the diffuse thalamic projection system, rapidly spreading to involve all areas of the cerebral cortex, probably at the same moment. This results in a seizure which will present as laterally symmetrical with impaired consciousness from the onset. Evidence of a focal onset, or aura, will not be present, although the person may have complained of an ill-defined malaise before the attack.

The focal epilepsies

The seizure discharge will begin in one part of the cortex. This always implies the presence of a localized brain lesion. Focal symptoms in the form of an aura will precede the seizure. Precise symptomatology will depend on the area of the cortex in which the discharge originates and the direction of its subsequent spread. In conjunction with EEG findings, the aura which precedes the focal epileptic attack can give vital information regarding the site of origin of the disturbance within the cortex. It is possible for an aura to arise without progressing to a full seizure; this can be an indication of a lesion, or may occur when the epilepsy is partially controlled by medication. Other irregular symptoms may be overlooked or misinterpreted. There is always the possibility that a focal epileptic attack may lead to a generalized convulsion.

Jacksonian epilepsy is an example of a focal epilepsy with elementary symptomatology. This occurs when an attack fails to generalize to the remainder of the brain, so 'motor march' may spread down one limb and then recede, while the subject will remain fully conscious. In this instance, if a generalized convulsion does occur it will usually be asymmetrical in distribution, and later may be followed by focal functional defects such as a transient weakness of the affected limb, known as 'Todd's paralysis'.

Temporal lobe epilepsy is a focal epilepsy with complex symptomatology. This type of epilepsy is thought to include about one third of the epilepsies. In the past, much controversy has surrounded temporal lobe epilepsy. The temporal lobe is especially vulnerable to damage, and the psychic content of these discharges renders the subject particularly susceptible to misdiagnosis. Symptomatology can include somatic hallucinations, disturbances of memory, depersonalization and affective disorders. A syndrome has now been proposed that is thought to be characteristic of temporal lobe behaviour. This includes features such as hyper-religiosity, anger, labile emotionality and altered sexuality (Geschwind 1979). Until the subject can be clarified by future research, it appears that the controversy will remain.

SCHIZOPHRENIA

Generally, psychiatrists agree that schizophrenia refers to one disorder, or a group of disorders, which involves severe disruption of cognitive and affective interactions with the environment. This disruption is identified by symptoms of a unique thought disorder, delusions and auditory hallucinations. Schizophrenia can be grouped into catatonic, paranoid, hebephrenic and simple subtypes; although one patient can, at times, display symptoms from different groups on different occasions, indicating that the labels may not refer to separate disease processes.

During the last decade research into schizophrenia has concentrated on genetic, environmental and anatomical factors.

The first genetic studies were a comparison of the incidence in relatives of index patients compared with families without schizophrenia (Kallman 1938), which showed a higher rate in the relatives of index patients. In later twin studies this was again highlighted in monozygotic twins in comparison with dizygotic twins (Gottesman & Shields 1966, 1972, Kringlen 1967).

Although these studies strongly suggested a genetic influence, there still remained the possibility that environmental influences could determine the incidence of schizophrenia. Identical twins may be treated alike in dress and expec-

tations, or there could be intra-uterine factors.

Consequently, adoption studies were undertaken. Heston (1966) conducted a study of children who were adopted at birth from schizophrenic parents and reared by normal adoptive parents. Subsequently, a reverse study was conducted (Wender et al 1974) where the adoptive parents were schizophrenic and the children from normal biological parents. These studies showed a higher incidence of schizophrenia in the children from schizophrenic parents. There was no indication regarding the importance of which parent was schizophrenic. However, a greater risk was evident if both the parents were schizophrenic.

As a result of the development of neuro-imagining techniques, research into schizophrenia has now begun to explore specific regions of the brain.

Examples include evidence that damage to the temporal lobe and limbic system will produce language problems such as ungrammatical speech and an inability to comprehend: characteristics of the language and perception abnormalities which present in schizophrenia. The ganglia which are primarily involved with motor control may be implicated in catatonic schizophrenia. Symptoms of the frontal lobe syndrome include stereotyped thinking, and a lack of insight and initiative that causes self-neglect and social isolation, all of which are characteristic of the schizophrenic state.

Johnstone et al (1976) were the first to report ventricular enlargement by computerized axial tomography (CT scanning). Since then, many more studies have been conducted with CT scanning, confirming these significant findings. Although this ventricular enlargement is now accepted in schizophrenia, it is still not certain whether it is specific to schizophrenia, as similar findings have been reported in relation to manic-depressive illness (Standish-Barry et al 1982), as well as large ventricles being identified in families with no history of psychiatric disorder.

Although numerous studies conducted over the last decade have provided evidence that there are certain biological clues to schizophrenia, research still has some considerable distance to cover before a specific cause for schizophrenia can be identified.

DEMENTIA

To those caring for the elderly, this syndrome where the patient exhibits global disturbance of cognitive function is a familiar picture. Initially, diagnosis is difficult. Symptoms are vague, memory loss being attributed to old age by relatives of the elderly person. Consequently, when a patient does present for examination the condition may have been active for a considerable time. Even in the younger patient, memory problems may have been explained by reference to a busy life-style and stress.

A neurologist will often diagnose the dementia, after which the patient will be cared for by a psychiatrist and/or the general practitioner. Follow-up for this group of patients is difficult. Often a patient becomes lost to the services, dies or the relatives refuse further investigation to protect the patient from extended suffering.

Consequently, the many causes of dementia are identified on postmortem examination; most cases demonstrating a degenerative disease of the central nervous system.

Alzheimer's disease

Postmortem studies indicate that at least 70% of dementia in geriatric patients can be attributed to Alzheimer's disease. This disease can only be diagnosed with certainty by cortical biopsy, so most cases are diagnosed on postmortem. On examination of the cerebral cortex, a widespread senile plaque and neurofibrillary tangle can be demonstrated; these plaques and tangles can normally be seen only in the hippocampus of the intellectually normal old person.

It has been suspected for some time that there could be a genetic link between Alzheimer's disease and Down's syndrome, as children with Down's syndrome who grow to adulthood demonstrate a similar dementia process in their later years. Postmortem studies have also shown a resemblance in brains of people with Down's syndrome to those of people with Alzheimer's disease. Following on from this, resemblance studies have been conducted looking specifically at chromosome 21 of which there is an extra copy in children born with Down's syndrome. A gene has

been identified which includes the protein sequence that characterizes the neurofibrillary tangles in Alzheimer's disease and Down's syndrome. This gene has been located on chromosome 21. However, Alzheimer's disease does not always appear to run in families. One reason could be that in some people symptoms do not appear until they reach the late eighties, so it is possible that many people die before the disease becomes active.

There is no doubt that an exciting era of research for the dementias is emerging. As well as genetic theories, biochemical and immunological theories are also beginning to emerge, although no one theory can claim superiority at this time.

It is clear that as people continue to live longer life spans, Alzheimer's disease will become more prominent than it is today, placing a greater demand on the health services, until research can offer prevention or a cure.

Huntington's chorea

This rare disease was first described by Huntington in 1872. Since its first description cases have been documented world-wide, regardless of race or culture. Because of the specific combination of choreiform movements and dementia, it was soon recognized that Huntington's chorea could be inherited by the offspring of an affected person. It is now possible, with a detailed history of family members and examination of a fetus via chorion villus sampling, to detect if a fetus is at low or high risk for Huntington's chorea. Although the gene for Huntington's chorea has not yet been identified, it is recognized that it is carried on chromosome 4. Until such a time that the gene is identified, families who run the risk of Huntington's chorea can, for the time being, attend for genetic counselling and reduce the risk of transferring this disease to another generation.

ACQUIRED IMMUNE DEFICIENCY SYNDROME (AIDS)

Human immune deficiency virus (HIV) is frequently associated with neuropsychiatric disorders. Neurological complications will occur in up to

30% of patients; 10% will present with these complications causing them to seek medical advice (Grant 1988).

Neuropsychiatric syndromes refer to the central nervous system (CNS) diseases and organic mental disorders. These may be due to opportunistic infections, neoplastic processes or the primary effect that HIV has on the CNS. The opportunistic infections include fungal, viral and protozoal groups, many of which are responsive to treatment. Although the neurological problems may initially mimic functional psychiatric syndromes, a thorough physical examination should be conducted to exclude an infection that may respond to treatment.

These syndromes may appear soon after HIV infection, at the time of seroconversion, and may involve any aspect of the CNS, although cerebral involvement is the most common.

HIV encephalopathy

This encephalopathy, inaccurately known as AIDS dementia complex, is proving to be the most common neurological complication in people with HIV infection. It has been estimated to occur in at least one third of people with AIDS. The onset is insidious in nature, mimicking dementia initially. Evidence exists from postmortem studies that the virus invades the brain, spinal cord and the peripheral muscles.

Typically, a person with this rapidly advancing encephalopathy will initially present with headaches, motor slowing and generally a progressive loss of cognitive functions, including memory loss.

Investigations should include examination of the cerebral spinal fluid and a CT scan to exclude the presence of an opportunistic infection or a space-occupying lesion. At present, the picture is of rapid degeneration from the person experiencing difficulty with work and daily living tasks, to one who is incontinent and paralysed. Death will usually occur within one year of diagnosis.

Although the psychological and physical implications of this disease are still not fully known, and treatment may be effective, it is possible that in the future many of these patients will require the support of the mental health services.

ANXIETY

Anxiety is a term used widely by health professionals and lay people alike. It is a subjective experience which everybody at times experiences and can identify with, but not one that can be easily observed.

A personal description of anxiety may include a queasy feeling in the stomach, weak knees, light headedness and poor concentration. The observer may only be aware that the individual looks 'worried'.

Anxiety can be classified in a number of ways. Two broad groupings can be identified:

- **Normal anxiety** is experienced in threatening situations. The individual's behaviour and mental functions are not necessarily impaired, rather they may be heightened, as in the examination setting.
- **Pathological anxiety** appears to have no precipitating factors. Behaviour and mental functions will often be severely impaired.

However, a large number of people, both in the Western world and in the East, demand relief from anxiety. Until the functions of the mid-brain are fully understood, the biological description for anxiety is provisionally that it arises from electrical activity in neurons that is transcribed into conscious experiences and emotions.

A major brain dysfunction in man has never been demonstrated. Anxiety is part of a biological reaction preparing the individual for flight or fight. Normal anxiety may be considered an expected attribute of the individual, whereas pathological anxiety may simply exhibit an overreaction in otherwise normal neuronal circuits. The physiological findings in anxiety that can be observed and measured are directly related to neurotransmitters. These findings include raised pulse, increased blood flow in forearm, augmented sweat gland activity, a reduction in salivation and an increase in muscle activity. All these signs indicate altered activity in the autonomic nervous system, and probably reflect the secondary physiological expression of the condition.

In summary, anxiety denotes a response to threat or danger which is accompanied by physiological symptoms and it prepares the individual for flight or fight by altering the activity of the autonomic nervous system.

SLEEP

Sleep can be defined as a state of unconsciousness from which a person can be aroused by appropriate stimuli. It appears that human sleep is the only time when the body goes into near total inactivity, very similar to hiberation in animals, but in human sleep it is based on a 24 hour cycle. In the past, this rhythm has been explained by reference to the oceanic origins of human beings, when the moon and the tides had a greater influence on biological systems. Nature is seen to be regulated by rhythms, whether they are the ebb and flow of the tides or the alterations in light and dark, all creatures have a sleeping and waking cycle.

If sleep is a time of near inactivity, then wakefulness is a time when the individual is active and orienting to the outside world before resuming sleep for internal orientation and activity. Although the sleep/wakefulness cycle is usually assumed to be linked to a 24-hour cycle, most people, if isolated from the light/darkness cycle, will eventually begin to function on a longer cycle of 25 hours.

Mechanism of wakefulness

Stimulation of the medial portion of the reticular activating system, particularly in the region of the mesencephalon and the upper pons, will cause the state of wakefulness. This can also occur indirectly via the sensory nerves, the cerebral cortex and from the lateral regions of the hypothalamus.

Situated in the pons is an area known as the locus ceruleus, which plays an important role in maintaining activity within the reticular activating system. The locus ceruleus lies bilaterally, immediately beneath the floor of the fourth ventricle. It comprises a group of neurons which are thought to form part of the reticular activating system, although they also perform other specific functions. These nerve fibres secrete norepinephrine, which,

it is believed, plays an important role in the process of wakefulness. It has also been suggested that dopamine and epinephrine contribute to the state of wakefulness. These transmitters are secreted by neurons in close proximity to the locus ceruleus and appear to be active together with the norepinephrine system.

Mechanism of sleep

The raphe nuclei, a thin sheet of nuclei located in the midline of the pons and medulla, is responsible for causing natural sleep. These nuclei extend their nerve fibres up into the reticular activating system, into the thalamus, hypothalamus and most of the limbic cortex. They also extend downwards into the spinal cord and terminate in the posterior horns. The transmitter serotonin is secreted by these nerve fibres. It is assumed that this major transmitter substance is associated with the production of sleep. Stimulation of several other regions in the lower brain stem and the diencephalon will also lead to sleep.

Structure of sleep

Electroencephalograms (EEGs) taken during sleep identify four distinct stages of sleep, which form a pattern that repeats every 90 to 100 minutes.

Electric waves reflected by the EEG are described in two ways: by frequency, which refers to the tightness of the tracing and rapidity of impulses; and amplitude, which is the vertical height of the tracing, reflecting the amount of energy discharged on each impulse.

During stage I EEG tracings are nearly the same as in drowsy wakefulness, with very low amplitude tracings. In stage II small amounts of energy appear as the amplitude increases. Stages III and IV are characterized by lower frequency and increased amplitude. These last two stages are when night terrors will occur. (The drug diazepam may be prescribed for night terrors, as it suppresses stages III and IV.) Rapid eye movement (REM) sleep occurs at the end of the cycle, when all four stages have occurred; the EEG trace looks similar to stage I sleep.

Slow wave sleep

Slow wave sleep (SWS), or deep restful sleep, is the result of depressed activity in the reticular activating system; waves are extremely slow at this point. This type of sleep will occur within 30–60 minutes of the individual's falling asleep. It is an extremely restful, dreamless sleep associated with a decrease in peripheral vascular tone, a drop in blood pressure and reduction in the respiratory and metabolic rates.

Although this is a particularly restful time for the individual, internally it is a time when protein synthesis becomes optimal. The growth hormone is released and memories from the previous day are stored.

Rapid eye movement sleep

Rapid eye movement (REM) sleep, or paradoxical sleep, results from the abnormal channelling of signals in the brain, even though the brain activity may not be significantly depressed. REM sleep will occur on average every 90 minutes and last for 5–20 minutes. The first period will occur 80–100 minutes after sleep occurs, but if the individual is very tired then REM may be absent or very short; as the night progresses and the tiredness decreases, the REM will increase.

During REM sleep the individual is more difficult to arouse. Muscle tone is exceedingly depressed, indicating a strong inhibition of the spinal projections from the reticular activating system. The EEG tracing will show a pattern similar to that during wakefulness, indicating high brain activity. Dreams and nightmares occur. High alcohol consumption and malnutrition suppress REM. Complementary to the production of the growth hormone which occurs in SWS, cell division will occur during REM sleep.

It has been proposed that during REM the brain is updating itself by selective mobilization of personal and evolutionary data banks, and utilizing experiences from the previous day. It is thought that during this process social and sexual needs are integrated, in order to prepare the individual for the challenges of the day to come.

Sleep is intimately related to wakefulness. Oswald (1970) states that exercise promotes sleep, particularly SWS. Crisp (1980) states that anger and anxiety are incompatible with sleep. From these statements it may be argued that when a person presents to their general practitioner, as many do, complaining about their disrupted sleep pattern, the person could be complaining about their state of wakefulness. Crisp (1986) recognizes that, on waking, a severely depressed person is at their most helpless and hopeless, and goes on to suggest that this could be from an inability during the sleep process to prepare the person for an active solution to their problems on awakening the following day. Thus the problem of early waking becomes secondary to this disorder.

BIPOLAR AND UNIPOLAR AFFECTIVE DISORDERS

Bipolar illness was first described by Emil Kraepelin (1921). This description confined the illness to either depressive or manic episodes. This concept was redefined by Leonhard (1959), who classified patients with both manic and depressive episodes as bipolar (BP) and patients whose illness had always been of the depressive type as unipolar (UP). Since his definition, BP has come to include all patients with mania, regardless of whether or not they have ever been seriously depressed (Angst 1966).

Kraepelin (1921) later observed that in 80% of his patients hereditary factors were present. More recently it has been widely acknowledged that there is an important genetic role in the transmission of BP and UP illness.

Studies have shown that the relatives of unipolar probands will usually have the UP disorder, whereas relatives of the bipolar probands will present with either the UP or BP disorder. Most studies agree that there is an average risk of 19.2% (McGuffin & Katz 1989a, b). These studies are supported by a register-based twin study (Bertelsen et al 1977) and adoption studies which confirm the high genetic profile in BP disorder (Mendlewicz & Rainer 1977).

There are three possible explanations as to how genes may be involved. Firstly, there is a continuous distribution among the population of those individuals who, with contributions from genes and the environment, may at times exceed a certain threshold, and so manifest the disorder. A second possible explanation is that a single gene or several different types of genes will act together with the environment. The last explanation concerns that of a single gene, the dominant X-linked gene (Reich et al 1969). However, this only accounts for a minority of cases, where there is father-to-son transmission.

To date, most provocative findings have come from an investigation of the Old Order Amish in Pennsylvania, USA. In this study a major gene for BP has been identified as linked to the arm of chromosome 11 (Egeland et al 1987). However, this study still needs to be replicated in other populations, and the X-linked results need to be further repeated before either can be proven.

Apart from the genetic studies, it is evident that other biological factors also have a role in BP and UP disorders. Women with a predisposition to BP show a 20% risk of developing mania in the first two weeks after childbirth (Reich & Winokur 1970). These women will often remain symptom-free for longer intervals than patients whose illness is not confined to the puerperium (Katona 1982). A possible explanation for this concerns the oestrogen level in the first two weeks after childbirth. Normally, the oestrogens will reduce the neuronal responses to dopamine (Cookson 1981), but during the puerperium oestrogen levels fall dramatically. This suggests the possibility of a subgroup of women with a predisposition to BP, who only become ill during the puerperium. In mania that accompanies weaning it has been suggested that the drop in prolactin may play an important role (Cookson 1985), although this is still not proven.

SEASONAL AFFECTIVE DISORDER

Historically, it has long been recognized that the incidence of depressive illness and suicide is highest from autumn to the spring months.

Seasonal rhythms have also been demonstrated in birth rate and hormone concentration in plasma.

Rosenthal et al (1984) described seasonal affective disorder (SAD), or winter depression, as a syndrome that is characterized by recurrent depressive episodes that occur annually, usually starting in October to December and diminishing in March.

Most sufferers have a bipolar affective disorder, usually bipolar II; where the depressive element is characterized by hypersomnia, overeating and carbohydrate craving. From numerous studies it has been suggested that the syndrome may be related to the hypersecretion of melatonin from the pineal body.

The pineal body is attached to the rear of the third ventricle and lies directly midline of the cerebrum. It is associated with the endocrine system, containing melatonin, serotonin and other biologically active amines.

In animals, melatonin secretion is thought to play a critical part in seasonal behaviour, although removal of the pineal body in sheep does not affect the seasonal reproductive cycle. When melatonin is administered to these same sheep the seasonal reproductive cycle continues regardless of the season. Thus melatonin may not be necessary in normal biology, but it may manipulate neuro-endocrine function. However, it is not understood how the secretory profiles of melatonin differ between summer and winter in patients with SAD.

Another biological consideration in patients with SAD concerns the possible involvement of serotonin, also secreted by the pineal body. It has been hypothesized that serotonin deficiency is related to depression and carbohydrate craving, both symptoms that are present in SAD. Postmortem studies of brains of people who have died from non-neurological, non-psychiatric conditions reveal that the content of serotonin shows a marked seasonal variation which is lowest in the autumn and winter months.

SAD should be seen as a separate affective disorder which may have a severely debilitating effect upon the sufferer, although the symptoms differ from those of a major depressive illness, as shown in Table 14.1.

Table 14.1 Symptoms in SAD versus major depressive illness

	Seasonal affective disorders (SAD)	Major depressive illness
Appetite	Increased with carbohydrate craving	Decreased
Weight	Increased	Decreased
Sleep	Asleep earlier Waking later	Difficulty in getting off to sleep Early morning wakening Disrupted sleep

Rosenthal et al (1984) found in their studies that all patients treated with bright white light exhibited some relief of symptoms and lifting in mood within 3–7 days of commencing treatment with bright white full-spectrum fluorescent light (approximately 2500 lux at 90 cm), three hours before dawn and three hours after dark.

From this study the authors have drawn up a working definition of SAD:

1. A history of major affective disorder
2. At least two consecutive years in which depression develops during autumn/winter and is relieved by spring/summer
3. Absence of any other psychiatric disorder
4. Absence of any seasonally changing psychosocial variables, e.g. work stresses.

Up till now, studies appear to confirm that there is a relationship between the administration of bright white light and the suppression of plasma melatonin. It can also be suggested that some populations may be sensitive to the length of the natural photo-period and that melatonin may play an important role in their response.

REFERENCES

Alstrom C H 1950 A study of epilepsy in its clinical, social and genetic aspects. Acta Psychiatrica et Neurologica Scandinavica 63 (suppl): 5–284 (212, 215, 232, 241)

Angst J 1966 Zur Atiologie and Nosologie endogener Depressiver Psychosen. Monographer ans der Neurologie and Psychiatrie No 112. Springer, Berlin

Berger H 1929 Uber das Elektrenkephalogram des menschen. Funfte Mitterlung. Archives Psychiatric Nervenler 98: 231–254

Bertelsen A, Harvald B, Halige M 1977 A Danish twin study of manic-depressive disorders. British Journal of Psychiatry 130: 330–351

Cookson J C 1981 Oestrogens, dopamine and mood. British Journal of Psychiatry 139: 365–366

Cookson J C 1985 The neuroendocrinology of mania. Journal of Affective Disorders 8: 233–241

Crisp A H 1980 Sleep, activity, nutrition and mood. British Journal of Psychiatry 137: 1–7

Crisp A H 1986 'Biological' depression: because sleep fails? Postgraduate Medical Journal 62: 179–185

Egeland J A, Gerhard D S, Pauls D L 1987 Bipolar affective disorder linked to DNA markers on chromosome 11. Nature 325: 783–787

Geschwind N 1979 Behavioural changes in temporal lobe epilepsy. Psychological Medicine 9: 217–219

Gottesman I, Shields J 1966 Contribution of twin studies to perspective on schizophrenia. Academic Press, New York

Gottesman I, Shields J 1972 Schizophrenia and genetics: a twin study. Academic Press, New York

Grant S M 1988 The hospitalized AIDS patient and the psychiatric liaison nurse. Archives of Psychiatric Nursing 2 (1): 35–39

Heston L J 1966 Psychiatric disorders in foster home reared children of schizophrenic mothers. British Journal of Psychiatry 112: 819–825

Hill D 1981 Historical review. In: Reynolds E H, Trimble M R (eds) Epilepsy and psychiatry. Churchill Livingstone, Edinburgh, p 1–11

Jackson J H 1873 On the anatomical, physiological and pathological investigation of epilepsies. Reports of the West Riding Lunatic Asylum 3: 315–339

Jackson J H 1890 On convulsive seizures. British Medical Journal 1: 703–707

Johnstone E C, Crow T J, Frith C D, Husband J, Kreel L 1976 Cerebral ventricular size and cognitive impairment in chronic schizophrenia. Lancet ii: 924–926

Kallman F 1938 The genetics of schizophrenia. Academic Press, New York

Katona C L E 1982 Pueperal mental illness: a comparison with non-puerperal control. British Journal of Psychiatric 141: 447–452

Kraepelin E 1921 Manic depressive insanity and paronoia. E & S Livingstone, Edinburgh

Kraepelin E 1922 Manic-depressive insanity and paranoia. (Trans Barday R M.) E & S Livingstone, Edinburgh

Kringlen J 1967 Heredity and the environment in functional phychoses. Heinemann, London

Leonhard K 1959 Aufteilung der Endogen Psychosen. Academic Verlag, Berlin

McGuffin P, Katz R 1989a The genetics of depression: current approaches. British Journal of Psychiatry 155 (suppl 6): 18–26

McGuffin P, Katz R 1989b The genetics of depression and

manic depressive disorder. Review article. British Journal of Psychiatry 155: 294–304

Mendlewicz J, Rainier J D 1977 Adoption study supporting genetic transmission in manic-depressive illness. Nature 268: 3026–3329

Oswald I 1970 Sleep, the great restorer. New Scientist 46: 170–172

Reich T, Clayton P J, Winokur G 1969 Family history studies versus the genetics of mania. American Journal of Psychiatry 125: 1358–1369

Reich T, Winokur G 1970 Post partum psychoses in patients with manic depressive illness. Journal of Nervous and Mental Disorders 151: 60–68

Rosenthal N E, Sack D A, Gillin J C, Lewy J, Goodwin F K, Davenport G et al 1984 Seasonal affective disorders. Archives of General Psychiatry 41: 72–80

Standish-Barry H M A S, Bouras N, Bridges P K, Bartlett J R 1982 Pneumoencephalograpic and computerised axial tomography scan changes in affective disorder. British Journal of Psychiatry 141: 614–617

Wender P H, Rosenthal D, Kety S S, Schulsinger F, Welner J 1974 Cross fostering: a research strategy for clarifying the role of genetic and experimental factor in the aetiology of schizophrenia. Archives of General Psychiatry 30: 121–128

FURTHER READING

Ciba Foundation 1985 Photoperiodism, melatonin and the pineal. Symposium 117. Pitman, London

Ferry G 1987 The genetic roots of dementia (Alzheimer's disease). New Scientist 113: 20–21

Gyton A C 1981 Basic human neurophysiology, 3rd edn. W B Saunders, Philadelphia

Hinchcliffe S, Montague S 1988 Physiology for nursing practice. Baillière Tindall, London

Lishman W A 1987 Organic psychiatry, 2nd edn. Blackwell, Oxford

McGuffin P 1988 Major genes for affective disorder? Annotation. British Journal of Psychiatry 153: 591–596

Nichols S E, Ostrow D G 1984 Psychiatric implications of acquired immune deficiency syndrome. American Psychiatric Press, Washington DC

Oatley K 1985 The biological basis of schizophrenia. New Scientist 1472 (Sept 5): 52–54

Owen M J, Lewis S W, Murray R M 1989 Family history and cerebral ventricular enlargement in schizophrenia: a case control study. British Journal of Psychiatry 154: 629–634

Plumlee A A 1986 Biological Rhythms and affective illness. Journal of Psychosocial Nursing and Mental Health Services 24 (3): 12–17

Royston R 1989 Schizophrenia, genetics and analytical psychology. British Journal of Psychotherapy 6 (1): 50–61

Silverstone T, Romans-Clarkson S 1989 Bipolar affective disorder: causes and prevention of relapse. Review article. British Journal of Psychiatry 151: 321–335

Snyder S H 1982 Neurotransmitter and CNS disease: schizophrenia. Lancet 2: 970–973

Thomas B 1989 HIV and encephalopathy. Nursing 3 (46): 4–7

Thompson C, Franey C, Arendt J, Checkley S A 1988 A comparison of melatonin secretion in depressed patients and normal subjects. British Journal of Psychiatry 152: 260–265

Warriner S 1990 Predictive testing. Nursing Times 86 (4): 49

Wurtman R J, Baum M J, Potts J T 1985 The medical and biological effects of light. Annals of the New York Academy of Sciences 143

15

The contribution of pharmacology

J. K. Davies

Psychotropic drugs produce their characteristic effects by altering the mechanisms by which nerve cells, or neurones, communicate with each other in the brain. The problem of defining how they produce these alterations has aroused the interest and exercised the ingenuity of pharmacologists since the therapeutic value of the drugs was first recognized. From their investigations, it has emerged that the fundamental mechanism of action of psychotropic drugs has much in common with that of drugs with peripheral sites of action, even though their effects are quite distinctive.

DRUG INTERACTIONS WITH CHEMICAL MESSENGERS

Modern drugs of all types tend to be synthetic chemicals, and are not naturally-occurring in animal organisms. Yet animal tissues are a source of pharmacologically active substances which certain types of cell (e.g. nerve and gland cells) have the capacity to synthesize and release, and which other cells (e.g. muscle cells) can identify and respond to. These natural substances comprise neurotransmitters, endocrine and local hormones and growth factors, and represent the chemical messengers which maintain functional contact between different cells and regulate virtually every bodily function.

The transmission of 'messages' between cells by chemical vectors is vulnerable to external interference, for example by foreign chemicals which are mistakenly identified, either by the transmitting or receiving cell, as being a natural messenger or one of the starting materials, or precursor substances, from which the messenger is produced.

'Mistaken identity' for a natural messenger appears to be a frequent mechanism of drug action. It explains why the action of individual drugs, instead of being exerted indiscriminately, tends to be localized onto types of cell which are also sensitive to a particular chemical messenger. (It is from this selectivity of action that drugs derive their usefulness as medicines.) Since the characteristics which identify drugs to cells are likely to be particular features of their structure, it also explains why drugs with similar chemical structures often have similar pharmacological properties.

The brain is an example of a physiological system whose functions are regulated by chemical messengers: in this case, by the neurotransmitters released at the synaptic junctions between different nerve cells. The 20-or-so central neurotransmitters which have been identified so far may represent only a small fraction of the number actually present, and the final tally may run into 100 or more different types, each operating in a distinctive manner and making its own contribution to the integrated function of the brain.

The potential for manipulating brain function by introducing foreign substances is considerable, and has already been exploited to some extent by existing psychotropic agents. To explain the mode of action of any of these drugs requires the identification, firstly, of the neurotransmitter and, secondly, of the particular component of the transmitter system with which the drug interacts. In relation to the second requirement, a variety of possible target sites for drug action exist, and are represented diagrammatically in Figure 15.1.

The 'receivers' for chemical 'messages' are specialized protein molecules located in the membrane of the target cell (Fig. 15.1(5)) to which transmitter molecules become temporarily attached following their release from the presynaptic terminal. Binding to these so-called 'receptors' occurs over an area of the molecule whose surface contour appears to complement that of the transmitter — a 'lock and key' analogy is often used to visualize the attachment of the transmitter to the receptor. Each transmitter has its own distinctive type, or types, of receptor, which are concentrated in large numbers at synapses where the transmitter is active.

The responses of target neurones to different neurotransmitters vary in size and duration, but basically represent either a stimulation or an inhibition of the functional activity of the cell. In most cases, the events which intervene between the binding of the transmitter to its receptors and the resultant cellular response are poorly understood, although it is likely that receptors which recognise different transmitters are also linked to different control mechanisms within the target cell.

A single neurone may receive chemical signals from numerous other cells and carry the receptors for a variety of transmitters. Each neurone also transmits a chemical signal to other cells and, in some instances, to itself. Thus, some transmitters are able to inhibit their own release from the presynaptic nerve terminal by acting on so-called autoreceptors located close to the release site (Fig. 15.1(6)).

The receptor site which 'identifies' a particular transmitter may also identify a drug molecule with similar structural characteristics. The binding of drug molecules to receptors may generate a similar response as is produced by the natural messenger. On the other hand, some types of drug can occupy receptors without generating a response from the target cell. These drugs are referred to as antagonist or blocking agents and produce pharmacological effects by inhibiting the normal physiological actions of particular chemical messengers. Note that neuronal autoreceptor blockade results in augmented transmission between cells by preventing the inhibitory effect of a neurotransmitter on its own release.

Receptors are not the only possible sites of drug action within control systems operated by chemical messengers. The release of neurotransmitters at synaptic junctions, for example, occurs in brief pulses, and the effect of each pulse on the target cell may be extremely transient. Transmitter

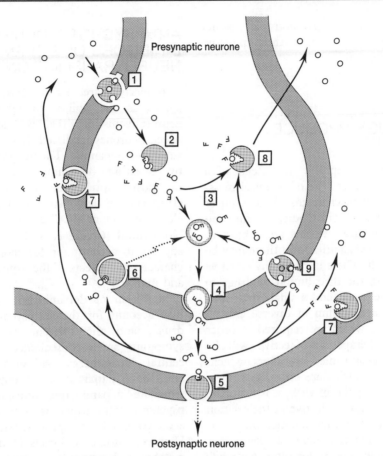

Presynaptic neurone

Postsynaptic neurone

Fig. 15.1 Potential sites of drug action at a synaptic junction. Key: (1) intraneuronal uptake of neurotransmitter (NT) precursor, (2) enzyme-catalysed synthesis of NT, (3) uptake and storage of NT in intracellular granules, (4) release of NT into synaptic cleft, (5) binding of NT to postsynaptic receptor initiates response of target cell, (6) binding of NT to presynaptic receptor inhibits further NT release, (7) enzyme-catalysed inactivation of NT in extracellular compartment, (8) enzyme-catalysed inactivation of NT in intracellular compartment, (9) intranueronal uptake of NT.

molecules can be inactivated within a fraction of a second of their release by two alternative mechanisms. Some transmitters are rapidly destroyed by enzymes which are strategically situated at the transmission site (Fig. 15.1(7)). Other transmitters are removed from the target area after attaching themselves to carrier proteins (Fig. 15.1(9)) which transport them intact, either into glial cells or back into the nerve cells from which they were originally released.

Drugs can both intensify and prolong the effects of neurotransmitters by inhibiting their inactivation. The mechanism of action involves binding of the drug, in preference to the transmitter, to the relevant enzyme or carrier molecule in a similar manner as to receptor molecules.

In general, a single neurone produces only one neurotransmitter which is synthesized in a sequence of enzyme-catalysed reactions within the cell (Fig. 15.1(2)). The newly-synthesized transmitter is held in storage pending its release (Fig. 15.1(3)); the accumulation of excessive amounts of transmitter is prevented by various means, including the action of degradative enzymes within the nerve terminal (Fig. 15.1(8)). Intracellular enzymes concerned with transmitter production or destruction are also, of course, potential sites of drug action, as are components of the systems concerned with neurotransmitter storage and release.

The pharmacology of psychotropic agents provides examples of several of these possible mechanisms of drug action.

WHY DO DRUGS PRODUCE SIDE-EFFECTS?

Drugs can intensify or inhibit the effects of a neurotransmitter, or other type of chemical messenger, by a variety of mechanisms. As a result of the interaction, the drug will modify the function of whatever physiological systems are subject to the influence of the transmitter, and these may be numerous and varied. There is rarely any effective means for localizing the distribution of drugs to specific areas of the body, and a single drug may therefore produce a spectrum of diverse effects. Any of these effects which are required in order to achieve some therapeutic objective will be almost invariably accompanied by others, which, to a greater or lesser extent, are not.

From a therapeutic point of view, it is fortunate that many drugs are more selective in their action than are the transmitters they interact with. For example, there is now convincing evidence that receptors for a single transmitter often have different properties according to the types of cell in which they are found and the type of response which the transmitter elicits. The binding sites on these different types of receptor have similar recognition properties as far as the natural transmitter is concerned, but drugs capable of binding effectively to one form of the receptor may be less well adapted to bind to another. As a result, such drugs may modify certain effects of the neurotransmitter while leaving others essentially unaffected, i.e. their ability to produce side-effects will be reduced.

It appears that chemical messengers rarely, if ever, cross-react with each other's receptors. The same is, unfortunately, not true of many drugs, including several used in psychiatry, which often interact with more than one type of messenger. This naturally widens the spectrum of activity of the compound and increases the variety of side-effects which are encountered in its use.

ANTIPSYCHOTIC DRUGS: INHIBITORS OF DOPAMINERGIC NEUROTRANSMISSION

A property shared by all classes of antipsychotic agents is the ability to inhibit dopaminergic neurotransmission, that is, communication between neurones mediated by the neurotransmitter substance dopamine. The majority of the drugs act by blocking dopamine receptors located on the postsynaptic neurone (Fig. 15.1(5)). This effect can be demonstrated experimentally using electrophysiological (Bunney et al 1973) and biochemical (Creese et al 1978) techniques, and appears to account for the more prominent and characteristic effects of the drugs, both in animals and man.

Inhibition of dopaminergic neurotransmission may account for the antipsychotic effect of the drugs, and the inference that schizophrenic symptoms are a consequence of overactivity in central dopaminergic pathways seems a natural one. Indeed, toxic doses of amphetamine, which stimulate dopaminergic transmission, induce a psychotic state which is indistinguishable from acute paranoid schizophrenia (Griffith et al 1972). However, studies of levels of dopamine and its metabolites have produced little or no evidence of an increased turnover of the transmitter in the brain of schizophrenic patients (Post et al 1975), although the recent application of radioisotope tracer techniques indicates a possible abnormality in the concentration of central dopamine receptors (Wong et al 1986).

Dopaminergic nerves project from nuclei in the brainstem to a variety of brain regions, both cortical and subcortical. Attention has focused on structures within the temporal and prefrontal lobes of the cerebral cortex, innervated by dopaminergic nerves of the mesolimbic and mesocortical systems, as a possible locus for the antipsychotic action of dopamine antagonist drugs (Anden 1972). In addition, there is substantial evidence that blockade of dopaminergic neurotransmission in the basal ganglia accounts for the extrapyramidal (parkinsonian) side-effects associated with antipsychotic drug treatment. Degeneration of dopamine nerves observed in actual parkinsonian patients produces a similar deficiency of dopaminergic neurotransmission as is produced by dopamine receptor blockade. The nerves affected are those of the nigrostriatal pathway projecting from the substantia nigra in the brainstem to the caudate nucleus and putamen. Examination of these regions in the postmortem brains of parkinsonian patients reveals substantial losses of dopamine (Price et al 1978). Moreover, the dopamine precursor substance, L-dopa, has been successfully used to treat Parkinson's disease, presumably because it is able to replenish depleted neuronal stores of dopamine. Centrally acting antagonists of the neurotransmitter substance acetyl choline (ACh) have also been found effective, and probably act by redressing an imbalance between the inhibitory effects of dopamine and the excitatory effects of ACh in the corpus striatum (Calne 1978). Consistent with this idea, antipsychotic agents which have pronounced ACh-antagonistic activity (see below), notably the phenothiazine derivative thioridazine, also produce the lowest incidence of extrapyramidal side-effects.

Dopaminergic nerves of the tuberoinfundibular pathway in the hypothalamus exert an inhibitory influence on the release of prolactin from the anterior pituitary gland. Quite low doses of antipsychotic agents are capable of removing this restraint and promoting secretion of the hormone. Dopamine receptors are also found in the chemoreceptor trigger zone of the medulla, and blockade of these receptors by antipsychotic drugs produces an antiemetic effect which has a number of clinical applications, including the control of nausea and vomiting produced by narcotics, general anaesthetics and cytotoxic agents.

Antipsychotic drugs antagonize the receptor binding of neurotransmitters other than dopamine, including that of noradrenaline, Ach and histamine. These additional blocking actions of the drugs produce a variety of side-effects, shown in Table 15.1. The potency of drugs in respect of these actions varies considerably in relation to their antipsychotic activity. Thus, autonomic side-effects are commonly seen with phenothiazine drugs, like chlorpromazine and thioridazine, used in therapeutic doses, but less frequently with

haloperidol and diphenylbutylpiperidines, like pimozide.

Table 15.1 Effects of psychotropic drugs resulting from blockade of specific neurotransmitter receptors

Neurotransmitter receptor	Effect of blockade
Dopamine	antipsychotic (?) extrapyramidal hyperprolactinaemia antiemesis
Noradrenaline	orthostatic hypotension miosis sedation (?)
Acetylcholine	dry mouth
	visual disturbances midriasis constipation urinary retention tachycardia
Histamine	sedation (?)

ANTIDEPRESSANTS: DRUGS WHICH MODIFY NORADRENERGIC AND SEROTONERGIC NEUROTRANSMISSION

Noradrenaline (NA) and serotonin (5-hydroxytryptamine, 5-HT) are transmitters employed in neural pathways which project from the brainstem to the cerebral cortex, limbic system, basal ganglia and other brain regions. Antidepressant drugs can modify the function of these messengers in a variety of ways. Most heterocyclic antidepressants inhibit neuronal uptake mechanisms (Fig. 15.1(9)). Some, like desipramine and maprotiline, have a preferential effect against NA uptake, while the action of amitriptyline and trazodone is directed primarily against that of 5-HT (Ho & Estevez 1982, Tyrer & Marsden 1985). Most other compounds of this type are less discriminating in their inhibitory effect. The tetracyclic drug mianserin has little effect on either NA or 5-HT uptake, but shows appreciable antagonist activity at presynaptic NA receptors (Fig. 15.1(6)) (Harper & Hughes 1979, Raiteri et al 1982).

The mitochondrial enzyme monoamine oxidase (MAO) regulates intraneuronal stores of the transmitters (Fig. 15.1(8)) and prevents excessive accumulation of NA and, 5-HT pending their release from nerve terminals. It is the site of action of the MAO-inhibitors phenelzine, isocarboxazid, iproniazid and tranylcypromine (Zirkle & Kaiser 1964, Biel et al 1964).

All of these drugs, acting in their various ways, would be expected to enhance central noradrenergic and/or serotonergic transmission, and there is some experimental evidence to this effect. Chronic treatment of animals with heterocyclic antidepressants, for example, produces changes in the brain which are consistent with increased synthesis and release of NA from adrenergic neurones (Sugrue 1981). At the same time, changes appear in the target cells for NA which represent typical adaptations to chronic over-exposure to a transmitter — the development, in fact, of a form of tolerance. This involves a reduction in the number of available NA receptors, particularly those of the β-type, and decreased sensitivity of the cells to the messenger (Wolfe et al 1978).

Significantly, similar changes in β-receptor number can be detected following the chronic application of virtually every form of antidepressant treatment, including electroshock, in animal experiments (Sulser 1982).

It is not known how effectively such an adaptive mechanism, often referred to as 'receptor down-regulation', could compensate for a drug-induced increase in neurotransmitter activity. It may be relevant, however, that the β-receptor population declines only during the first week or so of treatment, after which it stabilizes at about two-thirds of its former level (Wolfe et al 1978). Little or no effect is seen in patients during the first week of antidepressant treatment, and it is possible that during this interval the system compensates more than adequately for the increased activity of NA, and that only after the defences are overwhelmed, as it were, is any enhanced effect of the transmitter seen.

According to this version, the symptoms of depression are the result of a deficiency of central NA function. The opposite view, that depression is the result of overactive noradrenergic neurotransmission, has also been expressed (Sulser 1982). This attributes the antidepressant effect of drugs precisely to the down-regulation of NA β-receptors, and presumed decline in neuronal responsiveness, that their chronic use entails. The latter theory raises the interesting possibility that centrally-acting β-blocking drugs might prove to have antidepressant properties. Based on evidence currently available, this prediction seems unlikely to be borne out (Petrie et al 1982).

In respect of 5-HT activity, long-term antidepressant treatment both increases the responsiveness of brain neurones to the transmitter (Menkes et al 1980) and down-regulates 5-HT receptors in the brain, particularly those of the 5-HT2 subtype (Peroutka & Snyder 1980).

In terms of clinical effectiveness, there seems to be little to choose between drugs interacting mainly with the noradrenergic system and those interacting mainly with the serotonergic. It is possible that a deficiency of either or both of these monoamine transmitters could account for the symptoms of depression. Consistent with this idea, low levels of metabolites of NA and 5-HT have been detected in body fluids of depressed patients in some clinical studies (Sugrue 1981). At the same time, certain apparent inconsistencies have appeared, including the observation that cocaine, which has a powerful stimulant effect, particularly on noradrenergic neurotransmission, has proved to be of little or no value in the treatment of depression (Sulser 1982). Moreover, it should not be overlooked that a significant proportion of depressed patients appear to receive little or no benefit from any current form of antidepressant medication.

As shown in Table 15.2, the actions, particularly of heterocyclic drugs on presynaptic structures, is compounded by actions on the postsynaptic cell. These latter actions take the form of blockade of receptors, not only for NA and 5-HT, but also for Ach and histamine. These actions are reminiscent of those of the phenothiazine antipsychotic agents to which several antidepressants are chemically related, and result in similar side-effects.

The toxic interaction which occurs between monoamine oxidase inhibitors (MAOI) and certain foodstuffs (the 'cheese reaction') has contributed to a decline in their clinical use. The

Table 15.2 Pre- and postsynaptic effects of heterocyclic antidepressant drugs. (Refs: Peroutka & Snyder (1980), Hall & Ogren (1981), Ho & Estevez (1982).)

Drug	Presynaptic effect			Postsynaptic effect			
	Uptake inhibition		Receptor blockade	Blockade of receptors for:			
	NA	5-HT	NA	NA	5-HT	Ach	Histamine
Imipramine	++	++	−	++	+	++	++
Nortriptyline	++	++	−	++	++	++	++
Desipramine	+++	−	−	+	+	+	+
Amitriptyline	++	+++	+	++	++	++	+++
Mianserin	−	−	++	++	+	+	+++
Iprindole	−	−	−	−	−	−	+
Maprotiline	++	−	−	+	+	+	++

symbols indicate concentration ranges
over which 50% maximal effects are observed in vitro
+++ <10 nmol/l
++ 10–100 nmol/l
+ 100–1000 nmol/l
− >1000 nmol/l

postsynaptic receptor types:
NA — α_1
5-HT — 5-HT_2
Ach — muscarinic
Histamine — H_2

offending foodstuffs contain tyramine and other sympathomimetic amines (agents which stimulate noradrenergic neurotransmission), which are normally detoxified in the gut and liver before they enter the general circulation. The enzyme involved in this process is MAO, which is inactivated by the enzyme inhibitors, thus leaving the patient exposed to the action of the drugs, notably on the cardiovascular system. MAOIs with a selective action against the enzyme in brain cells are currently under development (Benedetti & Dostert 1985).

BENZODIAZEPINES: MODULATORS OF GABAERGIC NEUROTRANSMISSION

GABA (γ-amino butyric acid) is the major inhibitory neurotransmitter in the brain (Turner & Whittle 1983). GABAergic neurones are abundant in all brain areas and, in the main, form connections between other nerve cells over relatively short distances. GABA renders the target neurone less susceptible to excitation by other transmitters by two distinct actions, mediated by two different types of receptor. Receptors of the GABA-A type, located principally on the cell body of the target

neurone, operate a selective ion channel in the membrane which admits chloride into the cell, while those of the GABA-B type are located in the cell dendrites and operate a channel which allows the efflux of potassium ions from the cell. Both actions of GABA tend to increase the electrical potential difference across the cell membrane (hence the inhibitory effect of GABA on neuronal function), but the latency and duration of the effects are different (Newberry & Nicoll 1985). There is now abundant evidence that drugs of the benzodiazepine type (diazepam, lorazepam, oxazepam, etc.) enhance the inhibitory effect of GABA on neuronal function mediated by the GABA-A receptor subclass.

It is accurate to describe benzodiazepines (BZs) as modulators of GABAergic neurotransmission, since no detectable effect of the drugs is seen unless they are given concurrently with the transmitter (Gallager et al 1980). On the basis of electrophysiological evidence, it appears that in the presence of a BZ, chloride channels open and close at a faster rate in response to GABA, allowing a larger amount of the ion to enter the cell within a given time (Study & Barker 1981). Under the same conditions, barbiturate drugs, which exert a similar potentiating effect on GABAergic neurotransmission, increase the duration of time for which individual channels remain open.

BZs inhibit neither the uptake nor the metabolism of GABA (Gallager et al 1980), suggesting the site of action of the drugs lies on or close to the GABA receptor itself. This has recently been confirmed by the use of molecular biological techniques. Two different proteins have been isolated from brain tissue, one capable of binding to GABA, the other to BZs. It is likely that in the natural state of the nerve membrane, these proteins are the building blocks from which the GABA-operated chloride channel is formed, through the linking of two molecules of the GABA-binding protein with two of the BZ (Schofield et al 1987). It seems clear that the binding of BZ drugs to their receptors in some way facilitates the opening of the channel by GABA, but the mechanism remains to be elucidated.

BZs form a comparatively stable complex with their binding protein (Braestrup & Squires 1978), and their structure clearly complements that of the binding site admirably. The question of whether the BZ receptor is 'designed' to accept a GABA modulatory substance of natural origin has not been resolved, although some promising candidates for this physiological role have come to light (Alho et al 1985). Numerous non-BZ drugs also form stable complexes with the receptor, but, curiously, not all have BZ-like pharmacological properties, Flumazenil (RO 15–1788), for example, has little or no independent pharmacological activity, but is an antagonist of BZs (Hunkeler et al 1981) and has recently been introduced into clinical practice for this purpose. A further group of drugs, the β-carbolines, produce pharmacological effects which are diametrically opposite to those of BZs (Braestrup et al 1983). Such drugs show therapeutic potential for increasing vigilance and improving cognitive function.

The interaction of BZs with the GABA-A receptor appears to account for their characteristic effects of relieving anxiety, causing sedation and muscle relaxation and inhibiting seizures. The sedative effect of the drugs is a drawback in their use as anxiolytics and anticonvulsants; there is some optimism that future developments will produce similar drugs whose sedative effects are minimal.

CONCLUSION

The vital role played by neurotransmitters in regulating brain function provides the key to understanding the mechanism of the action of psychotropic drugs. The list of examples described in this chapter is far from exhaustive, but illustrates the variety of means by which drugs can enhance or inhibit the activity of particular messenger substances. The effect of a drug on the amount of transmitter released from a nerve terminal or the amount removed from the synaptic cleft by inactivation mechanisms or on the responsiveness of the target cell to the transmitter, effects which contribute to the drug's characteristic profile of activity, all have a fundamental chemical basis. The occupation of specific recognition sites on enzymes, carrier molecules and receptors by drug molecules alters the amount of natural transmitter that can be processed by these same species, and amplifies or attenuates the chemical signal that links the activity of one nerve cell to that of another.

Understanding the mode of action of psychotropic drugs can provide a valuable insight into the causes of psychiatric illness. Drugs which modify specific aspects of thought, mood and behaviour have not only revolutionized the treatment of mental illness. When used in conjunction with the instruments of modern technology they have also provided fundamental research with powerful tools for studying the involvement of particular messenger substances in physiological and pathological processes.

Needless to say, it would be premature to attribute, for example, schizophrenia to an abnormality of dopaminergic neurotransmission, or depression to a noradrenaline disturbance, solely on the basis of drug studies. Drugs might alleviate the symptoms of a disease by producing a lesion in one system which compensates for a lesion existing in another. Furthermore, a drug which has 'antipsychotic' or 'antidepressant' activity in 70% of patients, may have no such activity in the remaining 30%, so that any conclusions drawn from the mode of action of the drug regarding the aetiology of the disease might have, at best, restricted applicability.

Most drugs suffer from limitations, not only in terms of clinical effectiveness, but also because of their tendency to produce unwanted actions. Information concerning the mode of action of the drug may provide a clue as to how it could be modified in order to minimize or obviate its less desirable features, while retaining the desirable ones.

Finally, it must be remembered that some forms of mental illness have a basis in some organic, possibly congenital, abnormality, which no present or future drug, acting in the manner of those described in this chapter, could be expected to correct, however effectively it alleviated the symptoms of the disease.

REFERENCES

Alho H, Costa E, Ferrero P, Fujimoto M, Cosenza-Murphy D, Guidotti A 1985 Diazepam binding inhibitor: a neuropeptide located in selected neuronal populations in cat brain. Science 229: 179–182

Anden N E 1972 Dopamine turnover in the corpus striatum and the limbic system after treatment with neuroleptic and antiacetylcholine drugs. Journal of Pharmacy and Pharmacology 24: 905–906

Benedetti M S, Dostert P 1985 Stereochemical aspects of MAO interactions: reversible and selective inhibitors of monoamine oxidase. Trends in Pharmacological Sciences, 6 June: 246–251

Biel J H, Horita A, Drukker A E 1964 Monoamine oxidase inhibitors (hydrazines). In: Gordon M (ed) Psychopharmacological agents, vol 1. Academic Press, New York, pp 359–443

Braestrup C, Nielsen M, Honore T, Jensen L H, Petersen E N 1983 Benzodiazepine receptor ligands with positive and negative efficacy. Neuropharmacology 22: 1451–1457

Braestrup C, Squires R F 1978 Pharmacological characterization of benzodiazepine receptors in the brain. European Journal of Pharmacology 48: 263–270

Bunney B S, Walters J R, Roth R H, Aghajanian G K 1973 Dopamine neurons: effect of antipsychotic drugs and amphetamine on single-cell activity. Journal of Pharmacology and Experimental Therapeutics 185: 560–571

Calne D B 1978 Parkinsonism: clinical and neuropharmacologic aspects. Postgraduate Medical Journal 64: 82–88

Creese I, Burt D, Snyder S H 1978 Biochemical actions of neuroleptic drugs: focus on dopamine receptor. In: Iversen L L, Iversen S D, Snyder S H (eds) Neuroleptics and schizophrenia. Handbook of Psychopharmacology, vol 10. Plenum Press, New York, pp 37–89

Gallager D W, Mallorga P, Thomas J W, Tallman J F 1980 GABA-benzodiazepine interactions: physiological, pharmacological and developmental aspects. Federation Proceedings 39: 3043–3049

Griffith J D, Cavanaugh J, Held J, Oates J A 1972 Dextroamphetamine: evaluation of psychotomimetic properties in man. Archives of General Psychiatry 26: 97–110

Hall H, Ogren S 1981 Effects of antidepressant drugs on different receptors in the brain. European Journal of Pharmacology 70: 393–407

Harper B, Hughes I E 1979 Presynaptic α-adrenoceptor blocking properties among tri- and tetra-cyclic antidepressant drugs. British Journal of Pharmacology 67: 511–517

Ho B T, Estevez V S 1982 Molecular aspects of 5-HT uptake inhibitors. In: Ho B T, Schoolar J C, Usdin E (eds) Serotonin in biological psychiatry. Advances in Biochemical Psychopharmacology, vol 34. Raven Press, New York, pp 199–218

Hunkeler W, Mohler H, Pieri L et al 1981 Selective antagonists of benzodiazepines. Nature 290: 514–516

Menkes D B, Aghajanian G K, McCall R B 1980 Chronic antidepressant treatment enhances α-adrenergic and serotoninergic responses in facial nucleus. Life Sciences 27: 45–55

Newberry N R, Nicoll R A 1985 Comparison of the action of baclofen with γ-aminobutyric acid on rat hippocampal pyramidal cells in vitro. Journal of Physiology 360: 161–185

Peroutka S J, Snyder S H 1980 Long-term antidepressant treatment decreases spiroperidol-labelled serotonin receptor binding. Science 210: 88–90

Petrie W M, Maffucci R J, Woosley R L 1982 Propranolol and depression. American Journal of Psychiatry 139: 92–94

Post R M, Fink E, Carpenter W T, Goodwin F K 1975 Cerebrospinal fluid amine metabolites in acute schizophrenia. Archives of General Psychiatry 32: 1013–1069

Price K S, Farley I J, Horneykiewicz O 1978 Neurochemistry of Parkinson's disease: relation between striatal and limbic dopamine. In: Roberts P J, Woodruff G N, Iversen L L (eds) Dopamine Advances in Biochemical Psychopharmacology, vol 19. Raven Press, New York, pp 293–300

Raiteri M, Maura G, Cerrito F 1982 Effects of some atypical antidepressants on catecholamine synthesis and release. In: Costa E, Racagni G (eds) Typical and atypical antidepressants: molecular mechanisms. Advances in Biochemical Psychopharmacology, vol 31. Raven Press, New York, pp 199–209

Schofield P R, Darlinson M G, Fujita N, et al 1987 Sequence and functional expression of the GABA-A receptor shows a ligand-gated receptor super-family. Nature 328: 221–227

Study R E, Barker J L 1981 Diazepam and (-)pentobarbital:

fluctuation analysis reveals different mechanisms for potentiation of γ-aminobutyric acid responses in cultured cell neurons. Proceedings of the National Academy of Sciences of the USA 78: 7180–7184

Sugrue M F 1981 Current concepts on the mechanisms of action of antidepressant drugs. Pharmacology and Therapeutics 13: 219–247

Sulser F 1982 Antidepressant drug research: its impact on neurobiology and psychobiology. In: Costa E, Racagni G (eds) Typical and atypical antidepressants: molecular mechanisms. Advances in Biochemical Psychopharmacology, vol 31. Raven Press, New York, pp 1–20

Turner A J, Whittle S R 1983 Review article: biochemical dissection of the γ-aminobutyrate synapse. Biochemical Journal 209: 29–41

Tyrer D, Marsden C 1985 New antidepressants: is there anything new they have to tell us about depression? Trends in Neurosciences, 8 October: 427–431

Wolfe B B, Harden T K, Spawn J R, Molinoff P B 1978 Presynaptic modulation of beta adrenergic receptors in rat cerebral cortex after treatment with antidepressants. Journal of Pharmacology and Experimental Therapeutics 207: 446–457

Wong D F, Wagner H N jr, Tune L E, et al 1986 Positron emission tomography reveals elevated D-2 dopamine receptors in drug-naive schizophrenics. Science 234: 1558–1563

Zirkle C L, Kaiser C 1964 Monoamine oxidase inhibitors (non-hydrazines). In: Gordon M (ed) Psychopharmacological agents, vol 1. Academic Press, New York, pp 445–554

16

The contribution of clinical psychiatry

S. Turner

This section of the book is designed to introduce those disciplines most relevant to psychiatric nursing. Already, there have been contributions from a sociologist, a clinical psychologist and a medical scientist. The present chapter is written by a psychiatrist. Inevitably, each comes to the problem of understanding mental illness with a different perspective and it will be necessary to address some of the differences between these approaches. In this chapter, the concept of disease will be considered and an approach to classification with brief descriptions of the main syndromes will be presented. Common terms used in describing the features of mental illness (descriptive phenomenology) will also be defined.

ABNORMALITY AND MENTAL ILLNESS

The challenge

The concept of mental illness has been dismissed as no more than a modern myth. Szasz (1974) suggested that mental disorders are not illnesses so much as forms of expressing 'man's struggle with the problem of how he should live'. Laing (1965) has written of 'our present pervasive madness that we call normality, sanity, freedom'. In this inversion of the usual way of understanding the illness state, Laing asserts that those described as mentally ill may have an enhanced mental life with experiences of 'other dimensions' of living. In our society of 'one-dimensional men', someone with experiences of these 'other dimensions', other possibilities in life, is faced with a conflict in which he is either destroyed by others or forced to betray what he knows to be true. In either case he runs the risk of being described by society as mentally ill.

This issue is not just of theoretical interest. It is crucial to the practice of psychiatry. Szasz has suggested that just as the 'demonological' understanding of psychology led to treatment along religious lines (e.g. exorcism), so a belief in mental illness 'requires therapy along medical or psychotherapeutic lines'. In other words, by dismissing the concept of mental illness, he is also rejecting the validity of these forms of treatment. In his view, the primary effect of diagnosis is political rather than medical; he sees the enforced hospitalization of the mentally ill as serving 'moral and social, rather than medical and therapeutic, purposes'. This is a challenge which must be faced by those who believe in the value of medical or psychotherapeutic treatments, and therefore must accept to some degree the illness model.

Abnormality

Since the fundamental question being considered concerns the nature of the abnormal state, it would be natural to start with an attempt to define what is meant by the term abnormal. There are two basic categories of abnormality. In the first case, an amount is unusual (quantitative abnormality); in the second there are irregular or non-standard features (qualitative abnormality).

Quantitative abnormality

Many biological variables conform to a typical ('normal') distribution in the population, the great majority of measurements falling within the middle of the range (Fig. 16.1). Those values at the extremes are unusual and therefore statistically ab-

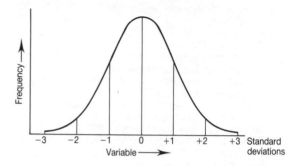

Fig. 16.1 Normal distribution curve.

normal. For example, people come in all sorts of shapes and sizes. There is a wide range of variation in weight, but some have such extreme obesity or thinness that they would be generally described as abnormal.

Similarly, biochemical results are often displayed with normal ranges; in one laboratory the range for blood potassium levels is 3.8–5.0 mmol/litre. These levels are derived from measurements of the normal population in such a way as to include about 95% of apparently healthy people. This means that about 5% of the 'normal' population have 'abnormal' results on each of the assays.

In the same way, intelligence is measured on a continuous scale. The scores are usually standardized so that the average (mean) value is 100. Approximately 68% of people have IQ scores between 85 and 115; about 95% have values between 70 and 130.

As the range of scores is widened, so the percentage falling outside that range decreases. At some point in this process it may be decided that people with such extreme scores are so unusual as to be frankly abnormal. The first problem, therefore, arises from the arbitrary nature of the threshold. If scores below 70 are defined as abnormal, then an IQ of 69 is as abnormal as one of 50 and a value of 71 is as normal as an IQ of 100. This imposition of categories (normal versus abnormal) onto a continuously varying parameter is associated with grave practical and ethical difficulties, particularly in the selection of the criterion value. The other point to note is that an IQ of 130 is about as unlikely as an IQ of 70 and therefore statistically just as abnormal, although not necessarily as disadvantageous for the individual concerned!

Qualitative abnormality

Others may be abnormal by virtue of some difference which is either present or absent. A clover plant usually has three leaves; the presence of a fourth is abnormal. There can be no doubt about the threshold between the normal and the abnormal; there is a clear discontinuity between the two categories. Trisomy 21 (the presence of an extra chromosome 21) is a cause of Down's syndrome (one of the more common reasons for mental impairment). Here, too, there is a categorical or qualitative abnormality.

THE NATURE OF DISEASE
(PHYSICAL AND PSYCHOLOGICAL)

Introduction

Just because something is abnormal (quantitatively or qualitatively) does not necessarily mean that it is diseased. Such a view would condemn the most intelligent, the most creative, the most charismatic as being diseased, presumably in need of treatment. The definition of disease must rely on other features. Kendell (1975), in an excellent monograph on the role of diagnosis in psychiatry, reviewed several possible definitions of the disease state ranging from purely subjective criteria (suffering) to the purely objective (the presence of the pathological lesion).

Although it is appropriate to start this discussion with the subjective experience, the symptom, suffering alone is inadequate as a definition of disease. It fails to include hidden disease, for example the lung cancer which is present but which has not yet caused symptoms. On the other hand it will be demonstrated that the lesion model in which symptoms are seen entirely as consequences of some objective pathological process (lesion), for example the abdominal pain caused by an inflamed appendix, is also flawed. Indeed, any simple unidimensional model of disease (physical as well as

psychological) has limitations. It will be demonstrated that it is in the interaction of the various approaches that the most fruitful path lies.

Historical perspectives and the lesion model

Historically, all diseases were regarded as having an independent existence, as being objects, each with a natural history and the potential to spread within a community (Taylor 1972). (This is very different from the modern notion of infection; it was the autonomous disease itself, not its cause (the bacterium or virus), which was held to exist and to spread.) Diseases were to be classified in exactly the same way as plants or animals. As recently as the middle of the last century, it was highly controversial to write that diseases 'have no independent or isolated existence: they are not autonomous organisms, not beings invading a body, nor parasites growing in it; they are only the manifestations of life processes under altered conditions' (Rudolf Virchow 1847, quoted in Taylor 1972). Since then there has been a growing understanding of some of the physical mechanisms of disease. One of the main areas of development was provided by bacteriologists. They were able to demonstrate that some diseases had specific infective causes. It did not matter what form the illness took; if the tuberculosis bacterium was the cause then the disease was tuberculosis.

As more and more disorders were discovered to have a pathological basis, the importance of seeking specific causes increased. This has been a general trend in medicine, only to be increased by the later advances in biochemistry and physiology. Many seem to assume now that almost all physical diseases have been traced to a series of specific lesions, with the implication that each disease ultimately represents a qualitative abnormality. Most medical students are taught pathology (the study of lesions) before being introduced to a single patient. It may be surprising, therefore, to find that for many of the common physical conditions there is no certain underlying lesion. One example is essential hypertension (the most common form of high blood pressure). Although blood pressures which are unequivocally high are associated with premature deaths, largely from heart disease and strokes, the precise level at which treatment may be beneficial is still a matter for disagreement. There is no qualitative difference in blood pressure between the 'well' and the 'ill'; a small shift in the threshold value would move many people from one group to the other.

There are other disadvantages of this narrow disease model. Symptoms which do not match known lesions are often rejected. When a 'new disease' is described, this often means that a previously unrecognized lesion has been detected. Both the lesion and the symptoms were already present. The emphasis on the physical lesion may also contribute to the difficulties sometimes experienced in understanding the role of other factors. It may be easier for a cardiologist to consider the electro-mechanical function of the heart than to explore the relationship between major life events (e.g. bereavement or earthquakes) and heart attacks. Both of these have been shown to be precipitating factors (Parkes et al 1969 Trichopoulos et al 1983).

In spite of its limitations, this approach still has an important role in physical medicine. In psychiatry, although many may find it easier to examine the social environment or to speculate about intrapersonal conflicts, it has to be acknowledged that biological processes often make a major contribution. For example, in schizophrenia there is evidence of a genetic predisposition. Children born to schizophrenic mothers but who are adopted into other families very soon after birth (removing the psychological influence of the mother on the child) have a considerably higher risk of developing the illness than normal controls (Heston 1966, Gottesman & Shields 1982). This sort of evidence is now very firm and, together with work on neurochemicals (Johnstone et al 1976) and brain structure (Weinberger et al 1979, Crow 1980, Turner et al 1986), indicates an active biological process in the disorder. In the major mood disturbances (mania and psychotic depression), similar factors operate. Just because the lesion model has inadequacies (both in physical medicine and in psychiatry), it does not mean that it should be totally rejected in either situation. Particularly in the psychotic ill-

nesses, it has an important part to play in understanding the full complexity of the disorders.

Biological disadvantage

Scadding (1967) has taken a different view. He has defined a disease as the 'sum of the abnormal phenomena . . . by which (people) differ from the norm . . . in such a way as to place them at a biological disadvantage'. The concept of disadvantage is an important addition to the concept of abnormality but is still insufficient to define disease adequately. A celibate life is both unusual and associated with a biological disadvantage (prevention of procreation), yet it is not a disease. Similarly, there are some blood disorders such as sickle cell trait which offer a degree of protection against malaria but which in extreme cases may cause profound anaemia or even death. Here the abnormality has both advantages and disadvantages in biological terms. In addition, the problem of definition remains; how much disadvantage would be required to constitute a disease?

Social and political perspectives

Health has occasionally been described in political terms. Illich (1974) has written that 'longevity owes much more to the railroad and to the synthesis of fertilizers and insecticides than it owes to new drugs and syringes'. The incidence of tuberculosis was declining 'before either the tubercle bacillus had been discovered or anti-tuberculous programmes had been initiated'. Perhaps it should not be a surprise to chart the consequences of widespread unemployment or increases in street crime on the prevalence of psychiatric illness.

In an influential series of radio broadcasts (the 1980 Reith lectures), Kennedy set about the task of 'Unmasking Medicine', a thesis later to be developed in a book (Kennedy 1981). The concept of disease was described as something which doctors, perhaps acting on behalf of society, have established as a way of controlling social and political forces. The lady who comes seeking tranquillizers when living in an area of social privation is given as an example. If she feels miserable, is that a symptom of disease or of a social predicament? For many symptoms of the minor psychiatric disorders (the neuroses), there is no qualitative difference between the normal and abnormal.

To accept that political and social forces may also be important does not in itself negate the role of biological processes. Why should some people and not others develop recurrent panic attacks when faced with the same circumstances? If antidepressive medication helps to relieve suffering, as much clinical experience indicates that it does, surely it should not be withheld.

Another problem which often arises in this sort of work is the use of behavioural disturbance alone as an indicator of illness. To suggest that it is abnormal to commit murder would be statistically correct; to claim that all who do this are insane would be illogical. Some may indeed be suffering from mental illness but others are not. The difference must lie in the presence of *other* features (disturbances of specific psychological 'part-functions', Aubrey Lewis 1953), which are both independent of the behavioural disturbance and characteristic of a particular illness.

In the same way, a person deciding on suicide may have no other evidence of mental disorder. This has recently been the subject of a successful play 'Whose life is it anyway?' (Clark 1978) in which a previously creative man becomes paralysed and totally dependent on nursing care. He elects to discharge himself from hospital, knowing that he will die. At a judicial review, it is concluded that he is taking this step in an entirely rational frame of mind.

Social forces may operate in other ways. In labelling theory (Scheff 1974), it is suggested that the fate of a patient is determined by the preconceptions of others as much as by the patient's condition. One example often quoted concerns the admission of eight sane people to different mental hospitals in America (Rosenhan 1973). Following the initial assessment during which certain psychotic features were simulated, all subjects behaved normally. In all cases they had enormous difficulties later in convincing the staff that they were sane. The initial label had a powerful effect on later assessments. This theory was intended to

challenge and lead to a change in current views rather than to reject psychiatric formulations which serve 'useful functions in theory and practice concerning mental illness' (Scheff 1974).

Diseases as explanatory models

Perhaps because it is so difficult to produce an adequate definition of disease, it may be better to regard diseases as no more than useful concepts. Sometimes these will change and history contains many instances of this, for example the abandonment of the separate entity of phthisis (cavitating tuberculosis) in the reclassification of infections according to the bacterial agent responsible. In psychiatry, at different times, it has been held that all psychosis is unitary or that the psychoses should be divided into many subcategories. Disease types are in other words no more than expressions of a prevailing understanding. They have no material existence of their own but should rather be seen as explanatory models. They are useful only in so far as they aid comprehension of the process involved. In the case of infectious disease, to be able to look for and identify a specific bacterium will allow the appropriate antibiotic to be selected. In just the same way, to identify the syndrome of depression as opposed to dementia will enable the practitioner to choose the form of treatment most likely to be effective.

A synthesis

Probably the best approach is to separate out the different components of being sick and to examine the ways they interact. This is likely to be more effective than any simple mechanistic (linear cause and effect) model. To take an example, a person may have a heart attack as a consequence of arterial disease. However, the timing of the attack may be related to psychological stress (Mitchell 1984). It is impossible not to regard this as an interaction of different factors. In some cases, one of these factors may be of paramount importance and this will vary from instance to instance. Similar mechanisms operate in psychiatry. A person may be genetically predisposed to schizophrenia but the timing of a relapse may be influenced by the emotional life of the family (Leff & Vaughn 1981).

One author (Taylor 1979) finds a commendable solution to these difficulties; he divides the components of sickness into three categories:

1. diseases (the objective component)
2. illnesses (the process, the subjective experience) and
3. predicaments (the situation or system).

This schema demonstrates an important division between the bioscientifically respectable (the disease) which corresponds roughly to the lesion (as described above) and the other attributes of sickness. Illness is the subjective experience which may occur in disease. This concept is important as it allows a distinction to be made between the severity of disease and the severity of illness. Indeed, illness may occur in the absence of disease. Finally, the sick person exists within a predicament, the complex of psychosocial ramifications, contacts, meanings and ascriptions which bear upon the individual. Predicaments are highly charged with moral and ethical implications. They can be painful without disease or illness ('problems of living'). They contain scope for social and political remedy.

Conclusion

A simplistic disease model has limitations both in physical medicine and in psychiatry. There are many factors which operate in the development of all types of sickness. To declare that schizophrenia is not an illness would therefore make about as much sense as to claim the same for appendicitis or tuberculosis. The technological aspects of diagnosis are less sophisticated and possibly less relevant in psychiatry. It is therefore easier to attack the disease model. Nevertheless, it may have just as important a part to play as in the rest of medicine. To go back to the days before there were effective physical treatments for depression and schizophrenia would be as unthinkable as to return to the time before insulin was available for diabetes. Current interest has linked many of the major psychiatric disorders to chemical (neurotransmitter) changes in brain function. However, it also has to be appreciated that life events, certain types of highly emotionally charged environments or internal conflicts may all play a part in the development of illness. In just the same way, political pressures may influence the predicament of the person and hence their suffering, their presentation and their management. None of these aspects should be neglected or given undue importance in the total assessment.

CLASSIFICATION, RANGE OF DISORDERS AND DIAGNOSIS

Introduction to classification

The classification and correct diagnosis of mental disorders are essential if a rational approach to treatment is to be adopted. Just as it would be illogical to offer antibiotics for high blood pressure, it would be pointless to consider antidepressive drugs for someone whose mental state was disturbed as a consequence of a low blood sugar. The distinction between these two types of disorder should be clear from a diagnostic system. This should act as a guide to treatment. Even less biologically determined therapeutic methods are explicit in their limitations. For example, one standard reference lists 'exclusion criteria' in a chapter devoted to the selection of patients for group psychotherapy (Yalom 1975).

Kendell (1975) has some wise comments to make about the value of classification: 'Whatever the context, whether one is concerned with sickness or not, there are three aspects to every human being:

1. those he shares with all mankind
2. those he shares with some men, but not all
3. those which are unique to him.

The value of classification in any given context depends on the size of the second of these categories relative to the other two.'

The classification of psychiatric syndromes, therefore, can only ever rely on the features which are generally present in people with one syndrome but which are generally absent in people with others. There will inevitably be both many unique personal experiences and many universal aspects of the human condition not included in these descriptions.

Descriptive phenomenology

The description and analysis of the phenomena of mental illness are therefore essential parts of any cohesive system of classification. Although those features which help to distinguish different disorders will be given extra prominence in the descriptions which follow, there are a few commonly used terms which merit special explanation here.

Affect. Synonymous with emotion. (*Mood* refers to a sustained affective state.)

Cognitive function. Those aspects of higher mental function to do with memory, reason and intelligence. Impairment is characteristically associated with the organic states but may also occur with other major disorders such as the 'pseudodementia' of depression.

Delusion. A false belief which is firmly held against evidence to the contrary and which is out of context with the patient's cultural background.

Hallucination. A perception (in any sensory modality) in the absence of an external stimulus. May be normal immediately preceding or following sleep.

Illusion. A perceptual misinterpretation of a real sensory experience.

Passivity experiences. These are described by people with schizophrenia as the experience of an external (alien) force controlling some aspect of their mental functioning. Unlike some religious experiences, it is not self-enhancing. There is usually a secondary (explanatory) delusion.

Thought disorders. This term is usually applied to abnormalities in the form of thought as revealed in speech or writing. Examples include flight of ideas and pressure of speech in mania, retardation (slowing) in depression and the loosening of association (knight's move thinking), neologisms (new words) and, rarely, frank incoherence seen in schizophrenia.

These are some of the features which are looked for in the examination of the patient's mental state. People may present with similar complaints caused by different processes. Abnormalities in some of these areas but not others may help to distinguish between the different disorders.

Classification of mental disorders

In psychiatry, the classification is different from that used in most of general medicine. It is based on a hierarchical approach (Foulds 1965). Disorders from higher in the hierarchy may include symptoms from disorders lower in the hierarchy. This becomes obvious on closer inspection. For example, a person with a major depression may have symptoms of anxiety or may behave in an obsessional way. It is important to recognize these symptoms as manifestations of the higher disorder, depression, whose treatment may lead to their complete resolution.

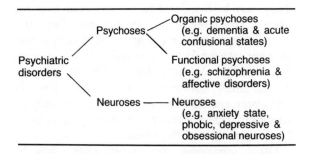

There are two diagnostic systems in common use. The World Health Organization (1978) has published an International Classification of Diseases, currently in its ninth revision (ICD-9) and shortly to be superseded by a tenth revision. In contrast to the descriptive approach of ICD-9, the American Psychiatric Association (1987) has published a Diagnostic and Statistical Manual (DSM-IIIR) in which a check-list approach has been adopted. To make a diagnosis, a specific set of criteria must be met.

The organic psychoses

These may be subdivided into three general categories: (a) acute organic reaction (acute confusional state), (b) chronic organic reaction (dementia) and (c) focal cerebral disorders, all described in detail in the standard reference book by Lishman (1987). (Acute and chronic are terms which relate solely to duration not to severity; acute implies a short duration and chronic a long duration.)

Acute organic reaction (acute confusional state)

This is a clinical syndrome in which psychiatric symptoms occur in association with an organic pathological process affecting the brain and (often) other systems; it is of abrupt onset and is characterized by impairment of consciousness. Minor impairment of consciousness may present as a difficulty in judging the passage of time, in focusing attention or in thinking coherently. People with this syndrome are often described as 'confused'. They may be disorientated in time (and later for place). The level of impairment may fluctuate, often being worst at night or in a darkened room. In more extreme forms, the patient may be drowsy and muddled. Memory deficits may be apparent at the time but are often more obvious in retrospect when the degree of impairment may be strikingly demonstrated by an inability to remember long periods of the illness.

Other symptoms may occur. There may be slowing or motor hyperactivity. Mood is often disturbed with features of anxiety or depression. (It is important to remember that people with acute organic reactions, experiencing bizarre and incomprehensible phenomena, may be frankly terrified and that this may explain some of their behaviour.) Vague persecutory delusions may be elicited. The patient may experience hallucinations (often these are visual and range from simple flashes of light to bizarre fantastic visions of scenes, people or animals) or there may be less marked perceptual distortions (illusions).

This is a syndrome (a constellation of symptoms); it is important to realize that there may be many underlying causes (diseases). In one hospital series (Cutting 1980), the two most common causes in adults were complications of alcohol abuse (intoxication, withdrawal or associated vitamin deficiencies) and intoxication with prescribed drugs (in therapeutic doses). Other causes include carcinoma, infection and head injury. With appropriate treatment it is usually fully reversible.

Chronic organic reaction (dementia)

This is another clinical syndrome; it may be defined as an acquired global impairment of intellect, memory and personality, but without impairment of consciousness (Lishman 1987). It is almost always of long duration, usually progressive and often irreversible. Memory impairment is often one of the early features, although this is usually noticed by friends or relatives rather than by the patient. Generalized cognitive deficits progressively become more obvious. The victim may revert to a rigid adherence to well-learned routines as a way of coping. If these break down or if patients are asked to do more than they can, a 'catastrophic reaction' may occur with an abrupt emotional expression of distress. Early in the illness, a degree of insight into the intellectual deterioration may lead to understandable anxiety or depression. Later in the illness, the patient may show self-neglect and appear to be quite indifferent to sloppy eating habits or even incontinence.

There is a subdivision into the presenile and the senile dementias. This is an arbitrary separation of those disorders which occur in the presenium (before the age of 65) from those which occur in the senium (after 65). To be senile strictly means no more than to be old, usually over 65 years in age.

Common causes of dementia include Alzheimer's disease (senile dementia of the Alzheimer type (SDAT) in those over 65), multi-infarct dementia, and a mixed form with features of both these syndromes. Alzheimer's disease appears to be a primary degenerative disorder; the cause is unknown although there is a familial predisposition. In multi-infarct dementia, the clinical picture is the consequence of multiple small strokes which have led to brain cell death. Sometimes these strokes may be apparent and then people are said to show a 'step-wise decline', each stage representing another small stroke. There are other causes of dementia, some of which are amenable to treatment. Although relatively uncommon, they justify further investigation of the patient.

Focal cerebral disorders

These take their characteristics from the region of the brain which is damaged. For example, thiamine deficiency (usually a consequence of alcohol abuse) may lead to a Wernicke-Korsakoff syndrome in which certain deep structures in the brain are damaged. There is a loss of recent memory and the production of coherent but false memories (confabulation). Other intellectual functions may be relatively normal.

The functional psychoses

These include (a) schizophrenia, (b) affective psychoses and (c) paranoid (delusional) disorders. They are mental disorders in which major disturbances of mental processes may be seen (e.g. hallucinations and delusions), but they differ from the organic states in that they are not caused by any identified physical disease.

Schizophrenia

In schizophrenia there may be disturbances of perception, beliefs, thought, behaviour, emotion and drive. Many of these symptoms are qualitatively abnormal (for example hearing voices in clear consciousness). It is helpful to divide the symptoms of schizophrenia into two classes (Crow, 1980).

Positive	*Negative*
Hallucinations delusions & thought disorder	Affective flattening, poverty of speech & loss of drive

The hallucinations in schizophrenia are usually auditory, although they may be present in other modalities. They may include voices talking to the person as well as voices talking about the person (although third person voices are often regarded as of diagnostic importance). There may also be primary delusions (not based on any other morbid process) and passivity experiences with secondary delusions. Illnesses characterized by positive features are said to have a good outcome, especially if they have an abrupt onset following a major life stress in a person who had been entirely normal beforehand. Positive symptoms respond well to antipsychotic medication (Johnstone et al 1978). On the other hand, the sort of patient seen in long-stay wards will often present with more chronic negative features. These can be very disabling. There is a loss of the normal range of emotional response (flattening or blunting); there may be a poverty of speech (where the patient says very little) or a poverty of the content of speech (where there is empty, meaningless speech). As well as loss of drive, there may be a deficit in attention and a tendency towards social isolation (Andreasen & Olsen 1982). These merge into the syndromes arising from 'institutionalization'. It has been demonstrated that social environment is important in reducing the impact of some of these processes (Wing & Brown 1970). A great deal of effort is now being put into early rehabilitation, active occupational therapy, day hospital care and social support in the hope of limiting as many of these features as possible. However, a small number of patients seems to show serious disabling symptoms whatever methods of treatment are adopted.

Some still distinguish three clinical variants of schizophrenia (paranoid, hebephrenic and catatonic). The paranoid type is characterized by stable delusions (*not* necessarily persecutory) and hallucinations; it is the most common. Hebephrenic schizophrenia is said to present in younger people. Here the mood is often shallow and inappropriate; behaviour may be irresponsible and silly; the stream of thought is frequently disorganized and hard to follow. In catatonic schizophrenia, the rarest form, the most obvious abnormality is in motor function. People may hold bizarre postures for long periods or there may be alternating stupor and excitement.

Although it is usually possible to say with confidence that there is a psychotic disorder, it may be more difficult to distinguish schizophrenia from one of the other psychoses. These may present with delusions or hallucinations as well. Following the demonstration in the 1960s and 1970s that there existed large discrepancies in diagnostic practice between American and British psychiatrists (Cooper et al 1972), increasing emphasis has been placed upon the use of specific diagnostic criteria. One of the best known of these is the list of first rank symptoms produced by Kurt Schneider (well described by Mellor 1970). He described 11 symptoms, each of which could be precisely defined, and suggested that the presence of any one of these in the absence of obvious physical cause would be sufficient to make a diagnosis of schizophrenia. (If a primary physical disease were present, the psychiatric syndrome would be reclassified as an organic schizophrenia-like psychosis. In practice, the abuse of amphetamines, which can lead to a psychosis indistinguishable from schizophrenia, is one of the more common reasons for reclassification.) These symptoms were:

- Audible thoughts (an hallucinatory voice speaking one's thoughts aloud)
- Hallucinatory voices arguing (two or more voices in disagreement or discussion)
- Hallucinatory voices commenting on one's actions
- Somatic passivity (the patient is a passive and invariably reluctant recipient of bodily sensations imposed on him by some external agency)
- Thought withdrawal (thoughts removed from the mind by an external force)
- Thought insertion (thoughts put into the mind by an external force)
- Diffusion or broadcasting of thoughts (thoughts are not contained within the mind; they may escape into the external world)
- 'Made' feelings (experiencing feelings which are not one's own)
- 'Made' impulses or drives (an impulse under the control of an external agency)
- 'Made' volitional acts (an action under the control of an external force)

- Delusional perception (an abnormal belief based on a normal perception). For example, a patient may say that because a chair is red (correct), the world is about to end (delusion).

Thus passivity experiences and certain types of hallucination and delusion were believed to be of high diagnostic importance. More recent systems have included other features of the illness. Feighner et al (1972) restricted the use of the term schizophrenia to chronic illnesses of at least 6 months duration. The American Diagnostic Manual (DSM-IIIR, American Psychiatric Association 1987) draws a distinction between schizophrenia (6 months duration) and schizophreniform disorder (an illness identical in appearance but of shorter duration). These differences will be considered further in the section on reliability and validity.

In practice, it is usually possible to make a firm clinical diagnosis, but this may have to depend on information gained from a careful period of observation and follow-up.

Affective psychoses

The primary disturbance is in mood which may be elated or irritable (mania) or depressed (psychotic depression). Other clinical features tend to be in keeping with the prevailing mood state (mood congruent). For example, in mania, there may be grandiose delusions, overactivity, overtalkativeness and a pattern of speech in which ideas run off one from another (flight of ideas). In this state the person is distractible and has impaired judgement. When hallucinations occur, they too have a grandiose quality. In psychotic depression, on the other hand, there is a mood of gloom and wretchedness. Other symptoms may include delusions of worthlessness or guilt; the person may have a conviction of severe illness such as cancer. There may be hallucinatory voices talking to the patient in an accusatory or persecutory fashion. Other bodily changes include sleep disturbance with early morning wakening, a mood worse in the morning, and loss of appetite and weight. Some patients may suffer extensive investigation for other causes of weight loss (for example, cancer) before referral to a psychiatrist or treatment for depression. (Unfortunately, it also has to be remembered that people with cancer may present with a depression!) Suicidal ideas are common.

These disorders have a tendency to recur. Some people only have one type of mood swing. They are said to have a unipolar affective disorder. Others have independent periods of mania and depression. They have a bipolar affective disorder (manic-depressive illness).

Mild forms of mania are sometimes called hypomania and this severe type of depression shades into neurotic depression, described later.

Paranoid (delusional) disorders

Some people have psychotic disorders which are often chronic and stable and in which they hold delusions restricted to one aspect of their life (see section on Delusional Disorders in DSM-IIIR, American Psychiatric Association, 1987). For example, these abnormal beliefs may concern the supposed unfaithfulness of a spouse (morbid jealousy syndrome) which, in extreme forms, may be a cause of domestic murder. The history of the paranoid disorders has been comprehensively reviewed by Lewis (1970).

The neuroses

In the neurotic disorders, symptoms such as anxiety, which are abnormal only in degree, are at the root of the problem. Individuals with neuroses are different from the general population only in the degree of their symptoms. To consider one example, a moderate amount of anxiety before a major examination is normal; to have severe pervasive anxiety and the maladaptive consequences of the fear are both important elements in an anxiety neurosis. Although a classification is still used, there is often a considerable amount of overlap between these disorders. For example, someone with a neurotic depression is likely to have anxiety symptoms as well. (One of the old terms for neurotic depression is 'anxiety-depression'.) The following will be considered: (a) neurotic depression, (b) anxiety state, (c) phobia, (d) obsessional neurosis, (e) hysteria and illness be-

haviour. This section is largely based on ICD-9, a diagnostic system still in common use. The reader is strongly advised to read more about the use of DSM-IIIR (e.g. Kaplan & Sadock 1988) which has many advantages over ICD-9. In particular it has much more relevance to work in liaison psychiatry (e.g. somatization disorder, somatoform pain disorder) and to understanding traumatic stress reactions (e.g. post-traumatic stress disorder).

Neurotic depression

In this disorder, although the mood is depressed, it tends to react to circumstances. It is easier to cheer someone up for a while than it would be in the more severe forms of depression. Delusions, hallucinations and (marked) bodily changes, such as weight loss, are absent. Sleep disturbance, if present, is more likely to consist of a difficulty in falling asleep; the mind is full of anxious ruminations. It has already been suggested that there is no firm division between the depressive syndromes. It should be emphasized that between this syndrome and the full psychotic depression described earlier, there is a range of intermediate disorders.

Anxiety state

Here the prevailing mood is one of fear. It may fluctuate in intensity but is not related to specific triggers. When present it is associated with over-activity of the sympathetic nervous system. Such symptoms as palpitations, butterflies in the stomach, a dry mouth and sweating of the palms are well known. Indeed, people may present with one of these as their main complaint; it is important to identify the underlying anxiety state before someone is subjected to unnecessary physical investigation.

Phobia

The symptoms are identical to those seen in anxiety states, but only occur in specific situations. For example, someone with a spider phobia will only feel anxious in the presence of a spider or in anticipation of such an event.

There are three classes of phobia. As well as simple phobias (e.g. animal phobias) there are social phobias and agoraphobias. In social phobia, the person experiences extreme anxiety (in thoughts and in sympathetic overactivity) in social situations. This may be crippling and often leads to avoidance behaviour or escape through drinking excessively. Agoraphobia is the most extensive of the phobias and most closely resembles the free-floating anxiety seen in an anxiety state. The person (usually female and often in early middle age) feels apprehensive going out of the house on her own. She will avoid travelling alone on buses (especially those with closing doors), trains or underground transport systems. Often the cause of most fear is standing in a busy supermarket, either well away from the doors or stuck in a long checkout queue.

Obsessional neurosis

This is a rare condition but one which can be extremely disabling. Although it may be normal for a person occasionally to return to his home once to check that a door is locked or a fire turned off, in an obsessional neurosis, the symptoms are much more pervasive. The normal sequence of events seems to start with a doubt. This is followed by an urge to check and increasing anxiety as this is resisted. Finally, the act of checking leads to a reduction in anxiety. In obsessional neurosis, similar phenomena are seen but in a magnified form. The obsessional doubt (perhaps a worry about contamination with germs) leads to an urge to carry out a ritualistic act (e.g. compulsive washing) or thought (a cognitive ritual with a superstitious element, e.g. repeating a sentence exactly nine times) which, when performed, results in anxiety reduction. This process is usually resisted by the patient but if repeated many times inevitably causes a marked interference in everyday functioning. In the assessment of a patient with an obsessional neurosis, the time spent carrying out motor and cognitive rituals and the degree of avoidance behaviour are usually good guides to severity and to degree of social handicap.

Hysteria and illness behaviour

Sometimes people present with physical symptoms but no underlying disease state seems to exist. Traditionally many of these were described as having 'conversion hysteria'. Others may present with amnesia or a fugue state (aimless wandering in a state of abnormal awareness), or rarely with multiple personalities; these are all examples of what has been called 'dissociative hysteria' in which it is hypothesized that conscious awareness is restricted by a psychological process, perhaps occurring as a reaction to an overwhelming stress.

A more recent contribution has been to consider the state in which physical symptoms occur in the absence of physical disease as an example of illness behaviour (reviewed by Kendell 1983) in which the sick role has advantages to the patient. However, there are probably complex interactions between physical disease, the experience of psychological difficulties and the development of physical (somatic) symptoms. Hysterical symptoms account for about 1% of a neurological practice; of these 60% will have a physical disease and perhaps as many as 50% will have a recognizable psychiatric illness (particularly depression) (Marsden 1986). It is important not to dismiss people presenting in this way; they often need full and careful investigation from physical and psychiatric perspectives.

Disorders of childhood and adolescence

No attempt will be made in this brief introduction to psychiatry to describe the specific conduct and emotional disorders of childhood and adolescence. Only one syndrome which commonly presents in adolescence or early adult life will be described in more detail.

Anorexia nervosa

To go through a period of preoccupation about weight and to react to this by abnormal eating or exercise behaviour is not unusual in adolescent girls. To go on to develop the full picture of anorexia nervosa is less common, although about 1 in 300 girls (aged 16–18) in the state educational system have the disorder (reviewed by Crisp 1980). This figure is higher in private and ballet schools. Relatively few boys or men have the disorder; the sex ratio is probably about 10 to 1.

There are three essential features, a profoundly low weight, an abnormal attitude towards eating (Crisp's 'weight-phobia') and a hormonal disturbance (in women this would be seen as loss of menstrual periods). Common ways of controlling weight include dieting, exercise, induced vomiting and abuse of drugs (e.g. laxatives). Frequently, the explanation for this state can be found within the family relationships or is in some other way related to the problems of maturation in adolescence. The full anorexia nervosa syndrome carries a not insignificant mortality (about 5%), but most people who go through a treatment programme in a unit specializing in the disorder have a good outcome.

The personality disorders

Finally, included in the International Classification of Diseases (ICD-9; World Health Organization 1978) are states called 'personality disorders'. Personality is a useful concept, one which most people use in their assessment of friends and colleagues. To say that someone is always cheerful/ miserable/friendly/shy is to say something important about his or her personality or character. Some people habitually behave in ways that lead them into conflict with society. Personality disorders are described as 'deeply ingrained maladaptive patterns of behaviour . . . continuing throughout most of adult life'. The definition specifically includes the concept that because 'of this deviation . . . the patient suffers or others have to suffer and there is an adverse effect on others or society' (World Health Organization 1978). The ICD-9 describes the following types of personality disorder: (a) paranoid, (b) affective, (c) explosive, (d) anankastic (obsessional), (e) hysterical, (f) asthenic (dependent, inadequate), (g) sociopathic.

This concept has been widely attacked. The types of personality disorder are not universally acknowledged. Diagnosis is very difficult and different psychiatrists will very often disagree. The inclusion of the effects on society in the definition of the disease state itself seems hard to justify. Although it is extremely important to know about the patient's premorbid personality in any assessment (to be able to make a judgement about the effects of the disease), it may be better to do this in a descriptive way.

However, with the increasing use of the new American diagnostic approach (American Psychiatric Association 1987), there has been renewed interest in certain well-defined conditions which appear to be chronic (may be life-long) and which may represent minor forms of disease states which are manifest as disturbances of personality alone. There is increasing evidence, for example, that schizotypal personality disorder is closely related to the clinical disorder of schizophrenia.

Reliability and validity of diagnosis

It is important that the classification system should have meaning (validity) and that there should be a high level of agreement in the use of the diagnostic criteria (reliability).

Reliability is relatively easy to assess and there are now scales for most of those phenomena which carry the potential for a high level of agreement between two or more raters. (Any scale can be used badly or without sufficient training.) Diagnostic criteria generally concentrate on symptoms which are easy to define and this has helped improve the reliability of diagnosis. However this can be taken too far. Some of the modern systems adopt a crude recipe list method to diagnosis, and although this is associated with good agreement, it does not inevitably mean that the correct diagnosis is being made. Validity of diagnosis in psychiatry is difficult to assess. The usual way is to compare the product of the procedure under scrutiny with an external criterion. For example, it is possible to compare the diagnosis of mitral stenosis, based on history and clinical examination, with the final diagnosis derived from cardiac catheter studies. In psychiatry, this external, independent reference is often lacking. Some have used outcome described in terms of social function, persisting symptoms, continued hospitalization and change in diagnosis in this way (e.g. Helzer et al 1981), but these are not altogether satisfactory. Diagnostic systems for schizophrenia which stipulate that symptoms must have been present for at least 6 months are relatively restrictive (missing out people whom many would diagnose clinically as having schizophrenia) but have a high rate of predictive specificity (including relatively few who later appear to have other diagnoses). However, perhaps it should not be too surprising that diagnostic systems which select patients with chronic disorders (with a duration of at least 6 months) are good at predicting chronicity and poor outcome.

Validity may also be investigated using statistical techniques. Everitt et al (1971) applied the method of cluster analysis to two unselected series of patients (500 in all). Their work supports the traditional distinctions between mania, schizophrenia and psychotic depression, although there was no evidence of a formal distinction between the neuroses.

CONCLUSION

In this chapter, a way of looking at the concept of sickness which incorporates elements of the disease model but also takes account of other complementary systems has been described. The view has been taken that a discussion of what it means to be sick must inevitably include subjective and social elements. However, the role of biological changes should not be underestimated. Particularly in the psychoses, these are likely to be of major importance. In the organic states, the mental disorders are secondary consequences of derangements of physical function. In the functional psychoses, people have such profoundly different experiences that they are categorically abnormal. In the neuroses, on the other hand, biological processes may be less central. Here it is the degree of anxiety or depression which is important. Social and psychological forces may be more fundamental. The disease model is probably least relevant in the 'personality disorders', although description of the personality in terms of traits or features is an important part of the whole assessment.

It is certain that any system of classification based on present knowledge is going to be a simplification. It may be that a multi-dimensional approach to the description of illness would be more valid than the categorical diagnostic method outlined here. However, that is the challenge for the future of psychiatry. There is scope for increased understanding and a need for the determination to achieve it.

REFERENCES

Andreasen N C, Olsen S 1982 Negative v positive schizophrenia. Definition and validation. Archives of General Psychiatry 39: 789–794

American Psychiatric Association 1987 Diagnostic and statistical manual of mental disorders, 3rd edn. American Psychiatric Association, Washington D C

Clark B 1978 Whose life is it anyway. Amber Lane Press, Ashover

Cooper J E, Kendell R E, Gurland B J, Sharpe L, Copeland J R M, Simon R 1972 Psychiatric diagnosis in New York and London. Maudsley Monograph No 20. Oxford University Press, Oxford

Crisp A H 1980 Anorexia nervosa: let me be. Academic Press, London

Crow T J 1980 Molecular pathology of schizophrenia: more than one disease process? British Medical Journal 280: 66–68

Cutting J C 1980 Physical illness and psychosis. British Journal of Psychiatry 136: 109–119

Everitt B S, Gourlay A J, Kendell R E 1971 An attempt at validation of traditional psychiatric syndromes by cluster analysis. British Journal of Psychiatry 119: 399–412

Feighner J P, Robins E, Guze S B, Woodruff R A, Winokur G, Munoz R 1972 Diagnostic criteria for use in psychiatric research. Archives of General Psychiatry 26: 57–63

Foulds G A 1965 Personality and personal illness. Tavistock Publications, London

Gottesman I, Shields J 1982 Schizophrenia: the epigenetic puzzle. Cambridge University Press, Cambridge

Helzer J E, Brockington I F, Kendell R E 1981 Predictive validity of DSM-III and Feighner definition of schizophrenia. Archives of General Psychiatry 38: 791–797

Heston L L 1966 Psychiatric disorders in foster home reared children of schizophrenic mothers. British Journal of Psychiatry 112: 819–825

Illich I 1974 Medical nemesis. Lancet: 918–921

Johnstone E C, Crow T J, Frith C D, Husband J, Kreel L 1976 Cerebral ventricular size and cognitive impairment in chronic schizophrenia. Lancet ii: 924–926

Johnstone E C, Crow T J, Frith C D, Carney M W P, Price J S 1978 Mechanism of the antipsychotic effect in the treatment of acute schizophrenia. Lancet i: 848–851

Kaplan H I, Sadock B J 1988 Clinical psychiatry (from synopsis of psychiatry). Williams & Wilkins, Baltimore, USA

Kendell R E 1975 The role of diagnosis in psychiatry. Blackwell Scientific Publications, Oxford

Kendell R E 1983 Hysteria. In: Russell G F M, Hersov L A (eds) Handbook of psychiatry, vol 4, The neuroses and personality disorders. Cambridge University Press, Cambridge

Kennedy I 1981 The unmasking of medicine. George Allen & Unwin, London

Laing R D 1965 The divided self. Penguin, Harmondsworth

Leff J, Vaughn C 1981 The role of maintenance therapy and relative expressed emotion in relapse of schizophrenia: a two-year follow up. British Journal of Psychiatry 139: 102–104

Lewis A J 1953 Health as a social concept. British Journal of Sociology 4: 109–124

Lewis A 1970 Paranoia and paranoid: a historical perspective. Psychological Medicine 1: 2–12 (also published in The Later Papers of Sir Aubrey Lewis 1979 Oxford University Press, Oxford)

Lishman W A 1987 Organic psychiatry, 2nd. Blackwell Scientific Publications, Oxford

Marsden C D 1986 Hysteria — a neurologist's view. Psychological Medicine 16: 277–288

Mellor C S 1970 First rank symptoms of schizophrenia. British Journal of Psychiatry 117: 15–23

Mitchell J R A 1984 Hearts and minds. British Medical Journal 289: 1557–1558

Parkes C M, Benjamin B, Fitzgerald R G 1969 Broken heart: a statistical study of increased mortality among widowers. British Medical Journal i: 740–743.

Rosenhan D L 1973 On being sane in insane places. Science 179: 250–258

Scadding J G 1967 Diagnosis: the clinician and the computer. Lancet 2: 877–882

Scheff T J 1974 The labelling theory of mental illness. American Sociological Review 39: 444–452

Szasz T 1974 Ideology and insanity. Penguin, Harmondsworth

Taylor D C 1979 The components of sickness: diseases, illnesses and predicaments. Lancet ii: 1008–1010

Taylor F K 1972 A logical analysis of the medico-psychological concept of disease Part 2. Psychological Medicine 2: 7–16

Trichopoulos D, Katsouyanni K, Zavitsanos X, Tzonou A, Dalla-Vorgia P 1983 Psychological stress and fatal heart attack: the Athens (1981) earthquake natural experiment. Lancet i: 441–444

Turner S W, Toone B K, Brett-Jones J 1986 Computerized tomographic scan changes in early schizophrenia — preliminary findings. Psychological Medicine 16: 219–225

Weinberger D R, Torrey E F, Neophytides A N, Wyatt R J 1979 Lateral cerebral ventricular enlargement in chronic schizophrenia. Archives of General Psychiatry 36: 735–739

Wing J K, Brown G W 1970 Institutionalism and schizophrenia. Cambridge University Press, Cambridge

World Health Organization 1978 Mental disorders: glossary and guide to their classification in accordance with the ninth revision of the international classification of diseases. World Health Organization, Geneva

Yalom I D 1975 The theory and practice of group psychotherapy. Basic Books, New York

17

The contribution of health education

S. Lask

The skills and abilities of the health educator are very similar to those of nurses working with people with mental health problems. These are skills which will enable people to take responsibility for their health, increase their autonomy and exercise their rights, and are concerned with:

- communicating effectively, facilitating and enabling learning, change and growth to take place
- promoting self-esteem
- teaching coping strategies and life-skills
- providing relevant information.

Mental health education has always been an integral and important part of mainstream health education. Shapland (1987) surveyed 50 health education units in England and asked them if their health education unit was involved, in any way, in education to promote mental health: 80% said they did have programmes for this. One unit summarized their philosophy on mental health education thus: 'In fact, anything that adds to understanding and lessens fear and doubts increases the mental health of the individual.'

Other interventions by health education officers described in this research included

- stress-management
- identification of life-crises
- life-skills and self-empowerment courses

- 'drinking-choices' courses
- racism and sexism awareness groups
- teaching and information packs on women's health, childbirth without fear, depression, child abuse.

Most, if not all, health education interventions take a holistic approach, where each component of health is considered in relation to the others.

There are a variety of strategies and approaches which have been found to be useful to health educators which are particularly relevant to the mental health nurse who wishes to develop her role as a health educator. These approaches are common in community and school health education initiatives and may also be familiar to many mental health nurses. Two of the most powerful approaches will be explored in examples later in this chapter:

1. The 'health careers' concept
2. Preventive educational programmes. The 'Kidscape' programme is taken as an example to illustrate the 'life-skills' and 'empowerment' approaches used to combat child sex abuse.

HISTORICAL DICHOTOMY

In health education, there has been an on-going debate as to whether the causes of ill health are 'deterministic' or 'voluntaristic'. This has led to a serious dichotomy within the discipline. The deterministic position, focuses on the *environmental causes of ill-health* and implies that the society in which we live is the main determinant of disease. The voluntaristic view focuses on the *individual*, and is concerned with attitudes and behaviour or individual choices.

A person who develops dependence on alcohol or drugs, for example, which leads to a disintegration in their normal everyday functioning, would be explained in terms of a personality weakness or deviance by the voluntaristic theorists, and by the overwhelming influences of a stressful society which condones such activities, by the determinists.

The latter group of health educators blames governments and feels that the responsibility lies with them. The charity Alcohol Concern (1987)

argues, for example, that in 1983 the government received £200 every second from tax revenue on alcohol, yet spent only one pence per second on health education and treatments for alcohol problems. This group sees the function of health education as raising public awareness and putting political pressure on government. It can support its arguments against the government with the following statistics which include evidence researched by orthodox and establishment bodies such as the Royal College of Psychiatrists (1986) who report that as a nation in 1983 we spent £13 billion on alcohol; by 1985 this had increased to £16 billion. In 1983 £11 billion was spent on the National Health Service, £10 billion on schools and £15 million on national defence. We spent £12 billion on clothing ourselves that year. The environmental perspective of health educators who criticize the government's priorities over expenditure on health is referred to by Tones (1981), Draper (1977), Ewles & Simnett (1985), Mitchell (1982) and many others as the radical or social model of health education, and has developed out of the public health movements of the 19th century.

Health educators who work within this framework often feel isolated and separated from those who work with individuals and who attempt to change each person in some way. Nurses usually work on a one-to-one basis with their patients and clients, and Lask (1987) analyses the dilemmas and difficulties which may occur in attempting to change peoples' attitudes and behaviour. This may partly explain why health education is not perceived as a priority and has attracted much comment from nursing researchers, including Macleod Clark & Webb (1985), Faulkner (1983) and Syred (1981).

The type of therapy, response or health education intervention which is taken by educators will depend on which philosophical perspective they have adopted. The health educational models which most commonly adopt the individual approach, which is concerned with changing the individual's attitude and behaviour, include the medical or behavioural model, the educational model and the life-skills or empowerment models. Adoption of the medical or behavioural change model has led to the concept of 'victim blaming' as described by Mitchell (1982), where the individual is held responsible for his own illness by health professionals, and a considerable amount of guilt is incurred and endured by the patient as well.

The philosophical debate about the nature of mental illness has long been a central feature of British psychiatry; in fact health education shares with the whole area of mental health the disagreements and difficulties which arise from a lack of conceptual clarity about the exact meaning of the term.

HEALTH CAREERS

The health careers approach attempts to reconcile these differences, and can provide a very useful model for nurses who work individually with patients and yet want to retain their political and social sensitivities. It is a concept borrowed by health education from sociology.

In sociology, a career line has generally been used to explore the social, environmental and personal influences on some aspect of social behaviour; it is a diagram which represents an individual's personal history over time. Figure 17.1 shows an example of an alcohol drinking

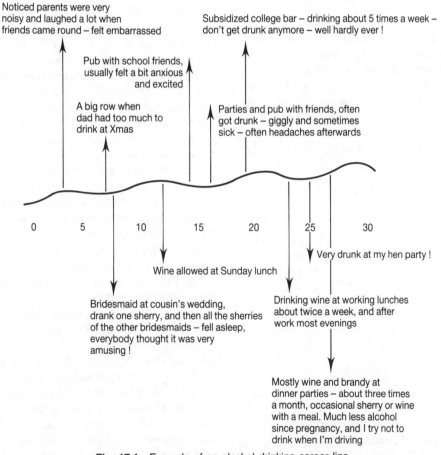

Fig. 17.1   Example of an alcohol drinking career line.

career line. The purpose of a career line is to show how patterns of potentially harmful behaviour can evolve through interaction with a person's social environment and through processes of socialization. It has been extensively used in school health education by the Schools' Council development teams (1979), and was developed for a variety of reasons, including the changing patterns of illness over the past 3 decades and the association of many of these diseases with life-styles adopted by individuals and groups. The Health Education Council's (1986) project identifies:

An inherent difficulty of many of our contemporary health issues is that they are rooted in the social and cultural life of society itself. Health education can, all too easily, be seen as a means of social first aid. . . . Health education is however now concerning itself with the natural history of some of these problems in an effort to identify their social antecedents — or, in sociological terms, their career-line patterns.

Everyone could draw his own eating, sexual, smoking or depression career lines, illustrating events which influenced his attitudes and behaviour; and how he felt or reacted to these influences may help his understanding of his current feelings and behaviour. Figure 17.2 shows the Health Education Council's (1986) example of the influences which may affect a person's smoking career. Even if people do not smoke or drink, they still have a history of influences which can be represented in a career line.

The career-line framework has been applied successfully to health education by Dorn & Nortoft (1982), who have developed teaching initiatives in drug education, but whose approach is applicable to mental health.

Problems addressed by the health careers approach

Dorn & Nortoft (1982) identify three problems with current health education which their programme addresses and overcomes. Firstly is the dilemma of whether to take the communal or the individual approach: they successfully combine both these perspectives.

The second problem is the inadequate portrayal of health-related issues facing women and girls, and of the relations between the sexes. Briscoe (1985) describes the differences in psychological problems and responses of women and men, with women consistently showing more psychological morbidity. Hunt (1986) also documents this and discusses the possible explanations and solutions. Yet this problem is not really addressed adequately by health care workers, and by continuing to neglect this aspect an unrealistic view of society is depicted for both girls and boys.

The third problem, identified by Dorn & Nortoft (1982), is the systematic neglect of 'youth culture'. Youth is divided into groups which have their own distinct variant of the broader culture. These groups can be according to gender, social class, occupation, ethnicity or region.

Class differences in health status have recently been acknowledged by nurses, but more specific variations, such as regional or cultural differences, have yet to be adequately explored.

Alcohol Concern (1987) describe different drinking cultures, where the psychological impact of alcohol is strongly influenced by culture. Cultures which define alcoholic beverages as a food, such as France and Italy, experience very few public disorder problems — i.e. there is less rowdy and aggressive behaviour despite high alcohol intakes — and alcohol problems can be regarded

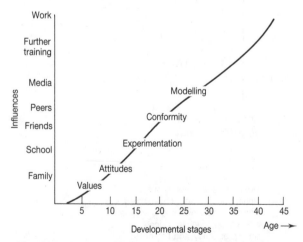

Fig. 17.2 Example of the influences which may affect a person's smoking career (Health Education Council 1986).

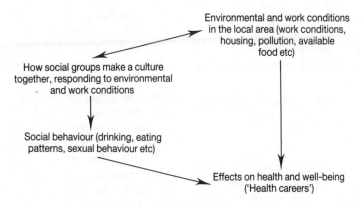

Fig. 17.3 Health careers (from Dorn & Nortoft 1982).

as similar to other dietary problems such as eating too much fat or sugar. Other countries have different cultural definitions: in Scandinavia there is a widespread tradition of binge drinking as a means of escape; and in Britain working class beer drinkers in the North have a Scandinavian style tradition whilst the middle class wine drinkers of the South are much closer to the French and the Italians.

A health careers perspective can be beneficial in attempting to understand an individual's behaviour and takes at its starting point the ways in which a person's relationship to his work affects his health. This will, of course, vary depending on whether the person is a housewife, mother, student, factory worker, shift worker, nine-to-five office worker or unemployed.

The health careers approach for the youth group examines the transition that young people have to make to the labour market and their subsequent relationship with it. It explores over time both the environmental and work conditions which are experienced by either the group or the individual, and simultaneously examines how that social group forms a culture, responding to these conditions, which of course will determine social behaviour such as drinking, eating and sexual behaviour. The individual's social behaviour and his psychological responses and coping strategies, together with the environmental and work conditions, are considered when looking at the effects on his health and well-being (Fig. 17.3).

The work we do defines the culture we make,

which in turn influences our social behaviour. How we spend our leisure time depends on whether we perceive it as a reward or a respite from work. Large sections of the population will be unable to view leisure in either of these ways, and this may influence to what extent they engage in potentially dangerous activities.

The concept of 'time off' from work is central to the health careers approach, as this can influence a person's chemical career. It is during time off that an individual usually engages in a leisure activity which may involve the use of chemicals in some way, for example: cigarettes and coffee in tea and coffee breaks, beer or wine at lunch, and more alcohol and possibly a variety of less socially acceptable chemicals after work. Those who do not have their work breaks defined by their employment may be at greater risk from abuse of alcohol or other chemicals. This group includes housewives and mothers, the unemployed, psychiatric patients, and those who can smoke and drink as they work, for example journalists and writers, and a proportion of the self-employed.

By analysing how an individual's life-style is determined by his employment, an understanding of his relationship to health-related behaviour is demonstrated.

Dorn & Nortoft (1982) suggest that a 24-hour day be divided up into the following categories:

- sleep
- work outside the home
- housework (cooking, cleaning, child-care,

shopping, looking after others in the family, washing clothes)

- body maintenance (eating, washing self)
- 'time off' (everything that a person regards as free time).

It may be useful to do this exercise several times and compare the relationships between each category for different individuals.

The career line approach can be used with most patients in an attempt to explore individual and personal influences in a systematic way. With experience, a skilled practitioner will facilitate a patient's understanding and aid him with insights into his own social behaviour.

PREVENTIVE PROGRAMMES

Many nurses implicitly believe that the purpose of health education is prevention. When they are confronted with a patient, either in hospital or the community, they assume that health education must have failed in some way, and either it is far too late to provide it (as the illness or accident has already occurred), or it is not appropriate when caring for the sick.

Holding this view demonstrates the pervading influence that medicine has on nursing, as a preventive approach is central to a medical model of health education. This model works as a deficiency model, i.e. it looks for deficits or problems, assesses them, prescribes a treatment, carries out that treatment, and evaluates its effectiveness. It is this empirical approach which the nursing process has emulated. This model is not the province of medicine alone; for example it is possible to take a 'medical model' approach to education. A problem can be identified — poor reading ability — a treatment can be prescribed and implemented — extra remedial reading lessons — and the programme can be evaluated.

Using a deficit approach may not be the most appropriate model for mental health nursing for a variety of reasons.

Firstly, it is difficult to define precisely what mental health is; it therefore follows that prevent-

ing something that is difficult to define and measure is equally difficult.

Secondly, using a deficit approach may create unnecessary feelings of negativity in both the patient and the nurse; identifying all the problems and attempting to provide treatments may seem too daunting. A model which identifies the patient's strengths and works to build on these is a much more positive and fruitful approach.

Finally, there are a variety of interpretations of what 'preventive psychiatry' is or could be, none of which offer the nurse a framework or theory base from which to practise.

Although the DHSS (1979) document 'A Service for Patients' recommended that health education should be emphasized in the forward planning for mental health by health authorities, and that priorities for the mentally ill should emphasize community care, there are no suggestions on how the nurse working with patients who have already suffered a crisis in their mental health status should incorporate this into her work.

Preventive psychiatry is usually referred to in the context of three issues. These are

- the removal of the stigma of mental illness from the population generally
- the early detection of mental ill-health
- the provision of the individual with better coping skills.

Public perceptions of mental ill-health

Recent work with school children has shown that positive attitudes to mental ill-health are developing. Leatherbarrow (1985) describes two recent teaching packs — one joint publication from MIND and Community Service Volunteers (1984), and the other from Wales MIND (1983) — which both acknowledge that being able to cope effectively with stress may be an important factor in preventing mental ill-health. In addition, stereotyped attitudes to mental ill-health are challenged.

That a considerable amount of wrong information is held by the public has been described by Skuse (1975), who has shown that in a group of psychiatric outpatients waiting for their first outpatient appointment there were a variety of misperceptions of what might take place, ranging from hypnotism and ECT to being 'taken back' to relive unpleasant childhood memories on 'the couch'. Other successful initiatives in promoting positive attitudes to mental ill-health in school-children have been described by Furnell (1985).

Work has also been accomplished by Pretty (1982) in changing attitudes to a more positive direction by using group work methods with home-helps.

Sauber (1973) identifies the nebulous concept of prevention when he describes it thus: 'Primary prevention needs to focus on both modifying the environment and strengthening individual capacity to cope with situations'.

Primary prevention

The programmes which develop out of holding a concept of primary prevention are ones which generally coincide with the socialization process of the community and are termed social action programmes. These include policies aimed at modifying the general attitudes and behaviour of the population by communication through the educational system, mass media and family, and interaction between professionals and the lay community. An example of a social action programme are the early programmes initiated by the Health Education Authority on AIDS prevention.

Caplan (1964) uses primary prevention to identify current harmful influences in the environment and resistance factors in the population. To enable this process to occur successfully, adequate psychiatric and psychological services must be fully funded and provided throughout the country, and many argue for this provision, including O'Donnell (1977) and Cole (1984).

Self-empowerment and life-skills training

The basic tenet of the approach used in preventive programmes is the development of self-empowerment. Table 17.1 lists some factors whose dimensions discriminate between those who demonstrate more or less empowered behaviour.

Table 17.1 Empowered behaviour

More empowered behaviour	Less empowered behaviour
Open to change	Closed to change
Assertive	Non-assertive or aggressive
Proactive	Reactive
Self-accountable	Blames others
Uses feelings	Overwhelmed by or fails to recognize feelings
Learns from mistakes	Debilitated by mistakes
Confronts	Avoids
Lives more in the present	Past or future-oriented
Realistic	Unrealistic
Thinks relatively	Thinks in absolutes
Sees alternatives	Tunnel vision
Develops commitments	Keeps obligations
Likes self	Dislikes self
Values others	Negates others
Alert to others' needs	Selfish
Interested in the world	Self-centred
Balanced life-style	One arena of life developed to the exclusion of others
Enhances the lives of others	Restricts the lives of others

Those with mental health problems behave in a very powerless way and illustrate how lack of empowerment can debilitate an individual's life. Nurses, too, are often unable to control aspects of their working life and have benefited from aspects of life-skills training (Hopson & Scally 1981) in their education, such as communication skills and assertiveness skills.

Life-skills programmes are most commonly used in secondary schools, but the behavioural aspects of the programmes have been successfully adapted to social skills training in mental health to increase self-empowerment.

The 'Kidscape' preventive programme

An unusual, yet welcome example of this progressive approach to education, used in a preventive way, is teaching children about child sex abuse in primary schools. One such programme is called

'Kidscape', and has been developed by Michelle Elliot (1986), an educational psychologist. The Kidscape approach involves the class teacher in some additional training provided by the Kidscape team. The teacher runs her own classes with the children who know her. Knowledge of the principles underlying these programmes and the implications to be drawn from them could benefit the mental health nurse when attempting to enhance her health educational skills.

Psychological damage?

Nelson (1987) describes how psychiatrists, social workers, marriage guidance counsellors and court workers will remark time and again how often they discovered a history of child sexual abuse in women and girls presenting severe psychological difficulties.

Lewis & Sarrel (1969) found anxiety symptoms of enuresis, speech problems, nightmares, and phobic and obsessional states in pre-pubertal victims. The Kempes (1978) found victims suffering from fear states, night terrors, clinging behaviour and developmental regression, insomnia and hysteria, in addition to running away from home and suddenly failing at school.

Depression, neuroses and suicidal tendencies are often the main causes of referral for adolescent or older survivors, and some American associations, such as Odyssey House, report a high correlation between abuse in childhood and drug addiction; some, such as John Silverston, suggest that as many as 70% of addicts have been abused (Nelson 1987).

Benward & Densen-Gerber (1975) found a strong association between incest and both promiscuity and prostitution. Incest survivors are also highly represented in compulsive eating self-help groups and amongst agoraphobics.

Elliot (1985) reports that at least seven out of ten child sex abuse assaults are perpetrated by either a relative, usually the natural father or stepfather, or by somebody already known to the child, so that warning children about taking care with strangers is like teaching them to cross the road, but only telling them to watch out for the red cars.

The Kidscape programme focuses on the concepts of 'Good sense defence', and 'Keeping safe', and is aimed at 5–11 year olds, their parents and teachers. It begins by concentrating on assertion and saying 'no' to bullying from peers; for example, it teaches children that adults can make mistakes and do things that are wrong. But most importantly it teaches them the difference between hugs and kisses and touches that they do like, and those that they don't, and that touches should never be kept a secret. So if an adult or an older child attempts to persuade them to keep a touch that they did not like a secret, the programme teaches them that it is right and proper to tell another adult.

The teaching pack is sensitive and child centred; it never uses the words child sex abuse, and it is carefully designed not to increase fear or suspicion, but to fundamentally raise the children's self-esteem, confidence and to increase their own self-empowerment. It includes a video, plus information booklets for the teachers and parents and charts for the children.

SUMMARY

Two major health educational strategies were explored and their usefulness to mental health education described. The first of these is the 'health careers' approach of Dorn & Nortoft (1982) which attempts to resolve the dichotomy of the individual behaviour change approach and the social, cultural or political view of health education. The second is the use of preventive programmes, an example being Michelle Elliot's Kidscape (1986), which incorporates the life-skills and self-empowerment ideals of Friere (1972) and Hopson & Scally (1981).

REFERENCES

Alcohol Concern 1987 The drinking revolution: building a campaign for safer drinking. Alcohol Concern, London

Benward J, Densen-Gerber 1975 Incest as a causative factor in anti-social behaviour: an exploratory study. Contemporary Drug Problems 4: 1977

Briscoe M 1985 Men, women and mental health. Health Education Journal: 44(3): 151–153

Caplan 1964 Preventive psychiatry. Tavistock Publications, London

Cole C W 1984 Community mental health — past, present and future. Health Education Journal 42(4): 99–101

DHSS 1979 Royal Commission Report: A Service for Patients. HMSO, London

Dorn N, Nortoft B 1982 Health careers. Teachers manual. ISDD, London

Draper P 1977 Health and wealth. Royal Society of Health. June

Elliot M 1985 Keeping safe: a practical guide to talking with children. Bedford Square Press/NCVO, London

Elliot M 1986 Kidscape primary kit. Kidscape, London

Ewles L, Simnett I 1985 Promoting health: a practical guide to health education. John Wiley and Sons, Chichester

Faulkner A 1983 Nurses as health educators in relation to smoking. Nursing Times Occasional Papers April 13 79(8): 47–48

Friere P 1972 Pedagogy of the oppressed. Penguin, Harmondsworth

Furnell J 1985 Doing more to promote positive mental health. Education and Health, November

Health Education Council 1986 Health education in initial teacher education. Southampton University, Southampton

Hopson B, Scally M 1981 Life-skills teaching. McGraw-Hill, UK

Hunt H 1986 Women's private distress — a public health issue: strategies for psychologists working in primary care. Medicine in Society 12(2)

Kempe R, Kempe C H 1978 Child abuse. Fontana, London

Lask S 1987 Beliefs and behaviour in health education. Nursing 3(18)

Leatherbarrow B 1985 Mental health education and the curriculum. Education and Health, January: 18–21

Lewis M, Sarrel P 1969 Some psychological aspects of seduction, incest and rape in childhood. Journal of American Academy of Child Psychiatry 4: 4

Macleod Clark J, Webb P 1985 Health Education — a basis for professional nursing practice. Nurse Education Today 5: 210–214

MIND/Community Service Volunteers (CSV) 1984 Insight: Mental illness in perspective. MIND, London

Mitchell J 1982 Looking after ourselves: an individual responsibility? Royal Society of Health 3

Nelson S 1987 Incest: fact and myth. Stramullion, Scotland

O'Donnell C R 1977 Behaviour modification in community settings. In: Progress in behaviour modification, vol 4, pp 69–117

Pretty P L 1982 An experiment in changing attitudes to mental disorder. Health Education Journal 41(1)

Royal College of Psychiatrists 1986 Alcohol our favourite drug. Tavistock Publications, London

Sauber S R 1973 Preventive educational intervention for mental health. Ballinger Publishing Company, Camb, Mass

Schools' Council 1979 Health education 5–13. Nelson, London

Shapland 1987 Unpublished MSc thesis. King's College, London

Skuse D H 1975 Attitudes to psychiatric outpatient clinics. British Medical Journal, August: 469

Syred M E J 1981 The abdication of the role of health education by hospital nurses. Journal of Advanced Nursing 6: 27–33

Tones B K 1981 Health education: prevention or subversion? Royal Society of Health 101(3)

Wales MIND 1983 An approach to mental health education. Wales MIND, Cardiff

Part 3

Principles of psychiatric nursing practice

18

Psychiatric nursing assessment

B. L. Thomas and J. I. Brooking

This chapter examines some of the benefits and
problems of making a psychiatric nursing assessment. The importance of a comprehensive
accurate assessment is discussed together with the
relevance of nursing models, assessment questionnaires and guidelines. Interviewing skills, issues
concerning the multi-disciplinary approach to assessment and making a nursing diagnosis are also
explored. No one would doubt the important part
assessment plays in the care of those who are mentally distressed. It is apparent from the amount of
prescriptive literature on the subject. However,
what else is apparent is the lack of nursing
research in this area.

THE PURPOSE OF NURSING ASSESSMENT AND MULTI-DISCIPLINARY ASSESSMENT

The importance of an accurate and systematic
assessment as a basis for planning care cannot be
over-emphasized. This first stage of the nursing
process is an essential prerequisite for carrying out
therapeutic nursing care. The nursing care plan
can only be as good as the assessment information
on which it is based.

Patient assessment has developed from the assumptions that individuals vary in their experience
of illness and in their responses to treatment and

care. Each person's problems and needs will differ, just as all humans differ in their genetic inheritence, constitutional factors, environmental experiences, physical characteristics, personality and emotional stability.

Patient assessment is carried out by all the professionals involved in care. Psychiatrists will carry out a full psychiatric and mental status examination culminating in a diagnosis. A psychologist will use a variety of standardized psychometric and/or projective tests to examine personality, intelligence and cognitive functioning. The neurologist will be interested in the effects of organic lesions in the central nervous system, the physician will carry out a medical examination. The social worker will assess the family and support systems, housing and finance. The occupational therapist will examine the extent to which the patient has the functional skills such as cooking and laundering and the ability to carry out daily living activities.

Nursing assessment focuses not on the psychiatric diagnosis but on the problems that arise from the illness, treatment and prognosis as well as the psychosocial components of the illness and its treatment. The patients' physical, psychological and social functioning are all assessed. Of course, with so many disciplines involved in the assessment process there may be areas of overlap. Duplication should be avoided whenever possible. A multi-disciplinary approach is common practice, in which psychiatric nursing assessment forms part of a joint enterprise. Its success depends upon collaboration, good communication and mutual recognition of the contributions made by all those involved.

Assessment should not consist of a random gathering of information but should have a specific purpose. The main aim is to understand the nature of the patient's problems and needs and to plan care to meet these needs and overcome identified problems. It is the collection of information with the intention of making a judgement about the care required. Nurses look at patients from the broadest possible viewpoint and will study assets as well as weaknesses, thereby enabling the patient to build upon his or her own resources. Nursing assessment may also have a more specific purpose:

for example, assessing suicidal intent, potential violence, and the need for rehabilitation or preparation for discharge.

An assessment interview also has a therapeutic function. Research to examine the efficiency of a nursing assessment guide found that patients frequently asked if they could talk with the interviewer again and stated how helpful they had found the process (Sanger et al 1988). The interview may be used as a means of initiating or fostering the nurse–patient relationship. Stockwell (1985) suggests that assessment is the means by which the nurse gets to know the patient and his or her problems. It is the basis on which all future care is planned and given. It is also therapeutic in that it may give the patient new awareness of his difficulties or ways of seeing them differently. A study by Sebastian (1987), assessing patients' perceptions of coming into psychiatric hospital, suggests that on admission the patients' highest priority is knowledge about their problems and the treatment process.

A nursing assessment is advantageous to the nurse. In the past, care strategies have been based chiefly on information obtained from doctors' notes. The use of a systematic continuous assessment enhances the nurse's autonomy as a professional and it broadens the base for care giving. The nursing assessment can also explore the role of the family and the community so that the nurse's perspective is broadened. The assessment process may be used to teach nurses interviewing skills, documentation of important information and record keeping, and the identification of patients' problems and needs. It may also be used for research purposes and for nursing and clinical audit.

SOURCES OF DATA

Data collected when assessing a patient's strengths, weaknesses, needs and problems may be obtained from a variety of sources, including observation, assessment interview and record review. One of the main instruments for data collection is the nursing history or patient assessment form compiled from information provided by the patient and or family and friends. The family may be an important source of data (Marriner 1979). Most assessment forms are produced at local level in response to organizational requirements. Most nursing textbooks include specimen history and assessment forms, e.g. McFarlane & Castledine (1982), Bauer & Hill (1986). Some forms have been developed specifically for psychiatric patients (Smith 1980, Tissier 1986).

Some hospitals have experimented with patient-completed assessment forms. In a comparative study, Aspinall (1976) found that data thus obtained compared favourably with data from a nursing interview. Apart from the inability of some patients to complete an assessment form, Crow (1979) commented that this would reduce nurse–patient interaction on admission, possibly stunting the development of a relationship. Rashidi (1975) reports that a self-administered psychiatric history form collects three times more information and twice as much significant data as traditional methods in medicine.

Contemporary nursing literature recommends a holistic approach to care (Schultz & Dark 1986). A holistic view during the assessment phase helps to ensure that important aspects are not overlooked. The introduction of the nursing process provides nurses with a systematic, problem-solving approach to care. By highlighting the importance of assessment, the nursing process enables nurses to recognize with the patient both potential and actual problems. However, the nursing process by itself does not provide guidance as to what to assess.

As a result the nursing process has often been used to assess patients' problems around a set of medical understandings of people and their needs (Aggleton & Chalmers 1986).

Nursing models

The introduction of nursing models provides nurses with various philosophies of care that can guide them in their use of the nursing process. Nursing models carry with them assumptions and underlying beliefs about individuals, health, society and nursing. These models also differ in terms of how they approach assessment. The assessment processes proposed are specific to that

model and they place different emphasis on what should be assessed. For example, according to Orem (1980) the healthy individual is a self-care agent. Therefore, assessment is governed according to the person's self-care requisites. Roper et al (1981) suggest that, in addition to the usual biographical and health data, the nursing history should include an assessment of each of the activities of living identified in her framework of nursing. Darcy (1980) prefers the term 'needs analysis' in preference to assessment. This he carries out in relation to Roper's (1976) activities of living, which are critically analysed against the background of the patient's illness, social circumstances, perception, personality, education, religion and treatment.

Darcy (1980) identifies three types of needs: those the patient can meet unaided; those he or she can meet with limited aid; and those he or she is unable to meet. Another basis for assessment is implicit in the Roy Adaptation Model. According to Roy (1976), people adapt to illness in four ways — physiologically, in terms of self-concept, in role function and in dependence. Nursing assessment should thus examine these four adaptations.

Nursing assessment will vary according to which nursing model is used. Not all psychiatric nurses use nursing models. Psychiatry also uses a number of models, including organic, psychotherapeutic, behavioural, cognitive, socio-therapeutic and medical models, and many psychiatric nurses prefer to work from one of these perspectives. Within each of these models there are similarities and differences, and some differ radically from each other.

DOCUMENTATION OF THE NURSING ASSESSMENT

There is much variation in the format and content of assessment documentation, depending on the model used in a particular ward or setting and on the individual nurse. In order to bring some conformity to this important task, a number of nurses have been concerned in the development of a comprehensive nursing assessment form. Two studies in general nursing found that the use of systematic assessment forms increased the number of physical and psychosocial problems identified (Hamdi & Hutelmyer 1970, Hefferin & Hunter 1975). A number of assessment forms have been specifically developed for use in assessing psychiatric patients.

Using a systems approach, Smith (1980) developed a form which was divided into sections relating to particular areas of a patient's life. An assessment guide aimed at developing nursing diagnoses has been tested with depressed patients and patients with thought disorders and manic conditions by Sanger et al (1988). In both studies, the guides were found to be useful in eliciting relevant information for the identification of nursing diagnoses but, as the authors point out, the guides were not intended to be a single source of comprehensive information. As well as the specifically designed forms, most psychiatric nursing textbooks make recommendations on what should be assessed. Darcy (1985) suggests that the assessment should include the background of the patient's illness, perception of hospital, personality, and social and family circumstances. Schultz & Dark (1986) identify 33 factors which are important when making a psychiatric nursing assessment. Tissier (1986) describes the development and testing of a patient assessment form designed to be used by psychiatric nurses in acute admission wards. Details of the complex steps involved in developing, testing and refining an assessment form are given below.

1. Literature search — to identify what nurse theorists suggest should be included in assessment forms
2. Examination of information collected by previous students in their assessments of psychiatric patients
3. Interviews with sisters charge nurses, and members of the multi-disciplinary team
4. Development of first draft of nursing assessment form
5. Validity testing — the first draft was sent to a panel of experts on psychiatric nursing and the nursing process for their comments on format design and content
6. Refinement of assessment form based on recommendations made by panel of experts

7. Testing of second draft for feasibility and inter-rater reliability. On the grounds of expediency and ethics this was carried out on pseudo-patients
8. The final draft was tested on a small group of patients on four acute psychiatric wards. A sample of student nurses were given either a conventional Kardex or an assessment form and asked to identify as many patient problems as possible.

The results showed that, overall, the number of problems identified increased by using the assessment form, especially psychological and social problems which had not been previously identified by using the Kardex. No firm conclusions can be reached from the study owing to the small numbers used. It seems that the form has potential in providing a systematic and concise instrument to assist nurses in the assessment process. Future testing of the form is required, using a larger sample and in different settings.

Content of the form

The form is divided into four stages:

- Stage 1 — Baseline admission information
- Stage 2 — Nurses' observations and additional information from relatives friends and other disciplines
- Stage 3 — Detailed assessment
- Stage 4 — Summary sheet.

The summary sheet provides a convenient, concise and immediate record of the patient's profile obtained within the first week of admission.

STANDARDIZED SCALES AND PSYCHOLOGICAL TESTING

To assist in making an assessment and providing baseline information from which the outcomes of nursing interventions can be measured, many psychiatric nurses are now using standardized rating scales and questionnaires. Nurses trained as behaviour therapists have been particularly influential in this movement where the accurate assessment of behaviour by measurement scales is common practice (see Gournay, Ch 43). Besides the rating scales which have been devised by behaviour therapists, a wide variety of other measurement techniques are now available. Many of these can be administered with little or no training, while others require specialist training. Whereas it could be argued that these techniques have not been specifically designed by nurses and are therefore limited in their appropriateness and application to nursing practice, many of them have been rigorously tested for validity and reliability and have become standard use both in clinical practice and in research.

There is a need for a greater use of standardized scales. This would determine their suitability for nursing assessment, discovering the best available techniques and providing comparable measurements using different interventions and in different settings. Unfortunately, descriptions of the development of such scales are widely scattered throughout a variety of academic journals, and keeping abreast of them is a difficult task. Like many researchers, nurses are often unaware of the numerous scales now available. Whereas individual initiative is to be encouraged, before devising their own measurement scales it would be more economical to search out and experiment with those already in existence. This approach seems particularly relevant in the areas of activities of daily living, social functioning, psychological well-being and quality of life, all of which fall under the remit of psychiatric nursing care. There are far too many measurement scales to review in this chapter and recently these have been well summarized elsewhere; for example, McDowell & Newell (1987). However, the use of rating scales, questionnaires and inventories in the assessment of patients is an area where much research is needed, particularly at a time when psychiatric nurses are continually being required to demonstrate the effectiveness of nursing interventions.

Interviewing

In assessing a patient it will be necessary to carry out an assessment interview. While many of the skills required for interviewing are similar to those used in other conversations that the nurse may have with the patient, interviews also required additional skills; for example, not only is the nurse expected to listen attentively to what the patient says but she has also to record the information. Such a situation is a dilemma for many nurses and they may become so concerned with recording accurately what the patient says that they neglect to observe non-verbal cues, fail to encourage the patient or come across as not being attentive and sensitive; that is, emphasis is placed on note-taking at the expense of the patient. Price (1983) has pointed out how such a situation can become depersonalized when the nurse hides behind standard questionnaires and documents. Nurses who experience such difficulties may find observation of more experienced staff useful and they should familiarize themselves with some of the literature available on interviewing, e.g. Cannell & Khan (1968), McFarlane & Castledine (1982).

An assessment interview is not a random discussion but a goal-directed method of communication, the purpose of which is to obtain comprehensive, accurate information in a systematic way. The type of assessment form used is often determined by local need. Sanger et al (1988) suggest the use of an assessment guide as opposed to a questionnaire, since they believe the former to be more appropriate and adaptable to different patients. In developing their assessment guide, they identified specific content areas to discuss with a patient. Whether an assessment form, guide or questionnaire is used, its purpose is to help to focus the interview. Where possible, open-ended questions should be asked and the patient given the opportunity to express himself spontaneously.

Interviews should take place in private, preferably in a room free from noise and distraction. It is important that the patient feels comfortable enough to impart personal information and to discuss his or her needs and problems. It may be necessary to rearrange the physical setting. Comfortable chairs of the same height and a coffee table within easy reach to hold coffee cups and ashtray are more conducive to creating a friendly and relaxed atmosphere than hard upright chairs placed on either side of a desk. This process must have adequate time.

An explanation of the purpose of the assessment

interview should be given to the patient, together with the reassurance that information disclosed will be treated confidentially within the confines of the care team. The success of the interview will depend on the nurse's sensitivity and ability to listen. The patient should be allowed to continue talking without undue interruptions. When introducing a new area to be discussed, it is best to begin with an open question. Closed and leading questions which indicate the type of answer expected should be avoided. Hargie et al (1981) has a good chapter on questioning which is particularly relevant for assessment interviews.

There has been little research into psychiatric assessment interviews. Price (1987) conducted research aimed at identifying the ways in which student nurses formulate an assessment for patients admitted to surgical and medical wards. The results led him to conclude that there is a need to review the reality of nursing assessment criteria, skills and protocols. He suggests that the way nurses are currently taught assessment strategies frequently leads them to minimize the subjective quality of the admission interview. He proposes that greater emphasis should be placed on the psychosocial areas of assessment. These include the nurse's own feelings of insecurity, control and reward in the assessment process, the negotiation of roles, status and exploration of the meaning of the health problems faced. Research into general communication patterns by nurses has also shown that questions to patients are nearly always closed or leading, with few examples of open questioning. Reinforcing or encouraging strategies were rarely used appropriately and there was evidence of a lack of listening and attending (Macleod Clark 1981, 1982).

Attention needs to be given to non-verbal behaviour displayed by the patient: for example, when exploring areas of information which may be particularly sensitive. The nurse must also pay attention to her own non-verbal behaviour: for example, facial expression may have the effect of encouraging or discouraging the patient. Similarly, appropriate use of head nods and silence may encourage the patient to continue speaking. Matarazzo et al (1965) found that when an interviewer did not respond immediately to a statement by an interviewee, almost 60% of the interviewees began to speak again.

In closing an interview, the nurse should thank the patient for cooperating and give the patient the opportunity to ask any questions or, alternatively, to make any further comments before the interview is terminated. It may be necessary to arrange a future time and date for a follow-up interview.

THE PROBLEMS OF BIAS AND MAKING INFERENCES

Just as patients are unique individuals, so each nurse will view a patient from his or her own perspective. Each nurse will be influenced by his or her own emotional or subjective response to different patients. Nurses are not value-free and may have individual biases in relation to numerous factors, including age, sex, race and religion (Field 1987), experience, memory and recency of experience (Tanner 1984). While it is accepted in psychiatric nursing that all are entitled to their own opinion, attempts are made during basic training and continuing education to raise awareness of such biases and prejudices. This is done in order that they do not interfere with clinical decision-making, reasoning and behaviour.

Attempts are made during assessment and observation to be as objective as possible by the use of questionnaires and other rating scales. However, the difficulty of achieving consistency between nurses has been highlighted by Wilkinson (1979).

In order to be as objective as possible, nurses are encouraged to provide factual descriptions of events and behaviour rather than subjective feelings or hunches. When personal opinion or subjective feelings are used, then they need to be clearly identified as such. Having collected this information, the nurse must reach an opinion about what is happening. The nurse makes inferences based on groups of cues revealed during data collection and classification. The significance of these cues must be interpreted in the light of the nurse's professional knowledge. Barker (1985) suggests that nurses have a tendency to devote too much energy to making inferences and not enough energy to collecting information. He points out the danger of making inferences and provides an example of how levels of inference can distort and generalize a basic observation. Crow (1979) gives the example of a patient who does not know what day it is and suggests that this does not mean that the nurse can infer from this information that the patient is confused. Inferences are drawn from a number of cues. Hein (1980) suggests that the more an inference is shared by other carers, the greater the likelihood that it is valid.

Having made an assessment, analysed all the available information and reached some conclusions, the patient's problems or needs are defined. It should be noted that a need is not necessarily a problem (Yura & Walsh 1983). The two are often misunderstood and used interchangeably. The word 'need' refers to a requisite for bodily or psychic functioning, as in Henderson's (1966) definition of basic human needs. A 'problem' arises when a 'need' is not met or is met inadequately. The terminology used will depend on local requirements, the nursing model used and the nurse's preference. Stuart & Sundeen (1983) use the term 'nursing diagnosis', Hunt & Marks-Maran (1980) use the term 'patient's nursing problems', while Wilson (1989) uses the term 'phenomena of concern'. The use of the term 'nursing diagnosis' is becoming more acceptable in the nursing literature. Before discussing the implications of this term, some of the remaining difficulties in making a psychiatric nursing assessment are briefly outlined.

REMAINING DIFFICULTIES

Overall, much progress has been made in the area of patient assessment in psychiatric nursing. In 1980 Smith suggested that the lack of a suitable vehicle for collecting a patient's psychiatric history may be one of the causes for the slow implementation of the nursing process in the psychiatric field. During the past decade numerous psychiatric nursing assessment forms have been developed. While the majority of these forms take a holistic approach, they all have their own particular orientation, strengths and weaknesses. The diversity of psychiatric nursing and the range of patients encountered raises doubts about the appropriateness of one universal assessment form. As already stated, the selection of a suitable form and the manner in which the assessment will be carried out depends on many variables, including the underlying philosophy of nursing, the patient's age group, level of disability and other characteristics and service requirements, including time restraints.

Despite assessment being carried out methodically, sensitively and systematically, a number of problems may still arise. These problems may be associated with or be a result of the patient's illness. Patients may be reluctant to provide the information required by nurses, for a number of reasons: for example, they may be suspicious, resistant, aggressive or mute. A full assessment may be prolonged until the nurse has had sufficient time to establish a trusting relationship with the patient and has gained his or her cooperation. In the meantime, information can be collected from other sources, such as observation and secondary sources, e.g. significant other medical and other informed professionals.

Sometimes patients may refuse to provide the information required on the grounds that they have already given similar information to other members of the multi-disciplinary team. In such circumstances, the nurse must be able to give an account of why such information is required for nursing care and acknowledge that there may be areas of overlap. This can be overcome by reducing the amount of biographical information or by asking the patient to fill in such details himself or herself in his or her own time. Technological developments such as computers and the instillation of 'patient information systems' have provided the means to reduce duplication and to increase continuity of care and inter-disciplinary communication.

NURSING DIAGNOSIS

Assessment of patients culminates in the identification of the patient's needs and problems, now referred to as 'nursing diagnosis'. While still in its infancy in this country, nursing diagnosis was described by Hornung in 1956 as 'an exercise in judgement'. As already described, there are a number of factors which may affect such a judgement and which may lead to different diagnoses. Such arguments are often used in opposition to the use of diagnosis in psychiatric nursing. Keane (1981) suggests that the possibility of inaccurate diagnoses in psychiatric nursing may occur because, unlike general medicine, signs and symptoms are not always elucidated and can be extremely difficult to observe. Similar arguments were made during the introduction of the nursing process in psychiatric nursing. Geach (1974) has highlighted the difficulties for psychiatric nurses when patients' problems are not always observable, e.g. disturbing thoughts, uncomfortable feelings, unusual ideas and beliefs. Schröck (1980) suggests that, while the majority of problems identified by general nurses are associated with observable physical problems, the problems of the mentally ill are not always so readily quantifiable.

These arguments are not new to psychiatric nursing. It has often been proposed that because general nursing deals with 'real' entities such as high temperature, raised blood pressure and pain it is scientific and value neutral, since a clear and objective norm of bodily functioning is determinable. Psychiatric nursing, on the other hand, cannot be value neutral because it involves the application of subjective judgement and reference to norms. However, all categorizations, including those made in general nursing, imply the application of norms and a judgement on the part of a nurse. Judgements by nurses are conditioned by prevalent social attitudes and beliefs and constrained by the criteria, training and practices of clinical nursing. The difficulty for psychiatric nursing is that it involves norms of mental processes, modes of reasoning, and socially acceptable forms of statement and behaviour. It is when these differ from what is currently acceptable that they may be identified as problems. However, what these arguments do not take into account is that the patient's behaviour may be problematic for himself or herself and for others precisely because it differs from expected norms of statement and behaviour.

It is because psychiatric nursing deals with such complex issues involving the psychological make-up of individuals that it needs a structured, systematic approach to documentation so that what it is doing or not doing may be sorted out. As Kendall (1975) pointed out, as soon as one begins to recognize features that are common to some people but not to all, and to distinguish those which are important from those which are not, one is classifying them, whether one acknowledges it or not. The only point at issue is what sort of classification to have. The purpose of diagnosis which involves categorization and classification is to organize the information collected during assessment in order that appropriate nursing interventions can be planned, carried out and evaluated. As with all classificatory systems, there is the danger that the uniqueness of individuals may be distorted by a standardized and fixed category — take, for example, the withdrawn, confused, aggressive or anxious patient. While these problems may be experienced by patients irrespective of the medical diagnosis, applying a nursing diagnosis is seen merely as substituting one label for another. It is on such grounds that the nursing diagnosis is often criticized, thought to be unnecessary and even harmful. Some American psychiatric nurses oppose such criticism, pointing out that in making a nursing diagnosis it is not the individual who is given a label but rather it is that person's human responses or behaviour which are named (West & Pothier 1989).

The identification of diagnostic concepts, their validation and the testing of their reliability is a major concern for many psychiatric nurses (McFarland & Wasli 1986, Thomas et al 1986, Whitney et al 1988). However, it must be remembered that among the most important functions for psychiatric nursing diagnosis is the determination of subsequent interventions and predictive statements about desired outcome. The problem for psychiatric nursing is that the interventions currently used are far from specific to the emerging diagnostic categories and in most cases have not been demonstrated to be effective.

REFERENCES

Aggleton P, Chalmers H 1986 Nursing models and the nursing process. Macmillan, London

Aspinall, M J 1976 Nursing diagnosis: the weak link. Nursing Outlook 24(7): 433–437

Barker P J 1985 Patient assessment in psychiatric nursing. Croom Helm, London

Bauer B B, Hill S S 1986 Essentials of mental health care: planning and interventions. Saunders, Philadelphia

Cannel T M, Kahn R L 1968 Interviewing. In: Lindzey G, Aronson E (eds) The handbook of social psychology. Addison Wesley, Menlo Park, Calif, vol 2

Darcy P T 1980 The nursing process — a base for all nursing developments. Nursing Times 76(12): 497–501

Darcy P T 1985 Mental health nursing source book. Baillière Tindall, London

Crow J 1979 Assessment. In: Kratz C R (ed) The nursing process. Bailliere Tindall, London

Field P A 1987 The impact of nursing theory on the clinical decision making process. Journal of Advanced Nursing 12: 563–571

Geach B 1974 The problem solving technique as taught to student nurses. Perspectives in Psychiatric Care 12: 9–12

Hamdi M E, Hutelmyer C M 1970 A study of the effectiveness of an assessment tool in the identification of nursing care problems. Nursing Research 19: 354–358

Hargie O, Saunders C, Dickson D 1981 Social skills in interpersonal communication. Croom Helm, London

Hefferin E A, Hunter R E 1975 Nursing assessment and care plan statements. Nursing Research 24: 360–366

Hein E C 1980 Communication in nursing practice, 2nd edn. Little Brown, Boston, Mass

Henderson V, 1966 The nature of nursing. Collier-Macmillan, London

Hornung G J 1956 Nursing diagnosis: an exercise in judgement. Nursing Outlook 4: 24–30

Hunt J M, Marks-Maran D J 1980 Nursing care plans: the nursing process at work. Wiley, Chichester

Keane P 1981 The nursing process in a psychiatric context. Nursing Times 177: 1223–1224

Kendall R E 1975 The role of diagnosis in psychiatry, Blackwell, Oxford

Macleod Clark J 1981 Nurse–patient communication. Nursing Times 77: 12–18

Macleod Clark J 1982 Nurse–patient interactions. An analysis of conversations on surgical wards. Unpublished PhD Thesis, University of London

Marriner A 1979 The nursing process: a scientific approach to nursing care. C V Mosby, St Louis, Mo

Matarazzo J D, Wiens A N, Saslow G 1965 Studies in interview speech behaviour. In: Krasner L, Ullmann L (eds) Research in behaviour modification: new developments and implications. Holt, Rinehart & Winston, New York

McDowell I, Newell C 1987 Measuring health: a guide to rating scales and questionnaires. Oxford University Press

McFarland G K, Wasli E L 1986 Nursing diagnosis and process in psychiatric mental health nursing. Lippincott, Philadelphia

McFarlane J K, Castledine G 1982 A guide to the practice of nursing using the nursing process. Mosby, London

Price B 1983 Just a few forms to fill in. Nursing Times 79: 26–29

Price B 1987 First impressions: paradigms for patient assessment. Journal of Advanced Nursing 12: 699–705

Orem D E 1980 Nursing: concepts of practice, 2nd edn. McGraw-Hill, New York

Rashidi N 1975 Psychiatry and self-administered data form. Journal of Medicine 75: 917

Roper N 1976 Clinical experience in nurse education. Churchill Livingstone, Edinburgh

Roper N, Logan W, Tierney A 1981 The elements of nursing. Churchill Livingstone, Edinburgh

Roy C 1976 Introduction to nursing: an adaptation model. Prentice-Hall, New Jersey

Sanger E, Thomas M D, Whitney J D 1988 A guide for nursing assessment of the psychiatric inpatient. Archives of Psychiatric Nursing 2: 334–338

Schröck R A 1980 Planning nursing care for the mentally ill. Nursing Times 76: 704–754

Schultz J M, Dark S L 1986 Manual of psychiatric nursing care plans. Scott, Foresman, Ill

Sebastian L 1987 Psychiatric hospital admissions: assessing patients' perceptions. Journal of Psychosocial Nursing and Mental Health Services 25: 25–28

Smith L 1980 A nursing history and data sheet. Nursing Times 76: 749–754

Stockwell F 1985 The nursing process in psychiatric nursing. Croom Helm, London

Stuart G W, Sundeen S J 1983 Principles and practice of psychiatric nursing. Mosby, St Louis, Mo

Tanner C A 1984 Factors influencing the diagnostic process. In: Carnevali D L Mitchell P H, Woods N F, Tanner C A (eds) Diagnostic reasoning in nursing. Lippincott, Philadelphia

Tissier J 1986 The development of a psychiatric nursing assessment form. In: Brooking J (ed) Psychiatric nursing research. Wiley, Chichester

Thomas M D, Sanger E, Whitney J D 1986 Nursing diagnosis of depression: clinical identification on an inpatient unit. Journal of Psychosocial Nursing and Mental Health Services 24: 6–12

West P P, Pothier P C 1989 Clinical application of human responses classification system: child example. Archives of Psychiatric Nursing 3: 300–304

Whitney J D, Sanger E, Thomas M D, Wolf-Wilets V C 1988 A validation study of the nursing diagnosis 'somatization'. Archives of Psychiatric Nursing 2: 345–349

Wilkinson T 1979 The problems and values of objective nursing observations in psychiatric nursing care. Journal of Advanced Nursing 4: 151–159

Wilson H S, 1989 Field trials of the phenomena of concern for psychiatric mental health nursing: proposed methodology. Archives of Psychiatric Nursing 3: 305–308

Yura H, Walsh M 1983 The nursing process, 4th edn. Appleton-Century-Crofts, New York.

19

Nursing care planning

R. G. D. Tunmore

This chapter examines some of the advantages and disadvantages of care planning in psychiatric nursing. Drawing from a range of literature and research, some general practical guidelines are identified for documentation of the care plan. Issues of responsibility and accountability for care planning, patient involvement and the multi-disciplinary approach to care are also discussed.

Planning incorporates setting goals for patient care and identifying alternative modes of action to reach those goals. It involves writing a clearly expressed, unique nursing care plan which can be understood by all staff in the multi-disciplinary team. The nursing care plan is both a permanent record of, and a guide to, the nursing care of the individual.

THE DEVELOPMENT OF CARE PLANNING

The development of nursing care plans has not been straightforward. As early as 1937 Henderson recommended that nurses make written plans for all patients, advocating a problem-solving approach in order to coordinate care (Henderson 1973). Others have argued vehemently against the use of care plans. For example, Palisin (1971) proclaimed them 'a snare and a delusion — a communications burden imposed on the practitioner by the theorist', asserting that they complicate the communication process and so confound the nursing care of the individual. Complication arises through lack of time and inadequate numbers of staff, together with a lack of appropriate writing and organizing skills.

Citing North American literature from the 1950s, Ciuca (1972) describes how early care plans derived from nursing care studies containing the patient's diagnosis and problems that affected nursing care. The care plan assisted communication and continuity of nursing interventions within the nursing care team. These interventions were evaluated and updated as the patient's needs changed. Decisions about patient care were based on nursing judgements and used information gathered from an admission interview. The care plan as a means of communication for nursing staff characterizes the first of three conceptual phases in Ciuca's review. The second phase, using the care plan as a professional assessment and diagnostic tool, reflects the growth of professionalism in nursing from the early 1960s. The literature on care plans began to emphasize the importance of nursing activities as a means of achieving specific objectives. Evaluation of the plan involved determining whether or not the objectives were therapeutic and realistic and whether the nursing interventions specified in the plan achieved the stated goals. Task-centred care was replaced with the concept of patient-centred care. Care plans reflected nursing objectives and interventions based on psychosocial as well as physical needs, included short-term and long-term objectives and were coordinated with medical treatment. Patient participation in planning care was also emphasized. Incorporation of the care plan into a multi-disciplinary approach to care is the third and most desirable phase of the 'evolution' of the care plan described by Ciuca.

McFarlane & Castledine (1982) suggest that care plans help nurses develop a critical problem-solving approach to the nursing care of the individual and should act as a clinical aid in communicating information. Daws (1988) found that qualified nursing staff may use care plans as a valuable teaching tool in the clinical setting.

Ciuca (1972) examined the use of the care plan in clinical practice. Taking a random sample of 235 care plans from six hospitals, notations from the plans were categorized into seven groups depending on their content. The groups related to medical treatment, preventative measures, infection control, elimination, physical comfort, emotional support, rehabilitation and discharge planning. Results indicated that care plans were used primarily for notation of functional, mechanical duties associated with medications, treatments and monitoring of vital signs. 75% of notations fell into this category. Under 6% were related to emotional support and less than 2% to rehabilitation. Ciuca reported that notations were brief and without rationale and it was not possible to distinguish medically prescribed treatment from nursing decisions. On the whole, the care plans did not reflect the patient as a 'total person', with little evidence of comprehensive care planning.

Case & Rooney (1982) indicate how the permanence of the written care plan could be threatening or intimidating for those nurses who, viewing it as a legal record, are reluctant to commit themselves to its use. The idea that there is a correct way to write a care plan or that a correct decision will result in the correct outcome — that there is one right solution to a problem — may discourage the use of the care plan through the nurse's fear of failure at not solving a problem the first time around. Stevens (1972) suggests this is a result of nurse training.

CARE PLANS AND STANDARDS OF CARE

The need for standards is indicated by literature and research on care plans. Implementation of the nursing process in the care of the mentally ill, by comparison with its use in general nursing, has been relatively slow. There is a lack of research on the use of care plans in psychiatric nursing. Most of the research has been based in general hospitals where physical illness is the focus of nursing care (DHSS 1986).

Stevens (1972) identifies some reasons stated in the literature to support the use of care plans:

1. Nursing as a profession needs to identify its own content beyond that of carrying out medical orders.
2. Agreement over the approach to nursing requires a written plan.
3. Continuity of nursing across different work shifts requires a written plan.
4. Formulation of a written plan helps nurses to identify clear nursing goals.
5. Clearly identified components of nursing highlight omissions in care.
6. The primary aim of the care plan is to promote communication and coordination of care to ensure patients' needs are met.

Grosicki et al (1967) summarize the needs of nurses in relation to writing care plans. These include:

1. A consistent approach in the preparation of care plans throughout the hospital, ward or department, so as to maintain continuity, interest in and appreciation of them
2. Assistance in developing skills in preparing care plans
3. Assistance in learning how to work from care plans.

The 1982 Syllabus of Training for Part 3 of the Professional Register (Registered Mental Nurse) includes planning nursing care as a skill required of the psychiatric nurse. It involves identifying individual needs, setting realistic goals and, using a problem-solving approach, identifying and implementing alternative interventions to meet the needs and evaluating the interventions (General Nursing Council 1982).

Standards to determine the quality of psychiatric nursing have been outlined by the American Nurses Association and adapted by the Royal College of Nursing. These standards aim to provide a structure for and improve the practice of psychiatric nursing. They include development of nursing care plans with specific goals and nursing interventions appropriate to the needs of each individual patient. These standards include the following criteria for planning care:

1. Nursing care plans are established through collaboration with patients, their significant others and other members of the multi-disciplinary team.
2. The nurse uses the care plan for:
   a. identifying priorities of care
   b. stating realistic goals in measurable terms
   c. identifying psychotherapeutic principles
   d. indicating which of the patient's needs will be the main responsibility of the nurse and which will be referred to other team members
   e. mutual goal setting and shared responsibility for goal attainment as appropriate depending upon the patient's abilities
   f. providing guidance for care activities performed by health workers under the nurse's supervision.
3. Altering the care plan as goals are achieved, changed or updated (RCN 1986).

The care plan is used to guide nursing intervention in order to achieve the desired outcome. The nurse will need opportunities to discuss the development of care plans with colleagues. The clinical environment can be adapted so that there is a system for care plans to be recorded and communicated to others, for example, in regular nursing reports or multi-disciplinary team meetings.

THE NURSING PROCESS

These standards place the written nursing care plan within the framework of the nursing process. Walton (1986) and De La Cuesta (1983) review critically the introduction of the nursing process emphasizing its complexity and the resulting confusion. They agree that most of this confusion stems from the documentation. The care plan is one of the two major documents in the nursing process, the other being the nursing assessment or history where relevant personal and demographic information is collected and recorded.

In an analysis of the implementation of the nursing process in the United States of America and the United Kingdom, De La Cuesta (1983) found that care plans were the common barrier to the full application of the nursing process despite differences in the structure and organization of nursing services between the two countries.

The success of care planning depends on nurses' problem-solving ability (Hurst 1985). Problem-solving skills for care planning in psychiatric nursing need to be develop and emphasized in training programmes (Geach 1974, Smyth 1983).

Four stages of planning care are described by Crow et al (1979): determining priorities, setting goals, selecting nursing actions and writing the care plan. These are identifiable within the problem-solving cycle of the nursing process (Fig. 19.1).

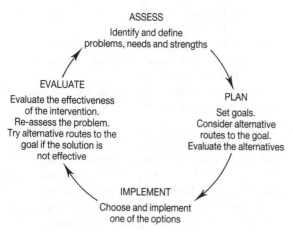

Fig. 19.1 The problem-solving cycle.

Assessment and planning

A nursing assessment is necessary in order to identify the patient's problem or problems. Comprehensive assessment may be guided by and based upon a particular model of nursing (Vincent et al 1976, Tissier 1986). Assessment involves making a variety of observations of the patient (see Ch. 18). Observations need to be stated as objectively as possible. Personal opinions or subjective inferences need to be identified as such. The assessment leads to the identification of actual and potential problems which are written in order of priority, indicating the cause if possible. Recording problems in writing requires precision, clarity and conciseness, identifying all the factors relating to the problem. Statements should include identification of the problem, identification of the

cause of the problem and identification of how the patient is behaving in relation to the problem (Hunt & Marks-Maran 1980).

Identification of patients' problems, needs and strengths

Walton (1986) highlights difficulties arising from interpretation and terminology. For instance, is it legitimate to describe as a problem some aspect of the patient's behaviour which is really a problem for the nurse rather than for the patient? Should the term 'needs' be preferred to 'problems'? Different guides to care planning use different terminology. Hunt & Marks-Maran (1980) identify 'patient's nursing problems' while Stuart & Sundeen (1983) use 'nursing diagnosis'. Sometimes the term 'problem' is interchangeable with 'need' within a care plan heading of Need/Problem (Bauer & Hill 1986).

French (1983) describes a need as factors or conditions necessary for maintenance of biological, psychological, social or spiritual functioning. Problems arise from unmet needs.

Patients' strengths and successful coping strategies are assessed along with their needs and problems (Bauer & Hill 1986). The plan of care can acknowledge and build upon these positive aspects in promoting mental health. Patients' problem-solving abilities, as well as their sense of perceived or actual control over a situation, could be incorporated into the plan. Few guides to care planning suggest how to incorporate strengths into care plans. Nurses tend to be concerned with what is wrong rather than what is right. While it is acknowledged that a problem-solving process will inevitably emphasize and identify problems, this should not be to the exclusion of patients' strengths and present coping strategies.

Planning in psychiatric nursing

Whyte & Youhill (1984) describe a prolonged assessment period during which 'primary information', derived from the patient's actions, words, appearance and behaviour, provides the basis of the nursing care plan. Information derived from other sources constitutes 'secondary information', i.e. from relatives, other health care workers and medical records. They state that psychiatric nurses are mainly concerned with the socio-psychological problems and needs of the patient rather than concentrating on or giving priority to physical needs. However, Schrock (1980) contends that psychiatric nurses have not used care plans in this way. There is a more general problem with the use of care plans for planning emotional or psychological care, and physical aspects of care tend to be emphasized (Pankratz & Pankratz 1973, Hefferin & Hunter 1975).

Geach (1974) identifies a source of conflict for psychiatric nurses in planning care. When the entities defined as problems are not visible at all times, for example, disturbing thoughts, uncomfortable feelings, unusual ideas and beliefs, to what should the nurse respond — to precipitates, symptoms, overt behaviour or its consequences? While the majority of problems identified by the general nurse are associated with observable physical problems, the problems of the mentally ill are not always so readily quantifiable (Schrock 1980).

Bauer & Hill (1986) see the observation of behaviour as a source for assessing an individual's needs. Wilkinson (1979) describes the difficulty nurses encounter in recording observations consistently. Krall (1976) contends that the basis of both written plans and goal attainment in psychiatric nursing is behavioural. Nursing interventions are directed towards identifiable behaviours. Using a behavioural framework Krall (1976) suggests a guide to care planning, including:

1. An awareness of the exact behaviour keeping the patient in hospital
2. Using behavioural terminology to write the care plan
3. Using terminology that the patient can understand
4. Ensuring that all nursing staff can understand the terminology used in the care plan
5. Ensuring that there is agreement over how the written care plan is to be used.

Setting and describing goals

The nursing care plan contains specific goals and interventions to guide nursing actions for each patient problem. Goals describe a desired change or improvement and may be long term or short term. Long-term goals are general, realistic statements. Short-term goals or objectives are specific, time-limited manageable aspects that form part of the more general long-term goal. Short-term goals may encourage the patient through achievement of early success. The problem statements, goals and interventions should be acceptable to the patient (Marriner 1979), as conflict may arise when the patient and nurse have different views.

Setting goals and documenting them is a difficult exercise. St John & Soulary (1973) report a lack of statements on treatment goals in an inpatient drug treatment setting. Hefferin & Hunter (1975) discovered a general tendency toward vagueness in making care plan statements. Grosicki et al (1967) found that two thirds of psychiatric nursing care plans either had no goals or unrealistic goals.

Goal statements should be written in specific terms that indicate the desired outcome or resolution for each particular problem. Goals specify the desired outcome in terms that are observable, measurable and time-limited. They are realistic, meaningful and achievable, and emphasis should be positive rather than negative.

Behavioural objectives

Specification of behavioural objectives involves a statement format consisting of components: Who (subject) — will do what (behaviour) — under what circumstances (conditions) — to what degree of success (criterion) (Anderson & Faust 1973, Sturmey et al 1988, McFarlane & Castledine 1982).

The subject of the statement is identified by name and is usually the patient, but may be a relative or friend who is involved in the care plan.

The behaviour is stated in terms of an observable response. Descriptions of behaviour using verbs such as 'sit', 'walk' and 'talk' provide a precise account of what is expected. Terms like 'normal', 'comfortable' and 'reassure' are open to different interpretations and lead to vagueness. Statements may also include an expected verbal response from the patient and clinical observations to be made by the nurse.

The conditions refer to the circumstances under which the specified behaviour will occur. They are realistic and take into account limitations and provisions of the ward or hospital environment.

The criteria are quantifiable and refer to frequency or amount expected of the behaviour; for example, specifying a time when the behaviour is to take place.

Example of a behavioural objective

'The patient (subject) will be up, dressed and washed (behaviour) by himself (condition) by 9.30 am Monday to Friday (criterion)', is preferable to 'The patient should get up at the normal time and not lie in bed all morning.'

Difficulties in using behavioural objectives are described by Tomlinson & Birchenall (1981). They suggest that it may be possible to assess an outcome without being able to specify with certainty the means by which it was achieved. This may occur when the nurse and the patient have a different view of a problem or place different value on the outcome. For example, the patient might conform to bathing three times a week and the goal in this case will have been achieved. However, the nurse may believe that the patient has learnt the principles of personal hygiene whereas the patient may only be bathing to please the nurse or avoid being confronted by the nurse.

Furthermore, the process through which goals are achieved may be more tangible than the goal itself. It is not always possible to express different facets of expected outcomes in words or quantify them accurately (Tomlinson & Birchenall 1981). This is particularly relevant to the more qualitative aspects of an interpersonal relationship, for example the development of trust by the patient through the nurse's demonstration of reliability and consistency. These qualities may be conveyed through behaviour such as being available to the patient at stated times and for specified periods. The development of trust in the nurse–patient relationship is part of an on-going process of which these behaviours are only a part.

Expressive objectives

Ward (1989) identifies expressive or experimential objectives as an alternative or complementary method of setting objectives (Box 19.1). These focus on the development of themes, skills and understanding associated with the problem-solving process. Expressive objectives emphasize the qualitative or subjective aspects of interactions within the context of the nurse–patient relationship. The aim of the expressive objective is to facilitate the process of problem solving, providing new or alternative ways of perceiving and conceptualizing events and experiences rather than providing a means for the resolution of the problem.

Expressive objectives may be written with a similar format to that set out for behavioural objectives. These objectives differ in their specification of the behaviour and criterion components and the way they are evaluated.

Verbs used to describe behaviour are replaced with those that describe a specific verbal or intellectual activity. For example, terms such as review, describe, discuss, explore and identify are used instead of verbs that describe the observable behaviour of the behavioural objective.

Outcome criteria that specify observable, quantifiable measures such as effect, frequency or amount are inappropriate for expressive objectives.

Box 19.1 Components of objective statements

Behavioural objectives	Expressive objectives
1. Who (subject)	1. Who (subject)
2. Will do what (behaviour)	2. Will do what (verbal/intellectual activity)
3. Under what circumstances (conditions)	3. Under what circumstances (conditions)
4. To what degree of success (criterion)	

Specification of expressive objectives involves a statement format consisting of three components: who (subject) will do what (verbal intellectual activity) under what circumstances (conditions).

Example of an expressive objective

I (patient as subject) will try to identify what I find most frightening about being in a crowd (verbal intellectual activity) when I meet with my primary nurse (condition).

While there are difficulties with documentation of goals in behavioural terms, the concept of care planning should not be dismissed simply because planning some aspects of psychosocial care appears problematic.

Implementation

Implementation of the plan depends upon clear, detailed and concise instructions. The nursing action or instruction describes the nursing care required by the patient in relation to each problem in order to achieve the desired outcome. As in setting goals, the nursing instructions need to specify who is expected to carry out the plan and what actions are expected of them at what times.

There are often alternative strategies for achieving a particular goal and these may be identified in the care plan. The nursing literature lacks adequate description of how alternative actions are generated or evaluated. Prescriptive accounts suggest that alternative actions should be identified before any are evaluated (Bailey & Claus 1975, Bower 1982). Each alternative should also be evaluated (Lancaster & Beare 1982, Yura & Walsh 1983) as one may prove more effective than the other and this can be documented in the plan as the rationale for its continued use. Corcoran (1986) provides evidence that the number of alternative actions and their evaluation is dependent on the complexity of the problem. Experienced nurses are likely to generate more alternatives, to be more specific in their evaluation and develop better plans than novices (Corcoran 1986).

In whatever way the alternatives are identified, Hunt & Marks-Maran (1980) state that nursing instructions must be based upon sound, scientific principles. This means selecting possible interventions and systematically implementing the alternatives until the required outcome is achieved. Interventions which are generally appropriate are adapted to the individual patient's particular strengths and weaknesses and directed towards a goal. For example, the nursing instruction 'reassure the patient' may be appropriate for a particular problem but is vague and conveys no clue as to the method of implementation. French (1979) examines the concept of reassurance and suggests several methods by which it may be achieved (Box 19.2). Identification of which specific actions are effective for a particular patient in a particular situation is a necessary component of the care plan, providing consistency and continuity of care.

Anderson (1983) provides a list of specific labels for interventions to be included in the care plan, for example seeking clarification and confrontation and reflection, suggesting that nurses document exactly what it is they do to, for and with the patient. Specific labelling of interventions documents the evaluation stage of the problem-solving process, enabling the nurse to identify which interventions have been tried or untried, which were successful or unsuccessful.

Evaluation

Evaluation involves assessing progress towards the goals identified in the care plan. When goals are

---

Box 19.2 Methods of providing reassurance

Explanation
Familiarizing an unfamiliar situation
Introducing a familiar element to an unfamiliar situation
Touch
Proximity
Conveying emotional stability through the nurse's manner
Counselling and use of the patient's own skills
Clarification of facts
Verbalization and ventilation of fears by the patient
Using diversional techniques

set they incorporate the date or time the actions or interventions should be reviewed or evaluated. The objective outcome measures included in the goal provide the criteria for evaluation. If the goal has been achieved and the problem resolved, the nursing action may be discontinued. If the actions have not achieved the desired goal this should be documented in the plan and alternative actions implemented, repeating the problem-solving process.

Evaluation of expressive objectives takes place during the nurse–patient interaction and is an analysis of that interaction (Ward 1989): for example, whether a review, description, discussion, exploration or identification ensues as part of the problem-solving process specified in the objective. An appraisal of the effect of this type of interaction on the patient and nurse in relation to the learning process would be part of the evaluation during the interaction. This would involve the use of facilitative interpersonal skills: for example, paraphrasing and checking for understanding as part of this process (Heron 1989). Writing in the care plan the main issues and concerns along with the activity through which they were expressed provides documentation of what has taken place. This account will be subjective and should be identified as such.

A further aspect of the evaluation is to determine whether or not goals remain realistic. For example, a goal may refer to the patient's rehabilitation and eventual discharge home from hospital. Circumstances outside the nurse's control, such as changes in family relations or accommodation arrangements during the patient's admission, may make the original goal inappropriate or unrealistic. Evaluation may result in an adjustment in the time scale for the original goal or it may be adjusted in line with changes in circumstances. Whatever evaluation is made, documentation in the care plan, along with the date and any relevant changes to the plan, ensure consistency in subsequent care.

CARE PLAN FORMAT

Kelly (1966) argues that an unstructured form for nursing care plans does not provide the nurse with any guidance and suggests that a structured form

with particular headings would ensure comprehensive care. Variation in authors' recommendations for sections in care plans are another possible source of confusion. The fact that no agreement has been reached on either the format or content of the written plan is a cause of consternation for some (McClasky 1975). However, the format of the care plan should reflect the stages of the nursing process following assessment, i.e. planning, implementation and evaluation (Stuart & Sundeen 1983). The general format incorporates space for the problem or need, the objective or goals of care, prescription of nursing action or intervention and evaluation. The stages of the nursing process offer a general format for care plans allowing for variation in the information recorded (Fig. 19.2). Such variation in care plan format is both necessary and appropriate and will depend upon the prevailing nursery models. Muhs & Nebesky (1964) found that many care plans were inappropriate for psychiatric nursing, focusing on aspects of treatment derived from a medical model. Schröck (1980) proposes that some conceptual framework or model is essential for planned nursing care. Collister (1988) describes a variety of models used by psychiatric nurses as the basis for nursing assessment and subsequent development of care plans.

STANDARD CARE PLANS

The standard care plan provides a checklist of routine care irrespective of specific individual needs (McFarlane & Castledine 1982) which can be used in conjunction with the problem-oriented care plan for the individual. Standard care plans detail nursing care and expected outcomes for specific diseases or conditions and the most common needs or problems associated with them. These are documented on a prepared form. Glasper et al (1987) argue that the time spent writing care plans is a lower priority than the actual provision of care. Standard care plans are a time-saving means of providing a patient-centred approach in busy clinical areas. Nichols & Barstow (1980) see them as useful guides to care. Ethridge & Packard (1976) promote the use of standard care plans as a tool to measure the quality of care.

Date: 20.6.89				Name: John Smith
Problem	Long-term target	Objectives	Nursing intervention	Evaluation Date: 27.6.89.
John says he 'just can't be bothered to get up in the mornings – there's nothing to get up for'.	Will John establish a routine start to the day?	John will be up, dressed and washed by himself by 9.30 a.m. Monday to Friday.	1. Ensure John has an alarm clock 2. Each night for the first week, remind John to set his alarm clock for 8.15 a.m. 3. When he is up on time give positive feedback to acknowledge this.	

Miller 1988

Problem	Goal	Nursing action	Outcome
John says he 'just can't be bothered to get up in the mornings – there's nothing to get up for'.	John will be up, dressed and washed by himself by 9.30 a.m. Monday – Friday.	1. Each night for the first week remind John to set his alarm clock for 8.15 a.m. 2. When he is up on time give positive feedback to acknowledge this. 3. If he is not out of bed at 9 a.m. give him one verbal prompt e.g. remind him of the time.	Evaluate by counting the number of days John was up, dressed and washed. Record whether or not he needed prompting each day.

Thomas 1988

Need/problem. John says he 'just can't be bothered to get up in the mornings – there's nothing to get up for'.	**Objective.** John will be up, dressed and washed by himself by 9.30 a.m. Monday – Friday.
What (patient) will do. John will set his alarm clock for 8.15 a.m. each night before he goes to bed and be washed and dressed by 9.30 a.m.	
What (nurse) will do. Remind John to set his alarm for 8.15 a.m. If he is not out of bed by 9.00 a.m. give him one verbal prompt, e.g. remind him of the time. When he is up on time give positive feedback to acknowledge this.	
Outcome. Note the number of days he is up on time and whether or not he needed prompting.	**Evaluation.** Evaluation after one week.

Ritter 1988

Problem No (1)	Nursing action	Result	
John says he 'just can't be bothered to get up in the mornings – there's nothing to get up for'. **Objective** John will be up, dressed and washed by himself by 9.30 a.m. Monday – Friday.	Each night for the first week remind John to set his alarm clock for 8.15 a.m. If he is not out of bed by 9 a.m. give him one verbal prompt, e.g. remind him of the time. When he is up on time, give positive feedback to acknowledge this.	Evaluate after first week by counting the days John got up, washed and dressed by 9.30 a.m.	

Green 1983

Fig. 19.2 Variation in care plan format.

The standard care plan is most useful for common procedures such as pre- and postoperative care or for specifying levels of safety in certain procedures. For example, Roper et al (1985) describe a standard care plan for restraint and seclusion. Additional space should be provided for the care of the individual patient.

PATIENT INVOLVEMENT

Involving patients and their significant others in care planning raises controversial issues associated with the traditional power of the professional to prescribe treatment and the power of the patient as a consumer of health care services. Fanning et al (1972) assessed the attitudes of 82 patients and 37 staff in a mental health centre to patients' participation in planning their own care. Staff expressed some reluctance in allowing patients to participate based on an assumption that they were incapable of safe or intelligent participation. However, there was agreement between patients and staff that care and treatment should be planned collaboratively from the time of admission. The main problem with joint patient and staff planning was in how it should be implemented.

Kramer (1972) recommends that one nurse is made accountable for both the patient's plan of care and involving the patient and family in planning care and developing a care plan. Changes to the plan are made in the presence of and in conjunction with the patient and family. Krall (1976) emphasizes the need for the patient to understand what is written in the care plan while patient involvement increases the likelihood that treatment goals and plans are emphasized (Willer & Santoro 1975).

Simonton et al (1977) conducted a study on the effects of giving patients in a small psychiatric unit their complete medical and nursing notes to read on a daily basis. The results from questionnaire responses indicated that both medical and nursing staff and patients found this an effective way of actively involving patients in treatment and provided opportunities for patient education. Other advantages included a lower rate of inaccuracies in the records and greater care in documentation by the staff. However, some infor-

mation about patients was not documented but was communicated by other means. On reading their notes, 30% of the patients became more pessimistic about their future, while about 70% felt more self-confident.

Another means of involving patients in care planning is described by Woodcock et al (1972). Here the care plan is written on a blackboard and provides the focus and structure for group therapy. Current goals and problems of each individual are reviewed and recorded by the group. A nurse copies from the blackboard into the appropriate nursing care plan, maintaining continuity between meetings. The blackboard method enhances concern for fellow patients, making patients able to respond to each other's needs during their daily interactions to a greater degree.

Difficulties may arise in planning psychiatric nursing care where the patient refuses or is reluctant to participate. Thomas (1988) gives the example of withdrawn patients who do not talk to their primary nurse. Careful consideration of whether or not it is appropriate or possible to involve all patients in all aspects of their care planning is necessary. While many patients may welcome the opportunity and develop a sense of self-control or self-confidence, others may be reluctant or unable to do so.

MULTI-DISCIPLINARY APPROACH

A multi-disciplinary approach is described by Ciuca (1972) as the most desirable approach to care planning. In a multi-disciplinary setting the nursing team is but a part of the total patient care team. Nursing care plans are established through collaboration with other health care workers including doctors, social workers, occupational therapists, psychologists and others. The care plan indicates who has primary responsibility for particular patient needs, depending upon who has the most appropriate expertise.

The success of this approach depends upon adequate consultation between disciplines and mutual recognition of contributions made by each professional group to patient care. Problems associated with rivalry and lack of clear role definition within multi-disciplinary teams (Marshall 1989) may be detrimental to such an approach.

Dunlap & Matteoli (1970) describe how the development of the nursing care plan in a psychiatric setting is a function of the multi-disciplinary team. A consistent approach by each member of the team with identified areas of responsibility enhances communication, increasing efficiency and quality of individualized care. In the nursing care plan, nurses identify their particular contribution to patient care as part of the total treatment plan produced by the multi-disciplinary team.

The reporting habits of psychiatric nurses and psychiatrists are described in a study by Willer & Santoro (1975). They found that nurses were more likely to discuss or record day-to-day patient progress than psychiatrists. Nurses' reports were mainly limited to behavioural descriptions, while psychiatrists gave more complete descriptions. Christopoulos (1970) asserts that the psychiatrist can obtain invaluable information from nursing records.

Nurses are not alone in emphasizing the need to develop care plans. Stevens (1989) states that the need for individualized care plans, containing clear goals, with specific carers having responsibility for various aspects of the plan, involving patients and their relatives in decision-making, is a dominant theme for psychologists working in the community. Training in appropriate skills necessary to implement the plan is required at both direct care and managerial levels.

ACCOUNTABILITY AND RESPONSIBILITY

Several authors address issues relating to responsibility and accountability in planning care. Most are in agreement that a qualified nurse is responsible for ensuring that each patient has a care plan that is adequately maintained and updated. Wagner (1969) is adamant that the care plan is the sole responsibility of the qualified nurse. Case & Rooney (1982) reported that qualified nurses regarded care plans as relatively unimportant and

that the task of writing them was delegated to student nurses. Many wards function with only one or two qualified nurses on each shift, making it unlikely that they would have time to write and update each patient's care plan. Harris (1970) suggests the nurse who admits the patient initiates the plan. Stevens (1972) suggests that any nurse may contribute to the plan under the direction of a specified qualified nurse. Mansfield (1967) argues that the nursing aide in a psychiatric setting can write and use the care plan.

Accountability for care planning has, until recently, received little attention. The Salmon Report (MOH 1966) made no reference to responsibility for planning care in the job description of the ward sister. The United Kingdom Central Council for Nursing, Midwifery and Health Visiting (1986) recommends that the registered nurse practitioner acquires the competencies required to 'identify physical, psychological, social and spiritual needs of the patient or client, be aware of and value the concept of individual care, devise a plan of care, [and] contribute to its implementation and evaluation by demonstrating an appreciation and practice of the principles of a problem-solving approach' (UKCC 1986 p. 41). The need for such administrative support and positive reinforcement for the use of care plans is widely acknowledged (Ciuca 1972, Clarke 1978, Shea 1986).

Nursing care plans are a means to an end, that of providing nursing care to individual patients. It has been suggested that there is a relationship between care plans and the quality of care (Ethridge & Packard 1976). However, it is not clear from the literature how care plans can be used to define or set standards by which the quality of care is then measured. A care plan with a clear description of the problem, well-defined goals and evaluation criteria does not necessarily ensure care of a particular standard or quality (Shea 1986). Care plans are a record of care and a guide for the provision of care. They may promote consistency and continuity of care for individual patients if their use is supported by nurses in the clinical area, administration and education.

REFERENCES

American Nurses' Association 1980 Nursing: a social policy statement. American Nurses' Association, Kansas City, Mo

Anderson M L 1983 Nursing interventions: what did you do that helped? Perspectives in Psychiatric Care 20(1): 4–8

Anderson R C, Faust G W 1973 Educational psychology; the science of instruction and learning. Dodd, Mead, New York

Bailey J, Claus K 1975 Decision-making in nursing, Mosby, St Louis

Bauer B B, Hill S S 1986 Essentials of mental health care: planning and interventions. Saunders, Philadelphia

Bower F 1982 The process of planning nursing care, 3rd edn. Mosby, St Louis

Case A C, Rooney D S 1982 Patient care planning strategies Nursing Management 13 (April): 23–26

Christopoulos A C 1970 Do you read the nurses' observation notes? Journal of Psychiatric Nursing and Mental Health Services (Jan–Feb): 24–25

Ciuca R L 1972 Over the years with the nursing care plan. Nursing Outlook 20(11): 706–711

Clarke M 1978 Planning nursing care: recent past, present and future. Nursing Times Occasional Papers 74(5): 17–20

Collister B 1988 Psychiatric nursing: person to person. Hodder & Stoughton, London

Corcoran S A 1986 Planning by expert and novice nurses in cases of varying complexity. Research in Nursing and Health 9: 155–162

Crow J, Duberley J, Hargreaves I 1979 Planning nursing care. In: Kratz C R (ed) The nursing process. Baillière Tindall, London

Daws J 1988 An enquiry into the attitudes of qualified nursing staff towards the use of individualized nursing care plans as a teaching tool. Journal of Advanced Nursing 13: 139–146

De La Cuesta C 1983 The nursing process: from development to implementation. Journal of Advanced Nursing 8: 365–371

Department of Health and Social Security 1986 Report of the Nursing Process Evaluation Working Group, Hayward J (ed). Nursing Education Research Unit, Department of Nursing Studies, University of London, DHSS

Dunlap L, Matteoli R 1970 A team function: developing a nursing care plan in a psychiatric setting. Journal of Psychiatric Nursing and Mental Health Services (Sept–Oct): 19–23

Ethridge P E, Packard R W 1976 An innovative approach to measurement of quality through utilization of nursing care plans. Journal of Nursing Administration (Jan): 25–31

Fanning V L, Weist Deloughery G L, Gebbie K M 1972 Patient involvement in planning own care: staff and patient attitudes. Journal of Psychiatric Nursing and Mental Health Services (Jan–Feb): 5–8

French H P 1979 Reassurance: a nursing skill? Journal of Advanced Nursing 4: 627–634

French H P 1983 Social skills for nursing practice. Croom Helm, London

Geach B 1974 The problem-solving technique as taught to student nurses. Perspectives in Psychiatric Care 12(1): 9–12

General Nursing Council for England and Wales 1982 Training Syllabus, Register of Nurses, Mental Nursing.

The General Nursing Council for England and Wales, London

Glasper A, Stonehouse J, Martin L 1987 Core care plans. Nursing Times (March 11): 55–57

Green B 1983 Primary nursing in psychiatry. Nursing Times (Jan 19): 24–28

Grosicki J P, Hagey M, Johnson I 1967 Nursing care plans: survey of status and opinions about current usage. Journal of Psychiatric Nursing (Nov–Dec): 567–585

Harris B L 1970 Who needs written care plans anyway? American Journal of Nursing 70 (Oct): 2136–2138

Hefferin E A, Hunter R E 1975 Nursing assessment and care plan statements. Nursing Research 24(5): 360–366

Henderson V 1973 On nursing care plans and their history. Nursing Outlook 21(6): 378–379

Heron J 1989 The facilitators handbook. Kegan Paul, London

Holden M, Bedgio R 1981 Kardex forms for psychiatric nursing. Journal of Psychiatric Nursing and Mental Health Services 19(5): 29–31

Hunt J M, Marks-Maran D J 1980 Nursing care plans: the nursing process at work. Wiley, Chichester

Hurst K 1985 Problem-solving tests in nurse education. Nurse Education Today 5: 56–62

Kelly N C 1966 Nursing care plans. Nursing Outlook 14(5): 61–64

Krall M L 1976 Guidelines for writing mental health treatment plans. American Journal of Nursing 76(2): 236–237

Kramer M 1972 Nursing care plans: power to the patient. Journal of Nursing Administration (Sept–Oct): 29–34

Lancaster W, Beare P 1982 Decision-making in nursing practice. In Lancaster J, Lancaster W (eds) Concepts for advanced nursing practice: the nurse as change agent. Mosby, St Louis

McClasky J C 1975 The nursing care plan: past, present and uncertain future — a review of the literature. Nursing Forum 14(4): 364–382

McFarlane J, Castledine G 1982 A guide to the practice of nursing using the nursing process. Mosby, St Louis

Mansfield E 1967 Use of nursing care plans by aids. Nursing Outlook 15 (April): 72–74

Marriner A 1979 The nursing process: a scientific approach to nursing care, 2nd edn. Mosby, St Louis

Marshall R J 1989 Blood and gore. The Psychologist 12(3): 115–117

Miller M 1988 Care plan for a suspicious person, using Roy's adaptation model. In: Collister B (ed) Psychiatric nursing: person to person. Hodder & Stoughton, London

Ministry of Health 1966 Report of the committee on senior nursing staff structure. HMSO, London

Muhs E J, Nebesky N T 1964 A psychiatric nursing care plan. American Journal of Nursing (April): 120–122

Nichols E G, Barstow R E 1980 Do nurses really use standard care plans? Journal of Nursing Administration 10 (May): 27–31

Palisin H E 1971 Nursing care plans are a snare and a delusion. American Journal of Nursing 71(1): 63–66

Pankratz D, Pankratz L 1973 The nursing care plan: theory and reality. Supervisor Nurse (April): 51–55

Ritter S 1988 Care plan for an anxious person, based on

Cawley's levels of psychotherapy. In: Collister B (ed) Psychiatric nursing: person to person. Hodder & Stoughton, London

Roper J M, Coutts A, Sather J, Taylor R 1985 Restraint and seclusion: a standard and standard care plan. Journal of Psychosocial Nursing 23(6): 18–23

Royal College of Nursing 1986 Society of Psychiatric Nursing. Standards of care. Royal College of Nursing, London

Schröck R A 1980 Planning nursing care for the mentally ill. Nursing Times (April 17): 704–706

Shea H L 1986 A conceptual framework to study the use of nursing care plans. International Journal of Nursing Studies 23(2): 147–157

Simonton M J, Neuffer C H, Stein E J, Furedy R L 1977 The open-ended record: an educational tool. Journal of Psychiatric Nursing and Mental Health Services 15 (Dec): 25–30

Smyth T 1983 SPECS — bridging a gap. Nurse Education Today 3(1): 4–7

Stevens A 1989 The politics of caring, the psychologist 12(3): 110–111

Stevens B J 1972 Why won't nurses write nursing care plans? Journal of Nursing Administration 2: 6–7, 91–92

St John D, Soulary E 1973 Introduction of goal-oriented record keeping in an in-patient drug treatment setting. Journal of Psychiatric Nursing 11 (Sept–Oct): 20–27

Stuart G W, Sundeen S J 1983 Principles and practice of psychiatric nursing, 2nd edn. Mosby, St Louis

Sturmey P, Newton T, Crisp A G 1988 Writing behavioural objectives: an evaluation of a simple, inexpensive method. Journal of Advanced Nursing 13: 496–500

Thomas B L 1988 Care plan for a withdrawn person, based on Orlando's psychodynamic model. In: Collister B (ed)

Psychiatric nursing: person to person. Hodder & Stoughton, London

Tissier J 1986 The development of a psychiatric nursing assessment form. In: Brooking J I (ed) Psychiatric nursing research. Wiley, Chichester

Tomlinson P and Birchenall P 1981 The intelligent use of educational objectives in nurse education. Nurse Education Today 1: 3, 5–11

United Kingdom Central Council 1986 Project 2000: A new preparation for practice. UKCC, London

Vincent P A, Broad J E, Dilworth L 1976 Developing a mental health assessment form. Journal of Nursing Administration (May): 25–28

Wagner B M 1969 Care plans — right, reasonable and reachable. American Journal of Nursing 69 (May): 986–990

Walton I 1986 The nursing process in perspective: a literature review. Department of Health and Social Security, London

Ward M 1989 Expressive objectives. Nursing Times 85 (51): 61–63

Whyte L, Youhill G 1984 The nursing process in the care of the mentally ill. Nursing Times (Feb 1): 49–51

Wilkinson T 1979 The problems and the values of objective nursing observations in psychiatric nursing care. Journal of Advanced Nursing 4: 151–159

Willer B, Santoro E 1975 The reporting habits of staff in a psychiatric hospital. Hospital and Community Psychiatry 126(6): 362–365

Woodcock E, McGehee T, Grub C 1972 The blackboard and care plan — nursing treatment tools. Journal of Psychiatric Nursing and Mental Health Services (Nov–Dec): 15–17

Yura H, Walsh M 1983 The nursing process, 4th edn. Appleton-Century-Crofts, New York

20

Communication

D. Skidmore

Communication may be defined as the action of transmitting information to others, either intentionally or unintentionally. When we refer to 'nurse–patient' communication, we normally tend to assume a controlled, intentional act; however, one should be aware that factors which defy control are also active. Communication may thus be considered in two broad categories: without words and with words.

NON-VERBAL COMMUNICATION

Communication cannot exist in a void, but requires two basic components — a transmitter and a receiver. Human communication is, indeed, very like the signals one receives through a radio set. For example, one can transmit forever and be unheard if there is no receiver. However, it is far more complex in that human communication contains more than one transmission outlet; that is, it involves various non-verbal, as well as verbal, signals. The term 'communication without words' is used to avoid confusion with the accepted interpretation of non-verbal communication: body language.

Person-to-person communication of all kinds is reciprocal and not one-way. It is thus as dependent on the condition of the receiver as it is on the message transmitted. One aspect of this is the

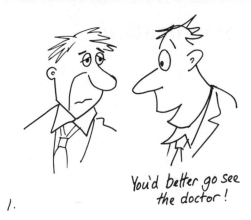

You'd better go see the doctor!

1.

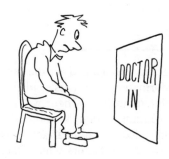

DOCTOR IN

2.

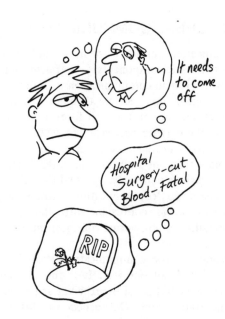

It needs to come off

Hospital Surgery—cut Blood—Fatal

RIP

3.

4.

phenomenon of 'selective attention', which relies very much upon receiver expectations and transmitter role display. As Lippman (1922) suggests, we tend to 'define first and then see'.

Consider going to see the doctor. Most people have expectations as to what doctors are and what they do, which are usually based on experience (good and bad) and social learning. Consequently, a form of communication has occurred before any medical encounter has even begun, in that a person has already constructed an image or definition of the doctor in his mind. This image functions very like a diagnosis, in that it informs not only what a thing is, but also what it does and how it should be dealt with. It is, in fact, a symbol and as such conveys far more information than mere words.

The cartoon illustrates the way in which a person makes associations when he defines a situation. The total symbol is not pure invention, but the result of communicated information from the individual's own past. It then forms the 'backdrop' which the receiver takes with him into the encounter, and which can distort or blind him to what subsequently occurs. In the cartoon, the patient's image of what the doctor is, is so strong in his mind, that he may not take in what actually occurs. This mechanism has been described previously by Skidmore (1980).

Let us follow the patient further into the encounter:

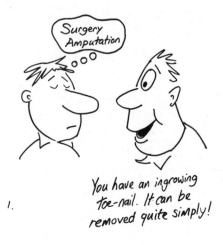

Surgery Amputation

1.

You have an ingrowing toe-nail. It can be removed quite simply!

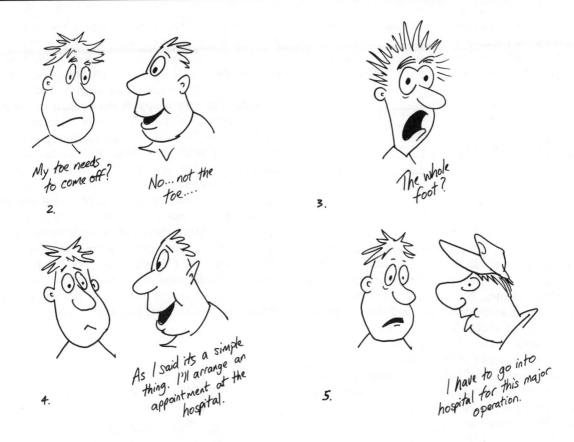

2. My toe needs to come off?

No... not the toe....

3. The whole foot?

4. As I said its a simple thing. I'll arrange an appointment at the hospital.

5. I have to go into hospital for this major operation.

In many ways, what happened to the patient in this sequence was the product of selective attention (or imagery deafness). He heard what he suspected he might hear. Rosenhan (1973) gives classic examples of the same phenomena, where nurses are deafened by the imagery of the diagnostic label. For example, when a pseudo-psychotic described his relationship with his wife as 'average . . . we do have the occasional angry outburst but nothing serious . . .', it is recorded by the nurse thus: 'This man has displayed considerable ambivalence in his relationships . . . his present relationship with his wife is punctuated by frequent angry outbursts . . .'

This is not what the man said; the key words 'angry outbursts' have been taken out of context, misinterpreted by the nurse because of what she expected to hear after hearing a diagnosis. She is first defining, then seeing.

The first component of communication without words, then, is the type of symbols that an encounter involves, prior to, during and after the encounter. It is essential to be aware of what has gone on in the head of both the transmitter and receiver prior to things actually being seen and/or heard.

Symbols are largely the product of our individual culture, in that their origins lie in a person's personal history. Certain words have very wide connotations; they are symbols of great depth, pictures with consequences. This is certainly true of diagnostic words. Davis (1963) suggests that 'polio' conjures images of callipers and iron-lungs; similarly 'psychotic' may well invoke in the layman the image of violent axe-men, whereas the professional will tend to construct a very different image. The crucial element is that of differing experience and knowledge. Marris

(1974) suggests that we all function by way of the conservative impulse:

Briefly, whenever we encounter a situation (B) we think back into our past (A) to gather relevant

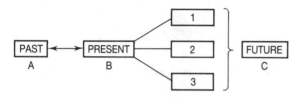

data that will help us to cope, look around in the present (B) to assess the reactions of others ('test the water'), and then act, with future effects (C) — which, in turn, become part of our past. If we experience 'normlessness', i.e. find that we cannot make sense of what is happening, then the conservative impulse leads us to rationalize the event. We base these rationalizations upon our expectations of what might, or should, have happened; however, if we do not have that basis of expectation, we tend to panic or enter a crisis state (Davis 1963, Roth 1963, Marris 1974).

Our images of people develop through our own personal history, nurtured by experience, hearsay and the media. Such images provide the foundation for all future communication. Thus the nurse will have developed an image of a patient, who, in turn, will have developed his own image of the nurse:

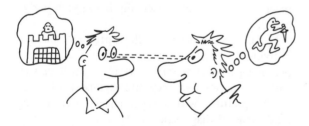

Such images can effectively block communication or cause it to be misinterpreted, as in the Rosenhan study cited above.

These images can be further reinforced by non-verbal cues — body posture, eye-contact, mannerisms — which can convey a message far more forcibly than words. Consider how actors can use their whole bodies to reflect a range of emotions without a word being spoken. They are merely controlling what we all do quite naturally. To state 'I'm very happy' is not enough unless it is accompanied by the correct body language (unless one plays for comedy), and our interpretation of the latter is strongly dependent on our social experience, which has taught us that certain postures have certain meanings. The more social experience we have, the more adept we become at reading the cues given off by another. Such meanings are very much culturally defined, so that any one gesture may have quite different meanings in different cultures (Morris et al 1979). It is thus crucial to understand the culture from which a person comes if one is to function as a successful transmitter to his or her receiver.

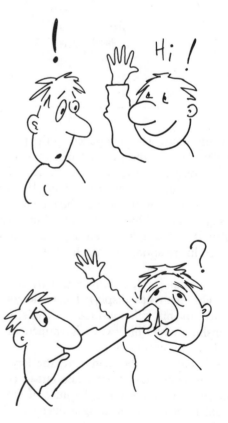

How, then, can the nurse transmit that she is interested in the person behind the patient? One cannot merely state interest, one has also to show it. The professional communicator has to become adept at controlling the transmission of body language in much the same way as the actor does. On one level, one receives information about any person or group of persons from the clothes they wear, their physical appearance, their demeanour and expressions. From this, one decides whether or not they are approachable, or likely to be aggressive. Often, one's decision will be incorrect, but nevertheless one remains reasonably confident in one's judgement. Indeed, a person's appearance tends to lead to his or her behaviour being stereotyped without negotiation, as occurs, for example, with punks, hippies, football supporters or motorbikers. It should be noted that even this type of communication is a dialogue. One's reaction to another's appearance can be perceived, and may lead to just the type of behaviour one anticipated, but because it was prompted not because it was in some way 'inevitable'. In other words, it is the 'give-a-dog-a-bad-name' phenomenon.

On a one-to-one level, one is able, without words, to express concern, interest and affection in many ways. For example, we display intimacy by penetrating body boundaries: we allow touching and are allowed to touch. In the United Kingdom, the act of holding hands, or hugging and kissing, communicates to each participant (as well as to an observer) that closeness is permitted and encouraged, since, in the UK, such behaviour is not encouraged with strangers. These are, of course, obvious examples, but analogous cues are delivered widely in everyday life. For example, eye-contact is important in terms of signalling lack of interest, interest and licence to reply; signals used in a similar way include yawning, fidgeting, looking blank and clockwatching. In short, a person starts to communicate before any words are uttered.

Barriers without words

Within the nurse–patient relationship, many barriers can arise that prevent effective communication. It should be remembered that a person's status as a patient means that all medical and paramedical staff hold power over him (Goffman 1969, Parsons 1951, Bradshaw 1978, Cassell 1978). Uniforms are particularly effective

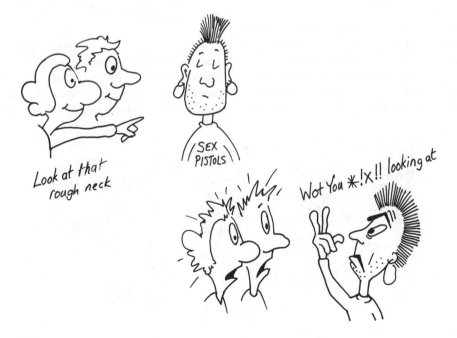

barriers, as are titles, since they reinforce status positions. Similarly, adopting certain expressions can prove effective (think of the type of look adopted for double-glazing salesmen and street interviewers). Another effective barrier often used by nurses and doctors is that of appearing to be busy; several studies have suggested that patients will not approach nurses when they seem busy.

To summarize, one can communicate effectively without words. Consider how one can greet, exclude, dismiss and intimidate someone without speaking. A little objective self-analysis can create awareness of the type of cues one offers to others in everyday encounters.

However, such explanations are strictly true only when considering the written word; the meanings conveyed by verbal communication are far more flexible. When a person speaks, it is not only the words that are heard, but also accent, tone and the level of vocabulary. After a few sentences are spoken, the listener tends to place the speaker in some form of imagined social framework which suggests, for example, his education, place of origin and present mood.

Often the non-verbal cues (our interpretation of which is often historically based) are reinforced by what one hears; to paraphrase Lippman (1922), we define first and then hear.

VERBAL COMMUNICATION

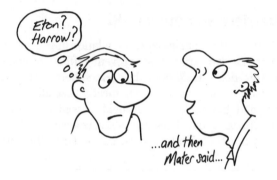

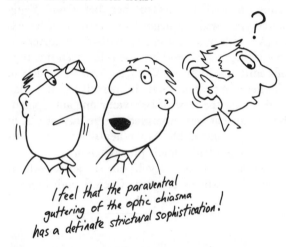

Verbal communication has been so well discussed in the literature, that an in-depth examination will not be made here. Briefly, we can suggest that language is also symbolic, in that a set of sounds are recognized as making sense, and there is a generally agreed meaning attached to each sound.

Most people tend to have confidence in the images and information conveyed by language. In many instances, however, one controls the way one speaks in order to create a false image (for example, to impress the opposite sex or prospective

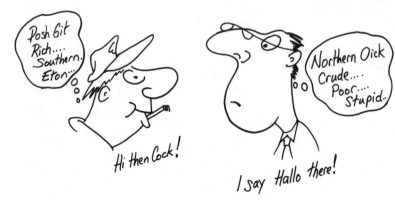

employers), or because we wish to include or exclude others. Various studies have illustrated how speech can be used to isolate a particular group from the general public; conversation in such groups is often disguised by way of codes (Duck 1983, Skidmore 1986). Thus, professionals use codes to include colleagues, who are party to the code, at the expense of excluding the client (Davis & Strong 1974, Stimson & Webb 1975).

Such a use of abstruse language is not always intentional. A good example of this in psychiatric nursing is the liberal use of terms such as 'delusion' and 'hallucination'. Over time, the nurse accepts such terms as part of her life and comes to assume that others understand them in the same sense. This is a common problem faced by researchers when designing questionnaires. Most professional groups have some form of jargon; it is both a shorthand way of communicating to colleagues, and offers a common identity, rather like the banter between RAF pilots during World War II. It can exclude others, although this is not always, or even often, intentional.

Similarly, in intimate circles, between friends or lovers, one word can convey paragraphs of information since the individuals concerned share common histories and find it unnecessary to explain the context of many remarks. Such a code includes them in the same group, strengthens their bond and advertises their affections, but it is not generally used at a conscious level to exclude others.

On a more general and less intimate level, groups devise codes to indicate their separate group identity. For example, many groups within youth culture use certain phrases to set them apart from the population at large and from other groups. Thus, words can be used deliberately to exclude others, to prevent outsiders from understanding the context or meaning of what is being said. This might be termed the 'Crisp syndrome' since it was Crisp (1976) who suggested that all foreigners secretly speak English in the confines of their own homes, using other language in public to keep Englishmen in the dark. Indeed, being an outsider within a group of colleagues or close friends, is rather like being in a foreign country.

Both the medical and psychiatric professions are guilty of using the techniques of inclusion and exclusion to the disadvantage of patients. Jargon is used to advertise one's status, to illustrate that one is staff; it gives one power and sets one apart from the rest. Such behaviour has been described by Illich (1976) as the 'priesthood syndrome'. Although it is often felt that if one parades one's knowledge by way of impressive language, the patient develops faith and confidence in the treatment, often the reverse is true. The patient is more likely to feel secure if he knows what is going on, no matter how unpleasant that information may be (Maslow 1963).

The feeling of power engendered by jargon can also encourage non-listening techniques, and influences verbal communication in terms of the informed interruption:

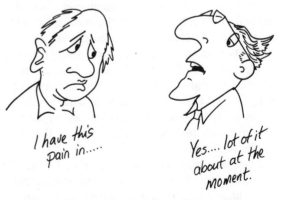

Listening is particularly important in psychiatry. If a patient believes that the nurse has no interest in him, he is unlikely to have confidence in any intervention she offers. Listening is also the principal means of gathering information about a client as an individual. Failure to listen encourages the situations illustrated by Rosenhan (1973) to emerge.

To summarize, what we say is related to how we are seen. Often, our demeanour can contradict the words we use, and verbal information alone is a poor transmitter of information.

COMMUNICATION AND THERAPEUTIC RELATIONSHIPS

It is argued that the most important aspect and foundation of any relationship is that of communication. Nurses and patients are also people and initially use the same skills as any other person. Unfortunately, they do not enjoy the equality of ordinary people at the onset of their relationship, as a great deal of information about one another has already been communicated by way of external sources.

From the patient's point of view, he may have gleaned information concerning psychiatry, nurses and hospitals from books and television. Such, often fictional, accounts tend to be inaccurate and grossly exaggerated. In addition, information derived from past experience can be, and folklore is usually, distorted over time. This information forms the database from which the patient constructs an image of the encounter before it happens. When he arrives at the encounter, things seen (e.g. uniforms) and heard (jargon) can strongly reinforce any negative image he has already formed. Because of this, it is often useful to invite patients to talk about what they expect to happen, and to offer their view of what psychiatry is about; in this way any myths can be tackled, although not necessarily dispelled, at the onset on the relationship.

The nurse may have been influenced in similar ways, her knowledge and expectations concerning psychiatric care and patients having been gathered from textbooks (often years old and outdated), teaching and experience, hospital folklore, labels

and the influence of credible peers. From such a database the nurse constructs her images prior to the encounter. During the encounter selective attention (discussed above) can reinforce that image. Consider, for example, the following hypothetical case:

Case example

Student John is having his Acute placement with Sister Susan; in school, he has been given glowing reports about Sister Susan's ability. At his first meeting with her he found her pleasant and attractive and this helped him to like her — a good basis for finding credibility in her actions. Because of her previous experience Sister Susan believes that puerperal psychosis cases are always violent and aggressive. Within John's first week of placement, a woman, Anne, is admitted suffering from post-natal depression (which is close enough to puerperal psychosis for Sister Susan). Susan gives John the benefit of her knowledge regarding post-childbirth disorders. At first, John is sceptical about the assertion that they are invariably violent. However, at medication time, Sister Susan and her staff gather outside Anne's room (it is Sister Susan's policy to nurse such cases in seclusion); at a given signal, the staff rush into the room and have to restrain Anne whilst administering the medication. John is amazed, and impressed, to discover that Sister Susan was absolutely right. What he does not consider is that he has been party to a self-fulfilling prophecy.

Let us now put ourselves in Anne's position: she is sitting on her bed, feeling miserable, wondering where on earth she is, when suddenly the door bursts open and in rush uniformed figures brandishing syringes; they seize and hold her whilst something is injected into her . . . she has no other choice but to fight because no one listens to her questions. What would you do in Anne's position?

The case has, of course, been exaggerated to exemplify how communication and misinterpretation can occur: all parties within the encounter were communicating with each other, but only in a negative sense. As a result, when Anne leaves the hospital, her negative views of psychiatry will be reinforced and passed on to others. Similarly, when John leaves the ward, his negative views about that particular condition will be retained and passed on to others.

This same mechanism occurs more generally, in both general and psychiatric treatment; if a treatment has been successful with one or two patients, it may happen that everybody within that diagnostic category receives the same therapy. Such an approach does not take into account the individuality of a person. Images tend to limit effective communication (which is always two-way) and the majority of psychiatric interventions rely on effective communication. A vicious circle ensues, because the images we have limit the communication one enters into, and this in turn reinforces one's previous image.

An extension of this is the situation where the therapist treats the patient for what she thinks the patient is suffering from, rather than for the actual problem. When the therapist realizes that the symptoms have gone (because they were never there) her original judgement is reinforced. These situations arise from limited communications, false images and informed interruptions. The extent to which society has been medicalized means that, with little effort, a diagnostic label can be provided for most conditions, and the label carries with it an indication of treatment. Unfortunately, the professional tends to be as impressed and as trapped by these labels as are her patients.

Naturally the therapist has the ultimate power and control since she can rationalize failure as the patient's fault. Even the textbooks inform her of the one-third who will not respond or refuse to be re-referred for further different therapy, but the therapist's failure to develop and maintain her part of the communication relationship is nowhere examined. Because a person is sometimes treated for something he has not got, he does not respond; the person then acquires a reputation for 'attention-seeking' and loses credibility in future encounters.

The above situation is assisted by the way such encounters are approached; the therapist does not communicate, she interrogates (Skidmore & Friend 1984). Certain questions have to be answered prior to treatment decisions, and it is the therapist, who may be blinded by her preconcep-

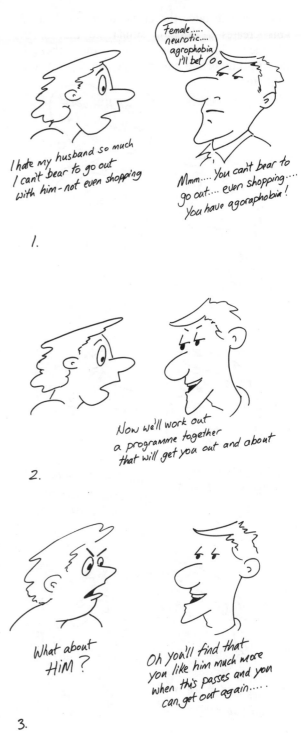

tions, who dictates the areas to be touched on. This creates a situation similar to that of the informed interruption, with the therapist interrupting before the patient can say what he wants to:

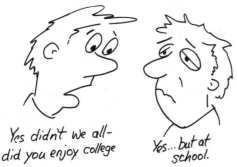

The therapist has to obtain certain information to complete the necessary documents (such as problem orientated records) and this tends to attain more importance than the patient. It is worth noting here that people tend to be constantly receptive to friendly approaches, regardless of the situation, and that it may therefore be more profitable to concentrate on this, rather than on pencil and paper exercises. At present, the primary interview to which patients are subjected is often less an exercise in communication than yet another way of not listening. Patients, like any other group of clients, prefer to test the water before plunging in. Within the nurse–patient relationship, the patient often tests the credibility of the nurse through a kind of verbal 'fencing' (Butterworth & Skidmore 1981). This is particularly marked within the area of sexual dysfunction when 'patients' will often disclose 'masking' problems, to test out the professional's ability, before disclosing the real issues. This is quite acceptable when people are revealing their inner selves.

Thus, one of the major principles underlying the therapeutic relationship is *reception*, which involves a full commitment on the part of the nurse to listen in full to what the patient is saying, and to accept that the patient is a person in his own right. Another important aspect is that of *understanding* what has been said by both parties.

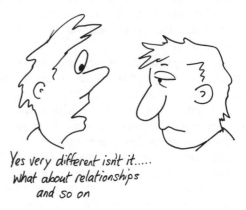

Finally, there is the time factor: both sides of a relationship must commit themselves in terms of time if they wish to communicate effectively. Effective communication cannot take place within severe time restraints, and no patient is going to be comforted by the nurse who interrupts his flow because of another appointment.

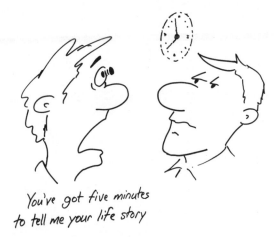

You've got five minutes to tell me your life story

REFERENCES

Bradshaw J S 1978 Doctors on trial. Wildwood, London
Butterworth C A, Skidmore D 1981 Caring for the mentally ill in the community. Croom Helm, London
Cassell E J 1978 The healer's art. Penguin, Harmondsworth
Crisp Q 1976 The naked civil servant. Penguin, Harmondsworth
Davis F 1963 Passage through crisis. Bobbs Merrill, Indianapolis
Davis A, Strong P 1974 Aren't children wonderful? Sociological Monographs. Sociological Review
Duck S 1983 Friends for life. Harvester Press, London
Goffman E 1969 The presentation of self in everyday life. Penguin, Harmondsworth
Illich I 1976 Limits to medicine. Pelican, Harmondsworth
Lippman W 1922 Public opinion. Macmillan, London
Marris B 1974 Loss and change. Routledge & Kegan Paul, London

Maslow A 1963 The need to know and the fear of knowing. Journal of General Psychology 68: 111–125
Morris D, Collett P, Marsh P, O'Shaughnessy M 1979 Gestures. Cape, London
Parsons T 1951 The social system. Free Press, London
Rosenhan D L 1973 On being sane in insane places. Science 179: 250–258
Roth J 1963 Timetables. Bobbs Merrill, Indianapolis
Skidmore D 1980 The hidden machine: medical encounters. Versus, Bournemouth
Skidmore D 1986 The sociology of friendship. PhD thesis, Keele University
Skidmore D, Friend W 1984 The effectiveness of CPNs. Unpublished research report, Manchester Polytechnic
Stimson B, Webb G 1975 Going to see the doctor. Routledge & Kegan Paul, London

FURTHER READING

Kagan C, Evans J, Kay B 1986 Interpersonal skills in nursing: an experiential approach. Harper & Row, London

21

Meeting physical care needs

B. L. Thomas

To be able to meet physical care needs enhances the quality of an individual's life by increasing the capacity for independent living and raising his self-esteem. When a person becomes mentally ill, the ability to meet his own physical care needs frequently diminishes. A deficit in meeting his own physical care needs is often important in making a psychiatric diagnosis. For example, one of the characteristic signs of people with schizophrenia disorders is deterioration in personal appearance and self-care skills. This deterioration stigmatizes them as having a mental disorder, interferes with their social relationships, prolongs institutional stays, and may endanger their physical health (Paul 1969). In depression, physical well-being, appearance and personal hygiene are often ignored and patients may not be capable of caring for themselves. Manic patients may be too busy to eat or take care of themselves.

Physical care needs cover a wide range of activities from very basic biological needs such as the need to eat and sleep, to very individual needs that contribute to giving us our unique identity, such as the clothes we wear, the way we style our hair and our own way of expressing ourselves. Many of these issues are discussed in other chapters of this book, for example the need for exercise is addressed by Brooking in Chapter 44. This chapter focuses on what are often regarded as the basic physiological and biological aspects of physical care needs, such as the need for air, nutrition, sleep and personal hygiene.

While mainly biological in origin, it must be remembered that these needs are inextricably bound up with psychological aspects, social expectations and cultural norms. Psychiatric nurses are often criticized for neglecting these physical care needs of patients. In this chapter, these critisims are addressed by reviewing the research and prescriptive literature available concerned with meeting psychiatric patients' physical care needs.

ASSISTING PATIENTS TO MEET THEIR PERSONAL CARE NEEDS

Regardless of arguments to the contrary, it is proposed that much of the psychiatric nurse's work is concerned with assisting individuals to maintain or increase the ability to meet their own physical care needs. In recent years the word 'assist' has taken on an important meaning in nursing literature, particularly in psychiatric nursing, where the emphasis has changed from taking over the complete care of patients to helping patients care for themselves. Contemporary psychiatric nursing focuses on 'doing something with patients' as opposed to 'doing something to patients'. This is evident in the move for psychiatric patients to be actively involved with nurses in planning their own care (Flanning et al 1972).

The turning point of this movement seems to have originated in the 1950s and 1960s when many of the most basic ideas of modern psychiatric nursing were formulated. These included: recognition of the dehumanizing effects on patients through institutionalization (Barton 1959, Goffman 1961, Miller 1970); the need for rehabilitation (Wing & Brown 1970), milieu therapy (Cumming & Cumming 1962), and therapeutic communities (Jones 1953) where the patients' social environment was to provide a therapeutic experience for them. Patients were to be active participants in their own care and to become involved in the daily running of the community. Emphasis was on the importance of the nurse–patient relationship and its therapeutic effect on patients (Peplau 1952, Orlando 1961).

Long-term confinement in a highly structured, controlled environment was indicated as demolishing personal identity and autonomy, leaving patients incapable of meeting their personal care needs and decreasing their ability for independent living and self-determination.

The answer to this problem was to change the place of treatment for patients from large, remote inpatient facilities to smaller, community outpatient facilities, or better still to the patient's own home (Cole 1984). However, it has become increasingly clear that institutionalization can occur anywhere (Underwood 1980). The cause of institutionalization is now recognized to be the type of care and treatment that prohibits or even decreases the patient's ability for meeting his own personal care needs and self-determination. The mass movement of psychiatric patients into the community has resulted in a smaller but often chronic hospital population (Hailey 1971). The prospect of these patients meeting their own personal needs and living an independent life is often regarded as an impossible proposition (Lamb 1981, Levine 1981). In the United States this has resulted in the setting up of advanced psychiatric nurse training for chronic psychiatric care (Krauss & Slavinsky 1982).

The need for this type of training is evident when considering the results of such studies as Towell (1975) and Savage et al (1979), who found that nurses spent most of their time in task-centred daily routines of physical care with no individualized care and little nurse–patient interaction. Armitage (1986), who describes the nursing care on a 20-bedded continual care ward, reports similar findings. He suggests that the nurse behaviour frequently observed related not to therapeutic activities but to administrative and maintenance activities. The maintenance activities included serving meals and drinks, ensuring that patients kept themselves clean and that their appearance was tidy, and ensuring that the patients' beds were made. Stokes & Keen (1987) present a similar picture of life on a long-stay ward in a psychiatric hospital. They state that nurses frequently resorted to nagging and cajoling patients to become involved in self-care and personal hygiene activities.

Psychiatric nurses have to be particularly skilled in continual monitoring and providing the various levels of care that are required. The level of care will vary at different times. It may involve providing complete care, including washing, feeding and toileting patients. It may involve teaching patients how to attend to their own physical needs, and it may occasionally include reminding patients about attending to their physical needs. Whatever the level of care being provided, psychiatric nurses must recognize that the assistance they give must not prohibit nor interfere with the individual's own ability to meet their own needs. This is particularly important with elderly patients when nurses have an urge to wash patients or dress them, or feed them because it is quicker than allowing the patients to do these things for themselves. Martin (1987) suggests that unless patients are allowed to maintain and practise self-care skills, they will become less independent and more dependent.

Whether or not psychiatric nurses are proficient in determining the level of assistance required is debatable. Pile et al (1968) suggest that psychiatric nurses are often unable to determine the kinds and amounts of care needed by psychiatric patients because nurses do not collect appropriate patient data with which to make realistic plans. Their solution to this problem was the development of a behaviour rating scale for assessing the nursing care required. The nursing assessment of psychiatric patients is fully discussed in Chapter 18. Its importance is mentioned here in the belief that the collection of information in a systematic and continuous manner is essential for the meeting of patients' personal care needs. While many such assessment forms are in existence there is a need for more research into their usefulness and applicability.

THE PRINCIPAL ROLE OF THE PSYCHIATRIC NURSE

The contemporary role of the psychiatric nurse is often prescribed as being mainly concerned with patients' socio-psychological problems and needs

rather than the physical needs of the patient (Whyte & Youhill 1984).

It seems that in an attempt to break away from a custodial caretaking role which characterizes institutionalized care, psychiatric nurses have been criticized for giving less attention to the more immediate physical needs of a patient than is warranted (Schröck 1980). Whether or not this is the case is debatable since the previously mentioned studies have demonstrated evidence to the contrary, at least on long-stay wards. The issue in question seems to be whether or not patients' physical and psychological needs are given the attention required. The introduction of the 1982 syllabus (see Ch. 5) was an attempt to redress the balance and ensure that psychiatric nurses acquired the necessary knowledge and skills to provide patients with comprehensive care. This was to be aided by the development of the skilful use of the nursing process.

THE INTRODUCTION OF THE NURSING PROCESS

The nursing process was to supply nurses with a problem-solving method for identifying the health needs of patients and provide individualized care (Ward 1984). While it has provided a problem-solving approach to care, the nursing process by itself has not provided nurses with the necessary theories on which to base their practice. For example, although the nursing process involves assessing the patient's needs, it does not tell the nurse *what* needs are to be assessed (Aggleton & Chalmers 1986). This has resulted in general nurses using the nursing process to organize care around a set of medical understandings of people and their needs, while psychiatric nurses have attempted to implement the nursing process in conjunction with the existing prevailing psychiatric ideologies (Cormack 1976). British psychiatry has traditionally functioned by using a combination of conceptual models, the most common being the medico-biological, psychological (including psychoanalytic and behavioural) and social models. Each model makes different assumptions about the nature of mental illness, its causes and effective treatment. Psychiatric nursing care varies according to the expectations set by the prevailing psychiatric ideology (Towell 1975, Cormack 1983).

To demonstrate this, Stockwell (1985) gives the example of an elderly schizophrenic patient who becomes intermittently incontinent. If nursing care is based on the medical model, the intermittent incontinence will be viewed as either a symptom of the person's mental illness or as a pathology of ageing. The nurse's intervention is to report the matter to the doctor for investigation and to carry out whatever treatment is prescribed. If nursing care is based on a behavioural model, then the nurse's intervention in conjunction with a behavioural therapist will be to implement a behavioural programme which will consist of timed toileting and a system of token reinforcement for periods of dryness (Pollock & Liberman 1974).

In reality, a combination of approaches is usually employed. King (1980) emphasized that in treating incontinence the physical, social, psychological and environmental approaches must be used in combination and that any treatment programme has to be tailored to meet the needs of the individual. For example, the physical approach may include helping a patient to be as mobile as possible. A social approach may involve encouraging the patient to bath regularly and to dress in his own clothes. An environmental approach may include access to toilets which are clearly marked. Psychological approaches may include acknowledging the distress caused by the incontinence, motivating and encouraging the patient to use the toilet and giving them praise when they do so. In tailoring these approaches to meet the needs of the individual, Turner (1986) suggests that the goal of total continence may often be unrealistically high. A more realistic gaol might be that the person should learn to indicate to a member of staff that he needs to use the toilet.

THE INTRODUCTION OF NURSING MODELS

One important move towards a more holistic view of patients and incorporating the various psychiatric approaches into the parameters of nursing, in such a way as to make them more relevant to nursing practice, has been through the medium of nursing models. Nurses are often criticized on this account — that is, that nursing models have simply reformulated existing models and theories from other disciplines. Maslow's (1954) hierarchical order of needs is an example of a borrowed theory which has been highly utilized by psychiatric nurses. To disregard the usefulness of knowledge from other disciplines is not very productive. As Fitzpatrick et al (1982) suggest, theories are not owned by any one discipline, but rather each discipline has a right and responsibility to select from the available knowledge and to modify and reformulate those theoretical positions for its own purposes.

The use of nursing models in going some way to meet patients' personal care needs is clearly demonstrated by the contributions made in such books as Martin (1987) and Collister (1988). In his review of the various models described Collister argues that two general types of nursing models were identified: holistic and reductionist. They are similar to the biomedical model except that biological parts are replaced by behavioural activities such as breathing, eating and eliminating, or wider concepts such as the biopsychosocial aspects.

In holistic nursing models sense is made of the person through identification of discrete elements which go together to make up the individual. However, rather than providing a holistic approach to care, the tendency seems to be to emphasize the separation of these elements and reduce the person to a series of fragments. Models of this type include those based on systems theory and those which incorporate activities of living or their equivalent.

The pursuit of holistic nursing has been undertaken by psychiatric nurses for some time. Oleck & Yoder (1981) suggest that psychiatric nurses often pride themselves on the ability to provide holistic care: for example, Lego (1970), White (1976), Harris & Solomon (1977). However, a closer look at what psychiatric nurses mean by the term holistic reveals the ability to integrate concepts from biological, physical, psychological and social sciences into their clinical practice. Whether or not such integration constitutes holism is debatable (Swanson 1981). Thomas (1987) found that student nurses identified holistic nursing in such a manner. The students' understanding of holistic nursing involved viewing the patient as a biopsychosocial being. According to Oleck & Yoder (1981), holistic care means a conception of man as composed of parts — biological, physical psychological and social. In a content analysis of articles published over a three year period in two American psychiatric nursing journals the authors tried to test the assertion that psychiatric nurses provide holistic nursing.

For an article to qualify as demonstrating integration the author or authors had to identify psychosocial and biophysiological needs and show that both were included in planning, implementing and evaluating nursing care. Unfortunately, of the 188 articles reviewed, only 18% met their stated critia and this led Oleck & Yoder to conclude that psychiatric nurses are only minimally reporting the integration of physiological and psychosocial knowledge in their clinical practice. Therefore, the degree to which psychiatric nurses provide holistic care is debatable.

Swanson (1981) is highly critical of Oleck & Yoder's (1981) methodology and, more importantly, the conclusions they draw. She suggests that their conception of man seems to focus more on totality than on wholeness. A similar argument is proffered by Collister (1988), who suggests that nursing models adopt such a reductionist view of man. Collister suggests that such models are unsatisfactory since problems are identified in isolation and care planned accordingly, which results in goals and interventions becoming routinized rather than individualized.

An alternative view is proposed by Torres (1986), who in reviewing the literature on the concepts of need suggests that nursing theories consistently identify the physical, biological and psychosocial needs of humans. Torres points out that nursing models which emphasize the concept of need are based on the original work of Maslow (1954), and incorporate his definitions of needs into their models.

Basic to all need-oriented nursing models is the assumption that nurses provide nursing care to individuals in terms of their specific needs (the parts) while viewing the individual as a whole organism. Maslow (1954) suggests that the individual is an integrated, organized whole. Torres (1986) argues that nurse theorists who have related their models of nursing to the concept of need all share a common frame of reference — that is, humans' universal needs. Nursing care can effectively be utilized from a framework of need. Whether this happens in reality is a moot point. Such models do, however, provide a check-list to guide nurses in their work and, as such, have the potential to draw nurses' attention to patients' needs which hitherto have been neglected: for example, sexual and spiritual needs. By emphasizing the psychological, social and physical spheres in the assessment of psychiatric patients such models may also prevent physical health problems being neglected (Holmberg 1988).

Another type of model identified by Collister (1988) tends to focus on the nurse–patient relationship. While both types of model employ a planned approach to care incorporating the nursing process, the difference between them lies in the process which is being addressed. Models which focus on the nurse–patient relationship have the process of evolution of the relationship as their theme, rather than the cyclical problem-solving process inherent in reductionist models. Smith (1986) suggests that the use of such models provides patients with the tools to alter their life situation rather than concentrating on providing solutions to problems. Using the non-reductionist models, care plans do include precise measurable goals. However, although these goals give direction they do not interfere with nor constrain the dynamics of the interaction. The means in human terms are of at least equal importance to the end result. The nurse can employ her skills in each intervention with a particular patient and, although the overall goal will remain the same, the uniqueness and individuality of both nurse and patient will be manifest.

The importance of examining the difference between reductionist and non-reductionist models resides in the underlying values implicit in each type. Within the reductionist model the 'worth' of a patient may partly depend on judgements about the progress he is or is not making in relation to care plan goals. The esteem in which the patient is held by the nurse is conditional upon the patient maintaining goal-directed progress and conforming to expectations. Failure to do so often results in frustration and a variety of undesirable behaviours (Stockwell 1972, Kelly & May 1982).

A non-reductionist model, by recognizing the patient as a person, acknowledges that progress does not always occur in a linear fashion but may proceed in a disjointed manner, regression often occurring before progress is made. These models have also much more potential for recognizing the meaning of the problem for the patient and the best means of solving the problem through the medium of the nurse–patient relationship.

Both types of nursing models, then, have provided some understanding and framework in which nurses can organize and deliver care. Aggleton & Chalmers (1986) suggest that while nursing models are useful in this respect they are nonetheless abstract representations of nursing, and what is needed are more concrete and specific theories which deal with a more limited number of events and situations. Meleis (1985) has advocated the pursuit of a theory–research–theory strategy for the development of nursing. This begins by recognizing that psychiatric nurses must work with some sort of theory 'making sense' of the work they do. As previously discussed, some of these theories may derive from psychological and social scientific understandings of individuals and their needs, while others may derive from nursing models. Hypotheses then generated can be tested in nursing practice, the outcome of which is the development of a more refined theory.

THE APPLICATION OF THEORY

The Royal College of Nursing (1986) describe the first standard of care in psychiatric nursing as being; 'The nurse applies appropriate theory as a basis for decision-making regarding nursing practice.'

A review of the literature on meeting patients' physical care needs has revealed very little theory which has been empirically tested. Research that has been carried out has been into specific aspects of patients' needs, such as sleep, nutrition and elimination. While not disputing the importance of this research, it often has little practical significance to guide psychiatric nurses in their daily work. For the most part, the information available remains anecdotal and prescriptive. The following sections examine the available nursing literature, both research and prescriptive, relating to the need for air, nutrition, elimination, sleep and personal grooming.

The need for air

The need for air includes the ability to breathe without difficulty. Underwood (1980) suggests that the need for air is rarely a problem with psychiatric patients. This claim is substantiated in considering both the dearth of psychiatric nursing research literature and prescriptive literature about psychiatric patients' need for air. Descriptions of nursing care using nursing models do occasionally mention breathing (Thomas 1988) but this need is usually expressed as 'breathing normally' or 'no evidence of ventilatory problem' (Martin 1987).

There are, however, numerous occasions when breathing can be problematic for psychiatric patients: for example, patients who are in a state of unconsciousness, such as after a general anaesthetic in the case of electroconvulsive therapy (ECT). During this period, patients require close observation and nurses must ensure a clear airway. Similar care is required by patients who suffer from epilepsy. Severely disturbed patients, particularly if being restrained, must also be protected from accidental aspiration or suffocation. Patients who are anxious and who experience panic attacks may also experience breathing difficulties; breathing becomes increased and over-breathing develops. Relaxation techniques using simple breathing exercises and muscle relaxation aid in ensuring an adequate supply of oxygen to the body and preventing over-breathing.

The other major effect on breathing is the large number of psychiatric patients who smoke. The prevalence of smoking among psychiatric inpatients has been reported by O'Farrell et al (1983). In their survey of a large psychiatric hospital they found that 82.9% of the patients were cigarette smokers, although only 16% of these patients were receiving anti-smoking treatment for addictive problems. Hughes et al (1986), in a comparison study of psychiatric outpatients and local or national population-based samples, found a higher prevalence of smoking among the psychiatric patients. Smoking was especially prevalent among patients with schizophrenia, mania and among the more severely ill patients.

There is a large volume of medical research on the effects of smoking and lung disease (Health Education Council 1983). However, research on schizophrenic patients who smoke found a lower rate of lung cancer in them than in non-psychiatric control subjects (Baldwin 1979, Tsaung et al 1983). A number of hypotheses have been suggested to explain these findings. The most obvious is that psychiatric patients die earlier from unnatural causes such as suicide and accidents (Martin et al 1984). Other hypotheses are that schizophrenic patients have a metabolic defect that protects them from cancer (Levi & Waxman 1975), that phenothiazines and other psychoactive drugs have antitumour effects (Driscoll et al 1978), and that social isolation and hospitalization protect schizophrenic patients from stress-induced cancer (Fox & Howell 1974). However, none of these hypotheses have been adequately tested.

Although psychiatric nurses have a large educative role to play in the smoking habits of psychiatric patients (Health Education Council 1983), there is little research or prescriptive literature available to guide nurses in dealing with the practical problems associated with the prevention of smoking and the dangerous smoking behaviours that patients exhibit, such as being forgetful and careless with lighted cigarettes.

Becker et al (1986) investigated the smoking behaviour and attitudes toward smoking among hospital nurses. Their results led them to conclude that nurses who continue to smoke may hold attitudes in conflict with their role in helping patients to stop smoking. Gaston (1982) describes a smoking programme which was successfully implemented in a ward for chronic schizophrenic patients. Dingman et al (1988) describes the effect of a non-smoking policy on an acute psychiatric unit. They conclude that hospitalized psychiatric patients can cope with a total ban on smoking. The lack of cigarettes as a source of conflict frees staff to deal with other patient issues and suggest that psychiatric facilities should promote healthy behaviour in their patients.

The need for nutrition

Psychiatric patients often have difficulty in meeting their need for food and fluid. This difficulty may be expressed in either excessive or diminished food and fluid intake (Ch. 33). Decreased nutritional intake may result from a number of reasons. Among those generally stated are being unaware of the impulse to eat or drink, an inability to go to the dining room or to sit with others, or the fear of being poisoned. Increased eating and drinking may be a function of anxiety, increased appetite owing to medication (Jackson & Haynes-Johnson 1988). Whatever the behaviour or its cause, patients may need various levels of assistance in order for their food and fluid intake to be sufficient. While there is much research on patients' nutrition (Kipp 1984) and not disputing the need for such research, the practical problems for psychiatric nurses remain unaddressed. These include how to motivate patients to eat, how to persuade patients to sit down at a table in the company of others and eat their food slowly. Should patients be allowed to prepare and cook their own food? What choices do patients have regarding the food they eat? It is difficult to control the types of food provided in a large psychiatric hospital; however, every effort should be made to provide nourishing meals, to offer varied menus which cater for the different ethnic groups and to present meals in an attractive manner.

The prescriptive literature advocates a number of approaches to be used when patients have difficulty meeting their need for nutrition. These range from verbally encouraging patients to eat (Darcy 1985) to physically spoon feeding and tube feeding patients (Martin 1987). The issue of force feeding patients, particularly demented patients, has received some attention. The literature discusses whether feeding should be regarded as an ordinary and mandatory treatment or whether it should be regarded as extraordinary (Watts & Cassel 1984). If feeding could be regarded as an extraordinary treatment the question is, when should it be withdrawn? Some moralists have stated that spoon feeding should never be withdrawn as it symbolizes love, care and concern, while artificial feeding by tube or infusions could be witheld (Lynn & Childress, 1983). Norberg & Hirschfield (1987) in an exploratory study of 60 health care workers in Israel found that when patients were force fed, care givers did not feel guilty for using force or accepting suffering, since they felt obliged to preserve life and thus their actions were right. This contrasted with previous studies of care givers in Sweden, who felt caught in a double bind conflict. While on the one hand wishing to feed patients, on the other hand they did not wish to use feeding techniques which they defined as force feeding (Norberg et al 1980, Akerlund & Norberg 1985).

The need to eliminate

Elimination concerns the ability to control bowel and bladder. There are many causes for deficits in these areas. These include the side-effects of psychiatric medication, which may produce diarrhoea or constipation and urinary frequency or retention. They may also be caused by physical impairment as in the case of elderly patients, or psychological distress as in the case of children. Whatever the behaviour or the cause, for the most part psychiatric nursing research in this area has focused on behavioural approaches to care (Hartie & Black 1975, Carruth 1976, Patrick & Raffety 1978, Linke 1982).

The use of nursing models in psychiatric nursing has also provided structure and purpose in dealing with patients' needs of elimination.

The example opposite (Fig. 21.1) of assessing a patient's need for elimination is provided by Roper et al (1981).

Nursing interventions vary according to the need: roughage, fruit and increased fluids being prescribed for some patients with constipation, while laxatives, suppositories or enemas may be prescribed for others. Bauer & Hill (1986) have listed various nursing interventions associated with the elimination needs of various clients with specific patterns of behaviour.

Anxious pattern of behaviour. Check daily weight, and intake and output of client who is vomiting. Poor nutritional intake may affect elimination; monitor daily.

Depressed pattern of behaviour. May forget to void. Check for distended bladder. Take to bathroom regularly; remind to void regularly. Check for constipation. Monitor toileting. Increase water, juices, fruit and activity.

Aggressive (manic) pattern of behaviour. Monitor elimination; may be too 'busy' for toileting.

Withdrawal pattern of behaviour (as observed in schizophrenia). May retain faeces and urine. Needs regular reminding and monitoring.

Overtly suspicious pattern of behaviour. Usually not a problem unless related to lack of food and fluids owing to delusions.

The need for sleep

Sleep as a personal need is another area which has received considerable attention. Bearing in mind that the actual length of time spent asleep may vary enormously between individuals (Jones & Oswald 1968), numerous aspects of sleep and its effects have been researched, including the factors which may affect normal sleep, such as gender, diet, temperature and drugs.

This research has covered such fundamental issues as attempting to find out why sleep is necessary and what precisely its functions are, nevertheless there still remains much controversy surrounding the subject. Closs (1988) suggests that there is a huge body of evidence which supports the hypothesis that sleep aids healing. Borkovec (1982) suggests that disturbed sleep may originate from a number of very different psychological and physical causes. Many insomnias are interpreted as being secondary to underlying psychiatric conditions and the initial treatment in these cases is directed at removing the primary cause. However, if the insomnias which are secondary to psychiatric conditions have been chronic for at least a few months, Borkovec suggests that a learned behavioural component often aggravates these insomnias. A vicious cycle then develops. This is depicted diagrammatically in Figure 21.2.

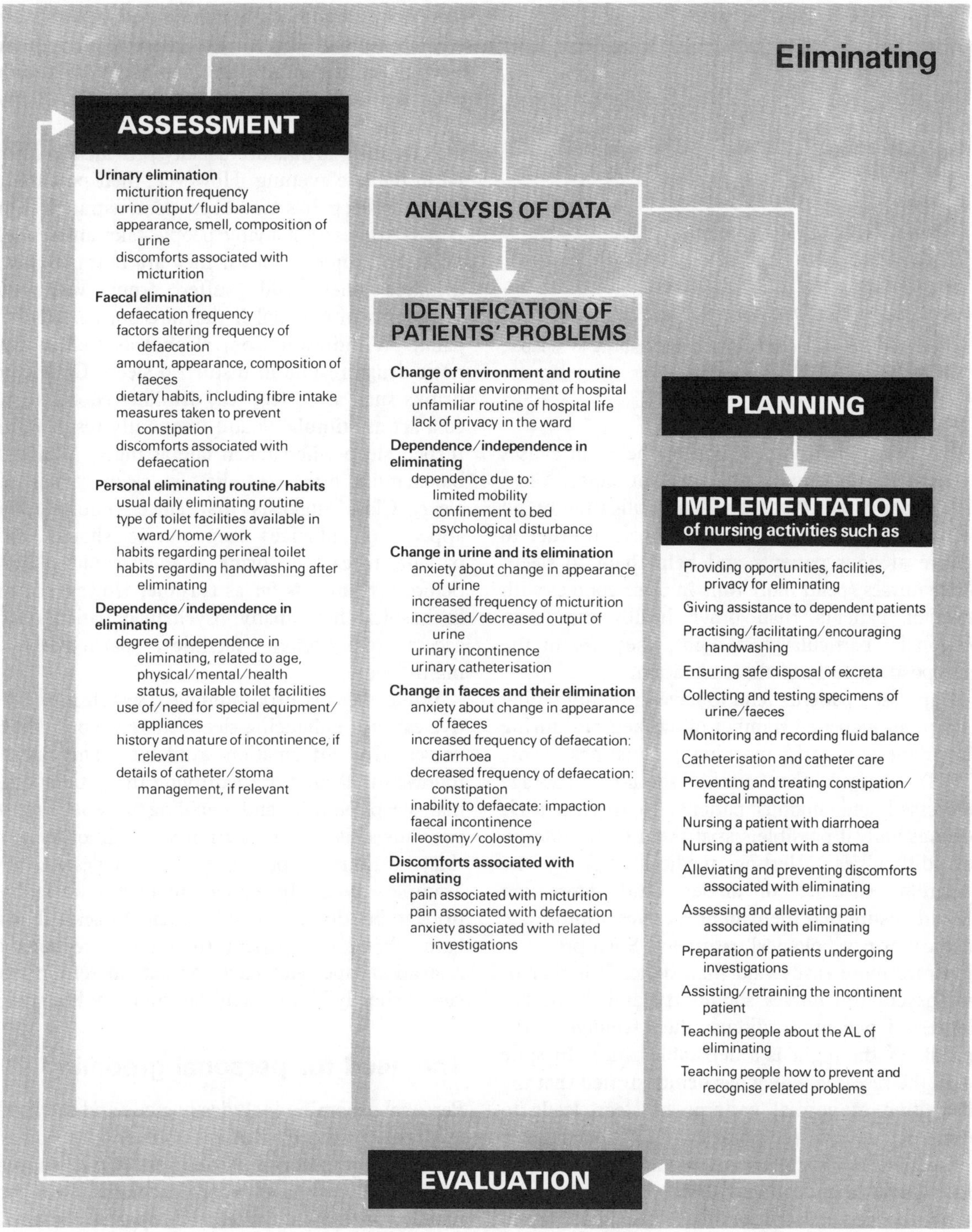

Eliminating

ASSESSMENT

Urinary elimination
micturition frequency
urine output/fluid balance
appearance, smell, composition of
urine
discomforts associated with
micturition

Faecal elimination
defaecation frequency
factors altering frequency of
defaecation
amount, appearance, composition of
faeces
dietary habits, including fibre intake
measures taken to prevent
constipation
discomforts associated with
defaecation

Personal eliminating routine/habits
usual daily eliminating routine
type of toilet facilities available in
ward/home/work
habits regarding perineal toilet
habits regarding handwashing after
eliminating

**Dependence/independence in
eliminating**
degree of independence in
eliminating, related to age,
physical/mental/health
status, available toilet facilities
use of/need for special equipment/
appliances
history and nature of incontinence, if
relevant
details of catheter/stoma
management, if relevant

ANALYSIS OF DATA

IDENTIFICATION OF PATIENTS' PROBLEMS

Change of environment and routine
unfamiliar environment of hospital
unfamiliar routine of hospital life
lack of privacy in the ward

**Dependence/independence in
eliminating**
dependence due to:
limited mobility
confinement to bed
psychological disturbance

Change in urine and its elimination
anxiety about change in appearance
of urine
increased frequency of micturition
increased/decreased output of
urine
urinary incontinence
urinary catheterisation

Change in faeces and their elimination
anxiety about change in appearance
of faeces
increased frequency of defaecation:
diarrhoea
decreased frequency of defaecation:
constipation
inability to defaecate: impaction
faecal incontinence
ileostomy/colostomy

**Discomforts associated with
eliminating**
pain associated with micturition
pain associated with defaecation
anxiety associated with related
investigations

PLANNING

IMPLEMENTATION
of nursing activities such as

Providing opportunities, facilities,
privacy for eliminating

Giving assistance to dependent patients

Practising/facilitating/encouraging
handwashing

Ensuring safe disposal of excreta

Collecting and testing specimens of
urine/faeces

Monitoring and recording fluid balance

Catheterisation and catheter care

Preventing and treating constipation/
faecal impaction

Nursing a patient with diarrhoea

Nursing a patient with a stoma

Alleviating and preventing discomforts
associated with eliminating

Assessing and alleviating pain
associated with eliminating

Preparation of patients undergoing
investigations

Assisting/retraining the incontinent
patient

Teaching people about the AL of
eliminating

Teaching people how to prevent and
recognise related problems

EVALUATION

Fig. 21.1 Assessment of a patient's need for elimination (Roper et al 1981).

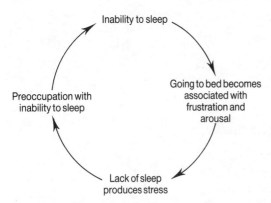

Fig. 21.2 A vicious cycle depicting the inability to sleep. (Adapted from Borkovec 1982.)

In a ward environment one of the main causes of sleep disturbance is the level of noise. Closs (1988) points out that there is an obligation on all who work in hospitals to reduce noise in order to relieve anxious patients and help them to sleep. Since nurses spend more time in close contact with hospital patients than other health care professionals, particularly at night, they are in the best position to fulfil this obligation.

Depressed patients tend to have difficulty falling asleep, an increased number of awakenings during the night and early morning awakenings. Closs (1988) suggests that nurses should encourage depressed and anxious patients to discuss their feelings and, if possible, assist them with underlying difficulties. Alerting medical staff to the apparent existence of anxiety and depression should ensure that the patient receives appropriate medical or psychological treatment. Such prescriptions are more easily said than done. Whether or not psychiatric nurses should try and encourage depressed patients to discuss their feelings in the middle of the night is a debatable point. In spite of all the research which has demonstrated that the disruption of normal patterns of sleep leads to numerous adverse physiological and psychological consequences, psychiatric nurses are still left with little guidance in dealing with people who have insomnia. Sleep-onset insomnia is one area which has received some attention from behavioural therapists. Borkovec (1982) suggests that behavioural techniques such as relaxation, bio-

feedback, paradoxical intention and stimulus control all contain ingredients effective in reducing sleep-onset insomnia. An example of a stimulus control procedure is given by Gournay in Chapter 43 of this book.

Hot milky drinks are usually provided in hospital in the late evening. However, their potential to enhance sleep has not been demonstrated. Closs (1988) argues that many people take an alcoholic nightcap at home, and if they are normally heavy drinkers they will suffer from withdrawal symptoms in hospital if they are not permitted to drink. Withdrawal from alcohol as well as hypnotic drugs results in disturbed sleep. Caffeinated drinks such as coffee, tea, drinking chocolate and cola act as stimulants and frequently result in disturbed sleep when taken late at night. While the biochemical effects of diet on sleep remain unclear, Closs suggests that since routine habits appear to enhance sleep nurses should allow patients to eat and drink as they would at home before bedtime, as far as feasible. However, while in hospital how many psychiatric patients have access to kitchen facilities, particularly at night-time?

While there is little nursing research into effective care for enhancing sleep, there is considerable prescriptive information available. This usually follows the format of identifying the patient's normal sleep pattern and enabling a return to the previous satisfying pattern of sleep. In order to do this, various approaches are suggested. For example, direct the patient to take a warm bath prior to bedtime, offer the patient a back rub after bath, direct the patient to follow directions on relaxation tape, and have the patient refrain from eating shortly before bedtime (Bauer & Hill 1986).

The need for personal grooming

Personal grooming includes hygiene and the ability to dress in accord with environmental needs and social cultural norms. Robinson (1982) suggests that cleanliness and good grooming are commended in most cultures and, apart from having pride in their appearance, people have a social responsibility to maintain personal cleanliness of body and clothing. The neglect of personal hygiene and personal appearance is a common occurrence among psychiatric patients. This neglect is often inextricably linked to whatever mental illness the patient is suffering. Patients require different levels of assistance in order to care for their personal cleanliness and appearance. Many of the techniques used to improve patients' personal grooming have been derived from behavioural learning principles. These include reinforcement, modelling and prompting procedures (Wong et al 1986). Tangible 'reinforcers' such as cigarettes and food have been successful in improving patients' grooming (Hollander & Horner 1975). The ethical implications are debatable (Bernie & Fordyce 1977), particularly since social 'reinforcers' have been shown to be just as effective in motivating patients to meet their personal grooming needs (Glickman et al 1973).

Token economy programmes have also been shown to be effective in increasing patients' personal grooming, such as face washing, shaving, tooth brushing, hair combing and dressing neatly. Desired behaviour was reinforced by praise and tokens exchangeable for edible items, clothing and privileges (Nelson et al 1979). That patients, particularly chronic psychiatric patients, improve when in a token economy programme is no longer in doubt (Elliott et al 1979). As a result, the use of token economy programmes has become an accepted procedure for improving personal hygiene and self-care (Barker et al 1977).

Such programmes have also provided nurses with a systematic and purposeful method to carry out their work and have led to valid and reliable methods of recording patients' behaviour. There are, however, two major criticisms of such programmes. Firstly, the research which has demonstrated that social reinforcement is as effective as token reinforcement (Barker 1982, Woods et al 1984) brings into question whether token reinforcement is the active ingredient responsible for patient improvement (Stokes & Keen 1987). Secondly, that patients require intensive supervision from nurses with little or no attempt to teach patients to become independent in meeting their own personal grooming needs.

A study by Wong et al (1988) described a practical and inexpensive programme for teaching independent grooming skills to hospitalized chronic psychiatric patients. The programme includes procedures for assessing a patient's appearance and pin-pointing deficits in grooming, training patients in specific grooming skills, motivating patients to monitor, evaluate and correct deficiencies in their grooming and dress, and maintaining acceptable grooming behaviour while gradually decreasing the involvement of the nurse.

Results of the study demonstrated that patients made vast improvements in grooming which were sustained for a six month period. Staff members indicated that the programme was highly acceptable to them and they considered it was beneficial for the patients. The authors suggest further controlled studies to validate the programme.

At the other end of the scale, many psychiatric patients have a preoccupation with dirt and are obsessional in daily washing and cleaning rituals. Again the research available in this area focuses on behavioural interventions (Farrington 1983, Barker & Wilson 1985). Although the prescriptive literature acknowledges that such rituals often result in damage to patients' skin, particularly when detergents are used, there are no descriptions available as to the treatment of such conditions and no psychiatric nursing research into its effectiveness.

CONCLUSION

This chapter has reviewed some of the psychiatric nursing literature relating to patients' physical care needs. It is evident that meeting these needs forms an important part of the psychiatric nurse's role. Meeting the physical care needs of mentally ill patients is often difficult and challenging for psychiatric nurses. Psychiatric patients are often admitted to hospital for many months. However, the facilities provided do not enhance their stay. For example, they have to sleep in dormitories, share washing and toilet facilities and have no choice in the food they eat. Such deficiencies call for ingenuity on the part of psychiatric nurses. For example, the health care setting should be representative of the community served, yet hospital kitchens do not usually cater for the needs of various ethnic groups.

The lack of research and theory development in psychiatric nursing has often been attributed to the difficulty of measuring outcomes. This argument cannot be substantiated when it comes to meeting patients' personal care needs: the results are observable and measurable events. Either the patients slept or they did not, either the patients cleaned their teeth or they did not, either the patients ate lunch or they did not. Of course, there may be a number of intervening variables in all of these examples, but the point being made is that clearly defined measurable goals can be specifically stated and evaluated.

The ability of a patient to meet his own care needs is often a deciding factor in being discharged from hospital. More than any other person who comes into contact with patients, the nurse has most influence in the area of assisting patients' to meet their physical care needs. It is therefore essential that nurses provide care that encourages the patient's ability for self-care in order that the length of hospitalization is minimized and the patient can regain independence.

REFERENCES

Aggleton P, Chalmers H 1986 Nursing models and the nursing process. Macmillan, London

Akerlund B M, Norberg A 1985 An ethical analysis of double bind conflicts as experienced by care workers feeding severely demented patients. International Journal of Nursing Studies 22: 207–216

Armitage P 1986 The rehabilitation and nursing care of severely disabled psychiatric patients. International Journal of Nursing Studies 23: 113–123

Baldwin J A 1979 Schizophrenia and physical disease. Psychological Medicine 9: 611–618

Barker P 1982 Behaviour therapy nursing. Croom Helm, London

Barker P, Hall J N, Hutchinson K, Bridge C 1977 Symptom changes in chronic schizophrenic patients on a token economy: a controlled experiment. British Journal of Psychiatry 131: 384–393

Barker P, Wilson L 1985 Behavioural therapy nursing: new wine in old bottles. Nursing Times 81: 31–34

Barton R 1959 Institutional neuroses. Wright, Bristol

Bauer B B, Hill S S 1986 Essentials of mental health care planning and interventions. Saunders, Philadelphia

Becker D M, Myers A H, Sacci M 1986 Smoking behaviour and attitudes towards smoking among hospital nurses. American Journal of Public Health 76: 1449–1451

Bernie R, Fordyce W E 1977 Behaviour modification and the nursing process. Mosby, St Louis

Borkovec T D 1982 Insomnia. Journal of Consulting and Clinical Psychology 50: 880–895

Carruth B F 1976 Modifying behaviour through social learning. American Journal of Nursing 76: 1804

Closs J 1988 Patients' sleep–wake rhythms in hospital. Nursing Times, Occasional Paper 84: 48–50

Cole C V 1984 Community mental health — past, present and future. Health Education Journal 42: 99–101

Collister B 1988 Psychiatric nursing: person to person. Arnold, London

Cormack D 1976 Psychiatric nursing observed. A descriptive study of the work of the charge nurse in acute admission wards of psychiatric hospitals. The Royal College of Nursing, London

Cormack D 1983 Psychiatric nursing described. Churchill Livingstone, Edinburgh

Cumming E, Cumming J 1957 Closed: an experiment in mental health education. Harvard University Press, Cambridge, Mass

Cumming E, Cumming J 1962 Ego and milieu. Atherton Press, Chicago

Darcy P T 1985 Mental health nursing source book. Baillière Tindall, London

Dingman P, Resnick M, Bosworth E, Kamada D 1988 A nonsmoking policy on an acute psychiatric unit. Journal of Psychosocial Nursing 26: 11–14

Driscoll J S, Melnick N R, Qinsen F R 1978 Psychotropic drugs as potential antitumour agents: a selective screening study. Cancer Treatment Report 62: 45–74

Elliott P A, Barlow F, Hooper A, Kingerlee P E 1979 Maintaining patients improvements in token economy. Behaviour Research and Therapy 17: 355–367

Fanning V L, Weist Deloughery G L, Gebbie K M 1972 Patient involvement in planning own care: staff and patient attitudes. Journal of Psychiatric Nursing and Mental Health Services. Jan–Feb: 5–8

Farrington A 1983 Obsessive-compulsive disorder. Nursing Mirror 157: 7–8

Fitzpatrick J, Whall A, Johnston R, Floyd J 1982 Nursing models and their psychiatric mental health applications. Robert Brady Co, Maryland

Fox B H, Howell M A 1974 Cancer risk among psychiatric patients: a hypothesis. International Journal of Epidemiology 3: 207–208

Gaston E H 1982 Solving the smoking problem on a chronic ward. Journal of Psychiatric Treatment and Evaluation 4: 397–401

Glickman H, Plutchik R, Landau H 1973 Social and biological reinforcement in an open psychiatric ward.

Journal of Behaviour Therapy and Experimental Psychiatry: 289–294

Goffman E 1961 Asylums. Penguin, Harmondsworth

Hailey A M 1971 Long-stay psychiatric in-patients: a study based on the Camberwell Register. Psychological Medicine 1: 128–142

Harris M, Solomon K 1977 Roles of the community mental health nurse. Journal of Psychiatric Nursing and Mental Health Services 1: 87–90

Hartie A, Black D 1975 A dry bed is the objective. Nursing Times 77: 1874–1876

Health Education Council 1983 The facts about smoking — what every nurse should know. Health Education Council, London

Hollander M, Horner V 1975 Using environmental assessment and operant procedures to build integrated behaviours in schizophrenics. Journal of Behaviour Therapy and Experimental Psychiatry 6: 289–294

Holmberg S 1988 Physical health problems of the psychiatric client. Journal of Psychosocial Nursing 26: 35–39

Hughes J R, Hatsukami D K, Mitchell J E, Dahlgren L A 1986 Prevalence of smoking among psychiatric out-patients. American Journal of Psychiatry 143: 993–997

Jackson R T, Haynes-Johnson V 1988 Nutritional management of patients undergoing long-term antipsychotic and antidepressant therapies. Archives of Psychiatric Nursing 2: 146–152

Jones H S, Oswald I 1968 Two cases of healthy insomnia. Electroencephalography and Clinical Neurophysiology 24: 378–380

Jones M 1953 The therapeutic community: a new treatment in psychiatry. Basic Books, New York

Kelly M P, May D 1982 Good and bad patients: a review of the literature and a theoretical critique. Journal of Advanced Nursing 7: 147–156

King M R 1980 Treatment of incontinence. Nursing Times 765, June: 1006–1010

Kipp 1984 Stress and nutrition. Contemporary nutrition 9: 7

Krauss J B, Slavinsky A T 1982 The chronically ill psychiatric patient and the community. Blackwell, Boston

Lamb H R 1981 What did we really expect from deinstitutionalization? Hospital and Community Psychiatry 32: 105–109

Lego S 1970 Nurse psychotherapists: how are we different? Perspectives in Psychiatric Care 16: 36–46

Levi R N, Waxman S 1975 Schizophrenia, epilepsy, cancer, methionine and folate metabolism. Lancet 2: 11–13

Levine M 1981 The history and politics of community mental health. Oxford University Press, New York

Linke S 1982 Behaviour analysis in the care of the elderly. Nursing Times 78: 656–658

Lynn J, Childress J F 1983 Must patients always be given food and water? The Hastings Centre Report 13: 17–21

Martin P 1987 Psychiatric nursing: a therapeutic approach. Macmillan, London

Martin R L, Cloninger C R, Guze S G 1984 Mortality in a follow-up of 500 psychiatric out-patients. II: Cause specific mortality. Archives of General Psychiatry 42: 58–66

Maslow A H 1954 Motivation and personality. Harper & Row, New York

Meleis A L 1985 Theoretical nursing: developments and progress. Lippincott, Philadelphia

Miller D H 1970 Worlds that fail. In: Strauss A L (ed) Where medicine fails. Transition Books, New York

Nelson G L, Cone J D 1979 Multiple-baseline analysis of a token economy for psychiatric inpatients. Journal of Applied Behaviour Analysis 12: 255–271

Norberg A, Norberg B, Bexell G 1980 Ethical problems in feeding patients with advanced dementia. British Medical Journal 281: 847–849

Norberg A, Hirschfield M 1987 Feeding of severely demented patients in institutions: interviews with caregivers in Israel. Journal of Advanced Nursing 12: 551–557

O'Farrell T J, Connors G J, Upper D 1983 Addictive behaviours among hospitalized psychiatric patients. Addictive Behaviours 8: 329–333

Oleck L H, Yoder S D 1981 Holism and hypocrisy. Perspectives in Psychiatric Care 15: 65–68

Orlando I J 1961 The dynamic nurse–patient relationship: function, process and principles. Putnam, New York

Patrick A, Raffety J 1978 Modifying behaviour in an institution. Nursing Times 74: 1840–1845

Paul G L 1969 Chronic mental patient: current status, future directions. Psychological Bulletin 71: 81–94

Peplau H E 1952 Interpersonal relations in nursing. Putnam, New York

Pile E N, Clark J R, Elder R D 1968 A behaviour rating scale for assessing nursing care requirements of psychiatric patients. Journal of Psychosocial Nursing and Mental Health Services, May–June: 150–153

Pollock D P, Liberman R P 1974 Behaviour therapy of incontinence in demented in-patients. Gerentologist 14: 488–491

Roper N, Logan W W, Tierney A J 1981 Learning to use the process of nursing. Churchill Livingstone, Edinburgh

Savage B, Widdowson T, Wright T 1979 Improving the care of the elderly. In: Towell D, Harries C (eds) Innovation in patient care. Croom Helm, Beckenham

Robinson L 1983 Psychiatric nursing as a human experience. W B Saunders, Philadelphia

Royal College of Nursing 1986 Standards of Care. Society of Psychiatric Nursing, Royal College of Nursing, London

Schrock R A 1980 Planning nursing care of the mentally ill. Nursing Times 76, April 17: 704–706

Smith L 1986 Issues raised by the use of nursing models in psychiatry. Nurse Education Today 6: 69–75

Stockwell F 1972 The unpopular patient. Royal College of Nursing, London

Stockwell F 1985 The nursing process in psychiatric nursing. Croom Helm, Beckenham

Stokes G, Keen I 1987 Developing self-care skills and reducing institutionalized behaviour in long-stay psychiatric populations: the role of the nurse in behaviour modification. Journal of Advanced Nursing 12: 35–48

Swanson A R 1981 Discussion. Perspectives in Psychiatric Care 15: 68–69

Thomas B L 1987 Are there any benefits? Interviews with general nursing students about their psychiatric nursing placement. Unpublished MSc dissertation, University of Manchester

Thomas M 1988 Care plan for a confused person, based on Roper's Activities of Living Model. In: Collister B (ed) Psychiatric nursing: person to person. Hodder & Stoughton, London

Turner R K 1986 A behavioural approach to the management of incontinence in the elderly. In: Mandelstam D (ed) Incontinence and its management. Croom Helm, Beckenham

Torres G 1986 Theoretical foundations of Nursing. Appleton-Century-Crofts, Norwalk, Conn

Towell D 1975 Understanding psychiatric nursing. Royal College of Nursing, London

Tsuang M T, Perkins K, Simpson J C 1983 Physical diseases in schizophrenia and affective disorder. Journal of Clinical Psychiatry 44: 42–46

Underwood P A 1980 Facilitating self-care. In: Pothier P (ed) Psychiatric nursing: a basic text. Little Brown, Boston

Ward M 1984 The nursing process in psychiatry. Churchill Livingstone, Edinburgh

Watts D T, Cassel C K 1984 Extraordinary nutritional support: a case study and ethical analysis. Journal of the American Geriatric Society 32: 237–242

White E A 1976 The clinical specialist on the mental health team. Journal of Psychiatric Nursing and Mental Health Services 14: 7–12

Whyte L, Youhill G 1984 The nursing process in the care of the mentally ill. Nursing Times 80, Feb 1: 49–51

Wing J K, Brown G W 1970 Institutionalism and schizophrenia. Cambridge Univ Press, London

Wong S E, Massel H K, Mosk M D 1986 Behavioural approaches to the treatment of schizophrenia. In: Burrows G D, Norman T R, Rubensteirn G (eds) Handbook of studies on schizophrenia. Elsevier, Amsterdam

Wong S E, Flannagan S G, Kuehnel T G, Liberman R P, Hunnicutt R, Adams-Badgett J 1988 Training chronic mental patients to independently practice personal grooming skills. Hospital and Community Psychiatry 39: 874–879

Woods P A, Higson P J, Tannahill M M 1984 Token economy programmes with chronic psychotic patients: the importance of direct measurement and objective evaluation for long-term maintenance. Behaviour Research and Therapy 22: 41–51

22

Social vulnerability

A. E. While

This chapter explores the effects of various disabilities on mental well-being and the importance of social life. An attempt is made to highlight those aspects of life which may make people more vulnerable to emotional ill health. Susceptibility to mental illness due to social, environmental and physical factors may be seen as social vulnerability. Four major topics have been selected for consideration in this chapter:

- physical illness and disability
- bereavement
- poor social circumstances, and
- membership of an ethnic minority group.

PHYSICAL ILLNESS AND DISABILITY

There is now a wealth of evidence that a serious illness is a crisis in any individual's life (Wilson-Barnett 1979). However, emotional responses to illness vary in intensity and duration and reflect not only the nature and degree of symptoms and disability but also the meaning of the illness to the individual and the amount of support he receives from others. Further, it seems that certain illnesses are more likely to produce emotional reactions and complications than others.

Castelnuova-Tedescu (1961) listed many disorders which are frequently complicated by

275

depression. These include: cardiac conditions, ulcerative colitis, endocrine disorders, hepatitis, asthma, anaemia and malignancies. Central nervous system disorders also appear to make individuals vulnerable to emotional disorders; indeed, epilepsy and multiple sclerosis have been found to be associated with emotional disorders by Merskey & Trimble (1979). More recent research involving school children also found that psychiatric disturbance was significantly more common among epileptic children than diabetic children, although both groups had a greater incidence of psychiatric problems than children in the general population (Hoare 1984).

Chronic ill health has been found to result in varying emotional reactions. While apathy and indifference have been found by some researchers, high levels of anxiety and depression have also been found by others. However, Kay et al (1964) demonstrated a significant relationship between physical and psychiatric disorders among elderly people, and Hafner & Welz (1989) have argued that chronic physical ill health and mental disorder interact.

Renal failure and its treatment with dialysis or transplantation put prolonged stress on patients and their families and can be expected to have pervasive effects upon everyday life. However, in renal failure organic factors also alter mood states, for example salt depletion. Neary (1976) in his review found that depression was a common reaction to renal failure and there is evidence that anxiety and irritability may occur in as many as a third of chronic uraemics. Neary also suggested that methyldopa (a hypotensive drug) may precipitate depression among chronic uraemics.

Organic factors may also play a role in diabetes mellitus. Poorly controlled diabetes, as evidenced by abnormal glucose levels, may impair performance and well-being (Holmes et al 1983). And there is some evidence that lower glycosylate haemoglobin concentrates are associated with depressive symptoms. Close et al (1986) have also suggested that maintaining good self-care with diabetes mellitus may predispose to feelings of depression because maintaining good control is much harder work than achieving poor control. Close et al, in their work with children, have

also argued that maintenance of good control may result in a degree of external positive regard by doctors, parents and perhaps others; however, internal personal rewards for the children are less readily apparent. For example, good control is not associated with a sense of well-being or greater social or personal opportunity. Further, poorly-controlled patients with diabetes are likely to receive more attention and enthusiasm from diabetic clinic staff — the well-controlled patient is more likely to receive routine care and have to attend the clinic less frequently. This lack of reward for coping may increase vulnerability by not enhancing the feeling of self-worth.

Prolonged physical disability is also associated with depression. Evans (1982) has argued that a depressive reaction is common, subsequent to a sudden reduction in ability caused, for instance, by a leg amputation or the formation of a colostomy, especially where the procedures have been carried out as emergencies so that there has been no time for proper psychological preparation. In such instances the patient may have to work through a bereavement reaction as intense and prolonged as that following the death of a spouse. The association between bereavement and depression has been found in numerous studies (e.g. Brown & Harris 1978).

The increased survival rate of individuals with severe physical handicap has resulted in increased amounts of research exploring how people with physical handicap face independence, work and sexual relationships. Dorner (1976) concluded from his study of adolescents with spina bifida that their lives were often difficult. Frequently the adolescents were severely socially isolated, miserable and depressed. He found that these problems were more acute among the girls in his study, who frequently had problems of finding satisfying work or indeed any work at all, and were often preoccupied by worries about their future and the prospect of unfulfilled wishes in relation to marriage and children. Of particular interest was Dorner's finding that only a very small minority of his sample had had the opportunity for skilled counselling which might have alleviated some of their anxieties. This lack of support has been found in other disability studies. It was also interesting that most of the teenagers expressed the wish for contact with able-bodied as well as handicapped people — in other words, they were aware of their exclusion from normal social life and desired to gain entry to social relationships beyond their disabled group.

It must be remembered that physical illness and disability affects both individuals and their families. Normal family relationships are obviously changed when a family member contracts an illness. Changes in roles of the remaining members inevitably occur, regardless of whether the patient is nursed at home or withdrawn from the family to be cared for in hospital. One consequence of ill health may be a change in financial status. In particular, self-employed earners are particularly vulnerable, although even employed earners suffer a reduction in earnings after 6 months, and overtime payments and bonuses cease with absence from work, so that long-term plans for expenditure may need adjustment. Financial uncertainty and shortage can be particularly disruptive to family life, and Lipowski (1975) among others has observed the relationship between long-term illness and family discord which is often associated with consequent financial problems.

The presence of a disabled member in a family also deserves consideration. As Taylor (1982) has pointed out, the parents of handicapped children have to adjust to a wide variety of emotional and psychological problems when first confronted with the failure of their reproductive expectations. While the experience of such a tragedy may bring out previously unknown resources and strengths within a family and within parental relationships in some instances, in others it may uncover or resurrect deep traumas and deficiencies previously undisclosed and thus cause a deterioration in mental health or manifest difficulties in general coping abilities. Taylor has argued that skilful counselling can help families to adjust and therefore reduce the incidence of psychopathology. However, while counselling may well assist families in their adjustment, the presence of disability in a family member may be a cause of ongoing psychological distress. Breslau et al (1982) found that mothers of disabled children (with cystic fibrosis, cerebral palsy, myelodysplasia or multiple physical handi-

caps) were significantly more distressed than mothers of normal children. The type of disability was unrelated to the mother's level of psychological distress; however, the more dependent the child regarding daily activities of living, the greater was the mother's distress.

One consequence of physical disability may be stigmatization, the process by which society sets aside a group or individual and accords them a devalued status. Goffman (1961) refers to it as 'shameful differentness'. Sensky (1982) has reviewed the research relating to family stigma in congenital physical handicap and has argued that the consequences of congenital handicap have to be borne by the whole family and are therefore best considered in this context. However, Sensky also acknowledged the fundamental problem facing the handicapped, which is the distorted perceptions of handicap adopted by society, so the stigmatization must eventually be tackled as a problem of society rather than of the stigmatized if long-term integration and acceptance are to occur. For it is only with a change in social attitudes that the handicapped will be able to enjoy normal social relationships and work opportunities.

BEREAVEMENT

When a loved one dies the formal bereavement period commences. However, the spouse/relative may have begun this process during the terminal period when he or she realizes how seriously ill the patient is. Many emotions are felt, although tension and depression are the most common as well as anger and guilt. Parkes (1975) noted that the recently widowed usually felt shock, pangs of grief and then depression and apathy. He also noted that they suffered a sense of mutilation and vulnerability and he described the most vulnerable as those who were young, left without adult family or those who felt ambivalent about their former marriage. Bowlby (1981) has referred to the loss of a loved person as an intensely painful experience which causes distress and emotional disturbance. However, Bowlby has argued that most do come to terms with bereavement, although the grieving process has a long duration and many difficulties may be encountered until adjustment is achieved.

The loss of a parent in childhood used to be considered of little importance. However, Bowlby (1981) and others argue that it has a more profound effect than previously thought. Bowlby has described how a child initially protests and makes urgent efforts to recover the lost figure before despair sets in. He has argued that the longing for the return of the lost figure does not diminish but hope of its being realized fades and with acceptance of the situation the child's misery slowly resolves. Walker (1985) has noted that a proportion of children referred to child guidance clinics will be those who have been bereaved and the majority of them will show depressive symptoms which require therapeutic intervention. However, the effect of parental loss may be long-term: Brown & Harris (1978) found an association between adult depression and the loss of a parent in childhood or adolescence.

Indeed, Brown & Harris in their study of women in Camberwell found that various life events were stressful and tended to precipitate depression. Loss of loved ones was found to be particularly stressful in their study, with two-thirds of psychotic patients having had a past loss compared with 39% of neurotic patients. When they distinguished past loss due to death from loss by separation (that is, absence) they found that the type of loss may be a powerful influence on symptom pattern when women do get depressed. Loss by death predisposes to psychotic depression and loss by separation predisposes to neurotic depression.

Parkes (1975) has found depression to be a common symptom among bereaved people, but he has argued that it is not necessarily a sign of pathology. Indeed, he has suggested that there are some grounds for regarding the absence of depression after bereavement as more 'abnormal' than its presence. In his work he found several differences between bereaved psychiatric patients and other bereaved widows: those who developed mental illness had more frequent ideas of guilt or self-reproach, a tendency for grief to be prolonged and a tendency for the reaction to bereavement to be delayed. Parkes (1975) identified three in-

dicators which may suggest that the reaction to bereavement may take a pathological course: extreme expressions of guilt, somatic symptoms and delay in the onset of grief of more than two weeks' duration. His research has also suggested that some people have a greater risk of getting into difficulties and should be offered counselling or other appropriate help after bereavement to prevent the development of pathological features. Indeed, Caplan (1964) has advocated prophylactic care and preventive measures as means of reducing the incidence of mental ill health. According to Parkes (1975) a young widow with dependent children and no relative living nearby is particularly vulnerable. A previous history of a depressive illness and timid personality, of difficulty with earlier separations, and of dependence upon her husband would exacerbate her vulnerability. The plight of such a widow would inevitably be worsened by the loss of income resulting from the death of the wage earner, changes of home and difficulties with children as they too cope with loss.

Elderly people experience multiple losses with their advancing years — lose of mobility, physical health, family home, work and loved ones. Bereavement may make an elderly person particularly vulnerable considering the many years that a couple may have lived together and the length of time devoted to building up the loving relationship. Most people who work with the bereaved agree that it usually takes about a year for the major part of the grief to resolve and that complete recovery is likely to take two to three years (Copperman 1983). However, for an elderly person the loss of a spouse may represent the last link with the outside world because failing physical health and poor mobility inhibit the development of new social relationships so that social isolation worsens the situation. Preventive care through helping people to cope with grief could perhaps reduce the incidence of abnormal grief reactions. It is noteworthy that the incidence of illness and death in surviving spouses rises markedly in the first 6 months following death, which suggests that individuals are particularly vulnerable during that period (Parkes et al 1969).

The needs of the dying are no less important. Robbins (1983) in describing the psychological and spiritual problems of dying patients has emphasized that many patients exhibit anxiety or depression. Fear of how the final phase of death will occur is common and may be associated with anticipation of intolerable physical events and uncertainty. Concern about finance and family well-being are other factors which should be considered by carers as these concerns may induce additional anxieties. However, Hinton (1972) has argued that although anxiety frequently occurs among the dying, depression is the most common form of emotional distress if those near to the dying are prepared to notice it. Sadness at the impending loss of life and all that is valued as an understandable response among the dying, and this makes it difficult to distinguish from depression. Any symptoms of depression such as loss of interest, incapacity to enjoy things and dulled emotion should be considered carefully since they are rarely entirely due to the serious physical disease. A number of studies have found that serious disease is associated with suicidal acts (Hinton 1972).

POOR SOCIAL CIRCUMSTANCES

Central to the work on inequality has been the development of the concept of 'social class'. A social class may be defined as a segment of the population sharing similar types and levels of resources and maintaining broadly similar life-styles (Townsend & Davidson 1982). Most evidence amassed in the Black Report (DHSS 1980) related to the increased physical morbidity and mortality rates of the lower social classes. However, there is also evidence that the incidence of mental illness is higher in lower social class groups, which in part may reflect less effective coping mechanisms of members of these groups (Pearlin & Schooler 1978). The work of Brown & Harris (1978) found that psychiatric disorder, and depression in particular, is much more common among working-class than among middle-class women. Further, it is well known that schizophrenia is commonest among unskilled occupations. However, this is probably because people handicapped by schizophrenia can only manage unskilled jobs

(Hare 1982). It seems that social factors may also play a part in precipitating an episode of florid schizophrenia. Wing (1982) has argued that a period of intense stress in an individual's life may well precede an acute episode of schizophrenia, and further factors in the social environment may increase or decrease the severity of long-term incapacity.

Associated with lower social class is unemployment. A lack of work skills means that an individual is unable to command a stable place in the employment market, and moreover unskilled labour is increasingly restricted to only a few industries as British manufacturers develop a more technological approach to production. The evidence linking unemployment to poor physical health is relatively weak. However, there is much stronger evidence linking unemployment with poor mental health, a relationship first noted by Jahoda et al (1960). Surveys have found that about one fifth of the unemployed report a deterioration in their mental health since becoming unemployed, with longer durations of unemployment increasing the likelihood of deterioration (Colledge & Bartholomew 1980, Jackson & Warr 1984). Some studies have measured the mental health of the unemployed and they too have found poorer mental health among the unemployed (Warr 1985). The unemployed tend to be more anxious, depressed, unhappy, neurotic, worried and dissatisfied, and have lower confidence and self-esteem. Jahoda (1982) has argued that work is not only important for its financial rewards but also because it provides social contact outside the family while imposing a time structure on the day and giving a purpose and a sense of achievement and its associated social status. Patmore (1983) has suggested that, in view of the evidence, the mental health services should be prepared to care for an increased number of distressed people who have been brought into the at-risk category by the dramatic increase in unemployment since 1979 (from 5.5% to 13%). However, current demographic trends may have an impact upon unemployment.

The relationship between unemployment and suicide and parasuicide has been extensively studied. Platt (1984) reviewed 156 studies which consistently found that the unemployed are over-represented among those who deliberately kill or injure themselves. Further, in his review of eight studies using a longitudinal design, he found significantly more unemployment, job instability and occupational problems among people who had committed suicide than among matched controls. Platt (1983) discounted the negative association between unemployment and suicide during studies of the 1960s and early 1970s as being a reflection of the unique decline of suicide rates in Britain due to the unavailability of the most common method of suicide (domestic gas poisoning). Since the early 1970s the relationship between unemployment and suicide among males has been positive and significant (Platt 1984). The evidence relating to unemployment and parasuicide has been consistent over time, with the parasuicide rate among the unemployed reported to be up to 30 times greater than the rate among the employed. There is further evidence that parasuicide rates tend to increase with lengthening durations of unemployment (Platt 1983).

A further consideration regarding unemployment and mental health is the reduced opportunities for rehabilitation of the mentally ill. British mental health services have long relied upon employment as a means of reintegrating people into the community and providing long-term psychological structure and support. As indicated earlier, employment offers daily social contacts, time structuring and routine, decision-making, social status and income for welfare and recreation. Patmore (1983) has argued that this neat, economical rehabilitation strategy is only possible when unemployment rates are between 2% and 3%, so that even very disadvantaged people have the opportunity of employment.

A further aspect of poor social circumstance is place of residence, especially when this means residence in an economically deprived inner city area. Blakemore (1983) has suggested that:

Enough is known about the decay, poverty and socially unstable nature of inner city environments for us to suppose that they can exert strangely negative influences on many of the people who live in them . . . (p. 82).

Madge (1982) concurred with this assertion in her review article. She noted in particular the environmental problems, not only the physical decay, pollution and noise, but also the nature of the housing stock and housing shortage which inevitably impinge upon the lives of residents. In reviewing the behavioural adversities Madge also highlighted the problems of crime and juvenile delinquency, as well as other psychosocial problems such as alcoholism, drug addiction, mental ill health, marital discord and family breakdown. Multiple and pervasive deprivation clearly has its effect upon inner city residents as they struggle through their lives, with the noise and pollution of dense traffic compounding the negative aspects of the physical environment. One of the costs may be a higher incidence of psychiatric disorder, a relationship first found by Faris & Dunham (1939). More recently Jarman's review (1981) of primary health care in London revealed an over-concentration of mental illness in the inner city districts as compared with London's suburbs. In 1970 the Psychiatric Rehabilitation Association commented upon the combination of social, physical and economic poverty in the East End of London as providing insuperable conditions for the mentally ill person. It is perhaps the case that the poorer communities are least able to offer help while also being those within which most people needing help are to be found.

However, one should be cautious about attributing the cause of mental illness to the environment or social circumstance. Muijen & Brooking (1989) have argued that both the social causation and social drift explanations have some validity. They suggested that it is most likely that both processes are operating simultaneously with varying impacts upon individuals depending upon their circumstances.

MEMBERSHIP OF AN ETHNIC MINORITY GROUP

There is abundant evidence that ethnic minorities in Britain are disadvantaged regarding every important socio-economic variable (Smith 1977, Community Relations Council 1977, Cross 1978, Scarman 1981). Many experience prejudice and rejection in everyday situations, examples of which include the allocation of poorer quality housing (Commission for Racial Equality 1984) and greater difficulty in gaining employment (Morris 1978). As a consequence of this many immigrants settle in inner city areas because the housing is cheaper and within their financial means, and, further, the large houses found in cities permit the closeness of extended families which would be unacceptable in the white suburbs. The multiple and pervasive deprivation of inner cities has already been mentioned, but it is noteworthy that immigrant residents are now accused of causing inner city decay although much dilapidation had occurred before their arrival. The plight of these families is further exacerbated by their attendance at ill-equipped schools, the continual difficulty in finding employment and the unceasing criticism that they are living on social security. It is easy to underestimate the extent of injustice suffered by minority groups and the sheer unpleasantness of a life of rejection.

Unlike the United States, British society is organized around exclusiveness so that speech, dress and habits are used as social signals. Membership of an ethnic minority is therefore stressful as such membership includes exploitation, deprivation and possibly also harassment. Recent immigrants face additional problems over and above the stigma of belonging to a despised group. While migration may appear to be an adventure, it is also a stressful undertaking. Everyone needs a sense of belonging, with the comfort of familiar landmarks and personal associations which are understood. Migration inevitably involves separation from both the familiar place and group, leaving immigrants both anxious and with a sense of loss. The stress is greatest, however, where the journey involved is long and complicated and where there are large differences in culture and problems of language (Rack 1982).

The stress of migration to a foreign land may cause relatively trivial incidents to be magnified into major issues so that slight setbacks and misunderstandings appear to be disasters. And even when initial settlement has been achieved, anxieties may be rekindled by new stimuli. Foster (1973) has suggested that most people take about

6 months to adjust to a new culture. Rack (1982) has argued that the loss of role identity compounds an individual's problems. Indeed, there is evidence that immigrants are more at ease in an alien environment when fulfilling a familiar role because it reaffirms their personal identity. However, difficulties in the new language alone can prevent the gaining of employment consistent with experience and previous status. Status and role loss is particularly important to men, and downward social mobility has been found to be a factor in the incidence of mental illness among immigrant groups.

Immigrants mainly travel to improve their economic and social situation. Therefore improvement of position relative to their peers in the country of origin and success are very important. However, it is frequently more difficult to gain employment than envisaged, not only because of greater competition but also perhaps because of prejudice; and although income may be higher, the cost of living is also higher, making support of family left behind difficult. The need to pretend success merely exacerbates the strain and sense of isolation. Royer (1977) described what he believes to be the situation of West Indian immigrants. He suggested that West Indians thought they were going to a land of Christians where they would be well received with compassion and respect and where they would adjust without much difficulty and seek their fortune through employment. These high expectations of welcome and standards of tolerance were not met and distress and disappointment resulted. Royer (1977) has argued that the chronic environmental stress experienced by West Indians may in part explain the higher incidence of schizophrenia, although difficulties in understanding the behaviour of a different culture may result in some diagnostic confusion. Rack (1986) has asserted that unusual behaviour is all too easily attributed to mental illness when it is in fact an expression of justified distress or anger.

The particular problems of three other social groups deserve comment. All political refugees are different, but all will have experienced the extreme trauma of enforced uprooting and the misery of permanent separation from loved people and places. Some refugees will also have experienced the horror of a concentration camp, torture, danger, hunger, feelings of despair and guilt; and the most unfortunate may have witnessed violent death and feared the same fate for themselves. Depression, paranoia and other psychotic and neurotic symptoms are common among refugees reaching safety (Baker 1983). There is now also a growing recognition of the long-term sequelae of being a refugee which may extend into old age. The particular situation of overseas students merits some consideration. Although their numbers in the United Kingdom have fallen dramatically in recent years, their number is still substantial, especially in the United States. As students, they are transient residents who are obliged to adjust quickly to a strange land while at the same time meeting special work objectives within a limited time period. Unlike other students they have additional anxieties which impinge upon their lives: the cost of examination failure is total humiliation and they have the constant uncertainty of arbitrary decisions of their sponsors. African students in the United Kingdom also find that language difficulties and unfamiliar study methods cause psychological stress (Cox 1986). The problems of expatriate workers are also worthy of comment, for it seems that they are particularly susceptible to family worries, alcoholism and psychiatric disorder (Cox 1986). However, it may be that expatriate workers have gone overseas in an attempt to escape problems in their home society and are therefore particularly vulnerable people.

CONCLUSION

The available evidence demonstrates that an individual's physical status and social situation are important contributors to mental well-being. It has been argued that physical illness and disability may increase vulnerability to mental illness. Further, the available literature regarding a recent loss or bereavement, poor social circumstance and membership of an ethnic minority supports the view that these aspects of an individual's social life may increase vulnerability to mental ill health. The psychiatric nurse should therefore consider her patients in the light of this evidence and in so doing improve the quality of the nursing care offered. A careful and competent approach to the taking of a nursing history should reveal relevant information upon which a nurse may formulate an appropriate and considered nursing care plan.

REFERENCES

Baker R (ed) 1983 The psychosocial problems of refugees. British Refugee Council, London

Blakemore K 1983 Ageing in the inner city: a comparison of old Blacks and Whites. In: Jerrome D (ed) Ageing in modern society. Croom Helm, London

Bowlby J 1981 Loss: sadness and depression. Penguin, Harmondsworth

Breslau N, Staruch K S, Mortimer E A 1982 Psychological distress in mothers of disabled children. American Journal of Disease in Childhood 136: 682–686

Brown G W, Harris T 1978 Social origins of depression: a study of psychiatric disorder in women. Tavistock, London

Caplan G 1964 Principles of preventive psychiatry. Basic Books, New York

Castelnuova-Tedescu P 1961 Depression in patients with physical disease. Cranbury Wallace Labs, New Jersey

Close H, Davies A G, Price D A, Goodyer I M 1986 Emotional difficulties in diabetes mellitus. Archives of Disease in Childhood 61(4): 337–340

Colledge M, Bartholomew R 1980 A study of the long-term unemployed. Manpower Services Commission, London

Community Relations Council 1977 Urban deprivation, racial inequality and social policy: a report. HMSO, London

Copperman H 1983 Dying at home. John Wiley, Chichester

Cox J L 1986 Overseas students and expatriates: sojourners or settlers? In: Cox J L (ed) Transcultural psychiatry. Croom Helm, London

Cross C 1978 Ethnic minorities in the inner city: the ethnic dimension in urban deprivation in England. Council for Racial Equality, London

DHSS 1980 Inequalities in health: Report of a Research Working Group (Black Report). DHSS, London

Dorner S 1976 Adolescents with spina bifida: how they see their situation. Archives of Disease in Childhood 51: 439–444

Evans G J 1982 The psychiatric aspects of physical disease. In: Levy R, Post F (eds) The psychiatry of late life. Blackwell Scientific, Oxford

Faris R E L, Dunham W H 1939 Mental disorders in urban areas. University of Chicago Press, Chicago

Foster G M 1973 Traditional societies and technological change. Harper & Row, London

Goffman E 1961 Asylums. Doubleday, New York

Hafner H, Welz R 1989 Social and behavioural determinants of mental disorders. In: Hamburg D, Sartorius N (eds) Health and behaviour. Cambridge University Press, Cambridge

Hare E 1982 Epidemiology of schizophrenia. In: Wing J K, Wing L (eds) Handbook of psychiatry, vol 3: Psychoses of uncertain aetiology. Cambridge University Press, Cambridge

Hinton J 1972 Dying. Penguin, Harmondsworth

Hoare P 1984 Does illness foster dependency? A study of epileptic and diabetic children. Developmental Medicine and Child Neurology 26: 20–24

Holmes C S, Hayford J T, Gonzales J L, Weydert J A 1983 A survey of cognitive functioning at different glucose levels in diabetic persons. Diabetes Care 6: 180–185

Jackson P R, Warr P B 1984 Unemployment and psychological ill health: the moderating role of duration and age. Psychological Medicine 14: 605–614

Jahoda M 1982 Employment and unemployment. Cambridge University Press, Cambridge

Jahoda M, Lazarsfeld P S, Zeisel H 1960 Die Arbeitslosen von Marienthal Verlag für Demonskopie. Allensbach, Bonn

Jarman B 1981 A survey of primary care in London. Occasional Paper No 16. Royal College of General Practitioners, London

Kay D W K, Beamish P, Roth M 1964 Old age mental disorder in Newcastle-upon-Tyne. British Journal of Psychiatry 110: 146–153

Lipowski Z L 1975 Physical illness, the patient and his environment: psychosocial foundations of medicine. America Handbook of Psychiatry 4: 1–42

Madge N J H 1982 Growing up in the inner city. Journal of the Royal Society of Health 102(6): 261–265

Merskey H, Trimble M R 1979 Personality and other factors promoting conversion symptoms. America Journal of Psychiatry 136(2): 179–182

Morris P 1978 Who'll be disadvantaged? Community Care 241, November 29: 16–19

Muijen M, Brooking J 1989 Mental health. In: While A (ed) Health in the inner city. Heinemann, Oxford

Neary D 1976 Neuropsychiatric sequelae of renal failure. British Medical Journal 1: 122–130

Parkes C M 1975 Bereavement: Studies of grief in adult life. Penguin, Harmondsworth

Parkes C M, Benjamin B, Fitzgerald R G 1969 Broken heart: a statistical study of increased mortality among widowers. British Medical Journal 1: 740

Patmore C 1983 Unemployment and mental health. Paper presented at Unemployment and Health Policy Seminar held at University of Leeds in November 1983

Pearlin L J, Schooler C L 1978 The structure of coping. Journal of Health and Social Behaviour 19: 2–21

Platt S 1983 Unemployment and suicidal behaviour. Paper presented at Unemployment and Health Policy Seminar held at University of Leeds in November 1983

Platt S 1984 Unemployment and suicidal behaviour: a review of the literature. Social Science and Medicine 19: 93–115

Psychiatric Rehabilitation Association 1970 Mental illness in city and suburb. PRA, London

Rack P H 1982 Race, culture and mental disorders. Tavistock, London

Rack P H 1986 Migration and mental illness. In: Cox J L (ed) Transcultural psychiatry. Croom Helm, London

Robbins J (ed) 1983 Caring for the dying patient and their family. Lippincott Series. Harper & Row, London

Royer J 1977 Black Britain's dilemma: a medico-social transcultural study of West Indians. Tropical Printers, Rosean, Dominica

Scarman the Rt Hon Lord 1981 The Brixton disorder 10–12 April 1981, Cmnd 8427. HMSO, London

Sensky T 1982 Family stigma in congenital physical handicap. British Medical Journal 285: 1033–1035

Smith D J 1977 Racial disadvantage in Britain. Penguin, Harmondsworth

Taylor D C 1982 Counselling the parents of handicapped children. British Medical Journal 284: 1027–1028

Townsend P Davidson N 1982 Inequalities in health. Penguin, Harmondsworth

Walker R 1985 Cot deaths: the aftermath. Journal of Royal College of General Practitioners 35: 194–196

Warr P 1985 Twelve questions about unemployment and health. In: Roberts R, Finnegan R, Gallie D (eds) New approaches to economic life. Manchester University Press, Manchester

Wilson-Barnett J 1979 Stress in hospital. Churchill Livingstone, Edinburgh

Wing J K 1982 Psychosocial factors influencing the onset and course of schizophrenia. In: Wing J K, Wing L (eds) Handbook of psychiatry, vol 3: Psychoses of uncertain aetiology. Cambridge University Press, Cambridge

23

Sexuality

C. Webb

Sexuality is not easy to define because it is a complex phenomenon having multiple interlinkages with all aspect of life, and Kuczynski's definition emphasizes that sexuality is much more than physical acts of sex:

Human sexuality is a complex attribute of every person, involving deep needs for identity, relationships, love, and immortality. It is more than biologic, gender, physiologic processes, or modes of behaviour; it involves one's self-concept and self-esteem. Sexuality includes masculine or feminine self-image, expression of emotional states of being, and communication of feelings for others and encompasses everything that the individual is, thinks, feels, or does during the entire life span. Sexual behaviour, more than any other behaviour, is intimately related to emotional and social well being, yet is misunderstood, feared, and misused (Kuczynski 1980).

Throughout the history of nursing, sexuality has generally been ignored both in relation to patient care and to nurses themselves, and the reasons for this lie deep in our cultural history (Hogan 1980). More recently, nurses have begun to see the importance of sexuality and how sexual functioning may be altered, inhibited or even ended for patients suffering from conditions such as arthritis, chronic obstructive airways disease, and after mutilating operations such as amputation, stoma formation and mastectomy. However, this broadening of perspective has usually been a relative matter, focusing on the biological aspects of sexuality and in particular genital sex and reproduction. For example, many nursing models have a predominantly biological emphasis and when completing assessment forms it is usually parity, menstrual details, contraceptive use and related information which are recorded under a heading such as 'Expressing sexuality' (Roper et al 1980).

Psychosocial aspects are at least as important, if not more so, in the experience and expression of sexuality (Webb 1985) and they are of major importance in psychiatric nursing because they have a profound influence on emotional health, both as cause and effect. For this reason, and because the biological and reproductive sides of sexuality have been discussed in books on physiology, reproductive medicine, and sexual disorders and therapy, this chapter will be confined to the psychosocial aspects of sexuality and their importance for psychiatric nursing. (A reading list for these other topics is given at the end of the chapter.)

Terminology can be confusing and so it is useful to clarify definitions before going on to examine ideas about sexuality, how patient/client care and nursing itself are affected by the way people think about these issues, and their implications for psychiatric nursing. 'Sex' refers to biological factors such as anatomical structures, genes and hormones, which are assumed to differentiate between the two categories of 'female' and 'male', although this is not always possible, as in cases of babies born with variations in their external genitalia, with or without accompanying internal malformations. 'Gender' refers to psychological characteristics which are socially constructed as 'feminine' or 'masculine' (Freimuth & Hornstein 1982). Defining sex and gender in this way clears up some difficulties but draws attention to new questions. Firstly, it is not always possible to assign sex unambiguously at birth and, when sex is unclear and children are reared in either the gender category 'feminine' or 'masculine', it is gender which becomes predominant. In cases where sex has later been found to have been mis-

takenly labelled, specialists advise continuing to bring up the child in the gender she/he is used to because this is how she/he and others perceive her/him (Archer & Lloyd 1982). Gender, once learned, is very resistant to change, suggesting that its influence and cultural norms and expectations are deeply embedded in thinking and behaviour (Freimuth & Hornstein 1982).

'Gender identity' is a person's self-concept of femininity or masculinity, or how she/he sees her/himself. Gender characteristics and roles are the social expectations of how women and men will and indeed ought to behave and live their lives. 'Gender preference' refers to an individual's preferred sexual partners, and whether she/he prefers to have sexual relations with others of the same or different sex. 'Gender preference' is a better term than 'sexual preference' since people usually make this choice on the basis of potential partners' whole selves and not just according to what kind of genitalia they have. In fact, the latter is usually of much lesser importance in the decision than the former (Freimuth & Hornstein 1982), and most people will not know anything about another's genital organs when deciding whether to initiate a sexual relationship.

These definitions of sex and gender focus on a division into two mutually exclusive categories, but the case of misassigned sex at birth raises the question of whether in fact sex is a dichotomous (two-way) variable. With regard to gender, its dichotomous nature is even more open to argument. Psychologists have carried out extensive research into these issues of how people see themselves and others and social expectations of behaviour in relation to sexuality, and an evaluation of this work can throw light on important aspects of psychiatry and psychiatric nursing.

THINKING ABOUT GENDER

The classic study of sex-role stereotypes and self-concepts is that by Rosenkrantz et al (1968). Female and male college students were asked to complete a questionnaire consisting of 122 bipolar (opposite) items, each describing a behavioural trait or characteristic such as 'Very emotional/not at all emotional' and 'Very competitive/not at all competitive'. Subjects were asked to indicate those items on the list which matched their expectations of male behaviour, then their expectations of female behaviour, and then to respond in relation to themselves. On 41 items there was at least 75% agreement among both female and male respondents on which pole described females and males. Typical masculine attributes included independent, objective, dominant, competitive, adventurous, ambitious, able to make decisions easily and worldly; while typical female attributes were emotional, submissive, subjective, passive feelings, easily hurt, dependent, home-oriented, tactful and gentle.

Another group of students was asked to complete the same questionnaire, this time indicating which pole of the items referred to the more socially desirable behaviour. Both women and men rated more masculine traits than feminine traits as socially valued. The differences observed in the students' self-descriptions mirrored those for masculinity and femininity, indicating that sex-role stereotypes were incorporated into people's self-concepts. Because women categorized themselves and other women as having less socially desirable characteristics than men, Rosenkrantz et al (1968) concluded that 'women also hold negative values of their worth relative to men'.

A similar study was carried out by Broverman et al (1970) with psychiatrists, psychologists and social workers, asking them to describe a healthy, mature, socially competent man, a healthy, mature, socially competent woman, and a healthy, mature, socially competent adult of unspecified sex. Items from the Rosenkrantz questionnaire were used for this purpose, as shown in Table 23.1. These clinicians judged healthy or mature, i.e. socially desirable, traits in the same way as the students had done in the former study. Both female and male clinicians had different concepts of health for men and women, corresponding to sex-role stereotypes. Their concepts for a healthy man and healthy adult of unspecified sex were similar, but their concepts for a healthy woman differed significantly. Healthy women were described as being more submissive, more easily

Table 23.1 Stereotypic traits identified by Broverman et al (1968)

Male-valued traits		Female-valued traits
Aggressive	Feelings not easily hurt	Does not use harsh language
Independent		
Unemotional	Adventurous	Talkative
Hides emotions	Makes decisions easily	Tactful
Objective		Gentle
Easily influenced	Never cries	Aware of feelings of others
Dominant	Acts as a leader	
	Self-confident	Religious
Like maths and science	Not uncomfortable about being aggressive	Interested in own appearance
Not excitable in a minor crisis		Neat in habits
	Ambitious	Quiet
Active	Able to separate feelings from ideas	Strong need for security
Competitive		
Logical		Appreciates art and literature
Worldly	Not dependent	
Skilled in business	Thinks men are superior to women	Expresses tender feelings
Direct	Talks freely about sex with men	
Knows the way of the world		

influenced, less independent, more conceited, more emotional and less adaptive. The authors concluded that:

for a woman to be healthy from an adjustment viewpoint she must adjust to and accept the behavioral norms for her sex, even though these behaviors are generally less socially desirable and considered to be less healthy for the generalized competent mature adult.

(Broverman et al 1970.)

Fabrikant et al (1973) used a 100-item adjective check-list to study perceived sex-role attributes and sex-role expectations in relation to women patients. They found that psychotherapists' descriptions paralleled the sex-role stereotypes identified in the earlier studies. In addition, male and female therapists rated over two thirds of the male attributes as positive and over two thirds of the female attributes as negative. Fabrikant et al (1973) concluded that these clinicians accepted stereotyped definitions of women and they suggested that they are more likely to incorporate these judgements into their clinical assessments and treatment programmes for women. More recent research suggests that the position remained much the same over a decade later (Teri 1982).

A number of criticisms must be made of the methods used in sex-role stereotype research, however. The problems of self-report and questionnaire methods are well-known (Treece & Treece 1977), and in fact Fabrikant et al (1973) achieved only a 20% response rate to their questionnaire. This raises the question of bias, because those who responded may have had a particular interest in the topic, may have had a particular 'axe to grind', or may have differed in their biographical characteristics from non-responders. Perhaps more important is the fact that researchers have asked subjects to differentiate between female and male characteristics, thereby ensuring that two lists of differences were produced. Had they asked subjects to report similarities between women and men, it is likely that the results would have been different. Secondly, the research is specific to the culture of the USA. While it probably describes features which are similar in societies such as the UK, evidence from anthropologists studying very different cultures suggests that women and men are seen very differently in different societies. Some societies see men as more gentle, passive and nurturing, and less assertive and independent than women, while others conceive of women and men as equally possessing these characteristics (Oakley 1972). Therefore, findings from reseach into sex-role stereotypes are highly culture-specific.

Bem (1974) was unhappy with a dichotomous, or two-way, conceptualization of gender. Accordingly, she developed the Bem Sex Role Inventory (BSRI). This contains both a masculinity scale and a femininity scale. Each comprises 20 personality characteristics 'selected on the basis of sex-typed social desirability'. Table 23.2 shows the items on the BSRI. When completing the inventory, an individual is asked to indicate on a 7-point scale how well each of these masculine and feminine characteristics describes herself/himself. An 'androgyny' score is then derived for each subject, measuring the extent to which both feminine and masculine characteristics form part of the self-

Table 23.2 Items on the Bem sex role inventory (Bem 1974).

Masculine items	Feminine items	Neutral items
Acts as leader	Affectionate	Adaptable
Aggressive	Cheerful	Conceited
Ambitious	Childlike	Conscientious
Analytical	Compassionate	Conventional
Assertive	Does not use harsh language	Friendly
Athletic		Happy
Competitive	Eager to soothe hurt feelings	Helpful
Defends own beliefs	Feminine	Inefficient
Dominant	Flatterable	Jealous
Forceful	Gentle	Likeable
Has leadership abilities	Gullible	Moody
Independent	Loves children	Reliable
Individualistic	Loyal	Secretive
Makes decisions easily	Sensitive to the needs of others	Sincere
Masculine	Shy	Solemn
Self-reliant	Soft spoken	Tactful
Self-sufficient	Sympathetic	Theatrical
Strong personality	Tender	Truthful
Willing to take a stand	Understanding	Unpredictable
Willing to take risks	Warm	Unsystematic
	Yielding	

concept. Four types emerge from research using the BSRI, and these are: High masculinity–high femininity or androgynous, High masculinity–low femininity or masculine, Low masculinity–high femininity or feminine, and Low masculinity–low femininity or undifferentiated.

Having a mixture of both feminine and masculine characteristics, androgynous subjects are said to have better psychological health, based on evidence from a number of studies showing that:

● high femininity in females is associated with high anxiety, low self-esteem and low self-acceptance
● high masculinity in males is associated with high neuroticism, high anxiety and low self-acceptance

- sex-typed boys and girls have lower intelligence, creativity, and spatial ability
- androgynous subjects score high on spontaneity, self-regard, self-acceptance, feeling reactivity, and capacity for intimate contacts
- androgynous women and men have higher self-esteem scores than others.

Kravetz (1976) repeated the pattern of the Broverman et al (1970) study by asking 183 mental health professionals to indicate on the BSRI how well the characteristics described a healthy man, woman or adult of unspecified gender. Over half of the respondents endorsed both feminine and masculine characteristics as healthy, appearing to agree with Bem (1974) that 'for fully effective and healthy human functioning, both masculinity and femininity must each be tempered by the other, and the two must each be integrated into a more balanced, a more fully human, and truly androgynous personality'.

The remaining respondents retained the traditional view that male characteristics are healthier, and Kravetz (1976) concluded that 'traits that are stereotyped as feminine are not considered healthy unless there is the equivalent or greater presence of masculine personality characteristics'. While there was an increased acceptance of women and men who do not wish to conform to traditional sex-typed behaviour, clinicians seemed more willing to extend masculinity as an ideal to women rather than reconceptualize and redefine their standards of mental health. In other words, as the song from *My Fair Lady* says, 'Why can't a woman be more like a man?'

Gauthier & Kjervik (1982) carried out a study of female graduate nursing students using the BSRI. They found that High masculinity–high femininity and High masculinity–low femininity students had statistically significantly higher self-esteem scores than those in Low M–high F and Low M–low F categories. Once again, then, it was the possession of 'masculine' characteristics which seemed to give these nurses a positive view of themselves, suggesting that masculine attributes are more valued and contribute more to self-esteem than feminine characteristics.

Discussing the effects of sex and sex-role style on clinical judgement, Teri (1982) concluded that a bias still exists. Therapists in their study were asked to rate the health and functioning of clients in bogus case histories. Sex of client was varied in the stories although the characteristics remained the same. Both female and male therapists negatively evaluated stereotypical female behaviours. However, when rating clients' prognoses, female clients were thought to have a better prognosis, suggesting that therapists see women as more manipulable and amenable to treatment. This in itself reflects sex-role stereotypes. Despite warnings that what respondents say on questionnaires does not necessarily indicate their actual behaviour, and that responders (24% in this study) may differ from non-responders, Teri (1982) concluded that her 'findings support the existence of sex and sex-role bias in clinical judgement'.

Whether gender is conceptualized and measured as a dichotomy or as a combination of feminine and masculine attributes, the notion of two categories remains, for even androgynous subjects are said to have a mix of female and male traits. Thus true reconceptualization of gender as a unisex phenomenon is not considered. Whatever method of measurement is used, each with its limitations, people in general, and mental health professionals in particular, can be shown to possess stereotyped ideas of appropriate behaviour for women and men and to have different pictures of what is healthy behaviour for a woman and a man. Kjervik (1979) summed up this research:

The results of [these studies point] to a double standard of mental health for males and females, whereby a woman might have to give up her femininity in order to be considered mentally healthy. One wonders then what route a therapist will take in guiding her or his female client to mental health — a road to femininity or a road to adulthood?
Psychotherapists are very influential, not only with individual clients but also in directing societal notions of mental health. The Broverman study indicates a subtle form of sexism being supported by mental health professionals.

Other kinds of research confirm that doctors define women as emotional and assign negative effects to stereotypes of femininity. Lennane & Lennane (1982) show how doctors have tended to attribute psychological causes to conditions which have perfectly adequate physical explanations, including dysmenorrhoea, labour pain, and infant colic. Similarly, the medical literature has tended to discuss hysterectomy and recovery primarily in psychological terms and to report high levels of depression after hysterectomy, linked with grieving for the loss of menstrual and reproductive functions. In a nursing study, however, Webb (1987) reports that impaired recovery from hysterectomy was marked by physical complications, particularly iatrogenic infections. Where women were less satisfied with the effects of their operations and were feeling 'low', this was because persistent infections were 'getting them down'. Frank depression was rare, and this finding has been confirmed by Gath (1980) and Coppen et al (1981).

Psychotherapists, psychologists, psychiatrists and other doctors share sex-role stereotypes with the general population because they have been reared in the same culture and are not immune to its socializing effects. For the same reasons, it is likely that psychiatric nurses also hold to these stereotypes and that they influence the way patients are assessed, their problems are identified, and nursing goals and interventions are decided.

Psychosocial aspects of sexuality affect the incidence of different diagnosis in other ways, too. In the course of exploring these in the following section it will become apparent that sex-role stereotyping is detrimental to men too, because they are discouraged from expressing their emotions and trained to be striving and ambitious. The stressful effects of this socialization take their toll in different ways but are nevertheless as destructive as those which women experience.

PSYCHOSOCIAL HEALTH AND SEXUALITY

Different expectations and role prescriptions for women and men are reflected in different rates of psychosocial problems. Table 23.3 shows that women and men are admitted to psychiatric hospitals with different diagnoses, although whether this indicates a 'true' difference in the incidence of diagnosis or a difference in the way doctors label patients is not clear. Women are hospitalized for psychiatric reasons in greater numbers than men, and more often for depression and neurosis than men. Men are admitted in greater numbers for alcoholism, schizophrenia and personality dis-

Table 23.3 Admissions by sex and diagnostic groups to mental illness hospitals and units in England in 1977 (Department of Health and Social Security 1977)

Diagnosis	Female	%	Male	%	Total	%
All diagnoses	104 336	100	71 086	100	175 422	100
Schizophrenia	14 683	14	14 376	20	29 059	17
Depressive psychoses	15 378	15	7 065	10	22 443	13
Senile psychoses	7 111	7	3 134	4	10 245	6
Alcoholic psychoses	630	1	1 049	2	1 679	1
Other psychoses	8 872	9	5 298	7	14 170	8
Personality and behaviour disorders	9 887	10	8 393	12	18 280	10
Alcholism	2 955	3	7 667	11	10 622	6
Drug dependency	484	1	960	1	1 444	1
Psychoneuroses	14 886	14	6 887	10	21 773	12
Mental handicap	452	1	402	1	854	1
Other psychiatric conditions	3 065	3	2 112	3	5 177	3
All other conditions	25 933	25	13 743	19	39 676	23

Note: % columns do not total 100 due to rounding.

orders. As Table 23.4 illustrates, women and men are convicted of different kinds of criminal offences, men committing more offences involving violence against others and more serious types of stealing. More men than women commit suicide and they do so using more violent methods, whereas women have four times the number of unsuccessful suicide attempts compared with men (Garai 1970).

Table 23.4 Persons found guilty of indictable offences in 1977 (Social Trends No. 9 1979)

	Female	Males
	(Thousands)	
Murder, manslaughter, infanticide	–	0.3
Violence against persons	4.1	38.1
Sexual offences	0.1	9.2
Burglary	3.4	79.6
Robbery	0.2	3.1
Theft and handling stolen goods	80.2	242.0
Fraud	5.0	17.5
Criminal damage	3.6	46.4
Other	2.0	8.9
All indictable offences	98.6	445.1

It is difficult to interpret these figures because of differences in the way people and crimes are categorized, the kind of sentences considered appropriate for women and men, and indeed whether a custodial sentence is given at all. As a result, suggested interpretations of apparent statistical differences are also varied. Explanations focusing on the different ways women and men are socialized suggest that men turn their anger outwards and express frustration in the form of violence against others or themselves, whether this takes the form of alcohol consumption or suicide. Women, on the other hand, are taught that it is appropriate to express emotions freely and so they manifest higher incidences of depression, which includes turning hostility inwards rather than acting it out in the way that is more socially acceptable for men.

Marriage has different psychosocial costs and benefits for women and men. Men tend to be dissatisfied with marriage in the early years, pre-sumably resenting its restrictions and financial costs, but they are happier when they have been married longer and perhaps realize the benefits of having domestic needs taken care of by someone else. Women, however, become increasingly dissatisfied the longer they are married. Women are more happy when they live alone, when the responsibility for taking care of the physical and emotional need of others is less, while men have better health when they are married and have these needs catered for by a wife (Gove & Tudor 1972, Williams 1977).

Women who work outside the home have a lower incidence of depression than full-time housewives and experience fewer menopausal symptoms. The social contact and feelings of self-worth and relative independence which come from having paid work outside the home seem to account for this, because when men take on full-time housework and child care they report similar feelings of isolation, boredom, strain and lack of self-esteem as do women who are full-time housewives. Men who lose their jobs have higher levels of depression than women, who otherwise have the highest incidence of depression, as discussed earlier (Archer & Lloyd 1982).

Research concerned with the psychosocial effects of sex and gender role expectations, then, suggest that all people are more healthy when they have opportunities to gain the self-fulfilment that comes from social contact with others and from having a sense of independence. Everyone needs to share his life and emotions with others, but the way in which these needs are currently met in this society is detrimental to the health of both women and men, albeit in different ways.

As people living in the same society, psychiatric nurses are subject to the same influences and effects, and the following section will pursue the connections between sex-role stereotyping and psychiatric nursing.

SEXUALITY AND PSYCHIATRIC NURSING

Nursing is predominantly a female occupation, and Florence Nightingale established the profession specifically on this basis. Hogan (1980) suggests that it is precisely because of women's history of subordination to men in life in general and to men as doctors in working life that certain ways of thinking and behaving within nursing have continued for so long. Because women are socialized to be submissive, yielding and non-assertive, authoritarian social relations tend to be the norm in health care work. The costs of this have been well described by Revans (1964) and Menzies (1961), and others have drawn attention to high rates of drop-out during training, wastage from the profession after qualification, high job turnover and sickness rates, and high levels of stress within the profession. Since the mid-1960s, as management theory and practice have been increasingly introduced into the health service in Britain, there has been a marked change in the sexual division of labour within nursing. Men are being appointed to top management posts in health care and nursing education institutions (Nuttal 1983). For historical reasons to do with the staffing of asylums by male attendants, who were thought more capable of controlling violent patients before the age of pharmacological methods, there have always been more men in psychiatric nursing than in other branches of nursing. Nevertheless, the majority of psychiatric nurses are women. As in general nursing, however, men occupy a disproportionate number of top management posts in psychiatric nursing in relation to their numbers in this branch of the profession (Pollock & West 1984).

Differing interpretations by female and male psychiatric nurses of their nursing role are described by Pollock & West (1984), particularly at the charge nurse grade. They consider that being in the ward seems to be sufficient for male nurses, whereas women perform a doing role: 'Female nurses appear "busier", attend more to the "housekeeping" tasks, and relinquish to their male counterparts the more office-based functions of money, off-duty and form filling.'

Pollock & West (1984) also question the male nurse's supposedly superior ability to control aggressive behaviour, a myth which seems to persist even in the presence of more humanistic models of psychiatric nursing. Male psychiatric nurses

find it easier to be assertive and to make themselves heard at report time; because their socialization leads them to be relatively passive, to seek approval and to be 'other-centred', female psychiatric nurses find it hard to be assertive. Thus men's socialization prepares them to dominate the clinical setting and to advance in the institutional hierarchy.

This situation is likely to be detrimental to male psychiatric nurses and to patients too. Because of the way men are socialized, it is considered unusual for them to perform caring work either in the home with their own children or in paid work with children and sick people. This cuts them off from large sources of emotional satisfaction and pressures them into striving for career advancement when they might be happier in roles closer to patients and clients. Just as women's mothering gives children a particular picture of how women and men are supposed to behave and thereby separates them from their fathers (Chodorow 1978), so the division of labour in psychiatric nursing diminishes interpersonal contacts between patients and male nurses. Patients, too, are thereby exposed to a more limited range of female and male models than they might otherwise be.

The effects of this are summarized by Hull (1970), a philosopher who teaches nurses, in the following terms:

The tragedy of sexism in health care is that it is ultimately an iatrogenic phenomenon, self-confirming, not based on a realistic assessment of the potentials and possibilities for human growth and development that still remain unexplored promises of the free society. The terrible irony is that medicine and nursing, with the historically persistent commitment to the Hippocratic maxim *primum non nocere* — above all, do no harm — are structured in practice so as to preserve a set of assumptions that may well produce as much harm as any pathogenic agent.

SEXUALITY: IMPLICATIONS FOR PSYCHIATRIC NURSING

All the evidence reviewed in this chapter leads to a strong suspicion that psychiatric professionals of all kinds, whether doctors or nurses, women or men, are likely to share cultural expectations of different characteristics and roles for women and men, and to incorporate these in their judgements about relationships with patients and clients. Whether particular kinds of behaviour are regarded as unusual or pathogenic, what goals are set for recovery or progress, and the methods chosen to achieve these are likely to be affected by sex-role stereotypes.

What can psychiatric nurses do when faced with these kinds of issues? It is clear that fundamental social change will not be achieved overnight because the factors responsible are structural features of society. People are born into a culture which already has particular norms and values, and these are beyond immediate and individual influence. But it is just as pointless to sink into pessimism as it is to wait for the revolution to bring about new forms of social relations in which people relate to each other as unique individuals who express their gender in a myriad of different combinations. Change will never come about unless people themselves begin to relate to each other in new ways and work to change their own and other people's perspectives. Once change is begun, little by little, it will gain momentum. Just as an equal sharing by women and men of child care would create children with totally different conceptions of sexuality, so changes in the division of labour in psychiatric nursing would have profound implications for patients and professionals alike.

How can psychiatric nurses begin to change these aspects of their work? It seems obvious that medical models of psychiatry, with their primarily biological focus, will be of little value in helping to understand clients' behaviour and needs. By the same token, many nursing models cannot help, either because they, too, have a mainly biological and/or behaviourist orientation (for example, the models described by Roper et al 1980 and Roy 1980) or because they place the nurse in a controlling or 'expert' position. If it is the nurse who 'manipulates the stimuli' (Roy 1980) or 'designs the nursing system' (Orem 1980), then it is likely to be the nurse's judgement and preferences which

determine what is identified as a problem, which goals are set, and which interventions are used. Only a nursing model which places at least equal emphasis on social factors in comparison with biological and psychological factors, and sees clients' needs, hopes and expectations as paramount is likely to be useful. Such a model will also need to face up squarely to the importance of nurse–client relationships in psychiatric nursing, and give guidance in how to build on these in the therapeutic encounter. Such a model will help nurses to be non-judgemental towards clients (Goldsborough 1970), to recognize clients' individuality and their rights to live in ways which they themselves define as healthy, mature and socially competent rather than being subject to practitioners' preconceptions.

Nursing education has an important role to play in working towards greater openness and mutual acceptance among nurses themselves, between nurses and doctors, and between nurses and clients. As well as learning about the biological, psychological and social aspects of sexuality, nursing students need help in clarifying their own values and understanding their own feelings so that they can feel more comfortable in situations involving clients' sexuality (Payne 1976). Nurses also need to develop social skills, including assertiveness skills, which will enable them to express themselves and relate to clients and other professionals at a more open, relaxed and deep level.

CONCLUSION

The issues discussed in this chapter are profound in their present effects and their implications for the future of psychiatric nursing. In a limited space it is only possible to highlight some aspects of sexuality and its implications. Much more thought, study, research and practical work lies ahead if nursing practice is to become truly holistic and humanistic, and if nurses are to respect all facets of their clients' selves, as well as their own self-esteem as gendered beings and as nurses.

REFERENCES

Archer J, Lloyd B 1982 Sex and gender. Penguin, Harmondsworth

Bem S 1974 The measurement of psychological androgyny. Journal of Clinical Psychology 42: 155–162

Broverman I K, Broverman D M, Clarkson F E, Rosenkrantz P, Vogel S R 1970 Sex-role stereotypes and clinical judgements of mental health. Journal of Clinical Psychology 34: 1–7

Chodorow N 1978 The reproduction of mothering. University of California Press, Berkeley

Coppen B, Bishop M, Beard R J, Barnard G J R, Collins W P 1981 Hysterectomy, hormones and behaviour. Lancet i: 126–128

Fabrikant B, Landau D, Rollenhagen D 1973 Perceived female sex role attributes and psychotherapists' sex role expectations for female patients. New Jersey Psychologist 23: 13–16

Freimuth M, Hornstein G A 1982 A critical examination of the concept of gender. Sex Roles 8(5): 515–532

Garai J E 1970 Sex Differences in mental health. Genetic Health Monographs: 123–142

Gath D 1980 Psychiatric aspects of hysterectomy. In: Robins L, Clayton P, Wing J (eds) The social consequences of psychiatric illness. Brunner Mazel, New York

Gauthier J, Kjervik D 1982 Sex-role identity and self-esteem in female graduate nursing students. Sex Roles 8(1): 45–55

Goldsborough G D 1970 On becoming non-judgemental. American Journal of Nursing 70: 2340–2343

Gove W R, Tudor J F 1972 Adult sex roles and mental illness. American Journal of Sociology 78: 812–835

Hogan R 1980 Human sexuality. A nursing perspective. Appleton-Century-Crofts, New York

Hull R 1970 Dealing with sexism in nursing. Nursing Outlook, February: 89, 94

Kjervik D K 1979 The stress of sexism on the mental health of women. In: Kjervik D K & Martinson I M (eds) Women in stress: a nursing perspective. Appleton-Century-Crofts, New York

Kravetz D F 1976 Sex role concepts of women. Journal of Clinical Psychology 44(3): 437–443

Kuczynski J H 1980 Nursing and medical students' sexual attitudes and knowledge. Journal of Obstetric, Gynecological and Neonatal Nursing, Nov–Dec: 339–342

Lennane K J, Lennane R J 1982 Alleged psychogenic disorders in women. A possible manifestation of sexual prejudice. In: Whitelegg E et al (eds) The changing experience in women. Martin Robertson/Open University, Oxford

Menzies I E P 1961 The functioning of the social system as a defence against anxiety. Tavistock, London

Nuttall P 1983 Male takeover or female giveway? Nursing Times 79(2): 10–11

Oakley A 1972 Sex, gender & society. Temple Smith, London

Orem D 1980 Nursing: concepts of practice. McGraw-Hill, New York

Payne T 1976 Sexuality of nurses: correlations of knowledge, attitudes and behaviour. Nursing Research 25(3): 286–292

Pollock L, West E 1984 On being a woman and a psychiatric nurse. Senior Nurse 1: 10–13

Revans R W 1964 Standards for morale: cause and effect in hospitals. Nuffield Provincial Hospitals Trust, London

Roper N, Logan W W, Tierney A J 1980 The elements of nursing. Churchill Livingstone, Edinburgh

Rosenkrantz P S, Vogel S R, Bee H, Boverman I K, Brown D M 1968 Sex-role stereotypes and self-concepts in college students. Journal of Clinical Psychology 32: 287–295

Roy C 1980 The Roy adaptation model. In: Riehl J P, Roy C (eds) Conceptual models for nursing practice. Appleton-Century-Crofts, New York

Teri L 1982 Effects of sex and sex-role style on clinical judgement. Sex Roles 8(6): 639–649

Treece E W, Treece J W 1977 Elements of research in nursing. C W Mosby, St Louis, Mo

Webb C 1985 Sexuality, nursing and health. Wiley, Chichester

Webb C 1987 Defining women and their health: the case of hysterectomy. In: Orr J (ed) Women's health in the community. Wiley, Chichester

Williams J H 1977 Psychology of women. Norton, New York

FURTHER READING

Bancroft J 1983 Human sexuality and its problems. Churchill Livingstone, Edinburgh

Broome A, Wallace L (eds) 1984 Psychology and gynaecological problems. Tavistock, London

Godow A G 1982 Human sexuality. C V Mosby, St Louis, Mo

Kolodny R C, Masters W H, Johnson V E 1979 Textbook of sexual medicine. Little, Brown, Boston

Masters W H, Johnson V E 1966 Human sexual response. Little, Brown, Boston

Masters W H, Johnson V E 1970 Human sexual inadequacy. Little, Brown, Boston

Masters W H, Johnson V E 1979 Homosexuality in perspective. Little, Brown, Boston

Webb C 1985 Sexuality, nursing and health. Wiley, Chichester

Woods N F 1984 Human sexuality in health and illness. C V Mosby, St Louis, Mo

24

Organizing inpatient care

S. A. H. Ritter

ORGANIZATION OF A WARD

For the purposes of this chapter, the unit of organization is taken to be a hospital ward of about 25 beds, staffed by a charge nurse who is a registered mental nurse, up to six other first and second level nurses, one or two unqualified assistants, and a variable number of learner nurses. Other staff who provide professional services to the ward are one or more consultant psychiatrists, a senior registrar and another junior doctor, occupational therapist, psychologist, social worker, welfare officer and chaplain. Ancillary services to the ward include cleaning, rubbish disposal and other portering functions.

To speak of a ward is a convenient shorthand for an organization which is otherwise difficult to define, and it is acknowledged that attributing characteristics and motivations to organization risks distorting the parts played by individuals within them. Wards vary widely. Because the ward is 'the true unit of operation' of psychiatric hospitals, the discussion uses this unit to illustrate points and to make generalizations whose applicability will vary according to local environments (Hooper 1962).

There are a number of ways of attempting to define what a ward and its organization consists of. One way is to try to identify the ward's key objectives in terms of key activities. This results, for instance, in five categories: clinical practice, ward management, professional relationships, teaching, and theory and research (Ritter 1981). Another way is to identify key processes in the ward organization and give an account of the ward in terms of the relationship of these processes to each other and the organization as a whole (Beer 1967). This has become known as a systems approach.

Components of ward organization: a systems view

For a ward to be seen as a self-contained system it must possess certain elements. There will be a clear boundary differentiating it from the wider system, the parent institution or hospital.

Boundaries mark the places where the organization makes contact with its environment. Flows to and from the environment to the organization take place across its boundaries, and the ward needs to be able to control what crosses to and fro. Within the boundaries the ward will also have mechanisms for monitoring its own performance and the feedback it receives from the wider system. There will be mechanisms for making and implementing decisions. If the ward does not have control over these mechanisms, or its internal communication processes are not up to dealing with the input from the environment, its ability to maintain equilibrium and deal with disturbance is interfered with (Lockett & Spear 1980, Open Systems Group 1981, Bignell & Fortune 1984, Carter et al 1984, Paton et al 1984).

For example, many charge nurses do not have a say over the nursing staff who are sent to work in the ward, and so have to deal with what is often a transient and unpredictable work-force (Proctor 1989). The allocation of other professionals is outside the ward's control, as often are the allocation of resources and monitoring of their efficiency. The nursing staff may have little say routinely in decisions about admitting and discharging patients. They may not be informed of letters of praise sent to the hospital administrators, and conversely may hear without warning of complaints. As well as being subject to internal tensions, a ward may come into conflict with the parent institution because of the blurring of decision-making and perfomance-monitoring systems. A ward may practise primary nursing and be asked at a few minutes' notice to send a primary nurse to relieve in another ward. It may ask to initiate a project for pre-induction preparation of students allocated to the ward, and be refused on the grounds that it is unfair for students to have treatment in one ward that is different from other wards.

The final component of the ward system is its world-view (*weltanschaung*) or philosophy (Carter et al 1984). This can only be a rational one if the other components are present.

PHILOSOPHY

It is desirable that a ward has an explicit philosophy which informs its ethos, atmosphere and working methods. A philosophy provides a model of the ward system to which staff refer in order to regulate the values and attitudes which determine the ways in which they deliver their service to clients.

When constructing a model, consideration must be given to the concepts of right and duty. It is tempting to assume that patients have rights and the staff have duties. But staff and patients have a variety of obligations to each other.

When an individual joins a ward, he or she joins an organization which acts as an agency (Argyris & Schön 1978). The agency shares accountability for its work among the staff who comprise its work-force. In joining the organization the individual gives up a number of rights, in particular, the right to exercise personal control of information. Because of shared accountability, other members of the ward have a right to take part in the process of decision-making about the relevance or otherwise of information to their work. There is a tension between this shared accountability and the accountability which derives from an individual's duty of care or status as a practitioner or both. Such tension can be expressed in interpersonal conflict with colleagues. Other rights and duties which are complicated by the ward's function as an agency include privacy, veracity and consent. They generate similar tensions which impinge on staff morale (feelings of comfort) and confidence.

A common-sense view is that nurses who feel comfortable in their work will generate feelings of comfort in patients (Crammer 1984). For patients to feel comfortable and confident, then, the organizational philosophy of the ward has to be one which fosters such feelings in nurses.

Either a ward can create a model which explicitly allows for and provides strategies for dealing with tensions, or it can apply a model which covertly reduces tensions. An example of such a model is one which is based on custom and tradition. Another example of covert tension reduction is the 'routinizing' of information-giving activities. A multiplicity of meetings designed for sharing information range from 'hand-overs' to ward rounds. These routines give the appearance of a psychosocial, patient-centred emphasis, but can become appropriated into a defensive system which in fact prevents the sharing of information by being superficial, perfunctory, yet characterized by the number of staff talking and the length of time they take doing so.

Case example

Mr Smith hears voices constantly, behaves agitatedly, does not sleep at night and keeps leaving the ward. He is given increasing doses of neuroleptics and referred to the occupational therapy department. After a week in OT the therapist reports in a management round that Mr Smith's movements are slow and stiff, he sits but does not otherwise participate in group activities, he appears drowsy and does not talk much. For two weeks the therapist gives a similar report while other team members describe how much better Mr Smith is, how well he sleeps, and say that he does not complain of voices. After two weeks the consultant happens to visit the ward and sees the patient walking across the sitting-room. She is appalled by his Parkinsonian symptoms and gives instructions for his medication to be halved. The team does not question her decision, presumably because if they did, they would have to consider what was going on during the management rounds when they appeared to be talking to each other.

RULES

A ward has little choice about certain of the rules by which it operates. Above all are the statutory obligations imposed by legislation such as the Mental Health Act 1983, the Health and Safety at Work etc Act 1974, and the Nurses Rules (1983 c 20, 1974 c 37, Statutory Instrument 1983 873). Next are the Department of Health circulars and memoranda which explicate and provide detailed and compulsory guidance to legislation. Thirdly are the codes of practice laid down by each profession to guide its members. The United Kingdom Central Council for Nursing and Midwifery now has a variety of papers stemming from its core Code of Practice (UKCC 1985). Nurses who breach the Code may be liable to disciplinary action by the UKCC, which is concerned to 'uphold and enhance the good standing and reputation of the profession' (p. 2). Fourthly, the common law imposes a variety of duties on ward staff, in particular the duty of care. Individual clinical responsibility of each registered nurse is the end-product of these four sets of rules. It is a responsibility to maintain a standard which at minimum is, in the case of a nurse, that of a reasonable average competent nurse who is practising at the level required to pass the requirements for entry to the register.

Hospitals are governed by the same rules but, in addition, in order to regulate day-to-day running, each institution develops its own sets of rules and guidelines. These are contained in policies and procedures. A policy is a statement of who may do what, when they may do it, why they may do it, and where they may do it. A procedure gives guidance on how to do it. The institution has an obligation to make its policies both in accordance with higher authority and in consultation with staff, and so committees comprising representatives of the various staff organizations are often the vehicle for carrying out consultation. Similarly, a ward which devises its own policies and procedures is obliged to take into account the published policies of the parent institution.

An individual practitioner's duty of care and statutory obligations override his or her obligation blindly to follow instructions. A policy which says that the movements of patients should not be restricted unless they are detained under the Mental Health Act 1983 could not be used as a defence by a nurse who knowingly allows a patient to leave the ward and endanger himself or other people. On the other hand, a nurse who allows a potentially suicidal patient to go out unaccompanied because, in the nurse's judgement, the patient will return safely, does so accepting that he or she may be individually called to account for that judgement. The existence of rules does not free individuals from the responsibility of making decisions.

Existing legislation also obliges ward staff to cooperate with organizations which act as watchdogs. The Mental Health Act Commission monitors the Mental Health Act 1983, and must be given free access to wards and patients' records, as must the Health Advisory Service, which monitors standards of care in psychiatric hospitals.

DECISION-MAKING

The basic elements of decision-making are estimating for a given course of action the risk or cost, and the possible benefits; and working out a means of achieving a desired result with the greatest benefit and lowest risk possible. That is, can the desired aim be met with the means available? During the following discussion it must be borne in mind that unless a ward has autonomy over its decision-making systems, reponsibility for acts and omissions can be diffused between it and the wider institution.

Aids to decision-making

Various formal systems have been developed to minimize the risk involved in decision-making, to predict results, and to analyse the effects of the different available choices. Some mathematical models represent quantitatively the likely outcomes of different options (Leavitt et al 1973). In the ward setting, however, decision-making systems are likely to attempt to minimize the risk by processes such as negotiation and consensus, car-

ried out in formal and informal settings such as ward and management rounds. Additionally a number of constraints will limit choices. These constraints range from institutional policies and procedures to the skill mix of the ward nurses.

In what has become known as the Glacier research, Jaques (1956) identified what he termed discretionary content of jobs. In the absence of prescribed tasks, individuals can exercise discretion about how they carry out a given activity. Prescription may be accomplished through written procedures or through custom and practice (Hill 1956). Prescription, routine and tradition are all used to minimize the discomfort often associated with the exercise of discretion. On the other hand, prescription of medication aims to ensure that patients receive a known amount of a specific drug at set times, so that the drug becomes a quantifiable variable in the planning and therefore the evaluation of a person's treatment. The aim of routine is to prevent unnecessary duplication of effort by different nurses; and tradition provides a ward culture which can override disruption.

Problem-solving

Although quantitative methods exist of modelling uncertainty in human services which deal with open-ended problems (Levin et al 1976), the strategies used by nurses in the ward setting are encapsulated in the term 'nursing process'. More or less detailed assessment procedures are the prelude to negotiated setting of objectives. The planning stage may be characterized by attempts to cover all contingencies, thereby reducing the perceived risk. The interventions required to implement plans may be planned in groups and delegated either by the group itself (for example, the ward round), or by senior nurses to junior nurses, or by other professionals to nurses. A registered nurse may plan with the multidisciplinary clinical team a graded exposure programme for a patient while learner and other unqualified nurses actually carry out interventions. A social worker may ask a nurse to ensure that a detained patient receives a copy of the leaflet detailing his or her rights under the Mental Health Act 1983. In this way, responsibility for a plan is diffused in the group and responsibility for carrying it out is delegated.

Delegation is a form of decision-making in itself and involves some risk for the person who will remain accountable for the work delegated to others. Nevertheless, the retention by more senior members of staff of accountability for interventions is lightened by delegation, and the assumption of responsibility by more junior staff is lightened by the absence of accountability. While examples such as those given above are relatively common, they may be criticicized because of the blurring of accountability and responsibility. Organizational systems which involve individualized patient care attempt to bring the decision-making process back to the nurse who is actually nursing the patient. Because of the logistic difficulties in arranging for each primary nurse to meet with the multi-disciplinary clinical team, and because the hierarchy is no longer available to maintain control, there is apt to be pressure for elaborate institutional policies and procedures which will restore a way of minimizing risks in decision-making by individuals.

QUALITY ASSURANCE

The evaluation stage of the nursing process was at one time seen as merely the end-stage of a linear sequence of activities (De la Cuesta 1983). Implicit was a notion that the nursing interventions had been completed in some way. However, alongside the development of awareness for the need for quality assurance has been a recognition of the dynamic nature of the nursing process, and of the need for continuous evaluation at all stages. Hospitals and wards are developing structure, process and outcome criteria which are used to set standards (Donabedian 1966, Mason 1984, Kitson 1986, Marker 1988). Standards having been set it is then possible to monitor quantitatively a ward's performance. Done retrospectively, such activity is audit. Done prospectively it involves setting targets and monitoring progress. Wards may supply raw data to specialized units within the hospital for analysis and feedback at a later date, or they may set up concurrent performance monitoring systems which they use to adjust their approach.

As discussed at the beginning of this chapter, if the ward does not have control over its own performance-monitoring its stability can be quite seriously threatened. At simplest, the delayed feedback from an external quality-monitoring unit may result in corrective action which is too late, is inappropriate to circumstances that have now changed, or duplicates action taken already. If a mechanistic analogy is used, misplaced or overcorrection can cause an enterprise to crash. The natural inertia of a ward will prevent such an outcome, but resentment and confusion are likely and damaging results.

One widely used performance-monitoring system is quality circles. These provide little quantitative data but do provide opportunities for face-to-face contact, airing of differences, and generally facilitating the carrying out of interpersonal tasks; as well as for identifying actual and potential problems, suggesting solutions and innovations.

For teams, therefore, the development of standards and implementation of performance-monitoring require them to differentiate their roles and to divide work according to skills and capacities to accomplish the functions required to achieve the standards set. Together with activities like quality circles these efforts can actually enhance team-building, as the team works on a common task.

At the centre of any quality assurance enterprise is the patient. Traditionally, psychiatric hospitals and ward staff have neglected their responsibility to provide information to patients, to facilitate investigation of criticisms and complaints and to respect the rights of both informal and detained patients to consent to various treatments. (Consumers Association 1978, National Consumer Council 1983, Brazier 1987, Sinclair 1987) The Mental Health Act 1983 provides for a code of practice for detained patients. Attention to consumer relations in the form of information booklets, satisfaction questionnaires, advocacy and the 'ombudsmen' now being appointed by some hospitals is a major responsibility of a ward.

Berry & Metcalf (1985) suggest that when organizational systems of nursing change, the effect on patient satisfaction is relatively small in relation to the effect on nurses' satisfaction. One implication is that any change generates more favourable feelings in nurses towards their work, as shown in early organizational research (Mayo 1933, Roethlisberger & Dickson 1939). Another implication is that nurses' motivations in choosing particular ways of working have little to do with patients (despite what may be said) and a good deal to do with their own feelings of comfort or discomfort. As suggested in the section on ward philosophy, nurses' morale is likely to correlate with patient morale, but it is not known whether suicide, self-injury and violence rates in patients can be related to absenteeism, sickness or ill-temper and rudeness in nurses, although there has been some investigation of sickness and violence (Rix 1987).

RESOURCE MANAGEMENT

Accountability to the client goes in parallel to accountability to the wider institution. Until comparatively recently this accountability was seen mainly in terms of correctly carrying out procedures. A ward did not have a great deal of control over the resources allocated to it.

Productivity

Productivity can be defined as the degree to which the stated objectives of an organization are achieved. It involves managing tasks (by setting objectives) rather than human relations. That is, it focuses on results or outputs rather than processes. The output must be relevant and appropriate to the capacity of the staff and to the other resources available. In industry, productivity is related to profit. In a National Health Service (NHS) ward setting, productivity is in terms of serving the patients well (Gray 1976).

Ward objectives

The ward will set its objectives in the context of those of the wider institution; within the constraints of available resources; and having regard to the fact that it may not be able to identify what its primary task is, but instead has to fulfil a num-

ber of purposes depending on the skill mix of its staff and the case mix (needs) of its clients.

The complexity and magnitude of the task of first defining the ward's purpose(s) and then devising objectives to achieve it (or them) requires the resources of groups constituted from team members. The production of ward objectives is incidentally a team-building exercise which eventually results in enhanced efficiency of a team whose members are confident in each other's abilities and clear about roles, responsibilities and limitations.

Outcome criteria

A well-defined objective is a statement of desired outcome and provides a performance criterion. Thus the ward objectives themselves are the critera by which to measure the ward's output. Other measures for resource consumption include bed occupancy, length of stay or utilization patterns, which are relatively easy to measure. Problems occur with the attempt to use them as indices of work-load. While the advantages of quantifiable data are obvious, it is equally clear that they tell only part of the story. Other work-load indices include patient dependency, case mix and diagnostic-related groups (DRGs). With the devolution to ward level of responsibility for managing budgets there is a pressing need for rational and reliable measures which have a predictive ability.

Among the costs of running a ward, additional to the clinical ones, are those for clerical, domestic, portering and other services, along with supplies, mail, and graphics services. If the clinical services of other professionals are bought in the demand must be measured against the capacity of the ward's budget. In these circumstances the more that can be stabilized and made predictable the easier budgeting will be. Some costs are easier to determine than others. A variety of methods exist for calculating, say, ward establishments. However, the tools for calculating skill mix, especially in the psychiatric setting, are less developed. The transition of student nurses to supernumerary status creates more uncertainty. In the end, all calculations are based ultimately on an assumption which is more or less intuitive. The arguments for various work-load estimations may be entirely valid, but are vulnerable to the possibility that their original assumption is incorrect (Miller 1984, Bright 1985, O'Brien 1986, Essock-Vitale 1987).

Work scheduling

How the staff/work ratio is worked out may be more or less explicit. A task-based approach allows charge nurses to cope with the transience of many nurses (Proctor 1989). Thus the hierarchy can be used as a way of managing resources economically.

In a setting without such transient staff, the division of labour cannot so readily be carried out on the basis of hierarchy. Work assignment becomes less a matter of task-distribution than of screening patients for their suitability to be allocated to nurses who are then responsible for their care. The responsibility for scheduling work is thereby largely devolved to the individual nurse. In itself this system may not improve the work flow of a ward, as the case and skill mixes may be outside the control of the charge nurse, and there is also the question of how skilled individual nurses are at managing their work. However, it does allow the use of discretion by nurses, and in doing so introduces the possibility of monitoring the use of resources quite sensitively. Problems for the charge nurse or resource manager include collating the diverse material which accumulates in patient records, and ensuring that nurses use the various devices for collecting outcome data.

Time management

Work-flow and scheduling are not just a matter of allocating personnel, and require effective use of time. Timetabling and routine are traditionally seen as ways of regulating use of time in wards. However, some human relations theorists argue that instead of being used for the limited purposes of optimizing time, routine and timetables become an end in themselves, developing into defensive structures. The effect on resource management is deleterious because the primary task(s) of the ward becomes subservient to the task of making fixed

and rigid what is really in a process of continuous change. The use of routine as part of a 'protective bureaucracy' (Kernberg 1980 p. 231) is discussed later in the chapter in the context of caring activities within the ward.

Stock control

Because the link between productivity and profit has been absent from NHS hospitals, there has traditionally been relative inattention to regulating ward stocks. With the devolution of budgets this is changing, but it is a skill which requires training in order to sensitize individuals to the costs of maintaining unused stocks on shelves in the ward, without encouraging them to strangle supply sources. From the USA, where hospitals are run for profit, an extensive literature is available to guide nurses in available technique.

PERSONNEL PROCEDURES

The ward has been defined as a collection of individuals acting as an agency which to some extent shares accountability for the work of the ward. This raises problems of determining where authority lies, so that there can be conflict between that which is sapiential, or knowledge- and skill-based, and that which is role-based. At its simplest, this becomes a question of whether the manager of the agency (usually the charge nurse) will act as a negotiator, diplomat, arbitrator, or ruler (Leavitt et al 1973). The management style of the ward may oscillate between participative and democratic and autocratic and paternalistic, according to internal as well as external stresses. Careful attention must therefore be paid to the various procedures which regulate the individual's relationship to the agency.

Moving sequentially, the first factor to be attended to is that of observing equal opportunities and racial equality legislation when making appointments. The Health and Safety etc at Work Act 1974, as well as industrial relations legislation, governs much of the ward manager's responsibility toward staff members. Next, staff require an induction and orientation programme which delineates their place in the ward structure, their responsibilities for aspects of the ward's work, and similarly their place and responsibilities in the wider institution. It is hoped that the content of this programme does not differ too much from the informal socialization which takes place and which moulds the newcomer into a 'person like us'.

How the next phase is managed depends on the ward's model or philosophy. In a more bureacratic setting, the staff member will be allocated a supervisor who is seen to have some accountability for the 'supervisee's' work until he or she is deemed competent by the institution. The supervisor will negotiate with the nurse in order to plan for personal and career development within the ward, and set targets to be used as the basis of regular appraisal, carried out with the supervisor and the next nurse above in the hierarchy. The advantages of this system are that it allows the charge nurse to predict and cost, say, the demands on ward resources of allowing nurses to go on courses. Conversely, among the benefits of having nurses trained, say in conducting groups, will be the increase in the capacity of the ward to carry out various forms of treatment. The supervisors are also the first line in ensuring attention to staff welfare. Where a philosophy of organizational development informed by human relations exists, supervision will be less a matter of instruction than of dialogue.

Rostering

A fundamental procedure is that of ensuring that there is the required number and mix of nurses to meet the ward's demands. In the end it is the charge nurse who is accountable for rostering, and although the task of devising a duty rota may be delegated, the responsibility for ensuring safe cover cannot. Requirements for rostering include providing an equitable division of shifts; following guidelines about maximum stretches of days on duty; providing days off together; acceding to reasonable requests; sharing unpopular shifts (such as Friday and Saturday afternoons, Monday mornings); ensuring that nurses attend meetings they are committed to attend; providing opportunities

for supervisors and the 'supervisees' to work together; distributing competence, skills and experience; negotiating and planning leave requests so that there will be not more than a certain number of nurses away at one time, and so that nurses of the same grade are not away together.

Absence and leave records

Many wards have to submit returns of sickness absence, annual and other forms of leave such as compassionate leave, although this varies between hospitals. It is an area where problems of resource may become evident, since if a hospital requires a nurse to notify a certain administrative office of sickness, say, but does not require that the ward itself be notified, it may happen that a nurse in charge of an early shift will not know why a nurse has not turned up until the start of office hours.

Trade unions and other staff organizations

The charge nurse will want to ensure that all nurses belong to a trade union or other staff organization, and that they have the time off agreed by the hospital and joint consultative committee for union activities. Good industrial relations start at ward level, and the first line manager has a particular responsibility for facilitating them.

Disciplinary procedures

In cases of errors in the administration of medicines, the UKCC Professional Conduct Committee distinguishes between 'those cases in which there was serious pressure of work and immediate honest disclosure in the patient's interests and those in which there were no such pressures, the error was a result of reckless practice and the practitioner, though aware of the error, did not then take action in the patient's interests' (UKCC 1988). It stresses the need for all questions of misconduct to be thoroughly and carefully investigated before decisions are made to proceed.

Such decisions are, according to the UKCC, professional and managerial ones.

Registered nurses need to be thoroughly familiar with the UKCC code of conduct and related documents, local policies and procedures, and confident enough in the supervisory system of the ward to be able to report immediately any errors or omissions.

INFORMATION MANAGEMENT

The diverse aspects of information management in a ward can be represented diagrammatically (Fig. 24.1). Dependent on the ward's philosophy will be the emphasis placed on the various aspects of information management. A ward which is interested in its human relations will be interested in its own informal patterns of communication which are usually across the levels of the hierarchy rather than up and down. The more apparently irrational processes of interaction will receive attention, as will the influence of unpredicted and unknown factors. For instance, the disturbed behaviour of a young man who threatens the nurses, who in turn feel angry with him, may be discussed in terms of his primary nurse going away on holiday and an early childhood separation from his parents. There is likely to be a good deal of open discussion between staff and between staff and patients. The distortions in communication which can occur are readily acknowledged and in their turn are used as material for discussion.

A ward which operates from a more bureaucratic philosophy will be less inclined to speculate about unknown influences. Information is handled according to the competence and specialization of team members deemed responsible. Discussion will take place in closed meetings attended only by staff at the top of the hierarchy. Information is communicated up and down the hierarchy, largely on a need-to-know basis.

A third model is one which combines aspects of both the previous ones, embedding the ideal of free and open discussion in a setting where roles and boundaries are clearly delineated. Central to the model is the assumption that individuals feel freer and more able to exercise discretion in their work if they do so in the context of a 'well-defined formal structure' (Gray 1976 p. 428).

The form that data will take depends on its purpose. Functional analysis of a patient's behaviour will be set out in graphs and diagrams as well as a certain amount of narrative in the patient's clinical record. A process recording of a nurse's interaction with a patient will contain more narrative and look very different. A depression inventory will consist of statement choices and ticks.

Documentation

Since hospitals are bureaucracies, there is a great emphasis on documentation of nursing actions and the preservation of these documents, because by so doing consistency and predictability of performance are encouraged.

Computerization

A common myth is that data management can easily be transferred to computers. This is not the case, mainly because of the inexact and complex nature of much of the day-to-day discourse of nursing staff. It is a truism that stereotyping and jargon maintain consistency of terminology at the expense of accurate representation of reality and, conversely, the accurate representation of

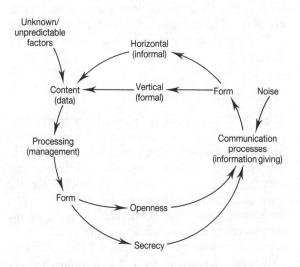

Fig. 24.1 Information management in a ward.

reality is too cumbersome, idiosyncratic and time-consuming to make it worth attempting to computerize. Extremely careful planning of an information management system is required, in order to take account of the psychosocial effects of introducing such technology to a ward, the relative needs of the different disciplines, the requirements of the wider institution, and the needs of the patients (Blois 1984, Forshaw and Roscoe 1988, Zuboff 1988, Bradley 1989).

MANAGEMENT OF RISK

As discussed earlier in relation to decision-making, wards with a bureaucratic philosophy will attempt to minimize risk-taking behaviour by adhering to a set of rules, by the exercise of authoritarian leadership, and by maintaining a fixed and rigid structure based on legitimation by qualification and status.

Two different approaches tackle risk head-on. The first stems from a view of the ward as a place where individual nurses adapt reciprocally with the organization. This gives them discretion in carrying out their role and therefore some discretion in deciding with a patient, say, the level of risk he or she will be assumed to present. The second stems from a view of the organization as a complex network of interlocking functions, processes and purpose. The individual nurse is supported by the structure which nevertheless allows discretion in his or her use of the support. Any policies and procedures are thus part of the supporting network, but the nurse's adherence to them is likely to vary with the nature of the support given by the rest of the matrix (Leavitt et al 1973).

Safety

Preventive measures

Self-injury. Prevention of self-injury requires a team approach in order to assess risk and plan interventions for self-injurious patients. Where possible, the patient is involved in assessing the risk, and all personal interaction between the nurses and the patient is documented and discussed.

The risk is classified and the team agrees on the level of supervision to be implemented (Ritter 1989).

Violence. Sclafani (1986) advocates what he calls 'therapeutic environment programming' to prevent violence. In essence this comprises attention to the morale of staff and patients; attention to the maintenance of the physical environment; and avoidance of protective routines. Stegne (1978) advocates regular update training for all staff, and hospital policies to be formulated after wide consultation and based on well-kept statistics. Owens & Ashcroft (1985) provide a full account of the origins and problems of violent behaviour by patients.

Fire. First-line managers (charge nurses) are commonly responsible for fire prevention and checking on hazards. In each ward the fire exits must be identified, precautions determined, action plans made, and regular checks of staff's knowledge carried out (Arscott & Armstrong 1976).

Management of self-injury and violence

It is essential that staff are trained in a variety of techniques to tackle aggressive or self-injurious patients or both. Sclafani's steps in managing violence apply also to self-injury. These involve early verbal intervention by nurses with patients who may relinquish control of their behaviour; a team approach if verbal interventions fail; pharmacological intervention when other measures fail; and physical restraint as a last resort (Sclafani 1986).

HOUSEKEEPING

Allen (1982) describes an 'identikit' portrait of the ward sister which emphasizes housekeeping responsibilities and which persists, especially in the minds of medical staff. She points out that charge nurses ceased to be responsible for the work of domestic staff in the late 1960s. However, the charge nurse is accountable for some of the housekeeping responsibilities in the ward, an accountability which is complicated by the different staff and managers who are accountable for housekeeping as a whole. These include domestic supervisors, stores managers, works managers, catering managers, and portering managers.

The underlying rationale for housekeeping responsibilities is that of maintaining a safe environment for staff and patients. The Health and Safety at Work etc Act 1974 requires all employees 'to take reasonable care for the health and safety of themselves and any others who may be affected by what they do'. Cleanliness and tidiness are important in prevention: preventing accidents and misuse by patients who wish to harm themselves or others, and maintaining hygiene. The charge nurse is also responsible for promoting environmental health in his or her ward. This may entail balancing the patients' demands against housekeeping restraints. In many hospitals, patients are locked out of ward kitchens except for a few brief periods each day, in order to prevent access to potentially harmful equipment, to conserve ward supplies of tea, milk and other rations, and to prevent squalor. Such a regimen characterizes an approach which puts the requirements of the institution above the needs of the patient. It can be tedious and frustrating helping patients to cooperate with each other in not wasting rations and keeping facilities clean, but there is a pay-off therapeutically in that apparently trivial issues of day-to-day living with other people can be used as the basis for, say, rehabilitative work, or relatively non-threatening group discussion.

The charge nurse is certainly accountable for arranging swift attention to repairs in the ward. These range from defective electrical fittings to broken or dilapidated furniture. Where the ward ethos is that therapy matters above material surroundings, this must be made explicit, its rationale set out, and the agreement of patients and team members sought. There is some evidence that attention to the ward environment improves ward atmosphere and so, it is reasoned, therapeutic outcomes (Baldwin 1985).

Feeding arrangements for patients are largely outside the control of the ward-based nurse, as domestic staff are responsible for bringing, serving and clearing away food. However, nurses are accountable for monitoring patients' nutritional status. Liaison with catering staff is necessary to ensure that patients are fed adequately.

The right of patients to have private, lockable storage facilities is one that is still neglected, despite the existence of standards for personal space and storage in psychiatric hospitals (DHSS 1980). The hospital will have a policy which disclaims responsibility for property not handed in for safe-keeping and a receipt obtained in exchange. Routinely depriving patients of articles such as belts or scissors, which are kept in communal cupboards, is not an acceptable alternative for arranging safe personal storage. Where patients may be admitted at any time, the ward nurses need 24 hour access to safes and receipt books for the large amounts of money and valuable objects that patients sometimes bring with them.

Supplies

The need for stock control was mentioned in the context of resource management. Although the process of stock checking, ordering and accepting delivery can be delegated, the charge nurse or resource manager will want to set stock levels himself or herself, having monitored these in consultation with other staff, so that the rationale for a particular ordering system is clear to the person responsible for ward stores.

ADMINISTRATIVE AND CLERICAL ACTIVITIES

In many wards, the charge nurse is tied to clerical and administrative tasks which do not intrinsically require his or her skills, even though the person dealing with them may wish to consult the senior nurse on duty. Such tasks include answering the telephone, redirecting calls, and maintaining a telephone communication book which is used by all staff to monitor and respond to messages left for them. Visitors to the ward, whether they are friends or relatives of patients, or other staff, need to be received and offered assistance. This function does not require a nurse, but the charge nurse does require a system of monitoring access to the ward and of ensuring that visitors are treated courteously.

Errands

Running errands may be regarded, among other things, as a form of time wasting by qualified nurses, of displacement activity to put off doing another less pleasant job, or as a means of maintaining informal contacts and systems of communication round the hospital. Whichever of these is the case, the charge nurse will be interested to know how much of them goes on. It is desirable therefore that errand-running is systematized with reception and other communication activities.

Clerical tasks

A variety of documentation is required from a ward, ranging from bed-state returns to staff rosters and leave sheets. The medical records of patients who have been admitted or discharged need to be kept safely, and in order, and returned for central filing as soon as possible. Again, these are tasks which do not require nursing skills, but which can seriously hamper nurses' efficiency if they are carried out negligently or haphazardly or both.

TEAMWORK

Teamwork is discussed in detail in the chapter on the role of the nurse in the multi-disciplinary clinical team. The problems of developing a model for teamwork spring from the same complex roots as organizational theory, and individuals in the same ward are apt to have different views about how best to work with other people.

Teamwork aims to manage complex relationships between staff and between staff and patients. Collaboration between colleagues in a ward, and liaison between colleagues within and outside a ward are often conducted through working groups, and all team members need to be trained and experienced in aspects of group dynamics in order that they may prevent group processes from interfering with the accomplishment of tasks. A number of models of group dynamics range from Bion's theory of basic assumptions to Heron's categories of intervention (Bion 1961, Heron 1986). Given the existence of such theories and available training, teams have a clear responsibility to make decisions on leadership; to make group norms explicit; to delineate the structure and function of different groups; to make tasks and goals explicit; and to agree on ways of managing conflict.

The quality of teamwork in the organization interconnects with the ways in which it manages information, whether face to face in meetings and 'hand-overs', or in writing in reports and record-keeping. Secrecy and withholding are commonly used strategies of controlling information in order to reinforce authority. On the other hand, diffuse oral sharing of information appears to reinforce democratic working relationships. Both tendencies impair the safe transmission of relevant material.

CARING ACTIVITIES

Pembrey (1980) used the work of Jaques (1956), Brown (1960) and Burns & Stalker (1961) in an innovative analysis of the processes of nursing in general hospital wards. She found that the management of nursing work (the 'daily management cycle') was made especially difficult where ward sisters neither had autonomy over management activities nor perceived the relevance of management to nursing care. The daily management cycle comprised nursing rounds of patients, prescribing work to nurses, and receiving reports from nurses on the work delegated to them. Pembrey found that where the daily management cycle was completed, her criteria for individualized patient care were fulfilled (Pembrey 1980). Pembrey's work strongly influenced the revival by King Edward's Hospital Fund of London of its ward sister training scheme, evaluated by Allen (1982). This scheme categorized the role of the ward sister under four headings: management of patient care; teaching; ward management; personnel management. Management of patient care in this chapter will be discussed under Pembrey's (1980) definition of the 'daily management cycle', consisting of nursing rounds, prescribing work, and accountability reports.

Daily management cycle

Nursing rounds of patients

In the psychiatric ward 'rounds' are out of place. Yet the principle — that the charge nurse has daily face-to-face contact with all the patients in the ward — is not. While individualized direct patient care will be delegated to other nurses, and the charge nurse will largely be engaged in indirect and associated patient care, she is responsible for supervision of work, and so needs to have a working knowledge of individual patients that is derived from a personal relationship. How the charge nurse accomplishes this is a matter of the philosophy of a given ward. One strategy is to hold regular groups conducted or facilitated by the charge nurse, preferably focused on practical issues, providing a supportive atmosphere without coercing patients to attend (Vaglum et al 1985, Ritter 1989). Given a demonstrable commitment by the charge nurse to attend reliably, these groups can become a forum for monitoring patients' satisfaction with their care and with the ward environment, assessing progress and mental states, and forming an impression of the quality of nurses' care.

Prescribing work

In a ward where primary nursing is used to deliver care, prescription of work necessarily leaves a margin of discreation for individual nurses. Jaques's theory of 'discretionary content' of work was touched on in the earlier discussion on decision-making (Jaques 1956). Jaques developed from his theory of discretionary content a complex model in which the 'potential capacity of [an] individual' is correlated with the 'level of work he can achieve' as measured by 'time-span' ('the length of time for which [individuals] are able to tolerate the effects of exercising discretion on their own account in pursuit of a living') (p. 90). Jaques has developed this theory further (Jaques et al 1978), but as a whole, it has not received wide acceptance (Gray 1976).

Planning meetings

However, the concept of discretion has heuristic value, as Pembrey (1980) has shown, in discussing the work of nurses. Part of the charge nurse's responsibility is negotiating with nurses the amount of discretion each nurse can exercise in his or her work with patients, which is, in its turn, negotiated with the patients concerned. Thus at the beginning of a shift a nurse may discuss with a patient his or her current care plan in order to determine what activities will occupy them that day, before meeting with the nurse-in-charge and other nurses on duty to agree a general plan of work.

Nursing process

The following diagram (Fig. 24.2) of learning outcomes for the nursing process illustrates the levels of skill (thereby increasing the discretionary content of their work) through which psychiatric nurses may be expected to progress. Benner (1984) provides another way of conceptualizing the same issues. She uses the notion of discretionary judgement to distinguish between novice and expert nurses. Expert nurses are able to respond to risk-laden situations with 'orderly, reasonable behaviour' without reference to the rules and procedures upon which novice nurses depend.

Primary nursing in a psychiatric ward has to be based on sound case management skills. From a carefully documented adherence to the sequence of assessment, planning implementation and evaluation, under close supervision, the nurse progresses to a flexible implementation of goals which can be changed in response to constraints and unpredicted changes, as well as emergencies. In the first place there is little discretion about the means of devising and achieving the goals of nursing care. In the second, there is a good deal of discretion.

Accountability reports

Pembrey (1980) observed that there was very little attempt by ward sisters to obtain reports from nurses on the work they were prescribed. Essentially, such a report is an account of the nurse's exercise

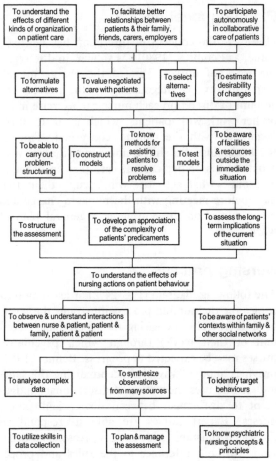

Fig. 24.2 Clinical learning outcomes for the psychiatric nursing process.

of discretion. However, in the absence of evaluative data it is not clear, firstly how this account is normally rendered, secondly how it is best rendered, and thirdly whether it has any relation to patient outcome. Nevertheless, it seems likely that failure to monitor nurses' use of discretionary judgement will miss those nurses whose capacity (whether for reasons of education or training) for discretion is insufficient, and who are thereby put under stress, and who thereby endanger patients' safety. There is speculation that increasing rates of suicide among inpatients is linked with the use of inexperienced or unqualified staff for the nursing of suicidal patients: that is, staff who are given discretion beyond their capacity (Hessö 1977).

Pitfalls in managing nursing work

Psychiatric nurses see themselves as to some extent 'living with' patients, sharing everyday activities such as talking, shopping, watching television or playing games. The ebb and flow of daily life may, as has been suggested, be tackled in different ways. Towards one end of what seems to be a continuum is the kind of therapeutic milieu where structure is valued as a means of opening participants' eyes to the dynamic process of social interaction and to the links with psychodynamics. Staff and patients are strongly differentiated. Timetabled groups or individual sessions are used to explore the internal world of patients as it is played out in the social context of the ward (Rapoport 1960). Towards the other end of the continuum is the setting where spontaneity and non-differentiation of staff and patients are valued as means of getting alongside or into the patient's world and, by directly sharing, contributing to the problem-solving abilities of the patient. However, beyond each of these trends, at one end of the continuum is the rigidly structured environment where the timetable and the booked activities are ends in themselves, where flexibility is absent and where the structure has become reified. At the other end, the undifferentiated tangle characteristic of therapeutic communities in collapse has resulted from the staff's inability or unwillingness to intervene to shift the direction of the community's activities (Baron 1987).

It was suggested earlier that nurses' motivations in choosing particular ways of working have less to do with patients than with their own feelings of comfort or discomfort (Berry & Metcalf 1985). Psychiatric hospitals have traditionally been characterized by 'rigid structures of treatment' (Leuschner 1985). If a ward abandons these structures in an attempt, say, to apply psychosocial principles of management, the staff are apt to be threatened by an upsurge of conflict within the unit, as tensions are openly expressed. One way of dealing with this conflict is by a Messianic impulse to convert the rest of the institution. Conflict with the parent institution ensues, and serves temporarily to distract attention from conflicts within the ward. However, the tensions become so intolerable that new bureacratic structures are introduced to manage them. These new structures form another 'protective bureaucracy' (Kernberg 1980 p. 231) which performs a similar function to the traditional bureaucratic structures of psychiatric hospitals (Leuschner 1985).

Another way of dealing with conflict between staff and between staff and patients is often demonstrated in the kind of handover which extends beyond the time allocated for it, and which concentrates on a minority of patients of the total in the ward or department. This spilling over the time boundaries suppresses open conflict whose consequences are feared disproportionately.

Vaglum et al (1985) identify similar processes at work in staff–patient groups in wards where milieu therapy is the philosophy. In an attempt to identify the variables that lead to poor outcomes for patients, they suggest there there is a phenomenon which they call 'pseudo-groups' and which are characterized by a high level of confrontation, a high level of compulsion to attend (which does not necessarily lead to high attendance levels), by an absence of practically oriented interventions, and by a low level of perceived support (Vaglum et al 1985).

The one-to-one relationship of nurse and patient can be very disturbing. If explained by reference to psychoanalytic concepts, it will be seen in terms mainly of the primitive defences used by the patient. These defences include acting-out of unconscious conflicts, concrete thinking, primary process thinking, projective identification, multiple transference, repetition compulsion and other forms of confusion of past and present. These defences lead the patient to behave in ways appropriate to the experience, but not to the reality of his or her situation (Rycroft 1968, Lego 1980, Jackson 1988). A protective bureacracy evolves partly as an institutional defence which is so successful that its original purpose (of escaping from the close contact with psychotic mental processes and primitive psychological defences of patients) is obscured (Leuschner 1985, Hinshelwood 1987).

CONCLUSION

The discussion in this chapter has been based on 12 aspects of organizing inpatient care. The pitfalls which have just been described are a natural hazard of the work — they arise from the very nature of the enterprise. It is clear that the 12 aspects discussed cannot have equal effect on the outcomes of care, although the contribution of each is difficult to quantify, and in a systems approach it is assumed that the whole is greater than the sum of its parts. Nevertheless, if the processes of decision-making, quality assurance, personnel procedures, information management and teamwork are working satisfactorily, it is likely that the whole system will be working satisfactorily.

REFERENCES

Allen H O 1982 The ward sister: role and preparation. Baillière Tindall, London
Argyris C, Schön D 1978 What is an organization that it may learn? Addison-Wesley, Reading, Mass
Arscott P, Armstrong M 1976 An employer's guide to health and safety management. Kegan Paul, London
Baldwin S 1985 Effect of furniture rearrangement on the atmosphere of wards in a maximum-security hospital. Hospital and Community Psychiatry 38 (5): 525–528
Baron C 1987 Asylum to anarchy. Free Association Books, London
Benner P 1984 From novice to expert. Addison-Wesley, Menlo Park, Calif
Beer S 1967 Management science. Aldus Books, London
Berry A J, Metcalf C L 1985 Paradigms and practices: organization of the delivery of nursing care. Journal of Advanced Nursing 11 (5): 589–597
Bignell V, Fortune J 1984 Understanding systems failures. Manchester University Press, Manchester
Bion W 1961 Experiences in groups. Tavistock, London
Blois M S 1984 Information and Medicine. University of California Press, Berkeley, Calif
Bradley G 1989 Computers and the psychosocial work environment. Taylor & Francis, London
Brazier M 1987 Medicine, patients and the law. Penguin, Harmondsworth
Bright J A 1985 A critique of methods for determining nurse staffing levels in hospital. DHSS Operational Research Service, London
Brown W 1960 Exploration in management. Heinemann, London

Burns T, Stalker G M 1961 The management of innovation. Tavistock, London

Carter R et al 1984 Systems, management and change. Harper & Row, London

Consumers Association 1978 A report on NHS complaints procedures. Consumers Association, London

Crammer J L 1984 The special characteristics of suicide in hospital in-patients. British Journal of Psychiatry 145: 465–476

De la Cuesta 1983 The nursing process: from development to implementation. Journal of Advanced Nursing 8: 365–371

DHSS 1980 Organizational and management problems of mental illness hospitals. Department of Health & Social Security, London

Donabedian A 1966 Evaluating the quality of medical care. Milbank Memorial Fund Quarterly 44 (2): 166–203

Essock-Vitale S 1987 Patient characteristics predictive of treatment costs on in-patient psychiatric wards. Hospital and Community Psychiatry 38 (3): 263–269

Forshaw D, Roscoe J J 1988 Personal communication

Gray J L (ed) 1976 The glacier project: concepts and principles. Crane Russak, New York

The Health and Safety at Work etc Act 1974 c 37

Heron J 1986 Six category intervention analysis. University of Surrey, Guildford

Hessö R 1977 Suicide in Norwegian, Finnish and Swedish psychiatric hospitals. Archiv für Psychiatrie und Nervenkrankheiten 224: 119–127

Hill J M M 1956 The time-span of discretion in job analysis. Human Relations 9 (3): 295–323

Hinshelwood R 1987 What happens in groups. Free Association Books, London

Hooper D F 1962 Changing the milieu in a psychiatric ward. Human Relations 15 (2): 111–122

Jackson M 1988 Psychiatry, psychodynamics and psychotherapy. Bronderslev Psykoteraputische Workshop, Denmark

Jaques E 1956 Measurement of responsibility. Tavistock, London

Jaques E, Gibson R O, Isaac D J (eds) 1978 Levels of abstraction in logic and human action. Heinemann, London

Kernberg O 1980 Internal world, external reality. Aronson, New York

Kitson A 1986 Standards of care in psychiatric nursing. Nursing Times 82 (52): 51–54

Leavitt H J, Dill W R, Eyring H B 1973 The organizational world. Harcourt Brace Jovanovich, New York

Lego S 1980 The one-to-one nurse–patient relationship. Perspectives in Psychiatric Care 18 (2): 67–89

Leuschner W 1985 Psychiatrische Anstalten — ein institutionalisiertes Abwehrsystem Teil 1. Psychiatrische Praxis12 (4): 111–115

Levin G et al 1976 The dynamics of human service delivery. Ballinger, Cambridge, Mass

Lockett M, Spear R S (eds) 1980 Organizations as systems. Open University Press, Milton Keynes

Marker C G 1988 The marker model for nursing standards: implications for nursing administration, Nursing Administration Quarterly 12 (2): 4–12

Mason E J 1984 How to write meaningful nursing standards. Wiley, New York

Mayo E 1933 (1966) The human problems of an industrial civilization. Viking, New York

The Mental Health Act 1983. c 20

Miller A 1984 Nurse/patient dependency — a review of different approaches with particular reference to studies of the dependency of elderly patients. Journal of Advanced Nursing 9: 479–486

National Consumer Council 1983 Patients' rights. HMSO, London

O'Brien G 1986 The intuitive method of patient dependency. Nursing Times 82 (8): 57–61

Open Systems Group 1981 Systems behaviour. Harper & Row, London

Owens R G, Ashcroft J B 1985 Violence: a guide for the caring professions. Croom Helm, Beckenham

Paton R et al 1984 Organizations: cases, issues, concepts. Harper & Row, London

Pembrey S 1980 The ward sister — key to nursing. Royal College of Nursing, London

Proctor S 1989 The functioning of nursing routines in the management of a transient workforce. Journal of Advanced Nursing 14: 180–189

Rapoport R N 1960 Community as doctor. Tavistock, London

Ritter S 1981 Ward Objectives. Unpublished project paper

Ritter S 1989 Bethlem Royal and Maudsley Hospital Manual of clinical psychiatric nursing principles and procedures. Harper & Row, London

Rix G 1987 Staff sickness and its relationship to violent incidents on a regional secure unit. Journal of Advanced Nursing 12: 223–228

Roethlisberger J F, Dickson W 1939 Management and the worker. Harvard University Press, Cambridge, Mass

Rycroft C 1968 A critical dictionary of psychoanalysis. Penguin, Harmondsworth

Schwartz S 1982 Is there a schizophrenia language? Behavioural and Brain Sciences 5: 579–626

Sclafani M 1986 Violence and behaviour control. Journal of Psychosocial Nursing and Mental Health Services 24 (11): 8–13

Searles H 1965 Collected papers on schizophrenia and related subjects. Hogarth Press, London

Sinclair L 1987 Proper channels: a practical guide to complaints about medical treatment. MIND, London

Snyder S 1986 Drugs and the brain. Scientific American Library, New York

Statutory Instrument 873 1983 (The Nurses Rules). HMSO, London

Stegne L 1978 A positive approach to negative behaviour. Canadian Nurse 74(6): 44–48

Strauss J S, Carpenter W T, Bartko J J 1974 Speculations on the processes that underlie schizophrenic symptoms and signs. Schizophrenia Bulletin 1(11): 61–75

Sullivan H S 1953 The interpersonal theory of psychiatry. Norton, New York

Taylor E, Rutter M 1985 Sex differences in neurodevelopmental and psychiatric disorders: one explanation or many? Behavioural and Brain Sciences 8: 460

Turner T 1987 Rich and mad in Victorian England. In: Murray R M, Turner T H (eds) 1990 Lectures on the history of psychiatry: The Squibb series. Gaskell, London

UKCC 1985 The administration of medicines (Circular no. PC/88/05). United Kingdom Central Council for Nursing and Midwifery, London

Vaglum P, Friis S, Karterud S 1985 Why are the results of milieu therapy for schizophrenic patients contradictory? Yale Journal of Biology and Medicine 58 (4): 349–381

Wing J K 1982 Handbook of psychiatry psychoses of uncertain aetiology, vol 3. Cambridge University Press, Cambridge

Wing J K, Brown G W 1970 Institutionalism and schizoprenia. Oxford University Press

Yalom I D 1983 Inpatient group psychotherapy. Basic Books, New York

Zuboff S 1988 In the age of the smart machine. Heinemann, Oxford

25

Day care

M. F. Muijen

Day care is an essential component of community care, ideally providing structured and individualized care close to the client's home. It bridges the gap between the institutional setting of an inpatient unit and the often inadequate support of an outpatient clinic. Three distinct groups of day-care users can be distinguished:

1. patients suffering from a serious mental illness, attending day hospitals as an alternative to inpatient care
2. patients suffering from mild to moderate neurotic disorders, attending day hospitals as an alternative to outpatient care, and
3. the long-term mentally ill, who attend day hospital or day centres for support and prevention of further deterioration.

However, among these three groups, many patients are unsuitable for treatment in a day-care setting. Some may need admission to an inpatient unit (a) because of severity of symptoms, (b) because they are a danger to themselves or others, or (c) because they need further assessment. For others day care may be unnecessary or even contraindicated, and outpatient or home care may have to be considered (a) because the symptoms are too mild, (b) because of the risk of dependency or (c) because of family needs.

The limitations of inpatient and outpatient care

are also well recognized (Bierer 1951). Disadvantages of inpatient care include:

1. the stigma of the mental hospital
2. the development of institutionalization
3. separation from the home environment
4. the lack of transferability of skills acquired in the hospital to the home, and
5. the high cost.

The two main disadvantages of outpatient treatment are:

1. the treatment offered is often inadequate, and
2. the lack of day-time support.

Several important issues will be examined in this chapter, such as organizational patterns, the efficacy of day care for different patient groups, and the demands on staff.

HISTORICAL DEVELOPMENT OF DAY HOSPITALS AND DAY CENTRES

The National Health Service Act of 1946 allocated the responsibility for treatment to the Ministry of Health, while prevention, care and after-care had to be provided by the local authorities (Editorial 1987). Since then a split has existed between day hospitals, which are financed by the health service, and day centres, which are financed by the local authorities.

The first day hospital in Britain was opened in 1946 (Bierer 1951), offering a variety of therapies ranging from individual, group and occupational therapy to treatments such as ECT. Antipsychotic drugs were only marketed 10 years later. It is interesting that it also offered 'social club therapy', which was considered enough of a contradiction to warrant a somewhat defensive statement: 'The social club is part of the day hospital and no day hospital is complete without it. The therapeutic social club can, however, exist without a day hospital and can serve on its own many useful purposes' (Bierer 1951).

Day hospitals increased gradually in number, even before the 1959 Mental Health Act which stimulated the move towards community care (Farndale 1961, Vaughan 1985).

'The Hospital Plan for England and Wales' (Ministry of Health 1962) suggested relatively small-scale psychiatric units. 'As the majority of patients in such a unit will not require nursing in bed, their treatment and rehabilitation proceed more favourably if they can go in and out of hospital during the day and so participate in the various activities of the general community.' It was expected that these combined inpatient and day hospital units would lead to the closure of many large mental hospitals.

Although the number of day hospitals continued to grow in the following decades, their aims diversified, and day hospitals took on varying roles (Vaughan 1985), often based on local needs and initiatives. The relative under-utilization of their potential was illustrated by the number of places in England in 1974 (Table 25.1): 11 200 day hospital places as compared with 104 400 hospital beds (Audit Commission 1986).

Table 25.1 Progress to White Paper targets for mentally ill people (England only) (from Audit Commission 1986)

	1974	1984	Target	Progress to target %
Hospital (available beds)	104 400	78 900	47 900	45
Residential places (local authority, private and voluntary)	3 500	6 800	11 500	41
Day hospital places	11 200	17 000	45 800	17
Day centre places (local authority and voluntary)	5 400	9 000	28 200	16

Day centres, meanwhile, had not been established in any number, in spite of recognition of their essential role in after-care (Farndale 1961). As the distinction between day centres and day hospitals had been tenuous from the outset, many functions were taken on by the day hospital. From 1971, since the creation of the local authority social services departments, the number of day centres began to increase noticeably (Vaughan 1985). However, only 5 400 places were available in 1974 (Table 25.1).

Only in 1975 with the publication of 'Better Services for the Mentally Ill' (DHSS 1975) was the philosophy of community care put into practice with the provision of target numbers for hospital beds and day-care places and a description of their role within the general psychiatric service. The Report distinguishes between day-care places as part of the inpatient unit — half of which should be used by inpatients, the other places being filled by patients attending the unit on a daily basis (0.65 places per 1000 population) — and a separate day hospital serving the local community (0.3 places per 1000 population).

The emphasis of day hospitals is clearly on treatment. In contrast, the objective of day centres is to alleviate the need for shelter, occupation and social activity. It is recognized that for some clients day care will lead to eventual discharge, while for others day-care attendance is a long-term need which may prevent institutionalization. Day centres should be easily accessible within the community, and ought to receive multi-disciplinary input, including input from nurses and psychiatrists. The planning figures for day-centre places are 0.6 places per 1000 of the population.

Since the publication of 'Better Services for the Mentally Ill' (DHSS 1975) the psychiatric services have gradually become more community based. Unfortunately, the reduction in the number of hospital beds has not been compensated for by an increase in day places, which means that some discharged patients are unlikely to receive adequate care. (Table 25.1). The number of hospital beds has been reduced by 25 500, but day places have only increased by just under 9000 (Audit Commission 1986).

These national figures, low as they are, hide local variations. The mean number of day places for chronic patients in units serving 56% of the Scottish population was 0.15 per 1000 of the local population, but the range was 0 to 0.4 per 1000! (McCreadie et al 1984). Even more worrying was the lack of correlation between the number of hospital beds and community facilities in the UK (Hirsch 1988), suggesting poor coordination of planning and an inequality of services.

A concerted effort between the health services and local authorities is required to provide an acceptable quality of day care, the more so because of the increasing dependence of psychiatric patients on these services as a consequence of the gradual closure of many large mental hospitals.

PATTERNS OF USE OF DAY CARE

It might be expected that day hospitals would serve a more acutely ill and more disturbed group of clients than day centres and that clients would attend for a relatively short period before returning to their pre-morbid roles or receiving rehabilitation in day centres. This does not seem to be the case. Day hospitals and day centres are often very similar, both providing care for the chronically mentally ill. About half the clients tend to be diagnosed as suffering from schizophrenia. Attendance can vary from a day a month to 5 days a week, with a somewhat higher turnover in day hospitals than in day centres. More than half the clients at day centres but less than one third of the day hospital patients in a large national survey had attended for over 2 years (Edwards & Carter 1980).

Several factors are positively correlated with duration and frequency of attendance, such as older age, duration of illness and treatment and length of unemployment (McGrath & Tantam 1987). This suggests that chronic patients make the most intensive use of day care, which seems appropriate, provided that over-dependency of patients and lack of flexibility in care can be avoided.

Unfortunately, this lack of flexibility can be present in day care. It is rare for clients to be referred from day hospital to day centres. Reasons for referral to one service or the other are less as a result of client characteristics than of professional background of the referrer. Psychiatrists, general practitioners and community psychiatric nurses tend to refer to day hospitals, while social workers tend to refer to day centres (Teasdale 1987).

The characteristics of clients selected for day care will depend to a large degree on the setting of the centre. In inner cities a high proportion of people suffering from schizophrenia or living in deprived circumstances can be expected. Day hospitals connected to large mental hospitals treat older and more chronic patients who attend for many years, while day hospitals at district general hospitals cater for younger patients with neurotic conditions (Gath et al 1973).

A major issue in day care is the high drop-out rate which can be as much as 50% after the first visit (Baekland & Lundwall 1975). This may be due to the limitations of the service or to patient characteristics. If day care does not offer the range of interventions the patient expects, he is unlikely to return. The severely mentally ill can be put at great risk as a consequence of dropping out of treatment, which is easier in day care than as an inpatient. Outreach, including home visits, may limit this, but is not a widely available component of day care. Another essential service is transport, without which the long-term mentally ill are particularly unlikely to attend (Lamb 1979).

Patient characteristics which predict drop-out from day care are depression and low self-esteem, a diagnosis of personality disorder, living in a hostel and poor employment history. Age, sex, a diagnosis of psychosis and chronicity of illness are not related (Bender & Pilling 1985). This means that a vulnerable group which could benefit from day-care facilities remains isolated and may be lost to psychiatric services. Assertive attempts to engage this group, especially at the first few visits, could improve attendance and clinical outcome.

EFFICACY OF DAY CARE

Day care is not a homogeneous treatment, but a form of care with many variations for different groups of clients in different settings. As a consequence, no simple statement can be made about efficacy. Before conclusions can be drawn from the various evaluative studies, criteria such as what care was provided for whom, leading to what results must be established in each case. For example, a study on intensive day hospital care for agoraphobics in a rural area provides no answer to the question of whether day care can offer an alternative to hospital care for a psychotic population in an inner city.

Three groups of studies need to be distinguished:

1. day hospital care as an alternative to hospital care
2. day hospital care as an alternative to outpatient care
3. the efficacy of day care in the maintenance of chronic mentally ill patients.

Day care as an alternative to hospital care

Studies evaluating the feasibility of treating patients with a mental illness in a day-care setting took place as early as the late 1950s, coinciding with the emergence of psychotropic drugs (e.g. Craft 1958, Smith & Cross 1957). In these studies patients suffering from neurotic conditions who were not considered to be a risk to themselves but considered to be in need of intensive psychiatric care, were allocated to day care. A control group was selected from matched inpatients. Little difference in outcome was found between the two groups, although the day-care group had a briefer follow-up period and made a slightly better adjustment after 12 months. Whether this was a genuine advantage of day care or a result of selecting patients with a better prognosis for day care is unclear and is an inherent disadvantage of retrospective matching of groups. A more valid method is the process of randomization in which patients who fulfil the entry criteria are allocated blindly to the two treatment conditions at the start of the study. This tends to be the design used in more recent research, although one study compared day care available to patients from one area with a matched control group from a neighbouring area which did not possess day-care facilities (Michaux et al 1973).

All these studies indicated that day care is a valid alternative to hospital care for a significant group of patients, but not for all. Two American studies (Herz et al 1971, Wilder et al 1966) found that about 40% of all seriously mentally ill patients admitted to an inpatient unit could be cared for in a day hospital setting without further need of inpatient care. Half those patients had been diagnosed as suffering from schizophrenia. In the UK the emphasis has been on the potential of day care in the treatment of neurotic disorders. Again, about 50% of emergency admissions could be transferred to day hospital care (Dick et al 1985a).

When clinical and social outcomes were compared, psychopathology was not strikingly different at the end of the treatment phase or at follow-up, but social functioning had improved significantly more in the day-care group and remained at a higher level at follow-up, even a year after discharge (Michaux et al 1973). In a similar study, patients in the day-care group managed to stay out of further contact with the psychiatric services for longer periods than the inpatients, and had a lower readmission rate (Herz et al 1971).

These results argue strongly in favour of an expanded role for day care, but have to be interpreted cautiously. Not all patient groups benefited equally from day hospital care. For example, patients suffering from schizophrenia may gain most from an initial period in hospital followed by day care, while the advantage of day care for affective and neurotic disorders is much stronger (Wilder et al 1966, Michaux et al 1973, Dick et al 1985a).

Patients for whom day care is not deemed to be suitable are those with very disturbed or suicidal behaviour, alcohol or drug abuse, physical problems or those patients whose relatives demand admission (Dick et al 1985a, Herz et al 1971). Other factors indicating inpatient care rather than day care are older age, a diagnosis of schizophrenia and a perceived lack of social support (Bowman et al 1983). Interestingly, the most powerful determinant of place of care is not clinical factors but the preference of the psychiatrist (Platt et al 1980). This confirms the idea that new forms of treatment need powerful advocacy before they will be adopted as they will have to replace trusted and familiar interventions.

An important advantage of day care is that both clients (Dick et al 1985a) and their relatives (Michaux et al 1973) prefer it. This is likely to mean higher compliance, and may be an important factor in achieving good treatment results. In addition, cost effectiveness studies indicate that day hospital treatment is significantly less expensive than inpatient care (Fink et al 1978, Dick et al 1985a).

In summary, day care can offer an alternative to hospital care for patients with a serious mental illness. It appears at least as effective, is appreciated by patients and relatives, and offers good value for money. However, a substantial group of patients require inpatient care. Day care and hospital care should be considered as complementary rather than antagonistic and mutually exclusive.

Day care as an alternative to outpatient care

Day hospitals can provide more intensive treatment than an outpatient setting, and if this leads to a faster and more persistent improvement in symptoms and functioning, the inherently higher costs of day care can be justified. However, according to a study by Tyrer et al (1987), this does not always seem to be the case. Patients suffering from repressive, phobic or anxiety neuroses were randomly allocated to day hospital treatment or outpatient care, and no consistent differences between the groups were found after 4 months, 8 months and 24 months (Tyrer et al 1987).

Although this suggests that day hospitals have no role in the treatment of mild to moderately neurotic patients, this may be an oversimplification. It is possible that patients with specific conditions can benefit from day care and further studies are required, as well as a replication of Tyrer's work.

The efficacy of day care in the maintenance of chronic mentally ill patients

The gradual closure of hospital beds has resulted in an increasing number of people with long-term mental illness living in the community. This is a very vulnerable group often living in deprived circumstances either alone or with an older relative. They tend to have little initiative and poor social skills and, as a consequence, can be easily neglected (Lamb 1979). The majority of people attending day centres and also many day hospitals fall within this category. The aims of attendance are maintenance and rehabilitation rather than cure, although the distinction is somewhat artificial, as successful maintenance will prevent deterioration and consequently preclude the need for further hospital admissions.

Unfortunately, facilities for this group are often poorly coordinated and lacking in provision. The organization of day care is not always based on the needs of the local community, and the referral and attendance of patients is often determined by availability rather than suitability (Dick et al 1985b). A survey of day-care facilities found deficiencies in leisure activities, a lack of emphasis on rehabilitation and inadequate support of relatives (Wing 1982). This is probably partly due to a lack of flexibility in the programmes of many facilities, which require a regular attendance and continuing involvement in activities which demand either too high a degree of assertiveness or too low a level of stimulation. Individualized treatment objectives are required, but are difficult to implement because of the pressure on staff. Some day centres allowed patients to use the centre as a social meeting place, and the value of this for patients is expressed by an improvement in attendance. Staff can be reluctant to let people attend in this unstructured way because of their fear of creating dependence in patients, and a choice has to be made between this risk of dependency and the risk of neglect if patients stop visiting.

Programmes not only affect attendance but also outcome, although very little research has been done in this area. Milne (1984) compared two neighbouring day hospitals with similar staffing levels and chronicity of patients, but differences in their approaches: one offered therapeutic activities of a directive, behavioural kind; the other had a non-directive, social interaction programme. Only the problem-solving, behavioural programme proved effective, although to a

limited extent, as would be expected with this difficult patient group.

The combination of day care with home care may be of particular advantage to the long-term mentally ill. Many of the skills acquired in day hospitals or centres do not transfer to the home, and some additional sessions at home could compensate for this. Home visits also increase the attendance at day-care facilities (Beard et al 1978). Home care has been evaluated against day care. Patients were referred at random to either an assertive outreach programme, with an average of twice weekly home visits, or to a drop-in centre (Bond 1987). Patients in the outreach programme had significantly fewer readmissions and days in hospital. However, this could be due to the poor quality of care and the lack of follow-up in the drop-in centre. After-care is important for the long-term mentally ill and reduces relapse (Kirk 1976, Winston et al 1977). But outreach alone did not improve the quality of life as compared with the drop-in centre. The combination of good day care and active outreach seems to be optimal.

STAFF ORGANIZATION

Day hospitals, being part of the National Health Service, are more medically orientated than day centres, which are funded by social services. Surveys have found major differences in programmes, staff employed and facilities, not only between day hospitals and day centres, but also within these services (Edwards & Carter 1980). An illustration is a comparison of two day hospitals in Nottingham (Tyrer et al 1987). The first was a specialized day hospital with a psychotherapeutic orientation, treating neurotic patients. The unit consisted of six beds and 10 day-patient places. It was staffed by a part-time senior psychiatrist, two trainee psychiatrists, a part-time psychologist and three nurses. The second unit, more typical of day hospitals, had an eclectic orientation, accepting a maximum of 40 patients suffering from a range of conditions, and was staffed by one psychiatrist, a trainee psychiatrist, a part-time psychologist and four nurses. It is interesting that outcomes were similar for the neurotic patients in spite of all the variations.

In general, day hospitals are staffed mainly by psychiatric nurses, with some occupational therapists, a clinical psychologist and a trainee psychiatrist. A consultant psychiatrist usually visits once or twice weekly in an advisory role. Social workers are often, but not always, part of the multi-disciplinary team. Staff–patient ratios are about 1 to 15.

Day centres are less predictable in their staffing, but generally include a clinical psychologist, occupational therapists, a social worker and psychiatric nurses; but there are proportionally fewer members of staff than in day hospitals and often some of them are unqualified. Medical input is rare and staff–patient ratios can be as low as 1 to 40.

Nurses occupy a central role in day care. Not only do they form the majority of staff in most day hospitals, but also they often have the most intensive contact with patients. Consistent with this is the finding that clients rated their therapeutic relationship with the nursing staff higher than their relationship with the doctor or social worker (Ferguson & Carney 1970). This puts demands on nursing staff, and specific skills need to be incorporated into their training to prepare them for their role in day care (Teasdale 1987).

The skills required for day care are listed in the following headings.

Assessment of patients

Staff have to decide whether patients are appropriate for the facility, and what services will be of benefit to them. An adequate knowledge of the presentation of psychiatric conditions is essential.

Treatment planning

The most effective form seems to be a problem-solving approach (Milne 1984). This means that the client's problems are defined, preferably as agreed with the client. Goals are set, and interventions selected which aim to achieve those goals. After a period of time the outcome is evaluated, and if required, new problems and goals can be added and interventions can be changed. It is a common misunderstanding that a problem-solving approach implies behavioural interventions only, probably because the problem-solving approach developed from behavioural treatment. However, problem-solving can be used for the planning of various interventions and treatment of most patients.

Application of treatment techniques

A wide range of approaches and therapies may be required, such as an individual or family approach, medical or rehabilitative therapy, psychotherapies or counselling.

Crisis intervention skills

Good use of these skills can prevent further deterioration and offer the opportunity for therapeutic interventions. However, staff are dealing with disturbed people who can be at risk, and close liaison with the patient's support system, including relatives, friends and GP is important.

Knowledge of local resources

Ideally resources are complementary and comprehensive, but this is rarely the case. The service can only function optimally if all health workers have a clear understanding of the system and if good collaboration exists. This should include the health service, local authority and voluntary services.

Understanding the potential and limitations of the long-term mentally ill

This is a group of patients requiring continuing effort, leading to limited gains. This can be very demoralizing, resulting in staff burn-out, unless the staff can take pride in maintaining the independence of those clients achieving objectively small goals over long periods (Stern & Minkoff 1979). Otherwise there is the risk that staff may begin to treat patients with minor rather than major psychiatric illnesses. A shift of interest can take place, and the chronic patients will be replaced by clients with relatively minor emotional problems who offer an opportunity for high status interventions such as family and marital therapy, with much personal gratification for the therapist (Langsley 1980).

No single individual or profession can expect to cover all the areas. Teamwork — relying on the skills of several different professions — is essential, with regular staff meetings to discuss treatment plans and allocate relevant tasks to team members, based on their interests and skills.

Teams in day hospitals and day centres are mostly multi-disciplinary. If functioning well, the various disciplines can complement each other, but frequently tensions arise, as each profession within a team regards itself as more important than it is thought to be by others (Watts & Bennett 1983). This is caused by a poor understanding of the skills other disciplines can contribute. More destructive can be inter-disciplinary rivalry, resulting in an unwillingness to accept that others possess skills unique to their background. A solution to this is regular staff support meetings, preferably with a facilitator, to discuss disagreements, and a continuing multi-disciplinary training programme at the day hospitals and day centres to foster good understanding of each other's potential.

The leadership role is central to the functioning of a team. Traditionally the leader in a psychiatric team was the consultant psychiatrist, but this is changing with the increasing independence of parts of the service, and day care has been in the forefront of this development.

Leadership is not a one dimensional role but consists of many functions which can be taken on by different members of the team (Watts & Bennett 1983). For example, the nurse manager may be responsible for organizing the staff and the budget, the psychologist for chairing the care plan meetings and the psychiatrist for supervising treatment. Leaders need to provide structure and support, and have to vary the degree of each, which will depend on the needs of the team. It is important that leaders are perceived as part of the team by sharing an involvement in the clinical work, rather than spending most of their time in meetings which seem to have little relevance to the clinicians. Leaders tend to be senior staff with

experience, and a clinical input will give them the opportunity to be a role model and to teach effective interventions.

Keyworker role

It is important for both clients and staff to know who is responsible for the care of specific patients. Clients can easily 'fall between the cracks of the service' unless someone coordinates their care. For example, an appointment card needs to be sent after discharge from hospital and this may have to be followed by a home visit in the case of non-attendance. Contacts may need to be made with the housing department and benefits provided if required; and the general practitioner needs feedback. From the client's perspective an identifiable, supportive staff member is a resource he can rely on in times of crisis, and this is likely to result in increased satisfaction and compliance. The staff member who takes this central place in the care of the patient is called the keyworker, a word which is gradually being replaced by its American equivalent 'case manager'.

According to Intagliata (1982), the functions of a keyworker are:

- to remain aware of the comprehensive needs of clients
- the coordination of services
- to monitor that services are provided
- a personal commitment to the patient, including advocacy.

Advantages of the keyworker system for patients are continuity of care, accessibility and efficiency. A consequence of the close and continuing contact between patient and staff member is the role modelling that case management offers. It is rational, integrative, individualized and uses problem-solving, all qualities of value to the long-term patient (Harris & Bergman 1987).

But this closeness between patient and staff is a two-edged sword. Dependency can easily develop, with patients reluctant to be seen by anyone but their own keyworker, not dissimilar to psychotherapeutic relationships. At times of staff holidays, and especially when the keyworker leaves the job, clients are at high risk of relapse.

Teams using the keyworker model tend to be very positive about this approach. Staff enjoy their responsibility and direct care involvement. However, this close involvement can become counter-productive if no progress seems to be made or if setbacks occur. Suicide in particular can be a severe personal trauma to staff who feel responsible for the care of the patient and who are likely to know the relatives and friends. As a result, case management can lead to the burn-out syndrome, characterized by lack of interest, tiredness and irritation.

For these reasons some sharing of tasks is important. Case management does not mean an exclusive relationship with a client, but means that one staff member is accountable for the implementation of the programme, the various parts of which can and should be allocated to different members of the team. This will not only alleviate the pressure on the keyworker, but also improve the quality of care and diminish the danger of burn-out.

CONCLUSION

With the growth of community care, increasing demands will be made on day care. The discharge of long-term patients from mental hospitals will continue. Many patients who were formerly admitted to hospital are now cared for in the community, and people who have made no demands on psychiatric services for fear of hospitalization will come forward. This chapter has illustrated that day care is capable of treating and supporting many of these potential clients, if only sufficient day hospitals and day centres were available, offering a range of activities suited to the varying needs of clients.

But the shift from hospital care to community care is not only structural, it will also require an investment in staff training. Nurses who have been working in institutions cannot be expected to transfer to working in day care without acquiring new skills. New demands will be made on them, and unless they are prepared for this, day care is unlikely to succeed.

It is surprising that day care has been implemented very cautiously in Britain. Studies indicate that it is effective, preferred by patients and relatives and good value for money. Factors which are likely to slow down the growth of day care are reluctance of clinicians and managers to change old habits and the absence of a network of services offering a comprehensive support system to clients living in the community. Day care cannot exist in isolation, and unless facilities like hostels, drop-in centres, and crisis units are established, coordinated by keyworkers, day care will not be able to fulfil its potential.

REFERENCES

Audit Commission for Local Authorities in England and Wales 1986 Making a reality of community care. HMSO, London

Baekland F, Lundwall L 1975 Dropping out of treatment, a critical review. Psychological Bulletin 82: 738–783

Beard J H, Malamud T J, Rossman E 1978 Psychiatric rehabilitation and long-term rehospitalization rates: the findings of two research studies. Schizophrenia Bulletin 4: 622–635

Bender M P, Pilling S 1985 A study of variables associated with under-attendance at a psychiatric day centre. Psychological Medicine 15: 395–401

Bierer J 1951 The day hospital. Lewis, London

Bond G 1987 A controlled study of the Thresholds Bridge, an assertive case management program. Presentation, American Psychological Association, New York

Bowman E P, Shelley R K, Sheehy Sheffington A, Simanan K 1983 Day patient versus inpatient: factors determining selection of acutely ill patients for hospital treatment. British Journal of Psychiatry 142: 584–587

Craft M 1958 An evaluation of treatment of depressive illness in a day hospital. Lancet ii: 149–151

Department of Health and Social Security 1975 Better services for the mentally ill. HMSO, London

Dick P, Cameron L, Cohen D, Barlow M, Ince A 1985a Day and full-time psychiatric treatment — a controlled comparison. British Journal of Psychiatry 147: 246–249

Dick P, Ince A, Barlow B 1985b Day treatment: suitability and referral procedure. British Journal of Psychiatry 147: 250–253

Editorial 1987 Psychiatric day hospitals for all. Lancet ii: 1184–1185

Edwards C, Carter J 1980 The data of day care. National Institute for Social Work, London

Farndale J 1961 The day hospital movement in Great Britain. Pergamon Press, Oxford

Ferguson R, Carney M 1970 Inter-personal considerations and judgments in a day hospital. British Journal of Psychiatry 117: 397–1103

Fink E B, Longabaugh R, Stout R 1978 The paradoxical under-utilization of partial hospitalization. American Journal of Psychiatry 135: 713–716

Gath D, Hassal C, Cross K W 1973 Whither psychiatric day care? A study of day patients in Birmingham. British Medical Journal i: 94–98

Harris M, Bergman H C 1987 Case management with the chronically mentally ill: a clinical perspective. American Journal of Orthopsychiatry 57: 296–302

Herz M I, Endicott J, Spitzer R L, Mesnikoff A 1971 Day versus inpatient hospitalization: a controlled study. American Journal of Psychiatry 127: 1371–1381

Hirsch S R 1988 Psychiatric beds and resources: factors influencing bed use and service planning. Royal College of Psychiatrists, Gaskell

Intagliata J 1982 Improving the quality of community care for the chronically mentally disabled: the role of case management. Schizophrenia Bulletin 8: 655–674

Kirk S A 1976 Effectiveness of community services for discharged mental hospital patients. American Journal of Orthopsychiatry 46: 646–659

Lamb H 1979 The new asylums in the community. Archives of General Psychiatry 36: 129–134

Langsley D G 1980 The Community Mental Health Centre: does it treat patients? Hospital and Community Psychiatry 31: 815–819

McCreadie R G, Robinson A D, Wilson A O A 1984 The Scottish survey of chronic day patients. British Journal of Psychiatry 145: 626–630

McGrath G, Tantam D 1987 Long-stay patients in a psychiatric day hospital: a casenote review. British Journal of Psychiatry 150: 836–890

Michaux M H, Chelst M R, Foster S A, Pruim R J, Dasinger E M 1973 Post-release adjustment of day and full-time psychiatric patients. Archives of General Psychiatry 29: 647–651

Milne D 1984 A comparative evaluation of two psychiatric day hospitals. British Journal of Psychiatry 145: 533–537

Ministry of Health 1962 A hospital plan for England and Wales. HMSO, London

Platt S D, Knights A C, Hirsch S R 1980 Caution and conservatism in the use of a psychiatric day hospital: evidence from a research project that failed. Psychiatry Research 3: 123–132

Smith S, Cross E G W 1957 Review of 1000 patients treated at a psychiatric day hospital. International Journal of Social Psychiatry 2: 292–298

Stern R, Minkoff K 1979 Paradoxies in programming for chronic patients in a community clinic. Hospital and Community Psychiatry 30: 613–617

Teasdale K 1987 Day services. In: Malin N (ed) Reassessing community care. Croom Helm, London

Tyrer P, Remington M, Alexander J 1987 The outcome of neurotic disorders after outpatient and day hospital care. British Journal of Psychiatry 151: 57–62

Vaughan P J 1985 Developments in psychiatric day care. British Journal of Psychiatry 147: 1–41

Watts F, Bennett D 1983 Management of the staff team. In: Watts F (ed) Psychiatric rehabilitation. Wiley, Chichester

Wilder J F, Levin G, Zwerling 1966 A two year follow-up evaluation of acute psychotic patients treated in a day hospital. American Journal of Psychiatry 122: 1095–1101

Wing J K 1982 Long-term community care: experience in a London borough. Psychological Medicine, Monograph Suppl. 2

Winston A, Parides H, Papernik D S, Breslin L 1977 After-care of psychiatric patients and its relation to rehospitalization. Hospital and Community Psychiatry 28: 118–121

26

Nursing in therapeutic communities

G. E. Chapman

The organization of care in a therapeutic community is concerned with recognizing the value of a normal domestic environment within which people with disturbances in mood or behaviour may develop trusting relationships with care workers out of which healthy mental functioning may develop. The different ways in which this is achieved will be the subject of this chapter.

The therapeutic community movement had its genesis this century in the ideas and discoveries of a group of army and civilian psychiatrists in the Second World War. However, the basic principles of therapeutic communities were understood and emerged earlier in the history of mental health care. Most writers in the field acknowledge this continuity of theme over the centuries (Brown & Pedder 1980, Clarke 1981, Kennard & Roberts 1983). It is helpful, therefore, firstly to outline the historical antecedents of the approach before discussing specific issues of nursing in therapeutic communities.

The chapter will take the following form: firstly the historical developments in the approach; secondly the current range, variation and characteristics of therapeutic communities in Great Britain; followed by evaluation studies; and finally a discussion about nursing in therapeutic communities.

HISTORICAL DEVELOPMENTS

Scull (1979) and Baruch & Treacher (1978) have noted that the care of the mentally ill prior to the middle of the 19th century was combined with ways of solving society's difficulties with a range of socially disadvantaged groups. The poor, disabled, unemployed and minor criminals were contained, together with the mad, in locally-based facilities. These included relief in the community, the local gaol or parish-funded, privately-owned 'madhouses'. Historians are agreed (Jones 1972, Scull 1979) that conditions within these small houses were degrading, repressive and cruel. Mostly, lunatics, as they were called, were physi-

---

Box 26.1 Types of therapeutic community

Genuine therapeutic community (Clarke)
Democratic/analytic (Kennard)

These are communities, such as the Henderson and the Cassel, where all the material and human resources in the hospital are actively engaged in the therapeutic programme. Usually sited in small residential buildings, the residents collaborate with staff in the day-to-day decision-making and running of the organization.

Therapeutic Milieu (Clarke)
Institutional (Kennard)

These are units in which some but not all aspects of the genuine therapeutic community have been used. The settings range from wards and small units in orthodox psychiatric settings (like the Atkinson Morley Hospital Unit), to units and departments in other social welfare settings. Patients and staff have less control over the domestic and administrative decision-making of the organization.

Social therapy (Clarke)
Concept-based therapy (Kennard)

Social relationships and social environments are the main focus of care. Settings range from voluntarily-run hostels, such as the Richmond Fellowship, to special hostels for alcoholics or drug addicts. Often residents have less control over the values which permeate the organization than the previous two.

---

cally restrained in chains or manacles. The occasional treatments consisted of purges, vomits and bleedings. The rationale for organizing custody in this way arose out of the ideologies, beliefs and values in society as a whole about human nature, and particular beliefs about how and why the insane behaved in ways which contradicted these ideas. The nature of these beliefs is complex, and detailed descriptions and analyses of society's perception of the mad and its relationship to broader social values can be found in Foucault (1967), Rothman (1971) and Szasz (1973).

As these values changed, in association with changes in the social organization of the economy, so attitudes to the insane changed. Social reformers, appalled by what they observed in the madhouses, were to influence the setting up of supervisory boards to monitor the care of the mad. By 1845 this led to a statutory requirement that local facilities should be provided for the care of pauper lunatics. Thus began the development and growth of the county asylums. The model of care upon which these asylums were originally based was that provided by Tuke, a Quaker. He established a hospice in York for the mad called The Retreat in 1792, following the death of a Quaker in a charity madhouse. Intended for only 30 residents, Tuke based the therapeutic programme on ideas pioneered by Pinel in Paris. Believing that much of the madness and deranged behaviour of the mad was directly attributable to the way in which they were cared for, he put into practice the principles of moral therapy. The 20th century heirs of these ideas were to be the founders of the modern therapeutic community ideal. Fears (1977) describes how Tuke replaced physical restraints with moral restraints, by organizing care which would appeal to and foster the insane's capacity to reason. This was achieved through purposeful work and social and educational activities in a normal domestic environment. It was felt that by stressing the value of work and discipline the insane would be better equipped to deal with the exigencies of social life outside the Retreat.

In Great Britain the attempt to base the county asylums on this model failed. Scull (1979) analyses the complex reasons for this failure. Firstly, the presence of institutions in which to put the mad led to increased numbers of people being diagnosed as such. This, together with the longer life span enjoyed by the mentally ill as a result of better treatment, led to overcrowding in the asylums. Furthermore, increasing medical dominance in the field stressing organic causation, together with medical failure to cure the insane, led to therapeutic pessimism and underfunding of the asylums. These factors contributed to the moral therapy movement lasting only about 50 years. The legacy of the failure was the large, overcrowded custodial 'warehouse for the mad' which stressed bureaucratic organization of patients' lives and the rigid doctor, nurse, patient hierarchies found in the asylums in the middle of the 20th century.

From the point of view of the emerging therapeutic community movement in the 1940s, the early advocates of moral therapy shared more than therapeutic optimism and a belief that planned social environments can be effective in ameliorating madness.

They challenged medical dominance in the field of insanity, arguing that professional medical expertise had not only produced abuses in care, but was unnecessary if care staff were selected on the basis of attitude and personality. Furthermore the early reformers believed that the newly emerging industrial society was the source of mental instability and its cure was to be found in mini-societies in which 'order, calm and productive work would replace the chaos and competitiveness of the new world' (Scull 1979 p. 17).

The institutions in which the pioneers of the 20th century therapeutic community approach worked still retained the custodial structure of the large asylums. By the 1940s, however, some classical research studies started to appear pointing to the damaging nature of the asylum. Goffman's (1970) description of the underlife of total institutions was based on an American asylum. In 1959 Barton published his material on institutional neurosis, arguing that the apathetic and withdrawn nature of the long-term mentally ill was a direct result of the way care was organized. It was, however, the Second World War which acted as a catalyst for the development of therapeutic communities in Britain. The American experience was slightly different. Bion, Foulkes and Main in Northfield Hospital, and separately Maxwell Jones in Belmont, developed ideas from different theoretical standpoints which were to influence institutional psychiatry for the next few decades.

Main and Maxwell Jones

Main coined the phrase 'therapeutic community' to describe the work he, together with Bion and Foulkes, achieved at the Northfield Military Hospital in Birmingham. Faced with poor morale amongst soldiers and staff, persistent absenteeism, and a high rate of returning late from leave, they devised ways to encourage soldiers to take on the responsibility themselves of solving these problems (Main 1946, 1980). Relinquishing his role of expert Main drew on the functioning capacities of soldiers to organize and be responsible for the daily events and programmes. A series of discussion groups and meetings supported this activity along with psychoanalytical group therapy sessions. Noting that some of these changes caused resentment and conflict amongst the staff, which he and the administrator were called upon to resolve, he began to realize how vital open communications were if the therapeutic programme was to be effective. Staff review meetings were set up to support an atmosphere of enquiry into differences of view and conflicts. Main stressed the importance of working with, not for, patients and developed means of increasing patient autonomy and participation in decision-making. To do this it became clear how important clarity of organizational structure and staff roles are. These ideas were taken with him when he became medical director of the Cassel Hospital in 1948, and together with the then matron it was developed as a therapeutic community in which psychotherapy was offered to troubled families and adults in the context of a social milieu facilitated and maintained by nursing staff. A post-registration training for nurses was established.

Maxwell Jones' ideas derived from his work with patients exhibiting 'effort syndrome' (Kennard & Roberts 1983). This is a condition where patients suffer palpitations, dizziness and breathlessness on exercise. These symptoms were a function of the anxiety which patients felt about cardiac problems. From his background in psychological and physiological research Maxwell Jones developed a series of lectures and discussion groups to explain to patients the physiological processes involved in their condition. This proved beneficial and soon patients began discussing and sharing this information with each other. Maxwell Jones took the idea, that sharing knowledge provided a valuable learning experience for patients, to the Belmont Hospital in 1947. There he developed a programme of socially-based therapy for behaviourally disturbed young people. In the following decades his name was to be associated with the therapeutic community movement as he took his ideas to Dingleton Hospital in Scotland, then America, and published a series of books and papers (Jones 1968). During his time at Belmont, later to be called the Henderson, a team of social scientists studied the way the therapeutic community functioned. Their findings, published by Rappoport (1960), have become synonymous with what are generally understood to be the characteristics of therapeutic communities. These will be discussed in the next section.

CHARACTERISTICS, RANGE AND DIVERSITY OF THERAPEUTIC COMMUNITIES

The therapeutic community approach was taken up by a range of organizations. The basic ideas have been modified and adapted to suit different client groups and differing types of institutional setting. Three writers, Clarke (1964) and Kennard & Roberts (1983), have provided typologies which describe this diversity. Clarke argues that there are three main types of therapeutic community, listed in Box 26.1; Kennard & Roberts' reformulations of this typology add further precision.

The shared characteristics of all types of therapeutic communities are that they attempt to:

- respect the individual client as a citizen with the capacity for autonomous action

- share decision-making with residents about the day-to-day life of the community
- use the mechanism of meetings and groups to develop openness of communication about problems, feelings and conflicts
- stress an ordinary domestic environment in which clients can engage in meaningful, purposeful activity.

Communities differ with respect to the therapeutic focus of the programme. For example, at the Cassel, psychotherapy in the context of a therapeutic community is offered; at the Henderson, the social group itself is the prime therapeutic tool; and in some settings drug therapy may be continued. In some hostels a rigid set of rules and expectations of residents' behaviour may be formulated as part of the therapeutic contract with patients. An example of this would include units caring for anorexic patients or drug-addicted patients. Many units aspire to the attributes of the Henderson, described by Rappoport (1960) and outlined in Box 26.2. Overall the ideals are thought to be beneficial because together they provide a 'living learning' situation for those with impoverished social skills and capacities.

Box 26.2 Rappoport's attributes of therapeutic communities

Permissiveness. This is a tolerance, even invitation, of disturbed feelings and relationships so that they can be open for community discussion and examination.

Reality confrontation. This is an insistence on feedback to members of the community about the consequences of their actions in practical and emotional terms.

Democracy. This is a flattening of the medical, nursing and patient hierarchies where all have the right to be heard and participate in decision-making. Role blurring and dissolution of professional boundaries and techniques flow from this.

Communalism. This is a stress on the shared and cooperative nature of the task which all participants face.

EVALUATION STUDIES

A review of the literature demonstrates that evaluation studies of therapeutic communities fall into three categories. The first consists of descriptive accounts of the way a community functions from the point of view of its participants. These include reports by nurses, doctors, care assistants and residents. The second category consists of accounts of the way a therapeutic community works from the point of view of outside researchers. The third consists of studies evaluating the effectiveness of the programmes in terms of patient outcome or financial savings. Each category will be discussed in turn.

Three collections of papers (Barnes 1968, Hinshelwood & Manning 1979, Jansen 1980) provide descriptive accounts and theoretical discussions about the nature of the participants' experience of community life. From these it becomes clear that all types of people suffering from a range of conditions, from the neuroses, behaviour disorders and addictions through to chronic schizophrenics, are deemed able to benefit from the approach. Most age ranges are considered to be suitable too. Shoenburg (1972), for example, describes the changes in Fulbourne Hospital, Cambridge, as it transformed orthodox methods to therapeutic community methods. The self-reflective and committed nature of staff working in these settings is also revealed as they examine the problems and difficulties the method poses. Janovsky & Atkinson (1982) note, for example, that nurses' creativity and innovation are increased in the therapeutic community context, and examine the conflicts of role and authority generated between registrars and nurses as a result. Rose (1983) discusses the problem of overcoming resistance to treatment amongst adolescents who fear the insight it engenders, and Hinshelwood (1982) notes that community meetings evoke the fear of individual psychotherapy in public. Others have looked at the possibility of using this approach in psychogeriatric units (Divine 1982, Chapman 1985). Residents report mixed reactions to the experience. For some it was puzzling and painful, confusing but ultimately rewarding, while for others it appears to have been an intrusive and unhelpful experience.

The second category of studies are those undertaken by social scientists. Systematic research programmes are undertaken by researchers using participant observation methods (Bellaby 1972, Manning 1979). Ethnographic accounts support the claim that everyday activities constitute the main therapeutic focus. Examples of contradictions between the ideology of therapeutic communities and the actualities of practice are, however, noted (Bloor 1980,1981). They challenge, for example, underlying assumptions about the client's autonomy; clients' accounts about the everyday experience are often subsumed beneath staff's accounts. The intrusive nature of an atmosphere in which every activity may be construed as being indicative of underlying pathology is noted by Baron (1984). McKegany (1983a, 1983b) challenges the notion of open communications in situations where there are 'front stage' (to clients) and 'back stage' (between staff) accounts of events in the community. The contrast between the ideology of democracy, equality and openness between staff and patients, and the underlying reality of their difference in status, is identified. Staff and patients are different; the former get paid for being in the community, for example, and it is usually staff who construct the rules and expectations of community life.

Contradictions between ideology and practice notwithstanding, other writers have sought to establish whether therapeutic communities are effective treatment. In this final category of studies the impetus for research often seems to have come from a politico-economic environment in which therapeutic communities are obliged to justify their existence. The approach is often viewed ambivalently and sometimes receives a hostile reaction from those adopting more orthodox methods. In such an atmosphere quantitative rather than qualitative assessments are undertaken.

Bouras et al (1982) looked at the impact of different milieux on disturbed behaviour. They found that in a modified therapeutic community dissatisfactions were more likely to be followed by behaviour disturbance than on a ward run on medical model lines.

Moos (1974) and later Verhaest (1983) used a 'ward atmosphere scale' to measure behavioural changes in patients arising from changes in emphasis in the therapeutic programme. They found associations between ward atmosphere and the capacity of residents to develop interpersonal relationships, autonomy and spontaneity.

Kutner (1983) explored the relationship between clients' self-concept and participation in a 60-day therapeutic programme with drug addicts. She notes that there was a significant difference between pre- and post-treatment scores. All post-treatment scores moved positively towards scores associated with normalization of self-concept. In short, clients were more likely to see themselves as being 'normal' after treatment.

Caine & Smail (1969) compared the number of symptoms and personality features of therapeutic community patients with those on a conventional hospital ward. At follow-up one year and 5 years later they found a significantly decreased number of symptoms and changes in personality amongst therapeutic community patients but not in the conventional ward group.

Evison & Trauer (1983) similarly found that therapeutic community patients, on discharge, had significantly reduced scores on measures of work problems and social anxieties compared with their outpatient department contemporaries. On follow-up they had significantly changed personality and social scores as well.

Finally, Griffin (1983) undertook an exploratory cost-benefit analysis of a drug addiction programme based on therapeutic community lines. She argued that the programme led to a saving for the government of some $3 million if the absence of criminal costs were taken into account.

These evaluation studies are small in scale; most therapeutic communities offer treatment for only 30 to 40 patients, and follow-up studies reflect this. The range of therapeutic communities is wide and comparisons between similar types are difficult. Similarly, the client groups being tested vary, and comparisons between treatments for these different groups are problematic.

Finally, a problem acknowledged by many in this field is associated with the nature of change. Usually the aims of the programme are to produce qualitative changes in the client's life. These are difficult to measure, and there are no universally agreed criteria for establishing success. Furthermore it is difficult at times to establish a causal link between life change and therapeutic programmes. It is sometimes argued that spontaneous remission may account for any improvements identified.

NURSING AND THERAPEUTIC COMMUNITIES

Only a few psychiatric nurse textbooks (Kalkman & Davis 1974, Lego 1984, Mereness & Taylor 1974) give anything but passing reference to the skills and techniques of nursing in therapeutic communities. This absence is generally reflected in the nursing research literature. There may be three main reasons for this. Firstly, the number of genuine therapeutic communities in Great Britain is small. Secondly, the way in which therapeutic communities developed may have influenced this trend. As noted earlier, there were two perspectives from which the approach developed in this country. Main's approach led to a psychoanalytically-based therapeutic community in which nurses and doctors' roles were sharply defined. Stress was placed on the importance of nurses developing a relationship with the patient; and, through the understanding of this relationship, the patient would gain insight and confidence in his or her capacity to function.

The more influential Maxwell Jones tradition stressed a different approach. He viewed the nurse's role as primarily concerned with limit-setting, social interaction and the maintenance of the community structure. Individual relationships with patients tended not to be encouraged (Kalkman & Davis 1974). The democratic element of the culture stressed role-blurring. Nurses began to refer to themselves as therapists or key workers. This tension between nurse as therapist, undertaking tasks often carried out by doctors, and psychosocial nursing which emphasizes the distinct set of skills nurses as nurses contribute, should be understood in the light of the professionalization debate. For many nurses, demonstrating they have the same set of skills as a higher status profession is seen as a means of personal and professional development. For others, revaluing and articulating a body of knowledge and skills specific to nursing is seen as the way forward.

Finally, the focus of the therapeutic community ideal has probably been subsumed in the literature on halfway houses, community homes and hospital hostels now being set up in the larger community outside hospitals.

Principles of care

The most useful way of outlining the principles of care is to refer to a typical therapeutic community programme. Figure 26.1 is a composite picture derived from nurses' descriptions of their work in two communities (Francis 1975, Chapman 1974, 1984, Macklin 1979, Mills 1977, Kynaston et al 1981). Each therapeutic community will of course have its own programme reflecting its basic philosophy.

The first thing to note is that patients and nurses move in and out of contact with each other throughout the day in individual and group interactions. It is during these interactions that relationships are developed and the nurse gains understanding about patients' strengths and weaknesses. Nurses' observations and insights become the foundation of individual care plans which are discussed and coordinated as part of an ongoing learning and discovery process with the patient/resident and the multi-disciplinary team, and, where appropriate, with the whole community of patients. These care plans not only identify patients' difficulties in psychological, social and physical functioning, but also identify patients' strengths and capacities. The latter are used imaginatively to help resolve problems associated with the former.

For example, a young socially-isolated man with low self-esteem and a depressive illness who also enjoys cooking may be encouraged to play a key role in the patients' cooking rota and catering meetings. Thus it is his own creativity which

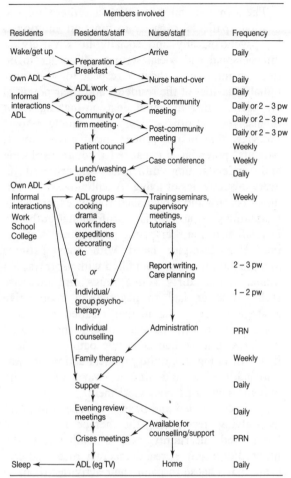

Fig. 26.1 Therapeutic community programme (a composite).

provides him with the opportunity to collaborate with other patients and staff and become a valued member of the community. On the other hand a suicidal patient may draw on the resources of the whole community at moments of crisis. Following a crisis meeting called by a nurse, the patient community may decide to arrange an all-night rota where one patient is always available for counselling and support to the suicidal patient. Such responsibility enhances patients' awareness of the strengths they have, and begins to lay the foundations of trust and effective concern. The nurse's task is to facilitate both these actions.

The aim of nursing care is, therefore, to facilitate patients' capacity to function emotionally, psychologically and socially in a variety of interpersonal and social settings. In order to do this the nurse must have a respect for the functional capacities of the residents and their potential for participating in sound decision-making about themselves and others. The nurse should respect the view that in the proper social environment, patients' potential is enhanced through exploring and understanding difficulties experienced in everyday activities of living. A willingness to relinquish control and a cherished role as expert while maintaining an appropriate professional authority in relation to the therapeutic programme is essential. For example, faced with four patients lounging around in a room filled with ashtrays, old dinner plates, dirty coffee mugs and cigarette stubs, a sister had to negotiate a cooperative strategy whereby she neither cleaned the room herself, ordered the patients to do it, nor ignored the mess, but worked alongside patients to clean it up. In doing this quite practical action she was also addressing and finding ways of helping patients solve a psychological mess.

An open-minded and flexible approach to problem-solving, recognizing the therapeutic value of failure and uncertainty, can be invaluable to the nurse. For example, real democracy means adolescents may choose to paint their activities room in purple and scarlet; the community meeting might recommend that mothers and children should not eat at the same time as the rest of the adults because the queues are too long and the children noisy. Living through and understanding the reason for these decisions and the results of implementing them are part of the nurse's task. It should be clear from these examples that the nurse also requires the ability to engage with difficult and painful issues. Working in this milieu puts the nurse in the position of having to develop tolerance towards disturbed behaviour and feelings and to display considerable personal integrity. Working in therapeutic communities can be painful and so professional supervision and support from colleagues in a variety of seminars and meetings are essential if the nurse is to sustain and develop skills. The nurse in this setting not only

needs good interpersonal skills, but also a willingness to have insight into and evaluate her own feelings and behaviour.

Ward-Miller (1984) discusses the personal attributes required of the nurse in a therapeutic community and includes the need to maintain contact and communications with patients' relatives, friends, lovers and key personnel, within and outside the hospital. The formal skills she lists are as follows:

- Sensitive observation of patients in their interpersonal and social relationships in order to inform care plans
- Individualized care planning, using imaginative ways of enlisting patients' cooperation in implementation
- Articulate and clear report writing and structuring of case notes
- Clarity of oral reporting (being able to distinguish between feelings, thoughts and actual observations)
- Listening and counselling
- Group techniques as leader, co-worker and participant
- Managerial, administrative and educational skills appropriate to own position and role in the community.

CONCLUSION

In this brief account of therapeutic communities I have outlined developments in Great Britain, tracing the continuity of themes from the 'moral therapy' of the 19th century to the genesis of the therapeutic community movement of the Second World War. The range and variation of therapeutic communities have been noted.

Characteristics of these organizations have been described, namely, permissiveness, democracy, reality confrontation and communalism. Evaluation studies have been discussed and some contradictions between ideology and practice noted together with assessments of their efficacy. A typical therapeutic programme has illustrated the lived experience in the community and traced the nurse's role and functions. Essential skills, attributes and attitudes have been listed.

It remains perhaps to identify the relevance of these specialist techniques to psychiatric nursing in general. Clearly, they are of direct relevance to those planning, designing and working in or with clients cared for in the halfway houses, community homes, group homes and hospital hostels currently being developed outside hospitals. Many workers have also modified these techniques and used them in rehabilitation wards, psychogeriatric wards and long-stay chronically mentally ill units. I would venture to suggest that the attitudes towards care of patients and the attributes listed as necessary for therapeutic community care should form the basis of sound psychiatric nurse practice in all settings.

REFERENCES

Barnes E (ed) 1968 Psychosocial nursing. Tavistock Publications, London

Baron C 1984 The Paddington Day Hospital: crises and control in a therapeutic institution. International Journal of Therapeutic Communities 5(3)

Barton R 1959 Institutional neurosis. Wright, Bristol

Baruch G, Treacher A 1978 Psychiatry observed. Routledge & Kegan Paul, London

Bellaby 1972 A sociologist. In: Shoenberg E (ed) A hospital looks at itself. Cassirer, Oxford

Bloor M J 1980 The nature of therapeutic work in a therapeutic community; some preliminary findings. International Journal of Therapeutic Communities 1(2)

Bloor M J 1981 Therapeutic paradox — the patient culture and the formal treatment programme in a therapeutic community. British Journal of Medical Psychology (54)

Bouras N, Trauer T, Watson J 1982 Ward environment and disturbed behaviour. International Journal of Therapeutic Communities 2(2)

Brown D, Pedder J 1980 Introduction to psychotherapy. Tavistock Publications, London

Caine T M, Smail D J 1969 The treatment of mental illness. University Press, London

Chapman G E 1974 Treating parents and disturbed adolescents. Nursing Times 70(5): 154–155

Chapman G E 1984 A therapeutic community, psychosocial nursing and the nursing process. International Journal of Therapeutic Communities 5(2)

Chapman G E 1985 New design for the old. Nursing Times 160(17): 20–22

Clarke D H 1964 Administrative Therapy. Tavistock Publications, London

Clarke D H 1981 Social therapy in psychiatry. Churchill Livingstone, Edinburgh

Divine B 1982 Milieu therapy: its growth, development and problems in Canadian institutions. International Journal of Therapeutic Communities 3(3)

Evison M, Trauer T 1983 An evaluation of outpatient group psychotherapy and therapeutic community treatment. International Journal of Therapeutic Communities 4(2)

Fears M 1977 Therapeutic optimism and the treatment of the insane. In: Dingwall R et al (eds) Health care, health knowledge. Croom Helm, Beckenham, Kent

Foucault M 1967 Madness and civilization. Tavistock Publications, London

Francis M 1975 Nursing: team work in action. New Psychiatry 2(7)

Goffman 1970 Asylums. Penguin, Harmondsworth, Middlesex

Griffen K S 1983 The therapeutic community: an exploratory cost benefit analysis. International Journal of Therapeutic Communities 4(4)

Hinshelwood R D, Manning N 1979 Therapeutic communities: reflections and progress. Routledge & Kegan Paul, London

Hinshelwood R D 1982 Complaints about the community meeting. International Journal of Therapeutic Communities 3(2)

Janovsky DS, Atkinson H 1982 Administrative democracy on the psychiatric ward: nursing and psychiatric resident issues. International Journal of Therapeutic Communities 3(3)

Jansen E 1980 The therapeutic community. Croom Helm, Beckenham, Kent

Jones K 1972 A history of the mental health services. Routledge & Kegan Paul, London

Jones M 1968 Social psychiatry in practice. Penguin, Hammondsworth, Middlesex

Kalkman M, Davis A 1974 New dimensions in mental health–psychiatric nursing. McGraw Hill, Maidenhead, Berks

Kennard D, Roberts J 1983 An introduction to therapeutic communities. Routledge & Kegan Paul, London

Kutner S 1983 The impact of a therapeutic community on the self-concept of drug-dependent males. International Journal of Therapeutic Communities 4(2)

Kynaston T, Meade H, Jackman K 1981 The Henderson Hospital: nursing in a therapeutic community. Nursing 2

Lego S 1984 The American handbook of psychiatric nursing. Lippincott, Philadelphia

Macklin D 1979 Trouble stirring in the kitchen. Nursing Mirror 148(21): 38–39

Main T 1946 The hospital as therapeutic institution. Bulletin of the Menninger Clinic 19(3): 66–76

Main T 1980 Some basic concepts in therapeutic community work. In: Jansen E (ed) Therapeutic community. Croom Helm, Beckenham, Kent

Manning N 1979 Evaluating the therapeutic community. In: Hinshelwood R D, Manning N (eds) Therapeutic communities: reflection and progress. Routledge & Kegan Paul, London

McKeganey N 1983a The social organization of everyday therapeutic work: making the backstage visible in a Camphill Rudolf Steiner school. International Journal of Therapeutic Communities 4(2)

McKeganey N 1983b Research note: the cocktail party syndrome. Sociology of Health and Illness 5(1): 95–103

Mereness D, Taylor C M 1974 Essentials of psychiatric nursing 9th edn. Mosby, St Louis, Mo

Mills V 1977 Mutuality in nursing leads to vulnerability for patient and nurse in a psychotherapeutic community. Journal of Advanced Nursing 2(1): 21–28

Moos R H 1974 Evaluating treatment environments. Wiley, Chichester, Sussex

Rappoport R N 1960 Community as doctor. Tavistock Publications, London

Rose M 1983 Fear of insight. International Journal of Therapeutic Communities 4(1)

Rothman D 1971 The discovery of the asylum. Little Brown, Boston

Scull A T 1979 Museums of madness. Penguin, Harmondsworth, Middlesex

Shoenberg E 1972 A hospital looks at itself. Cassirer, Oxford

Szasz T 1973 The manufacture of madness. Paladin, London

Verhaest S 1983 The assessment of the maturation of a therapeutic community. International Journal of Therapeutic Communities 4(3)

Ward-Miller S 1984 Therapeutic community meetings. In: Lego S (ed) The American handbook of psychiatric nursing. Lippincott, Philadelphia

27

Community psychiatric nursing

C. Brooker

The development of community psychiatric nursing (CPN) services over the last 30 years has been an undoubted success. This chapter will begin with an examination of the reasons for such progress from a historical viewpoint.

It will become apparent that expansion in CPN services, particularly over recent years, is related strongly to the community care policies of successive governments. As CPN teams have grown, so ultimately have individual teams changed the ways in which they operate. The organizational progression of CPN teams will therefore be discussed in some detail. It will be demonstrated that a reorientation of CPN service philosophy can have important implications for the role of each individual CPN.

Community psychiatric nursing shares, in common with other branches of psychiatric nursing, the need to identify the skills and elements of nursing practice that work to the client's best advantage. The process by which such aspects of good practice are identified systematically is, of course, research; thus a section is devoted to the current 'state of the art' in terms of the CPN and research.

Community care policies in England mostly centre around the closure of large psychiatric hospitals and the concomitant build-up of a network of community-based mental health services.

Most district health authorities' plans in this area have yet to reach fruition, so the opportunity has been taken to indulge in a little 'crystal ball gazing' and to speculate on how such planning decisions may affect the future role of the CPN.

Finally, the nursing education issues that affect CPNs are addressed. The impact of the 1982 Registered Mental Nurse (RMN) training syllabus on post-basic training for CPNs is considered and both sides of the debate concerning mandatory training are presented. There is also a commentary on the relevance of the relatively new English National Board Clinical Course No. 811 for CPNs.

COMMUNITY PSYCHIATRIC NURSING — A HISTORICAL REVIEW

The first CPN Service to be established in England was at Warlingham Park Hospital in Surrey in 1954 (Peat & Watt 1984). Here, nurses who were hospital based were employed in a full-time capacity on work with ex-psychiatric patients, attending outpatient clinics, evening social clubs and after-care groups.

Hunter (1974) has also described the origins of a CPN Service at Moorhaven Hospital, Devon, in 1957. Originally entitled the 'Nursing After-care Service', four nurses were employed to carry out a range of activities with discharged psychiatric patients.

The birth of community psychiatric nursing should not be divorced from the wider context of reforms that were occurring in most British psychiatric services in the 1950s. As the recent Social Services Committee Report (1985a) into community care states:

In the 1950s, the pace of reform gathered as a result of the introduction of drugs (such as Reserpine and Chlorpromazine), social treatments, and the Royal Commission on Mental Illness and Mental Deficiency of 1954–7, culminating in the 1959 Mental Health Act. The phrase 'Community Care' occurred in policy statements with increasing frequency. (para 13)

A Royal College of Nursing Report in 1966 concerned itself with the role of the psychiatric nurse in the community and the preparation required. The Working Party discovered that at this time a large number of hospitals were employing nurses to work in the community. Indeed, 26 nurses were

employed full-time and 199 nurses part-time and they were using 42 different hospitals as their base.

Perhaps the single most significant event that influenced the growth of CPN services at the end of the 1960s was the implementation of the Local Authorities Act (1968).

The Act implemented the main findings of the Seebohm Report which advocated absorbing specialized local authority mental health departments and mental welfare officers into generic social service departments. Thus, as Paykel & Griffith (1983) pointed out,

Specialized workers were temporarily replaced by relatively inexperienced generalist workers with different skills and priorities leaving a vacuum in follow-up care. (p. 10)

The Royal Medico-Psychological Association (now the Royal College of Psychiatrists) immediately saw the need for a new profession to fill the yawning gap that had been created,

It is likely that a new body of mental health social workers would have to be evolved to fill the gap left by the destruction of the present growing services, perhaps with an enhanced medical or nursing background.

(Royal Medico-Psychological Assn 1969)

This latter comment was certainly prophetic, and nurses were quick to rise to the challenge of 'undertaking the social rehabilitative roles previously seen as the function of the social worker' (Leopoldt 1973), as developments in the decade 1970 to 1980 were to demonstrate.

As the number of individual CPN services increased, peaking in the mid-1970s (McKendrick 1982), so did the diversification of the individual CPN role within teams. CPN services began to encompass a number of functions that differed markedly from those described earlier. The general approach could be described as environmental, interpersonal and social in nature within a broad network of aims. At this point, the change in CPN role was being accompanied by a change of work location or base. Corser & Ryce (1977), for example, describe a CPN's work based in the community within a multi-disciplinary team.

However, although such schemes were innovative in nature, the majority of CPN services were based either in a psychiatric hospital itself, a district general hospital or a day hospital. In this model of a CPN service a likely scenario would be for the individual CPN to be attached to a consultant psychiatrist, following up, in the main, this doctor's patients once discharged.

1980 was a watershed for CPN services and heralded some important developments. In the first instance the Royal College of Psychiatrists (1980) produced a document entitled 'The Role of the Community Psychiatric Nurse'. In this paper the Royal College of Psychiatrists noted that:

The move of specialist CPN services out of hospital into the community may raise problems concerning clinical responsibility. In particular it is important to determine whether the consultant psychiatrist or the general practitioner is controlling the prescription of drugs given to patients cared for by CPNs. (p. 3)

This comment formally acknowledges for the first time the movement of CPN services out of hospitals into more community-oriented services. The Royal College of Psychiatrists' policy statement also remarked upon the manpower requirements needed if CPN services were to expand more fully:

If it was hoped to develop a nationwide service of CPNs attached to primary care teams the numbers of CPNs would have to be trebled to meet this need alone. If, in addition, specialist units and services are to have their own CPNs, the manpower increase would have to be four or five fold. (p. 7)

Unfortunately, at the time this document was produced no-one knew exactly how many CPNs there were nationally. This was to change with the publication in 1980 of the first survey of CPN services in the United Kingdom (CPN Association 1980).

It can be seen that community psychiatric nursing has a history of isolated and experimental development which has led incrementally over the last quarter of a century to a nationwide provision. The establishment of new CPN services peaked in the mid 1970s at a time when government policy was becoming more directed than ever before to a philosophy of 'Care in the Community'.

Government mental health care policy

In England, since the late 1950s, there has been increasing discussion about running down large psychiatric hospitals. The catalyst for these proposals was undoubtedly the advent of phenothiazine drugs and the then radical 1959 Mental Health Act (see Ch. 11). In 1961, two government statisticians, Tooth and Brook, examined trends in the decline of psychiatric hospital inpatient populations and predicted that:

Between 1955 and 1959 the long stay population resident on 31 December 1954, was running down at a rate which, if continued, would eliminate it in about sixteen years. (p. 713)

Perhaps it was this vision of the future that prompted the 1962 government White Paper 'The Hospital Plan' (Ministry of Health 1962) which predicted a halving over 15 years of the number of mental illness beds and mooted for the first time the idea of a psychiatric unit attached to a district general hospital, supported by better services in the community, services which at this stage remained unspecified.

In 1963 the Department of Health and Social Security (DHSS) published 'Health and Welfare: The Development of Community Care' which outlined in more detail the implications of psychiatric hospital run-down for local authorities. This was followed in 1971 by another document 'Hospital Services for the Mentally Ill'. This, in essence, essence, again underlined the need to abolish large psychiatric hospitals and to develop community-orientated teams.

However, it had become clear that government policy statements between 1962 and 1971 were not changing the hospital basis of psychiatric care. Furthermore, during this period there were a succession of critical inquiries into individual hospitals.

The government response was to publish yet another White Paper, this time in 1975, entitled 'Better Services for the Mentally Ill' (DHSS 1975).

This document again underlined the desirability of changing the basis of care from hospital to community-based models.

Four specific aims for local development were stressed; an expansion in local authority personal social services to provide a range of community support; a relocation of specialist services into local settings; the establishment of the right organizational links between all those staff involved in the delivery, management and planning of mental health care; and finally, a significant improvement in staffing to allow for earlier intervention and preventative work.

The 1975 White Paper saw the first formal acknowledgement by the government of the role to be played by CPNs in the development of locally accessible comprehensive district mental health services. The document states:

The district psychiatric nursing service in the new pattern will be responsible for meeting all the psychiatric nursing needs of mentally ill people from the district. It will include community psychiatric nursing for patients living at home and specialist nursing advice to primary care teams.

'Better Services for the Mentally Ill' (DHSS 1975). recognized as a valuable attempt to determine the shape of a coherent mental health service that integrates hospital and community provision. The DHSS report 'Care in Action' (1981) reiterated these objectives and also supported the recommendations of the Working Party on the Organization and Management of Mental Illness Hospitals (Nodder Committee 1980). The main suggestions were that psychiatric hospitals should reduce their catchment areas to that of their own districts and that those institutions not well placed to develop in this way should plan for appropriate community services.

The Short Report (Social Services Select Committee 1985b) has readily acknowledged the developing role of the CPN in relation to government policy advocating community care over the last 20 years. The Report makes direct reference to the Director of the Health Advisory Service who has stated that:

The CPN is probably the most important single professional in the process of moving care of mental illness into the community. (para 192)

Further, the Report notes that there has been a gradual transfer of staff from wards of mental hospitals to community work, where CPNs carry a generic caseload, typically of 40–50 patients, a third of whom are probably aged over 65 years. The Select Committee see the role of the CPN as 'providing expertise in psychiatric care equivalent to the best nursing care available in hospitals'. However, the Report acknowledges a major deficiency in the existing knowledge concerning CPN services, particularly in the area of manpower:

Because of difficulties of definition and gaps in the Department's system of statistical returns nobody knows how many CPNs there are: the Department's estimate was 2000 while professional nursing opinion suggested a figure nearer 3500. However many, the figures are certainly not up to the guideline of one per 10 000 referred to by the CPNA and Royal College of General Practitioners. (para 192)

This relatively brief and selective review of government policy in relation to mental health care during the period 1962 to 1985 has attempted to highlight the trend in policy away from large outdated psychiatric hospitals to more local community care. Community psychiatric nurses have become an increasingly important component of a comprehensive district service, especially since 1970, when as a professional group they moved into the gap created by the abolition of the mental health welfare officer. This is a fact acknowledged by the Short Report (1985), the MIND Manifesto 'Common Concern' (1983), the Mallinson Report (COHSE 1983) and the Richmond Fellowship (1983), who in their Enquiry into Mental Health and the Community, described CPN services as 'a significant initiative'.

To summarize, CPN services nationally have been expanding since 1954 and, further, expanding firmly in line with government community care policies. The ways in which the organization of the CPN service altered during the period 1980 to 1985 will now be examined.

CHANGES IN CPN SERVICE ORGANIZATION

In 1980 the Community Psychiatric Nurses' Association (CPNA) carried out a national survey of CPN services, the aim being to understand how services organize their delivery of care. In 1985 the survey was repeated by the CPNA, with three main aims in mind:

1. To update the national profile of the total CPN workforce. This was felt to be especially important as many Regional Health Authorities had begun to adopt formal manpower planning targets, e.g. 1 CPN per 10 000 of the population, and it was important to assess progress in achieving these.
2. To examine comparative changes in the following aspects of organization: CPNs' main base and referral source. Anecdotal reports had suggested there was a trend away from traditional hospital-based modes of practice.
3. To ascertain the educational attainment of CPNs with specific reference to ENB Clinical Courses Nos 810 and 811.

The CPN workforce

Table 27.1 demonstrates how the total CPN workforce changed during the period 1980 to 1985. The results are given by grade of nurse and expressed in terms of whole time equivalents.

The most striking aspect of the table is the overall increase in CPNs by just over 65%, rising from 1667 in 1980 to 2758 in 1985. The growth is most noticeable in the charge nurse/sister grade 2 banding, a total of 940 in 5 years. In terms of management structure nearly all CPN services are now led by a senior nurse grade 7, whereas in 1980 the service manager would most likely have been a nursing officer grade 2. The reason for the turn around is undoubtedly the 1982 National Health Service reorganization which introduced a new management structure in England and Wales.

There was a small increase in the charge nurse/sister grade 1 banding of 27.5 whole time equivalents. It is worth noting that 12 of these posts were in one district health authority in Wales, where completion of ENB Clinical Course Nos 810/811 warrants automatic upgrading.

The increase in the total workforce is mirrored by the large numbers of CPNs who now work exclusively in a given specialty. Table 27.2 illustrates the total numbers of CPN by specialty in 1985, and it can be seen that in total 29% of all CPNs specialize. A further important finding is that 20% of all CPNs are working exclusively with the elderly, but perhaps a less reassuring finding, given community care policies, is that only 42 CPNs nationally specialize in rehabilitation.

Finally, Table 27.3 indicates how variable overall CPN team growth is nationally, using the concept of average team size within the English regional health authorities. There has been massive growth within the Trent, East Anglia and South Western Regions of 9.3, 8.9 and 9.3 whole time equivalent per team, whereas in the Northern Region increase has been in the order of 3.2 whole time equivalents per team. Small-scale research explaining this variation has been reported elsewhere (Brooker 1985). However, one vital factor has been the introduction of formal regional health authority manpower planning targets, usually recommending 1 CPN per 10 000 of the population. Progress towards achieving such targets can be assessed from Table 27.4.

Table 27.1 Total CPN work-force figures by grade and year (Source, CPNA Survey 1985. Reproduced by kind permission of the CPNA)

Grade	1980 total	1985 total	Change (1980–85) no	per cent
SN7/NO1/SNO	32.0	116.0	+ 84	+262.5
SN8/NO2	147.0	65.0	−82	−55.0
Charge nurse 1	58.5	86.0	+27.5	+47.0
Charge nurse 2	1144.0	2084.0	+940.0	+82.0
Staff nurse	137.5	206.0	+68.5	+50.0
SEN	130.5	163.0	+32.5	+25.0
NA	17.5	12.0	−5.5	−31.5
Total	1667.0	2758.0*	+1091.0	−65.5

* Total includes 26 'other' managerial

Table 27.2 National breakdown of CPNs who specialize by area of interest (Source: CPNA Survey 1985. Reproduced by kind permission of the CPNA)

Specialism	no	per cent
Elderly	505	64.0
Crisis work	100	12.6
Drugs/alcohol	72	9.0
Rehabilitation	42	5.2
Children	36	4.5
Behaviour therapy	36	4.5
Family therapy	2	0.2
Total	793	100.0

Table 27.3 Average CPN team size by Regional Health Authority (Source: CPNA Surveys 1980 and 1985. Reproduced by kind permission of the CPNA)

RHA County	Size (1980)	Size (1985)	Net change
Yorkshire	3.8	8.9	+5.1
Northern	5.8	9.0	+3.2
Trent	5.9	15.2	+9.3
East Anglia	4.6	13.5	+8.9
North West Thames	6.6	13.1	+6.5
North East Thames	8.2	13.5	+5.3
South East Thames	7.8	12.6	+4.8
South West Thames	9.5	14.2	+4.7
Wessex	9.0	16.7	+7.7
Oxford	10.2	14.5	+4.3
South Western	8.3	17.6	+9.3
West Midlands	7.0	12.2	+5.2
Mersey	6.6	12.1	+5.5
North Western	7.1	11.3	+4.2
Wales	—	16.7	—
Scotland	—	6.8	—
Northern Ireland	—	8.0	—
Mean	7.0	12.7	+5.7

Table 27.4 Regional population ratios per CPN (1980 & 1985) (Source: CPNA Surveys 1980 and 1985. Reproduced by kind permission of the CPNA)

Region	Ratio (1980)	Ratio (1985)	Change
Yorkshire	75 200	34 500	−40 700
Northern	53 300	21 300	−32 000
Trent	72 400	27 150	−45 250
East Anglia	74 000	20 000	−54 000
North West Thames	58 900	22 800	−36 100
North East Thames	31 700	19 000	−12 700
South East Thames	38 600	21 250	−17 350
South West Thames	60 000	18 130	−41 870
Wessex	38 300	17 800	−20 500
Oxford	39 500	21 300	−18 200
South Western	37 800	18 000	−19 800
West Midlands	42 000	22 300	−19 700
Mersey	42 300	24 200	−18 100
North Western	37 400	22 300	−15 100
Total	50 000	23 800	−26 200

It seems a fair conclusion to reach that if CPN growth 1980 to 1985 is maintained over the next 5 years then many regional health authorities will be meeting their targets. Whether or not this is an appropriate way to plan services will be examined later.

Referral patterns and base location

There would seem to be an important relationship between where CPNs are based, from whom they accept their referrals and ultimately their role. CPNs based in primary health care receiving most of their case referrals from a general practitioner are likely to be concerned with secondary prevention, that is decreasing the probability of hospital admission. Alternatively, CPNs working from a hospital with all referrals mediated by a consultant psychiatrist will be mainly concerned with tertiary prevention, that is follow-up and after-care. These two referral modes have been described as the 'open' referral system and the 'closed' referral system respectively (World Health Organization 1967).

Table 27.5 provides some evidence to suggest that CPN services are developing more and more 'open' referral systems. In 1980 three-quarters of all CPNs were based in hospitals; by 1985 this situation had changed with approximately half working in such an environment. To interpret this figure another way, approximately 750 CPNs turned their back on the hospital as a base and began working in more community-orientated settings.

But what evidence is there to suggest a relationship between CPN's work base and their referral patterns?

One study undertaken in a London health authority sheds some light on this question (Brooker & Simmons 1985). The research indicated that CPNs based in a day hospital received very different sorts of referrals from CPNs in the same team who were working from health clinics. Interestingly, however, contact with the inpatient services was higher in the health clinic based CPN team than with their counterpart based in the day hospital.

Larger scale research has shown that a similar

Table 27.5 CPNs by main base (1980 and 1985) (Source: CPNA. Reproduced by kind permission of the CPNA)

	1980 per cent	1985 per cent	1985 no	Change (per cent)
Psychiatric hospital	49.0	37.35	962	−11.65
Psychiatric unit (DGH)	28.0	19.1	492	−8.9
Health centre/general practitioner practice	8.0	17.5	442	+9.15
Day hospital	8.0	9.8	252	+1.8
Mental health centre (other)	7.0	16.2	427	+9.6
Total	100.0	100.0	2575	0.0

relationship exists between CPN base and source of referral (Skidmore & Friend 1984a, Simmons & Brooker 1986). Skidmore & Friend, in a survey of 12 CPN services, demonstrated that the self-referral of new clients was 500% more likely for the primary health care based CPN than the CPN based in a psychiatric hospital. It seems certain that a CPN service based in primary health care is perceived by the potential client as a great deal less stigmatizing than a first appointment at a large hospital.

The generic CPN versus clinical specialization

A generic CPN works with clients of all different ages and with any sort of problem, as compared with a specialist CPN who works exclusively with one client group such as the elderly. Here the arguments for and against CPNs being specialists will be discussed.

As Table 27.2 illustrates, approximately one-third of all CPNs specialize; however the proportion specializing varies immensely geographically. In Wessex 33% of all CPNs work exclusively with the elderly, compared with 10% in Trent. The importance attached locally to CPN specialization varies a great deal, and nationally the 'typical' CPN service is made up of very different proportions of generic and specialist CPNs.

Detractors of the development of CPN specialism argue that if CPNs are to specialize, resources would be better used if attention was focused on patients still in hospital (Mangen & Griffith 1982). On the other hand, these same authors propose that a generic role for CPNs reduces their efficacy

and in this event ward-based nurses should be encouraged to work in the community part-time. It is hard to take these arguments seriously, particularly the latter one which suggests a return to the situation of Warlingham Park Hospital in 1954!

Other recent research has suggested that specialists are seen to be arrogant, escapist and elitist (Skidmore & Friend 1984b). Their study warned of the danger of CPN teams developing into a plethora of exclusive therapists who then neglect clients who do not fit neatly into any of the specialist categories. Finally, Skidmore & Friend discovered that a large majority of the CPNs specializing in behaviour therapy had been unsuccessful candidates for the ENB Clinical Course No. 650 in behavioural psychotherapy. These CPNs described a feeling of being without direction when newly appointed, a situation which it is hoped will change when products of the new skills-based 1982 basic RMN syllabus emerge.

These then are the dangers of CPN specialization, but there are some positive advantages. Specialists who have been trained for their role have been found to be confident and responsive to particular local clinical problems. It is also true that the status of 'specialist' attracts CPNs to work in unglamorous fields, e.g. with elderly people, where previously they may not have been so committed.

To conclude, a number of CPNs within district health authority teams should undoubtedly work in specialist fields; just how many should be elicited by local service managers on the basis of locally researched 'need'. In order that a safety net is provided, however, it seems likely that specialists will work alongside other colleagues, the majority of whom will be generic CPNs.

EVALUATION OF THE CPN

There are a number of levels on which the evaluation of CPN teams might be discussed; these include organizational aspects of the service, the clinical outcomes of clients nursed by CPNs, and the satisfaction of clients who have direct experience of CPN care. Each of these major elements of evaluation will be discussed and illuminated with recent major studies.

There has been only one serious piece of research which has addressed the clinical outcome of clients cared for by CPNs in this country (Paykel & Griffith 1983). This study used a variety of measures to assess the outcome of two randomly assigned groups over a period of 18 months. The first group were allocated to CPNs; the second group were given routine appointments with a psychiatrist in Outpatients. It should be stressed that all clients in the study were assessed as having neurotic problems as defined by the International Classification of Diseases. In relation to effects of the two modes of care on clinical symptoms, social adjustment and family burden, the researchers elicited no significant differences. Perhaps the most interesting finding was that the CPN group expressed greater global satisfaction with care at 12 and 18 month follow-up. Of particular importance was being visited at home which, through the greater informality, allowed the clients to develop a more trusting relationship with the CPN.

Pollock (1986) has taken the concept of consumer satisfaction a little further by examining families' views of the outcome of CPN intervention. In particular the burden of caring for a family member with a mental health problem at home was studied. The sample of 24 families included in the research design found CPNs helpful when relatives were behaving oddly, expressing strange ideas, and being argumentative and aggressive. CPNs were found to be less helpful in preventing relapse or onset of illness; indeed 82% of those interviewed disagreed that CPNs prevented patients from being admitted to hospitals.

The psychological effects of caring for a relative at home have been studied from a different perspective (Simmons 1984). This study, which employed phenomenological research methods, showed that relatives are aware of how different their lives are from others' and of the responsibilities they assume. Some relatives had grown isolated, felt that a social life was beyond them, and that a holiday was out of the question. Indeed, for some the strain had greater effects and had caused both physical and mental health problems. The implications for CPNs of this study point to the need for a full assessment of the family system rather than solely the identified client. Clearly also, the effect of caring for relatives at home needs to be taken into account by the advocates of community care; finance is not the only important aspect of the equation.

The organizational aspects of evaluating CPN services have been, in part, referred to earlier, when the relationship between base, referral source and role was discussed. As CPN services look likely to grow in the future, it is worth commenting here on the 'top down' approach to planning that is being adopted by many regional health authorities in relation to the required size of CPN services. It is self-evident that if, say, a ratio of 1 CPN per 10 000 of the population is recommended, then little consideration is being made of local need in any one district. To assess local need for services is clearly the task of CPN service managers and will, in the future, require research in the following areas:

1. The characteristics of the area in which the CPN team is based. This may include incidence of mental health problems, patterns of unemployment, type of housing and age structure of the population served.
2. The effects on the CPN team of the individual district's strategic and operational planning proposals. This would seem especially important when the closure of a large psychiatric hospital is a local issue.
3. The range and extent of locally-assessed requirements for specialist CPNs. This may mean, for example, in the case of CPNs working with elderly people, that existing levels of services for this client group are

balanced with epidemiological research on the incidence of dementia and the district's age structure.

4. The appropriateness of the present style and organization of existing CPN provision. For example, research has shown that CPN services that are hospital based and consultant attached have a finite capacity for expansion when compared with community-orientated teams (Brooker 1985).

To summarize this short discussion of the CPN and evaluation it can be said that large-scale objective valid studies of CPN services are few. In the future 'consumerism' seems to be an issue that all services need to take seriously, particularly given the new general management arrangements in England and Wales and the report of the community nursing review (DHSS 1985). There are glimmers of light on the horizon and it is hoped that these glimmers represent the coming dawn of a new era in the field of CPNs and research.

THE CPN AND EDUCATION

At present there is uncertainty about the whole future of all basic psychiatric nurse training. The uncertainty is likely to continue in the short term whilst proposals for a restructuring of basic education are discussed.

However, one development in psychiatric nursing is clear, and this concerns the implementation of a new more community-orientated and skills-based curriculum for registration as a psychiatric nurse.

Whether or not post-basic training for community psychiatric nursing should be mandatory has been a contentious issue for many years now. Although, as has been noted, the call for mandatory training pre-dated the implementation of the new 1982 syllabus for RMN education (Brooking 1985).

In 1985 the proportion of all CPNs holding the post-basic qualification was 22%, compared with 24% in 1980. These figures are slightly misleading in that the number of places on ENB Clinical Courses Nos 810/811 has increased during this period, but not at the rate that the overall CPN workforce has expanded.

There are at the moment some 2000 untrained CPNs working in the United Kingdom, and nationally about 250 places are available annually on ENB Clinical Courses Nos 810/811 (and its equivalents). For all CPNs to complete a course would require the total workforce to remain static for a period of 8 years just to catch up on the backlog! Partly in recognition of this problem the English National Board has approved a short course, ENB Clinical Course No. 992, the length of which is 20 days. Whilst in the preamble to the course syllabus it states 'the course is not an alternative to courses Nos 810/811', it is difficult to see how enthusiastic general managers will not interpret it in this way, especially as it is shorter, cheaper and therefore imposes less demands on the existing service whilst the CPN is undertaking the educational experience.

It is important to note that more and more CPNs are being appointed with no previous community experience and many more will be before new products of the new 1982 RMN syllabus emerge in the early 1990s. In their response to the 1985 report into community care (DHSS 1985) the government stated:

the scale of proposed expansion in the number of CPNs makes action urgent. It is hoped that authorities will wish to make greater use of the ENB clinical course syllabi for nurse care of the mentally ill . . . in the community for registered nurses working in these fields. (para 77 p. 20–21)

The future training of CPNs remains an unresolved problem both for health authorities and statutory bodies such as the ENB. A coherent strategy for future CPN education must be seen as a priority otherwise services themselves will continue to 'muddle through'.

FUTURE DEVELOPMENTS IN COMMUNITY PSYCHIATRIC NURSING

When Lena Peat began work as the first CPN at Warlingham Park Hospital in 1954 she could never have envisaged the way community psychiatric nursing would develop over the next 30 years — from outpatient psychiatric nurse to community mental health worker, as CPNs based at community mental health centres in Exeter are now called. This change in name is not merely cosmetic, it represents a vast philosophical shift from treatment of psychiatric illness to promotion of mental health. The concept of 'community care' set in motion by Tooth & Brook's (1961) erroneous statistical prognostications seems to be coming of age.

So what does the future hold for CPNs apart from perhaps a change in name? One certainty is that CPNs are going to need to re-acclimatize to working within multi-disciplinary teams. The lone pioneering days are over; as hospitals gradually close in the next decade, territory formerly exclusively owned by the CPN will have to be renegotiated with others, such as psychologists and psychiatrists. For some CPNs a radical reappraisal of working practice and role is just around the corner. There will certainly be heated debates about accountability, sphere of competence, role overlap and perhaps referral patterns.

General management arrangements will add fuel to the fire of these debates: as district services are sectorized, the present role of the CPN service manager is threatened, as is perhaps the concept of a district CPN team.

Future flux in the organization of CPN teams may be spurred on by the government response to the Report of the Community Nursing Review (DHSS 1985).

Again the Cumberlege report (DHSS 1986) envisages CPNs working in multi-disciplinary teams but eventually with colleagues in primary health care rather than mental health professionals. These teams, based on the concept of a neigh-bourhood, would develop a high degree of professional autonomy with nurses not being subject to control of their work by doctors; a scenario many see as likely within the evolution of community mental health teams that include consultant psychiatrists.

To conclude this chapter inevitably involves a summary of the state of the art of community psychiatric nursing. CPN teams have developed at a frantic pace nationally, although within regional health authorities this is at a variable level. The CPN workforce looks set to grow even larger in the next decade. The role of the CPN has developed in relation to the way the service is organized and depends greatly on relationships with GPs and psychiatrists. CPN specialists and generic CPNs are both important and can live happily together within the same team. Research into community psychiatric nursing is gradually growing but much more effort is required into the local assessment of need for CPNs and in the whole area of consumer satisfaction and family burden. Perhaps the major areas of future concern are firstly the educational needs of CPNs — in particular a major commitment to the concept of special post-basic training is essential, and secondly, the way in which general management arrangements look likely to damage the coordination of CPN services within some districts.

The CPN child of the 1950s has come of age and developmentally is now perhaps just entering early adulthood — the next 10 years will be a fascinating period during which to observe further growth.

REFERENCES

Brooker C 1985 The 1985 national community psychiatric nursing survey: The evolution of a methodology. Unpublished MSc dissertation, Steinberg Collection, Royal College of Nursing

Brooker C, Simmons S 1985 A study to compare two models of community psychiatric nursing care delivery. Journal of Advanced Nursing 10: 217–223

Brooking J I 1985 Advanced psychiatric nurse education in Britain. Journal of Advanced Nursing 10: 455–468

Community Psychiatric Nurses Association (CPNA) 1980 The national survey of community psychiatric nursing. CPNA Publications, Leeds

Community Psychiatric Nurses Association 1985 The 1985 national community psychiatric nursing survey update. CPNA Publications, Leeds

Confederation of Health Service Employees (COHSE) 1983 The Mallinson report. COHSE, London

Corser C M, Ryce S 1977 Community mental health care: A

model based on the primary care system. British Medical Journal 2: 936–938

Department of Health and Social Security 1963 Health and welfare: the development of community care. HMSO, London

Department of Health and Social Security 1971 Hospital services for the mentally ill. HMSO, London

Department of Health and Social Security 1975 Better services for the mentally ill. HMSO, London

Department of Health and Social Security 1981 Care in action. HMSO, London

Department of Health and Social Security 1985 Neighbourhood nursing — a focus for care. Report of the community nursing review. HMSO, London

Department of Health and Social Security 1986 Neighbourhood nursing — a focus for care (Cumberlege Report). HMSO, London

Hunter P 1974 Community psychiatric nursing in Britain: an historical review. International Journal of Nursing Studies II: 223–233

Leopoldt H 1973 Towards integration (an experiment in psychiatric community nursing in group practice attachment). Nursing Mirror 136: 38–42

McKendrick D 1982 Statistical returns in community psychiatric nursing. Unpublished project, Manchester Polytechnic

Mangen S, Griffith J 1982 Community psychiatric nursing services in Britain: the need for policy and planning. International Journal of Nursing Studies 19(3): 159–165

MIND 1983 Common concern. MIND, London

Ministry of Health 1962 The hospital plan. HMSO, London

Nodder Committee 1977 Report of the Working Party on the Organisation and Management of Mental Illness Hospitals. DHSS, HMSO, London

Paykel E S, Griffith J H 1983 Community psychiatric nursing for neurotic patients: a controlled trial. Royal College of Nursing, London

Peat L, Watt G 1984 The Passing of an era. Community

Psychiatric Nursing (CPN) Journal 4(2): 12–16

Pollock L 1986 An evaluation research study of community psychiatric nursing employing the personal questionnaire rapid scaling technique. CPN Journal 6(3): 11–22

Richmond Fellowship 1983 The Richmond fellowship enquiry: mental health and the community report. Richmond Fellowship Press

Royal College of Nursing 1966 Investigation into the role of the psychiatric nurse in the community. Unpublished

Royal College of Psychiatrists 1980 Community psychiatric nursing: a discussion document. Bulletin of the Royal College of Psychiatrists. August: 117

Royal Medico-Psychological Assn 1969 Report of the committee on local authorities and allied personal social services. Royal Medico-Psychological Association, London

Simmons S 1984 Family burden — What does it mean to the carers? Unpublished MSc dissertation, Surrey University

Simmons S, Brooker C 1986 Community psychiatric nursing — a social perspective. Heinemann, London

Skidmore D, Friend W 1984a Should CPNs be in the primary health care team? Nursing Times (Community Outlook). 9 Sept: 310–312

Skidmore D, Friend W 1984b Specialism or escapism? Nursing Times (Community Outlook). 10 June: 203–205

Social Services Select Committee Report 1985a Care in the community. HMSO, London

Social Services Select Committee 1985b Community care: with special reference to adult mentally ill and mentally handicapped people. (Short Report.) House of Commons Paper 13, 1, vol 1. HMSO, London

Tooth G C, Brook E M 1961 Trends in the mental health population and their effect on future planning. Lancet. 1 April: 710–713

World Health Organization 1967 The psychiatric hospital as a centre for preventative work in mental health. 5th Report of the Expert Committee on Mental Health, Geneva

Part 4

Psychiatric nursing interventions for specific client groups

28

Nursing disturbed children and adolescents

R. Alstead

PHYSICAL DEVELOPMENT

History taking. The stages of a child's physical development are identified by taking a detailed history from a health clinic or medical records, or by obtaining information from the child's parents.

Measurement

A thorough medical examination will assist in identifying the stage of physical development reached by the child.

Measuring the child's height and weight are important indicators of the child's development, particularly when plotted on a growth chart which graphs height against age, weight against age and produces a point which can be placed on a percentile graph showing if the child is taller/heavier/smaller lighter than the average child.

The reasons why children fail to grow adequately include malnourishment, physiological illness and emotional distress or neglect.

PSYCHOLOGICAL DEVELOPMENT

Knowledge of childhood development is essential for psychiatric nurses working with children and families. An understanding of normal child development helps nurses to identify a child's needs and puts the child's developmental and situational difficulties in an appropriate context. Developmental stages or tasks can be broken down by age, or by the physical, psychological and social aspects in the child's own particular environment. Developmental 'tasks' identified by Erikson (1963) describe the child's progression from dependence to the autonomy of an independent adolescent.

Development of psychology incorporates a number of varying theories explaining human behaviour. Each theory sees the same set of events from different perspectives. These theories include psychoanalytic, learning, social and humanistic schools of thought.

Significance of early experience of attachment relationships

Bowlby (1969) identified a critical period in which it is essential for a child to form an intimate attachment relationship with a significant figure: this being crucial for the development of trust and formation of future relationships. Attachment experiences, or lack of, within the first 7 years of life set up defensive processes which affect the subsequent development of the child's personality.

Schaffer (1979), Clerke & Clerke (1976) and McGuck (1951) do not share Bowlby's (1969) view of the importance of the mother. They suggest that the child continuously interacts with its environment, so that children initially deprived of attachment figures may be less impaired than suggested by Bowlby. Clerke & Clerke (1976) outline other sensitive periods during which the individual is more susceptible to a particular life experience. They question whether infantile experience always predominates over experiences in later life. Rutter (1981) shows that attachment can be learnt at any time, given the right environment, but favours sensitive periods.

No one theory of development has been scientifically proved to be the only explanation and important issues arise from all of them. For example, learning processes are important at all ages. Twin studies seem to show clearly that individual differences are determined by inherited personality as well as social experience. Emotions are a form of social experience which are influenced by the presence or absence of attachment figures, separation and loss.

Facilities available in Britain for children and families with special (emotional or behavioural) difficulties

Facilities existing to meet children's needs are wide ranging.

Educational services

School medical officers and nurses routinely screen, examine and inoculate children at particular ages. They may see referrals in order to give advice, if teachers express a concern about a particular child.

Specialized services provided by education authorities include educational psychologists, who may see children, with parents' consent, following poor academic performance or behaviour which deviates from that child's usual behaviour in school. Education welfare officers may be concerned with similar referrals but would focus on children's attendance at school, and would work with families to ensure legal attendance or assess the children's special needs and assist in changing schooling facilities.

Community services

Less stigma is attached to community-based services as opposed to hospital services. Children with severe problems may be referred by a general practitioner to the hospital. Alternatively, families may seek out assistance from voluntary organizations, the Church, or their own local friends.

Local authority social services

Children deemed by social workers to be at risk can be taken into local authority care. Preferably, children are placed with foster families and may subsequently be adopted. This ensures continuation of a domestic family environment for the child to develop normally. Some local authorities have assessment centres where children taken into care may go initially; children's homes continue to exist but are reduced in number.

Child and family psychiatric services

These range from outpatient services to day attendance (9–5 p.m.), or nurseries (10–12 a.m.), or day units (12–2 p.m.) which would close at weekends and all children would be expected to return home for that time. Seven-day residential children's units also exist for children requiring continuous 24-hour hospitalization. The therapeutic orientation, or model, of hospital services varies throughout the country. Services are generally run by a multi-professional team, including nurses, psychiatrists, social workers, psychologists, teachers. These workers will possess a variety of general skills and also skills specific to their professional background. Specialized therapists such as art therapists, play therapists, and psychotherapists, may be full-time members of the team or are sometimes employed on a sessional basis. Most units are eclectic in orientation.

HOMELIKE ENVIRONMENT OF CHILDREN'S UNIT

All children are dependent on adults. If a child becomes a resident in hospital, the nurses who are with the children throughout the 24-hour period have an important role in fulfilling parenting tasks without taking over and becoming substitutes for the child's parents. The child's dependency needs and spontaneity facilitate development of transference relationships. The therapeutic value of this relationship with a nurse enables the child to express and to modify relationship difficulties which he experiences in life with others.

Identification of the normal developmental needs of children is essential, in addition to the management of the child's difficulties. Therefore, inpatient units are designed to look as homelike as possible. The design of the unit, and the provision of particular furnishings, play equipment and toys (with adequate indoor and outdoor activity space) are important. The maximum number of children who reside in a children's unit is approximately 10–12. Nurses need to create and maintain an atmosphere which promotes a feeling of caring, fun and activity, but which is structured enough to produce an awareness of clear boundaries, facilitating emotional growth and behavioural change. Some units have residential facilities for parents or for whole families. This usually occurs if a specific focus of family work is necessary.

Routines of residential units reflect those in family life. Children's units often have a specific timetable structuring most of the children's time. Interactions between the child and parent or nurse can be observed while the child is completing everyday routines: for example, observing how he washes and dresses, and participates in tasks such as assisting laying the table, cooking and washing up. The child's level of social interaction provides useful information about sociability and level of functioning.

Residential units also meet children's educational needs. Most units have classrooms attached. Daily attendance of the majority of children is expected, despite difficulties which may have led to poor school attendance at home. Teachers assess each child's individual education and social needs, and then provide wide curricular activities to meet these needs. Teachers liaise with the child's teacher in his own school to ensure continuity of work and to obtain reports of scholastic achievement. They also spend time reintegrating children back into their own school when ready.

The purpose of the initial assessment interview is to ascertain the difficulties identified by the family and the individual child, and their motivation to work to minimize the problems. In the initial assessment a plan of action is formulated between the family and keyworkers.* Work may continue on an outpatient basis. Alternatively, key workers may offer a home visit to gain a more accurate picture of family interaction and home environment.

---

* Keyworkers are one or two workers, often from different backgrounds, who will work specifically with the child and family. They will be chosen because their specialist skills meet the needs of the individual child/family.

Bruggen (1973) identifies specific measurable objectives for admission, the planned programme for the child's family and, in terms of changed behaviour, establishing the point at which the family will accept the child home: this is useful focusing.

ASSESSMENT

A detailed nursing assessment of the family and individual child is made, whether the child is receiving help in a community or hospital-based service. It is important to get the whole picture of what is happening within a family, so a detailed assessment of the family and individual child is necessary.

Assessment methods

Observation used by nurses

Observation can be carried out directly or indirectly. The individual observing can either be participative or non-participative. Nurses observe children in daily activities and while generally participating in activities. They look at behaviour and listen to interactions. Nurses use two methods of direct participant observation:

1. interviews
2. specific rating scales.

Interviews with children tend to be unstructured but those with families may be structured with a prepared format. These interviews can elicit information about historical background, individuals' feelings towards themselves/others/an event, attitudes towards being helped and so on. The interview may be structured by the interviewer asking a lot of specific open questions, or it may be spontaneous and free flowing, allowing individuals in the family to talk as they wish.

Rating scales can be used in assessment and also as indicators to progress in specific treatment programmes. Specific behaviours may be rated on a scale 0–8 by nurses or by families at home. The scores would be recorded in diaries or on assessment sheets. For example, a family may present with a child who is demonstrating antisocial

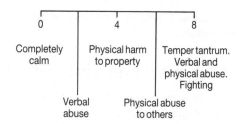

Record in the diary

1. Date and time and number of times in a daytime behaviour occurs
2. Any predisposing factors. What was child doing just prior to outburst?
3. Duration of angry behaviour
4. How resolved.

Fig. 28.1 Rating scale and diary used in assessment.

behaviour and is unable to control his anger (Fig. 28.1).

Self-assessment scales are often useful for older children or adults to rate/score their own behaviour at particular times of the day, and this involves them in their own care. It is important to use the language they would use to describe their behaviour on the scale. With a child who has anxiety about attending school, a family may be asked to rate themselves on a daily or less frequent basis (Fig. 28.2).

From these regular ratings a pattern may be established. For example, the child's anxiety is highest at break times when he is alone, having no close friends.

Subjective ratings of the nursing relationship formed with the child is a method used to back up nurses' more objective findings. For example, by examining the transference–countertransference relationship, nurses can identify how the child relates to them and work on their own feelings towards the child.

Psychiatric nurses in the USA have developed

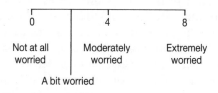

Fig. 28.2 A family rating scale.

well-researched and validated specific assessment formats in their work with children and families in psychiatric units. Most are little known in Britain (Brady et al 1984).

TRUST AND RELATIONSHIP BUILDING

Following the referral interview, the key workers with major therapeutic involvement for a particular child are identified. One of the two key people is often a nurse. These two people regularly see the family to review progress and discuss issues, initially attempting to form a relationship with the child and family by beginning to enlist their trust and confidence.

Building relationships with children takes time, particularly with younger children who have few significant relationships. Often being with the child, participating in play and daily living activities, assists in building relationships. Finally, the child may trust the nurse enough to play a game or read with her. This has to occur in the child's own time. Individual game playing or reading with a child may develop into more formal therapeutic sessions if the worker is suitably skilled and supervised, and this is regarded as desirable and helpful by the team.

Building relationships with families often results from regular information given in family sessions, so all members of the family hear the same information. By means of regular telephone contact and visits, families make known the child's likes/ dislikes, and family routines. The family, in return, receives regular information about the child's behaviour on the unit.

Intervention framework

Children's behaviour when playing reflects their personality and experiences. Individual children vary in their ability to concentrate on play alone.

Play is a medium through which children express their emotions. Nurses working in children's units may use play in a therapeutic way with a child. For example, they may encourage children who are physically violent towards others to take part in energetic games, and to express this feeling

verbally (or at times physically) with toys rather than with other people. Children can be encouraged to express their fears or worries through imaginative play and fantasy play. Some children have little previous experience of play and need to be encouraged and shown how to enjoy play.

MOTIVATING AND ENABLING SKILLS

Motivating skills involve having a positive objective in mind and shaping or reinforcing a child's behaviour so that it reflects the desired behaviour. Maintaining a positive attitude and being enthusiastic and consistent also help to motivate the child. If the child's behaviour shows no significant improvement or becomes worse, the nurse may use the skill of witholding social attention to behaviour.

Building up a child's self-esteem also helps to motivate him. This may involve working and developing something the child is already good at, rather than continually focusing on his faults.

LIMIT SETTING

Wilkinson (1983) defines a limit as, 'The point at which someone decides to stop certain behaviours in order to keep behaviour socially acceptable,' and suggests that the aim of limit setting is to teach the child socially acceptable behaviour while assisting in other areas of development. By having their behaviour limited, children are provided with freedom and security, enabling them to explore their environment and emotions safely and so have a wider experience from which to learn.

Components of limit setting

1. The child is given clear expectations for behaviour at all times. These expectations must be reinforced consistently by all adults associating with the child.
2. Confrontation over setting a limit needs careful consideration, and is resorted to only if it is over something adults can win. It is important to be reasonable and to value the child's sense of fair play. Adolescents in particular react to perceived injustice, and it

is important to state and restate the behaviour expectations.

3. The frequency of responses influences outcome. It is best to reinforce as near to the behaviour as possible and for reinforcement to occur as many times as possible.
4. Positive behaviour is praised, however small the change. Verbal praise is most effective. If given gifts, the child expects bigger and better gifts as improvement continues; this is not desirable.
5. Children's behaviour is influenced by behaviour displayed by parents, so role modelling of appropriate behaviour is important.
6. If the limit set is reasonable and the child makes no effort to behave in the expected way, realistic sanctions may be used. Sanctions help children to realize that there are consequences of their behaviour. If possible, it is helpful to relate the sanction to the expectation the child was unable to meet. For example, if the child is not out of bed by 9.00 a.m., he misses breakfast.
7. Follow-up or going through the incident with the child at a time well removed from the actual incident (at least 30 minutes later) is helpful in order to discuss insights gained, if any. With very young children a form of time out may be used in limit setting, removing the child from reinforcing situations without discussion to a quiet place, and taking him back almost immediately after he has calmed down.

Family work

Family work is not necessarily family therapy. A child is dependent upon adults, who are legally responsible for children and adolescents until the age of 16 years. It is important, therefore, not to view the child in isolation but as part of a dynamic system, the sum of which is greater than all the individual parts. The family rather than the child may become the focus for work when a child is experiencing difficulties. The child's needs are recognized by the parents, who follow through the referral process and decide whether or not to accept help as a family. The minimum expected from all families would be involvement in the initial assessment stage, attending regular family reviews or feedback concerning the child's progress from key workers, and attending discharge and follow-up meetings.

In a children's unit, informal meetings are also held with families or parents before a child goes on leave, so that discussion about continuing the child's therapeutic programme can take place. Occasionally, parental casework may be taken on where the problem identified lies mostly within the adults' relationships with each other. The child would then attend review meetings.

Family therapy approaches

Therapists from different theoretical backgrounds concentrate on different aspects of family functioning; these might be boundaries or communication. There are four stages which most therapists experience:

1. Entering the family system. The worker adopts a position where she is able to observe but is also partially involved in the family system
2. Putting the symptom back so the family own the problem
3. Facilitating communication of thoughts and feelings
4. Acting as role model, educator, and exploring family myths.

Examples of some specific techniques used by family workers:

a. Setting the family tasks — homework between sessions
b. Using a videotape to feed back issues to family
c. Role playing and psychodrama
d. Genograms — constructing family trees
e. Contract setting
f. Giving the family directives to achieve certain changes.

(Minuchin 1974, Hailey 1976, Palazzoli Boscalo et al 1980)

Specific behaviour programmes

Skills used to assist a child in changing undesirable behaviour include:

Ignoring, i.e. not responding either verbally or non-verbally to the child's undesirable behaviour, keeping a blank expression for 5–10 seconds, and carrying out this non-response consistently.

Time out from positive reinforcement involves removing the child from the situation immediately following the behaviour, and commenting as simply as possible or what was happening and why. Once the child's undesirable behaviour has stopped, the child is allowed to return to the situation he was in.

Desensitization techniques involve working with a child or his family gradually to reintroduce a child who is refusing school to school work, followed by hospital school and then his own school. The amount of exposure over a set period of time is increased steadily until the child becomes re-integrated. If this is not achieved, the child may have a home tutor, and work towards attending a specialized tutor centre for children with difficulties in attending normal school.

Group work

Group work in children's units varies according to the philosophy of the unit and the age of the child. It ranges from activity-centred play with young children, to social skills training groups, and peer support and community groups for adolescents.

Setting up group work with children requires careful consideration and agreement within the multi-professional team over the type of group to meet the children's needs, its defined aims and boundaries, and membership. There must be discussion of leadership style; the opportunity to evaluate the process of groups in supervision with an outside facilitator is necessary.

Normal group situations like meal times are used optimally with children to work through issues relating to individuals, for example the child may be asked to undertake simple chores such as laying the table. The nurse works with the child to elicit maximum participation and achievement of this task, for which he would then be praised.

Groups feature regularly in some children's units. These can either be verbal or activity centred. Activity groups are often smaller, family-sized groups, with 3–5 children and two facilitators. Children decide on activities, and facilitators examine interactions and social relationships experienced within the group, thereby promoting healthy participation and interaction. Facilitators need 5–10 minutes after the events in order to discuss and record the group processes and to plan the next meeting. Groups wherein there is greater emphasis on verbalizing thoughts and feelings are also included in the weekly timetable. They are used by their facilitators (nurses and other workers) to discuss how the children relate to each other as a community, encouraging independent contributions from children who may talk about their loneliness, frustrations and fears. Facilitators encourage other children to support their peers.

Some staff run relative support groups. These are not intended to replace family sessions but to focus on relatives' shared experience so that they can learn from each other, and gain insight into all aspects of parenting, their child's behaviour and the behaviour of other children.

Staff support groups are also essential. Working with children and young people is demanding and frustrating. Children's units often have a staff support group for which they engage a facilitator from outside the organization to explore working relationships between staff members and feelings towards particular children's incidents in the unit. The aim of providing this type of forum is to promote an environment conducive to optimum change in young people. This is particularly important for nurses.

Evaluation

Hunt & Marks (1981) define evaluation as, 'Essential for determining whether the interventions have been effective. It involves measuring how far the specific objectives have been met'.

Evaluation determines whether objectives have been met; provides information to reassess children's and families' needs; discovers which nursing actions are most consistently effective in solving particular problems and meeting needs;

and includes a written statement of what actually happened and how this was measured.

During the evaluation exercise, the child's and family's needs and difficulties are reassessed, and a decision made to continue with the plan of care and intervention outlined, or to plan a new intervention, setting another review date. If the patient's need has been met and new needs identified, a change of care plan is required.

If the family's objectives have been reached, then the child may be discharged home from the unit. Progress would be acknowledged, and the family may continue to visit the unit weekly or fortnightly for family sessions and discussions with key workers. If units have child nurses and family community psychiatric nurses as part of their team, these specialists may take over this work and follow the family's progress in their own homes, or in a local child and family centre.

Future developments in children's units appear to be directed towards efforts to reduce the need for children to be away from their families. Five-day wards are more common now than 7-day wards, ensuring that the family system adapts, with the child as part of the family at weekends. Many services only offer day care from 9 a.m.–7 p.m., with children going home every night. Community workers, particularly community psychiatric nurses, are taking on increasingly specialized roles, working with families in their own homes.

REFERENCES

Allen H 1981 The non-conformists. Nursing Mirror, May 20

Barker 1985 Assessment in psychiatric nursing. Croom Helm, London

Bollard & Nettleback 1982 A component analysis of dry bed training for treatment of bedwetting. Behaviour, Research and Therapy 20: 383–390

Bowlby J 1969 Attachment and loss. Hogarth, London

Bowlby J 1973 Separation and Anger. Hogarth, London

Brady et al 1984 Childhood depression — development of a screening tool. Paediatric Nursing 10(3)

Bruggen P et al 1973 The reason for admission as a focus of work for an adolescent unit. British Journal of Psychiatry 122: 319–329

Clerke A M, Clerke A D B 1976 Early experience, myth and evidence. Open Books, London

Erikson 1963 Childhood and society. Norton, New York

Eysenck H 1967 The biological basis of personality. Thomas, Springfield, Ill

Eysenck H 1971 Identity Youth + Crisis. Faber, London

Eysenck H 1973 The measurement of intelligence. MTP, Lancaster

Freud S 1962 Essays on theory and sexuality. Hogarth, London

Freud A 1974 Introduction to psychoanalysis and child analysis. Hogarth, London

Freud S 1986 Essentials of psychoanalysis. Hogarth, London

Glaser et al 1984 Focal Family Therapy. Journal of Family Therapy 6: 265–274

Heron J 1975 Category intervention analysis. Human Potential Research Project. University of Surrey, Guildford

Hunt J, Marks M 1981 Nursing care plans. HM & M.

Jensen 1968 Social class, race and psychological development.

Kamin et al 1981 Intelligence, the battle for the minor. Pan, London

Lorenz K 1970 Studies in animal and human behaviour. Methuen, London

McGurk 1951 Ecological factors in human development. Paper presented at Conf. July 13–17 Holland 1977. International Society of Human Development

Piaget J 1953 The dying of intelligence in the child. Routledge & Kegan Paul, London

Price R 1976 Abnormal Behaviour. Holt, Rhinehart & Winston, London

Reed & Shilitoe 1986 Dry at night. Nursing Times (Community Outlook), March.

Rogers C 1961 On becoming a person. Constable, London

Rogers C 1969 Encounter groups. Penguin, Harmondsworth, Middlesex

Rosen & Glasier 1983 Introduction to family therapy. Unpublished handouts, Guy's Hospital, Bloomfield Clinic, London

Rutter M 1975 Helping troubled children. Penguin, Harmondsworth, Middlesex

Schaffer 1979 Mothering. Fontana, London

Skeels 1966 (1938) A study of environmental stimulation. Child Welfare 15(5)

Stanberg 1986 (ed) The adolescent unit. Wiley, Chichester

Vygotsky 1962 Thought and language. Wiley, New York

Walff 1973 Language of the brain — an introduction to the psychology of language.

Wilkinson T 1983 Child and adolescent psychiatric nursing. Blackwell, Oxford

29

Depression and suicide

E. Minghella

Depression is the most common psychiatric disorder, comprising 35–40% of all those brought to medical attention (Linford Rees 1976). It is also a problem, which, to a greater or lesser degree, affects most people from time to time. It is therefore unsurprising that it is the subject of much debate.

This chapter presents a critical examination of some well-respected theoretical models of depression. It also discusses those treatment choices which have particular relevance to psychiatric nurses, both in hospital and the community. The problems associated with the experience of nursing depressed patients are often neglected, and a section in this chapter addresses this issue. Finally, there are sections on the special problems of suicide and parasuicide and developments in the psychiatric nursing treatment of patients who deliberately harm themselves.

THE NATURE OF DEPRESSION

Whilst the possible causes of depression are the subject of controversy, most practitioners and theorists agree on the general features. Clearly the most obvious complaint is of 'depressed' mood. However, it is worth noting that this is not always expressed, especially in the early stages, and sometimes the predominant feeling is of indifference rather than sadness; this is often described as 'masked depression' (Trethowan & Sims 1983). Nevertheless, depression is most commonly characterized by a depressed mood which is persistent and all pervading. Depression affects the whole person, including psychological, intellectual, social and physiological functions.

Other features of depression include disrupted sleep, reduced appetite and weight loss, lack of energy accompanied by retarded speech and motor activity, poor concentration and decreased libido. Thoughts are centred on the negative, and the sufferer often feels guilty, inferior and unworthy. There may be feelings of depersonalization, auditory or sensory hallucinations, and in severe depression, delusions in keeping with the content of these ideas. For example, the depressed person may believe that he or she has no internal organs, that he or she is being eaten away from the inside. There is a general feeling of hopelessness, and there is a grave risk of suicide. In some instances, agitation is present: the psychological aspects of depression exist without the physical retardation. The sufferer is highly anxious and tense, unable to keep still or sleep. Box 29.1 contains a summary of the common features of depression, according to the particular function affected. Further discussion of symptoms can be found in the next section, in particular in the analysis of the medical model of depression.

It is important to note that depression can occur in other conditions, and is sometimes an integral part of another mental illness, such as manic-depressive psychosis. Depression may also feature in physical illness.

Women appear to be more vulnerable to depression than men, although differences in research methods and diagnostic techniques reduce the reliability of the statistics. Goldberg (1983) cites several studies whose findings regarding the incidence of depression range from 2.6% to 16% of the male population, to 6.7% to 24% of females. Nonetheless, the sex difference remains fairly constant in the research, with women two to three times more likely than men to be diagnosed as depressed.

Recent trends in research suggest that social fac-

Box 29.1 Common features of depression and functions affected

Intellectual
Poor concentration
Impaired memory
Slow and impoverished speech
Thought processes slower

Physiological
Tiredness
Sleep disruption
Loss of appetite
Weight loss
Constipation
Restlessness/Tearfulness

Psychological/cognitive
Depressed mood
Apathy
Auditory hallucinations
Sensory hallucinations
Depersonalization
Suicidal ideas
Hopelessness
Guilt
Poor self image
Anxiety

---

tors may account for much of this discrepancy (Tennant 1985).

MODELS OF DEPRESSION

Four well-known approaches to the understanding of depression will be described. It will be noted that whilst all are relatively independent, there are clear points of overlap. Furthermore, there are often variations *within* the models which, through lack of space, will not be discussed here.

Medical model

Classically, the medical model of depression, described in many psychiatric textbooks, is the one accepted by nursing authorities and practitioners. This is a pity as other models have much to offer nursing, especially as a basis for nursing practice.

Traditional psychiatry divides clinical depression into two categories:

- reactive (neurotic/exogenous) depression
- endogenous (psychotic) depression.

Reactive depression, as the term suggests, is seen as an exaggerated reaction to an external stressor. That is to say, there is always a precipitating event (such as the loss of a loved one) or environmental factors which are instrumental in the development of the illness. Reactive depression is usually seen as less severe than endogenous depression.

Endogenous depression is generally described as dependent on genetic and/or other constitutional factors, *within* the individual. Little is known about the exact nature of any genetic predisposition to endogenous depression, which is seen as qualitatively different from reactive depression. Its onset may occur independently of external influences, and it is characterized by 'diurnal variation' of mood, where the patient feels worse in the morning, gradually improving as the day goes on. Waking early in the morning is seen as a symptom of endogenous rather than reactive depression. In endogenous depression, psychotic features are sometimes present. These include hallucinations and delusions, the content of which reflect the patient's depressed state and self-image; for example, the patient may hear voices accusing him or her of terrible sins or commenting on body odour.

There are claims that specific biological functions are altered in depression, and that these alterations are present only when the mental state is abnormal. Consequently, it is asserted that such 'biological markers' can be used in the understanding and diagnosis of depression. The 'Dexamethasone Suppression Test' (DST) has been hailed as an important 'marker' in this respect. Studies mentioned by Checkley (1985) report that the DST yields abnormal results in some depressed patients; when the patient recovers, the test results return to normal.

Slater & Cowie (1971), discussing the possible genetic bases of psychotic depression, assert that the question of genetic inheritance remains unsettled. They summarize various viewpoints from those who support the idea of a sex-linked dominant gene, to those who argue a multi-factorial inheritance, including constitutional personality factors; however, they suggest finally that there needs to be greater understanding of the biochemical and metabolic process of affective disorders before further progress along genetic lines is made.

The question of genetic influences in the causation of 'reactive' depression is even more undecided. Noting a number of studies which examined depressed patients' dizygotic and monozygotic twins, Goldberg (1983) argues that there is no evidence that genetic factors make a specific contribution to the aetiology of reactive depression. Instead, he suggests that there may be constitutional susceptibility to *general* anxiety and neurotic disorder.

Modern psychiatric textbooks no longer adhere to a strict division between the two entities of reactive and psychotic or endogenous depression, although the distinction continues to be made when describing symptoms.* Precipitating events can be identified in endogenous as well as reactive depression; a recent study could not confirm the hypothesis that endogenous depression is relatively independent of prior life stresses (Bebbington et al 1989). Increasingly, depression is seen as running along a continuum, from a mild disorder to the most severe and disabling. Within this formulation, the implication is that the cause or causes of depression remain the same, regardless of the severity of the illness, and in general, the nature of depression is seen as *both reactive and endogenous*. Linford Rees (1976), for example, states that 'depressive illnesses are the result of the interaction of genetic and constitutional factors on the one hand, with environmental and other exogenous influences on the other' (p. 186). Trethowan & Sims (1983) assert that a depressive illness can occur as a reaction to a wide variety of both external and internal circumstances in people who are genetically or in other ways predisposed to the disorder (p. 92). However, it is difficult to

---

* Interestingly, Brown & Harris (1978) note that, whilst early morning wakening is considered a symptom of 'psychotic' depression, one-fifth of their sample of *neurotic* patients also experienced this problem (p. 213).

ascertain precisely what these genetic or 'other' predispositions are.

The medical model, then, assumes a genetic or physiological basis to depression, whether this is seen as specific to depressive illness (endogenous depression) or general to neuroses (in reactive depression). Medical treatments such as antidepressants are therefore prescribed to alleviate, if not 'cure', depressive illness. However, this assumption has yet to be satisfactorily verified, despite a vast number of studies and continuing research. The main problems with the research are that: firstly, different studies use different criteria and methods for diagnosing depression; secondly, results are not consistent; and thirdly, it is impossible to control for external factors. Nonetheless, traditional psychiatry continues to look for an acceptable biological model of depression.

Linford Rees (1976) advises: ' . . . . we must look forward to the day when (we) . . . . will have had the time and opportunity to carry out long-term prospective genetic studies on patients selected on the basis of epidemiological criteria. These patients would have to be studied over a very prolonged period of time in order to ascertain their biochemical and physiological characteristics, to discover what factors influence the course of the illness, and finally to correlate these findings with the response to particular methods of treatment.'

Cognitive-behavioural model of depression

Cognitive-behavioural theories have developed from the simple behavioural approach to a more sophisticated attempt to explain the origins and maintenance of depressive symptoms.

The theories vary, but the central postulate is that abnormal 'cognitions' constitute the primary disorder of depressed patients. Cognitions can be defined as 'attending, perceiving, thinking and remembering' (Gelder 1985 p. 1). These cognitions arise from a person's particular circumstances and history. In depression, behaviour patterns are seen as a direct result of maladaptive thought processes which have distorted positive thoughts and experiences into negative ones.

Aaron Beck is one of the first and most import-ant exponents of cognitive behaviour theory and therapy (Beck 1967, 1976). His basic model, founded on clinical observations, posits the establishment of a 'cognitive triad' which forms the basis of the depressed person's negative view of self, his or her world (or current experience) and the future (see Fig. 29.1).

Underlying this cognitive triad are relatively stable ways of thinking, termed 'schemas' (Beck et al 1980) which distort the person's perceptions of reality. A schema may lie dormant for prolonged periods, only to be activated by a particular set of stressful circumstances, such as divorce. It is argued that negative schemas, underlying the depressive cognitive triad, predispose a person to depression.

Faulty information processing maintains the depressed person's distortion of reality, creating a vicious circle in which negative expectations are confirmed and consequently reinforced. Faulty information processing refers to four basic errors of thinking:

- 'selective abstraction', where the depressed person focuses on negative factors taken out of context and discounts the positive

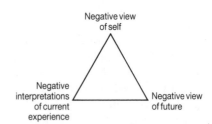

1. Negative view of self

The depressed person sees him or herself as inadequate, bad, sick. He or she is worthless, unattractive and full of self-criticism. These feelings correspond quite clearly with the symptoms of depressed mood as described above.

2. Negative interpretations of world/current experience

The depressed person experiences the world as a poor, deprived place in which impossible demands are placed upon him or her.

3. Negative view of the future

The depressed person expects the future to reflect his or her assessment of the present; in other words, he or she anticipates continued failure, hardship and suffering. The third angle of the cognitive triad, then, is an amalgamation of the first two, extended into the future.

Fig. 29.1 The depressed cognitive triad.

- 'arbitrary inference', in which the depressed person forms subjective conclusions without reference to the objective evidence and fails to consider alternative explanations
- 'over-generalization', where general inferences are made from a single instance
- 'minimization and magnification', in which evaluations about the self are underestimated, and problems grossly overestimated.

(These categories are clearly not mutually exclusive.)

Depressive thinking is characterized by self-blame and worthlessness, persistent hopelessness and helplessness. It is important to note that, in Beck's model, distorted cognitions are sufficient to cause depression, but may not be *necessary*; in other words, causation, and indeed depression, is seen as multi-faceted.

The cognitive-behavioural model of depression is persuasive because it takes into account the depressed person's thought processes, and describes how these might serve to maintain depression. However, the problem of causation is not adequately addressed; in particular, the concept of the 'schema' is a weak point in the model. How the schema develops, how its existence is maintained, its resistance to change and how and why it should be 'energized', as Beck puts it, are not fully explained.

The model can be seen as circular; as such it could be argued that traumatic events cause negative thought processes leading to cognitive distortions, rather than these cognitive distortions being the primary disorder. Nevertheless, its value is found in the development of clinical techniques and practices which will be mentioned briefly in this chapter.

Social models of depression

Social models of depression seek to produce an explanation of depression as a response to environmental conditions and experiences. In their book *Social Origins of Depression*, Brown and Harris (1978) set out to argue that, whilst there must always be a physical basis to it, 'clinical depression' is 'an understandable response to adversity' (p. 46).

They carried out a community study of 572 women in Camberwell, South London. Women were chosen rather than men, partly because they are more accessible, but primarily because clinical depression is considered to be more common amongst women.

Brown & Harris's findings, based on detailed interviews, produced a model of depression based on three main categories of causative social factors:

Provoking agents

These 'life events' or 'major difficulties' are seen to influence when depression occurs. Life events are defined as events which disrupt, or threaten to disrupt, normal activities: the life-threatening illness of a loved one, or a job loss, for example. The study found that 61% of depressed women had at least one severe life event before the onset of the illness, compared with only 20% of non-depressed women in a comparable 38-week period before interview.

'Major difficulties' constitute severe long-term problems, such as chronic, substandard, crowded accommodation. Again, Brown & Harris found that major difficulties were three times more common in depressed than in non-depressed women.

Vulnerability factors

Four factors were seen to affect women's vulnerability to depression. These were: the presence of 3 or more children under the age of 14 at home; the woman's loss of her mother before the age of 11; no employment outside the home; and the lack of an intimate relationship. In this model, vulnerability factors increase the woman's risk of becoming depressed in the presence of provoking agents. For example, nearly half of the women who had lost their mothers before the age of 11 developed depression, *but only if they experienced a life event or major difficulty as well*.

Intimacy (usually with a husband or boyfriend) was especially important, because it appeared to *protect* the woman from depression, even if other vulnerability factors were present.

The existence of vulnerability factors is crucial

to the model, because the authors argue that these factors lower self-esteem and explain why certain women are more prone than others to depression.

Symptom-formation factors

Brown & Harris found that psychosocial circumstances also affected the *severity* of the depressive illness. A severe event occurring after the onset of the illness, past losses and a previous depressive episode were all important. There is an overlap here with the vulnerability factor of the loss of mother before age 11; the results implied that the type of loss influenced whether the depression was 'reactive' or 'endogenous'. If the mother had died, then the depression was likely to be more serious (endogenous) than if the mother had left home.

Loss in general is crucial in this model. Brown & Harris argue that loss events produce hopelessness, and it is the generalization of hopelessness which is seen as central to the development of depression.

Social class was another important factor. Brown & Harris found that working-class women were more vulnerable and experienced more life events and difficulties than their middle-class counterparts. For example, working-class women with three or more young children at home were four times more likely to suffer from depression than middle-class women in similar circumstances.

The main criticisms of Brown & Harris' (1978) work are directed at details of the research design and statistical analyses; for example, Lawson (1978) raises the issue of defining events as 'problems'. The research team agreed, in certain instances, which events would be considered as stressful, even if these events were not presented as problems by the women concerned. This could be seen as imposing 'objective' meanings of events at the expense of a woman's 'subjective' experience, thus challenging the validity of these 'events' as a significant category.

Methodological issues notwithstanding, this model continues to be well respected and highly influential. It has prompted others to examine social factors in relation to depression. For example, Birtchnell et al (1988), in their study of

young married women living on a London housing estate, found that depressive symptoms were linked to poor housing. George et al (1989) found that there was a strong link between lack of social support and recurrence of depression at a 6–32 month follow-up of patients who had been admitted to hospital with major depression. Interestingly, the quality of this support was an important component; not all social relationships were seen as beneficial and supportive. Bebbington et al (1988) discovered a far greater than expected number of life events shortly before the onset of depression in a group of 130 depressed patients, and their results suggested a causal relationship between depression and life events.

Clearly, Brown & Harris's study has had major implications for the understanding and treatment of depression, and is of particular relevance for psychiatric nurses working in the community. Anthony Storr remarks: 'Every time I encounter George Brown's work on 'Social Origins of Depression', I blush for my profession. We have allowed a sociologist to discover what psychiatrists ought to have found out years ago, but failed to do because of their pseudo-medical assumptions' (Storr 1983).

Psychodynamic model of depression

In *Mourning and Melancholia*, Freud (1917) compared depression (or melancholia) with the normal affect of mourning. He described melancholia as painful dejection, loss of interest, loss of the capacity for love, inhibition and loss of self-esteem, all of which, except for low self-esteem, he argued are part of the normal experience of mourning.

In mourning, the loved one (loved 'object') has died, no longer exists, and reality demands that all attachment is therefore withdrawn from that object. However, naturally, the bereaved person resists this, and this can lead to a turning away from reality and clinging to the loved object through hallucination. The effect of this is to psychically prolong the existence of the loved one until there is a gradual return to reality. Freud noted that it is only because we know how to explain it, that mourning does not seem to be pathological.

Freud argued that melancholia is also a reaction to loss, but that it is not so easy to see what this loss is. Sometimes, it may be possible to know *who* the loss is, but not *what* it is. In other words, it is not always possible to understand, at first, the *symbolic meaning* of the lost object. This may be because the loss is withdrawn from consciousness, whereas in mourning, the loss is a conscious one.

Loss of self-esteem is seen as significant in distinguishing melancholia from mourning. As Freud put it: 'In mourning it is the world which has become poor and empty; in melancholia it is the ego' (Freud 1917, p. 246)*. Pedder (1982) describes self-esteem as a two-person relationship: 'the esteem in which one part of the self is held by another part of the self — or in other words an internal object relationship' (p. 333). For Freud, then, the self-abasement and self-reproaches characteristic of depression are reproaches against a loved object which have been shifted away from the object to the patient's own ego. This is followed by an identification of the ego with the lost object, so that both the ego and the object fall under the harsh scrutiny of the 'critical agency', an idea which was later developed into the concept of the 'superego'. Freud gives an example of a woman who expresses pity for her husband for being tied to such an incapable wife; in reality, he says, she is *accusing her husband* of being incapable (Freud 1917 p. 248).

Clearly, the notion of 'ambivalence' is important here. In object relationships, love is mixed with hate in varying degrees; occasions of being slighted, neglected or disappointed can create or reinforce an existing ambivalence. In depression, the stronger the feelings of hate, the more sadistic the internalized self-reproaches; suicidal, thoughts and behaviour, then, are seen in terms of internalization of murderous, impulses. Stengel (1964) expanded on this much later, in his influential work on suicide and attempted suicide.

---

* Here is an important difference from Beck's depressive cognitive triad, where both the self and the external world are seen as poor and deprived.

Freud's psychoanalytic theories have been widely criticized, on the one hand by those who refuse to accept the basic tenets of psychoanalytic theory (such as the posited existence of the 'unconscious'). This group tends to criticize on the basis of the 'non-scientific' nature of the theory, arguing that it cannot be observed or validated. On the other hand, later psychoanalysts have challenged or developed Freud's ideas. For example, Bowlby (1961) has criticized Freud's emphasis on depressive illness as opposed to normal mourning, and expanded on the notion of early maternal loss as a major contributing factor in the development of depression in later life.

Discussion of the models

There are clearly points of similarity and overlap between the models described. One of the central shared concepts is that of loss as a crucial factor in the causation of depression. A loss can be a concrete loss, such as a bereavement, or less tangible, such as loss of role. In the medical model, a loss counts as an environmental factor which may precipitate 'reactive' or even 'endogenous' depression. In cognitive theories, a current loss can reactivate the depressive cognitions associated with a past loss. Losses of many kinds, but particularly the loss of a woman's mother before the age of 11, is crucial to Brown & Harris's model. Finally, early psychoanalytic theory emphasizes loss in the form of a lost love 'object', in the explanation of melancholia or depressive illness, whilst later work suggests that early loss of the mother may make a child susceptible to depressive illness in later life.

Strongly connected with these environmental losses is the psychological loss of self-esteem. How this loss is conceptualized, and its status as either a symptom or as a causative factor, varies between the models. Indeed, this latter question is often blurred *within* models; for example, within Beck's model low self-esteem is seen as both a symptom and a cause of depression.

TREATMENT FOR DEPRESSION

Different theoretical frameworks implicate different treatment choices. However, it is worth noting that in psychiatry it is often the case that two or more models are employed at any one time; consequently, patients often participate in more than one type of treatment.

Many different professionals adopt differing or, indeed, similar approaches to the care and management of depressed people. Within the multi-disciplinary team, nurses' roles may vary widely, often depending on the therapeutic setting. Nursing intervention can range from basic, but no less important, 'caring' and monitoring of medical treatments, to implementing treatment programmes derived from psychological and social models of understanding depression. Perhaps too often, nursing intervention is entirely devoted to implementing treatment programmes instituted by other professionals, especially psychiatrists.

Psychological and social theories of depression have resulted in a plethora of therapeutic methods and approaches to the treatment of depression. Even if these are not formally adopted — for example, very few nurses are in a position to offer formal psychoanalysis — many of the concepts and techniques are invaluable in the formulation of nursing interventions.

Some commonly used approaches will be described in brief and general terms.*

Any discussion of therapeutic approaches will inevitably include medical treatments, but the emphasis is on the nursing role in the care of depressed patients.

Medical treatments and nursing intervention

Medical treatments, based around the medical model of mental illness, presuppose a biological basis to depression. There are two major types of medical treatment: antidepressant medication and electroconvulsive therapy.

---

* Further reading is recommended, and it is nearly always worthwhile pursuing further training if specializing in a particular approach. Adequate supervision is also important.

Antidepressant medication

Antidepressant medication can be split into two basic groups: tricyclics and monoamine oxidase inhibitors (MAOIs). Tricyclic antidepressants are used more commonly than MAOIs, mainly because they do not show the dangerous drug and food interactions associated with the MAOIs.

Drugs in the tricyclic group include amitryptiline, which has additional sedative properties and is often used when there is related anxiety, and imipramine, which is less sedating. There are sometimes adverse side-effects, such as dry mouth, drowsiness, constipation, blurred vision, urinary retention, cardiac irregularities, tachycardia and anorexia.

MAOIs, such as phenelzine, are usually used after tricyclic antidepressants have been tried unsuccessfully. There are numerous adverse side-effects, and the contraindications are hazardous. The most important problem is the dangerous interactions of MAOIs with foods containing tyramine. Cheese, food containing yeast extracts, such as Bovril, broad beans and alcohol (but red wine in particular), must be excluded, and all food should be fresh. If these rules are not observed, the reaction is likely to be severe and could be fatal. Such a reaction is characterized by severe, throbbing headache and a rapid rise in blood pressure, followed by cardiac failure or intercranial haemorrhage.

Another problem with MAOIs is that they interact adversely with a wider range of medication than any other class of drugs. For example, certain cough mixtures and common cold remedies, as well as tricyclic antidepressants, could prove extremely dangerous if taken at the same time as MAOIs, or within two weeks.

Because of these problems, a special treatment card (see Fig. 29.2) is usually issued when MAOIs are dispensed, and it is vital that patients know exactly what they can and cannot eat or drink, and that they do not take any other form of medication without prior discussion with the prescribing doctor. A further confounding factor for both tricyclic antidepressants and MAOIs, is that they do not produce an immediate therapeutic effect. It is likely to be about 2 weeks before the patient notices

TREATMENT CARD

Carry this card with you at all times. Show it to any doctor who may treat you other than the doctor who prescribed this medicine, and to your dentist if you require dental treatment.

INSTRUCTIONS TO PATIENTS

Please read carefully
While taking this medicine and for 14 days after your treatment finishes you must observe the following simple instructions:-

1 Do not eat CHEESE, PICKLED HERRING OR BROAD BEAN PODS.
2 Do not eat or drink BOVRIL, OXO, MARMITE or ANY SIMILAR MEAT OR YEAST EXTRACT.
3 Eat only FRESH foods and avoid food that you suspect could be stale or 'going off'. This is especially important with meat, fish poultry or offal. Avoid game.
4 Do not take any other MEDICINES (including tablets, capsules, nose drops, inhalations or suppositories) whether purchased by you or previously prescribed by your doctor, without first consulting your doctor or your pharmacist.
   NB *Treatment for coughs and colds, pain relievers, tonics and laxatives are medicines.*
5 Avoid alcoholic drinks.
Keep a careful note of any food or drink that disagrees with you, avoid it and tell your doctor.
Report any unusual or severe symptoms to your doctor and follow any other advice given by him.

| M.A.O.I. | Prepared by The Pharmaceutical Society and the British Medical |

Association on behalf of the Health Departments of the United Kingdom.

Fig. 29.2 MAOI treatment card.

any improvement, and if this is not fully explained, it can add to feelings of distress and hopelessness.

The nurse's role in relation to the prescription of antidepressants is manifold. Firstly, it is often the nurse who dispenses the drug, particularly for inpatients, but also for day-patients, and sometimes for outpatients. As such, the nurse will invariably need to explain about therapeutic effects, side-effects and precautions. Even if the prescribing doctor has already discussed these issues with the patient, it is worth remembering that the patient may not have absorbed or understood all the information.

The nurse also has a responsibility to look

for and report side-effects. When MAOIs are prescribed, it is crucially important that the nurse ensures that the patient is fully aware of the dietary restrictions and the consequences of failure to adhere to the dietary regime. In the case of inpatients, this will extend to ordering a special diet from the hospital kitchen and ensuring that it is received by the correct patient at each meal-time.

Very depressed patients may refuse medication as a consequence of self-destructive or suicidal thoughts, or because as part of their depressive psychopathology, they feel they do not deserve treatment. It may be necessary, then, for the nurse to take over responsibility for the patient, to persuade the patient to take medication, and to ensure that, once given, the drugs are swallowed (a suicidal patient may well be hoarding tablets to be taken as an overdose at a later stage). One way of easing this task is to ask the doctor to prescribe the drug in liquid form for vulnerable patients.

A further nursing responsibility is to monitor the therapeutic effects of the drugs, such as changes in appetite, sleep, self-care and mood. It is necessary to know if and how the treatment is working, and to observe whether the therapeutic effects are increasing the patient's vulnerability to suicidal behaviour.

Electroconvulsive therapy (ECT)

Electroconvulsive therapy (ECT) is most commonly used in the treatment of severe, intractable 'endogenous' depression, especially when this is characterized by marked physical and mental retardation.

ECT is generally given twice-weekly in a course of about four to six treatments. A major fit is electrically induced under anaesthetic; the fit itself is modified by the use of a short-acting muscle relaxant.

If it is to be effective, the results of ECT are often immediate and marked, with great improvement in the patient's symptoms. In this sense, it has advantages over the use of antidepressants, which take up to a fortnight before any therapeutic benefit is noted.

However, there are several problems with ECT. Firstly, there is an increased risk of suicide immediately after treatment because the patient is sufficiently better to act on suicidal feelings. Secondly, there is also the risk of precipitating mania in manic-depressive patients. Both of these risks demonstrate the importance of adequate supervision during and immediately after ECT.

Other problems are mainly associated with the ethical considerations regarding side-effects of the treatment. Most notably, memory impairment, especially the inability to retain recently learned material, has been well documented. Advocates of ECT argue that such damage is usually transient, and that most patients consider this a minor complaint compared with the suffering relieved by the treatment. Furthermore, it is argued that memory functions are often impaired in depression. This issue remains contentious.

Some critics have argued that ECT can cause permanent brain damage; indeed Clare notes that some commentators attribute the therapeutic effects of ECT to damage inflicted on sensitive nerve cells (Clare 1979). However, he concludes that the 'evidence does not support the belief that ECT, in the manner and frequency with which it is commonly administered to patients, produces brain damage as a matter of course' (p. 672).

Other problems include the risks involved in using muscle relaxants and anaesthetics; again, supporters of ECT would argue that many routine medical procedures involve the same risks.

Finally, it is not known how ECT works. Many would assert that it provides only temporary relief from symptoms, without dealing with the underlying problems or causes of the depression; as such, it is argued that ECT involves substantial risks without major therapeutic advantages.

One of the most important aspects of nursing a patient who is to have ECT is adequate preparation, both physical and emotional. Physical preparation includes ensuring that the patient does not eat for the required period before the anaesthetic is administered, and preparing the treatment trolley, which should always include resuscitative equipment. Emotional preparation is more difficult to define and gauge. Discussing the possible therapeutic effects and side-effects with the patient, encouraging ventilation of feelings — both hopes and fears — about the treatment, simply

spending time with him or her the night beforehand; these are all ways of helping to prepare the patient for ECT. Remember, too, that the patient is likely to be well aware of the controversy surrounding ECT and may wish to discuss it.

The importance of close nursing supervision *after* treatment and monitoring the effects of ECT have already been mentioned. This is essential because the sudden improvement may provide the patient with the energy and impetus — previously absent — to attempt suicide. Some patients are also vulnerable to manic episodes.

Ethical considerations have prompted some nurses to refuse to participate in the nursing tasks associated with ECT. However, this has been known to result in dismissal.

Psychological therapies and nursing intervention

There are several different psychological therapies used in the treatment of depression. As Peplau (1987) has stressed, nurses now have the opportunity to use psychotherapeutic skills as an alternative to biomedical psychiatric treatment. A brief outline of the more common approaches which have special relevance to nursing will be presented.

Cognitive-behavioural therapy

Cognitive change is the primary target of cognitive-behavioural therapy, but modification of behaviour is also seen as important, since the patient must learn from experience. Therapy is usually brief, focusing on current problems. The cognitive therapist works with the depressed person to test the validity of his or her thoughts by applying reason and logic; the patient is encouraged in this way to discover the relationship between his or her (maladaptive) cognitive processes and his emotional state. As well as identifying cognitions and challenging their validity, the therapist's role includes setting homework in between sessions. Homework typically involves the patient keeping a structured diary to record situations which provoke negative thoughts and feelings, and to consider alternative ways of thinking about and dealing with those situations.

There are inevitably difficulties in engaging in any kind of treatment with depressed people. One important problem with cognitive-behavioural therapy is that, as the patient perceives his or her life, world and future as utterly negative and hopeless, then the nurse/therapist may be drawn into this set of thoughts and feelings. This can act to prevent the therapist working effectively to help the patient consider alternative, positive thoughts and behaviours. Another problem is that the patient must be motivated in order to participate in therapy and, particularly, to undertake tasks set as homework; yet, lack of motivation is a central feature of depression.

✳Because cognitive therapy is essentially a problem-solving approach to treatment, it fits neatly within the framework of the nursing process. After exploring the problems with the patient, the therapist breaks down the information into a list of target problems (Assessment). The therapist then discusses ways of dealing with the problems (Planning). Both within the sessions and outside as homework, the patient works on tasks which centre around the selected problems (Implementation). Feedback and testing (Evaluation) are built into each session. The active participation of the patient is a vital part of the treatment.

Counselling

Counselling draws on various psychological theories and can involve a number of different therapeutic approaches ranging from simple advice-giving to more sophisticated client-centred or psychodynamic approaches. However, generally, therapeutic counselling is based on the development of an understanding relationship within which the patient or client can help him or herself to change.

Depressed people can work in a counselling relationship, although the problem of motivation remains. In particular, when *psychosocial*, rather than full-blown *psychiatric* problems are most prominent, focused, short-term counselling can be helpful. The development of a positive relation-ship can be instrumental in helping to improve the patient's low self-esteem.

Counselling involves patients taking responsibility for their own actions and lives; this can be a problem in the treatment of depression for both nurse and patient. Nurses often feel that they must take responsibility for the patient, and many patients may agree. In some instances this may be appropriate, for example when a patient is severely depressed and *unable* to take responsibility for even the most basic tasks of daily life. It is often difficult, however, for the nurse to break out of this traditional role. Suicidal thoughts, threats and actions exacerbate the problem and can contribute to the nurse feeling responsible for what happens to the patient.

It is important, as Nelson-Jones (1983) points out, that the question of responsibility is handled sensitively: 'The last thing that certain clients may be looking for from their counsellor is the suggestion that they may be contributing to their own and to other peoples' distress' (p. 102). He discusses the 'attribution' (and 'misattribution') of responsibility in the counselling relationship, and suggests ways in which counsellors can explore this issue by focusing on specific situations, offering feedback, and encouraging the patient to use the pronoun 'I' rather than 'it' or 'they'.

Another important, but often neglected, aspect of counselling is its termination. With depressed people, who are vulnerable to feelings of rejection and low self-esteem, this issue is even more crucial. Past experiences of separation and loss, as mentioned in the theoretical discussion, may have contributed to the development of the depressive episode. Endings should be discussed, preferably negotiated, and prepared for. In short-term therapy, it is often worth working towards the ending almost from the beginning. Indeed, the termination of counselling can itself provide an opportunity to focus on past losses.

Counselling is a particularly useful therapeutic approach for helping depressed patients in the community, where contact is limited and it is easier to maintain boundaries. Contact need not be long term, but there should always be clear aims and objectives.

Of course, counselling skills, such as listening,

observing, empathic responding, are very important in the practice of psychiatric nursing in general.

Group psychotherapy

Group therapy is an economical and powerful therapeutic method, although too often there is not adequate supervision and training for the therapists. There are several different approaches to group therapy, but in general attention is focused on the relationships of the group members with each other and with the therapist or therapists. A group also provides an opportunity for the members to share their problems and experiences with others in similar circumstances, and to learn from each other.

Having carried out research in both the United States and Britain, Gordon (1986) reported on the efficacy of nurse-led group therapy for depressed women. She echoed others' views that professionally qualified nurses could function well as group facilitators, and that because women are highly represented among nurses, they would be particularly appropriate as therapists in groups for women. Gordon's findings, based on the comparison of depressed women treated in nurse-facilitated groups and control samples, suggest that nurse-facilitated groups can be effective in the treatment of moderately depressed women. Feelings of self-esteem improved and depressive and hopeless feelings decreased in the group members. It is worth noting, however, that in this research the nurse therapists underwent special training before facilitating groups and were highly experienced; this highlights the need for adequate training and supervision for the good and effective practice of group therapy.

Hospitalization

For a minority of depressed patients, periods of hospitalization may be necessary. In such situations it is the nursing staff who have the most contact with the depressed person. Indeed, the therapeutic milieu of the ward itself relies heavily on the nursing staff. Ward nurses have the opportunity to make full and comprehensive personal assessments of the patient's problems and needs and to provide a safe and therapeutic environment for the patient. The chart in Table 29.1 highlights areas for nursing assessment of the possible problems and needs of the depressed patient in hospital.

Planning and implementing care should be based on the assessment, and it may be the very basic needs which need immediate attention. Fluid charts, monitoring food intake, regular weighing and encouraging personal hygiene are all fun-

Table 29.1 Nursing assessment for depressed patients in hospital. (Assessment of needs based on Maslow 1970)

Needs	In depression
Physiological	Common problems: appetite and sleep disorders, constipation, diarrhoea. Risk of infection. Antidepressant medication tends to exacerbate physiological problems.
Safety	Feelings of insecurity often associated with suicidal ideas. Assessment of suicidal risk extremely important; must be reconsidered at every review. Hallucinations and delusions can be very frightening.
Love and belonging	Self-condemnation and unworthiness common features. Inhibited communication, unresponsiveness and poor self-care can cause/increase social isolation. Complete social withdrawal not infrequent.
Self-esteem	Poor self-esteem central to depression. Can be accentuated by humiliation associated with physiological dysfunctions, dependency, lack of privacy in institution.
Intellectual	Impaired memory and concentration common. Reduced likelihood of intelligent and stimulating conversation from others. Lack of curiosity may mean patient not kept properly informed.
Aesthetic	Self-expression though work and art grossly inhibited.
Self-actualization	Self-realization, adaptability, independence, ability to form relationships spontaneously etc. — all absent in depression. Important to monitor any changes and improvements, but these goals can feel impossible to achieve for both nurse and patient.

damental considerations. The risk of suicide must be taken seriously. Some practitioners advocate continuous or close observation for suicidal patients. The patient sometimes resents this approach, but Altschul & McGovern (1985) point out that often it is a great relief for the patient to 'put his life into the hands of the nursing staff' (p. 161).

Particular attention must be paid to the availability of sharp instruments, cleaning fluids, any kind of medication or any other instruments which could possibly be used for a suicidal act. It is sometimes necessary to ensure a patient does not bath alone, even when continuous observation is not part of the care plan. Whatever precautions are decided upon, perhaps the most important factor is consistency of approach. This encourages a feeling of safety in the patient, and ensures that agreed policies and procedures are implemented.

A common misconception is that people who make suicidal gestures or threats are unlikely to commit suicide; however, a history of parasuicide actually increases the likelihood of eventual suicide (Ovenstone & Kreitman 1974). Morgan & Priest (1984) highlighted the problems of assessment of suicide risk in psychiatric inpatients. Misleading signs of improvement, strong reassurances from the patient of no suicidal intent and deteriorating relationships were amongst the factors in this study which inhibited an accurate assessment of suicidal risk in patients who eventually did commit suicide. Significantly, ward staff became critical of several of these patients, considering them provocative, unreasonable and over-dependent. The problem of inadequate surveillance was also mentioned. A more recent paper echoed these findings, and stressed the importance of clear communication between staff, particularly regarding the degree of observation of patients at risk of suicide (Goh et al 1989).

The relationship between nurse and patient is an invaluable tool in helping rekindle the patient's self-esteem and self-respect. One-to-one contact, encouragement of ventilation of feelings and the reassurance of a consistently reliable listener are all crucial aspects of this relationship. Gradually improving self-image can then precipitate increased socialization and participation in occupational and other therapies and activities. Progress is often slow and fraught with set-backs which can be discouraging. It is therefore important that there is regular evaluation and reassessment and that care remains flexible.

A note on the experience of nursing the depressed patient

Nursing depressed patients is never easy. The main problem is that, in a way, depression is 'catching'. Depressed people often 'project' their feelings, that is, attribute to others the bad and guilty feelings they have about themselves, e.g. 'You don't like me, nurse, do you'. A depressed mood is difficult to shake, and patients do not seem to respond to everyday, cheerful conversation. Depression lasts a long time, and the nursing staff, too, begin to feel hopeless. The patient says: 'You can't do anything to help me, nobody can. I'm not worth helping anyway.' and the nurse feels, 'No, nothing can be done.' The patient 'brings down' other people.

While it is possible to feel empathy and compassion for a while, these feelings are often difficult to maintain, and can be replaced with feelings of anger and dislike for the patient (i.e. the patient's own feelings about him or herself).

Very often, the nurse cannot, in fact, do very much. It may be necessary simply to sit with the patient, to remain a constant factor, showing concern and interest. (Altschul & McGovern (1985) note that recovered patients often recall their need for the nurse's attention at a time when, in deepest depression, this need could not be expressed.) This can be boring and frustrating. Furthermore, it takes a great deal of effort to show concern and interest in people who have no concern or interest in themselves.

Respect for the patient is important in helping him or her to re-establish self-respect, but it may be difficult to feel genuine respect when, for example, the patient has not washed for several weeks and needs to be coaxed, like a child, into having a bath, or even needs to be fed.

Such difficulties are compounded by the fact that the care plan for the severely depressed patient who is felt to be suicidal often includes continuous observation. This can be uncomfortable, tedious and embarrassing for both nurse and patient. The common practice of allocating this duty to student nurses, nurses borrowed from other wards or agency nurses, exacerbates the problem: not knowing the patient, the nurse has little or no incentive to remain interested; he or she is often resentful at being given the task in the first place, and an inexperienced student nurse may feel inadequate and insecure in such an intensive relationship with the patient. For the patient, it may well feel more of an invasion of privacy if the nurse is unfamiliar. By allocating the task of continuous observation to an unfamiliar nurse, its value in terms of continuity and the potential for recognizing important changes and developments is diminished. Goh et al (1989) argue that such special nursing observation should be a task for skilled, knowledgeable and experienced nursing staff only.

Demoralization and further frustration may arise when after considerable hard work the patient appears to improve, but then, suddenly, takes an overdose. This is classically the time when depressed patients are at grave risk of suicide because their increased energy and drive provide them with the capacity to make an attempt.

With depressed patients, the question of ECT is often raised, causing difficulties for nurses who are unsure of their feelings about the use of this form of treatment. Patients are usually very concerned about ECT, and often ask nurses about the possible effects and consequences. Frequently, the nurse has had no say about whether or not a patient is to be given ECT, yet is expected to perform an appropriate nursing role if the treatment is prescribed.

Generally, then, nursing depressed patients is fraught with a formidable mixture of distress, anger and frustration. Altschul & McGovern (1985) argue that 'the only comfort that can be given to the [depressed] patient is empathy, interest and appreciation of mood. The nurse continues this without ever giving the slightest sign of boredom or irritation and she responds to the slightest evidence of the depression lifting' (p. 158–159). While clearly well-intentioned, this prescription would appear unrealistic and, through

failing to acknowledge the difficulties discussed here, may also weaken good clinical practice. This is because the uncomfortable and unpleasant reactions which may be caused by working with depressed patients could inhibit the effectiveness of the nurse and undermine the therapeutic value of the nurse–patient relationship. For example, irritation and frustration with the patient could reinforce his or her own self-image as an unlikeable person; it may result in nurses being unwilling to spend time talking with or listening to the patient, and perhaps thereby failing to recognize suicidal risk.

On the other hand, difficult feelings are not simply obstacles. If nurses accept that they may reflect the patient's own internal state, it is important to monitor and use these feelings to help gain a deeper understanding and insight into how the patient is feeling. Therefore nurses' feelings and reactions should be included as an important part of a continuing nursing assessment. Here, clinical supervision is invaluable.

THE SPECIAL PROBLEMS OF SUICIDE AND PARASUICIDE

Suicide and parasuicide are both possible features of depression, and have already been mentioned in the context of nursing depressed patients. However, parasuicide, and to a lesser extent, suicide, are not necessarily accompanied by clinical depression, and require separate discussion.

Suicide

Suicide can be described as a deliberate and fatal act of self-harm (although it is worth remembering that this term is also used to mean a person who has committed suicide). Official statistics show that there are approximately 4000 suicides each year in England and Wales (Office of Health Economics 1981) but it is likely that this is a gross underestimation given the well-recognized unreliability of suicide statistics.★

More recently, McClure (1984) reported a significant increase in official suicide rates between 1975 and 1980, particularly in males who showed an increase of 21%. He found that the most common form of suicide was self-poisoning, comprising more than 36% of total suicides (1572 deaths) in 1980. More violent methods (hanging, strangulation and suffocation) were also common, accounting for nearly a quarter of suicides in the same year. Men over the age of 40 seem to be more at risk of suicide than women or younger age groups (Greer 1981).

Psychiatric illness, and depression is particular, is common: in a study of 100 suicides, 70% were depressed and a further 20% were diagnosed as having other kinds of mental illness (Barraclough et al 1974).

A history of parasuicide increases the risk of suicide: between a third and half of people who commit suicide have made previous attempts (Greer 1981, Ovenstone & Kreitman 1974).

Social factors also play a part in suicide. The rate is higher among social classes I and II, with doctors and dentists being over-represented. Social classes III and IV have relatively low suicide rates, but in class V the rate rises sharply (Stengel 1964).

Parasuicide

Parasuicide is a term used to describe 'any non-fatal act of deliberate self-injury or taking of a substance [excluding alcohol on its own] in excess of the generally recognized or prescribed dose' (Kreitman & Dyer 1980). It is important to note that the parasuicide act does not necessarily involve an intention to commit suicide; for this reason, the term 'unsuccessful suicide' is misleading and unhelpful.

At least 100 000 people in England and Wales deliberately harm themselves each year (Office of Health Economics 1981), although as in the case of suicide statistics, this figure is likely to be an underestimation. Kennedy & Kreitman (1973) reported that general practitioners might be seeing as many as 30% more parasuicide cases than those

who attend hospital from where statistics are usually obtained. Kreitman & Dyer (1980) point out that parasuicide is the commonest reason for emergency medical admission to hospital for women, and the second most common in men.

It has generally been reported that around twice as many women as men deliberately harm themselves (Bancroft et al 1977), although this ratio appears to be diminishing (Hawton & Catalan 1987, Brooking & Minghella 1987).

In contrast to the suicide statistics, parasuicide is more prevalent in younger rather than older groups: up to 75% of people who deliberately harm themselves are under the age of 40 (Greer 1981), and parasuicide is a major problem among adolescents (Hawton & Catalan 1987).

Psychiatric illness is less common than might be expected; for example, Newson-Smith & Hirsch (1979) found that only about a third of parasuicides could be diagnosed as mentally ill (in most cases, this was depression).

Social problems predominate. Amongst the many mentioned by various researchers are: low social class, social deprivation, marital difficulties (including violence in relationships), alcohol problems and drug addiction (Buglass & McCulloch 1970, Hawton & Catalan 1987). There also appears to be a strong relationship between male unemployment and parasuicide, and this correlation is strengthened if the man has been out of work for more than a year (Pratt & Kreitman 1984, Hawton & Rose 1986).

As discussed earlier, Brown & Harris (1978) argued that chronic problems plus one or more precipitating event could lead to depression in women; the current trend is towards a similar approach to the understanding of parasuicide. For example, Hawton & Catalan (1987) suggest that parasuicide patients' problems 'can be divided into problems which occur shortly beforehand, and which have often acted as precipitants, and longer-term or chronic problems in the context of which acute problems have arisen' (p. 26).

Bancroft et al (1977) found that crisis events involving a 'key person' (e.g. spouse, family member, boyfriend, girlfriend) were the most common kinds of crisis, occurring within the week prior to the parasuicide act. A major quarrel with

---

* The main problem with the statistics seems to be the legal constraints placed upon the coroner's verdict. However, other factors, such as a country's religious orientation creating a state opposition to the concept of suicide, may decrease the likelihood of a suicide verdict. For a full discussion of these issues, see Stengel (1964).

a key person was found to be the most likely precipitant.

An important point is that the characteristics of parasuicide patients at risk of suicide resemble those who have committed suicide (Michel 1987), although Stengel's (1964) influential work had emphasized the difference between those who die (suicide) and those who do not (parasuicide).

Table 29.2 shows common differences and similarities in the two groups. Where features of suicide and parasuicide overlap, then this constitutes a risk area. For example, a 50-year-old man who has tried to hang himself, is depressed and has a history of parasuicide, is at a higher risk of suicide than a 20-year-old woman who has taken an overdose, and who is distressed but not clinically depressed. It is important to recognize, however, that such examples are necessarily stereotypical, and that, as parasuicide itself is a risk factor, consequently *all* patients who have deliberately harmed themselves present a suicide risk.

The identification of further risk factors related to the circumstances of the act and the patient's own interpretation of the events has led to the development of suicidal intent scales for use in the clinical assessment of parasuicide patients (Beck et al 1974, Pierce 1981, Pallis et al 1984). The scales

Table 29.2 Summary comparison of suicide and parasuicide

Suicide	Parasuicide
Older — most over 40	Younger — most under 40
More men than women	More women than men (although gap closing)
Violent methods/self-injury common	Self-poisoning 90%
Psychiatric illness: majority	Psychiatric illness: minority
Alcohol and drug problems	Alcohol and drug problems
Physical illness common	Physical illness more prevalent than in population in general
Social isolation	Overcrowding
Upper > lower > middle socio-economic class	Lower > middle socio-economic class
Unemployment?	Unemployment
Previous parasuicide	

attempt to assess the degree of planning and preparation that have preceded the act. In addition, they consider the patient's motivation and own understanding of his or her intentions and expectations. For example, intent scale questions may ask whether or not a suicide note was written (high risk), whether somebody else was present or in contact at the time of the act (lower risk), whether or not the person expected the method to be fatal (high risk). Suicidal intent scales are extremely useful when used *as part of a comprehensive assessment.*

The assessment of parasuicide patients attending general hospitals has traditionally been the domain of psychiatrists, and, indeed, government guidelines recommended that all parasuicide patients should be admitted to a general ward and given a psychiatric assessment before they are discharged (Ministry of Health 1968). However in the last decade or so, research has indicated that specially-trained psychiatric nurses as part of a multi-disciplinary hospital team (Catalan et al 1980) or a relatively independent community psychiatric nursing specialist team (Brooking & Minghella 1987) can function as competently, safely and as effectively as psychiatrists in this field. More recent government guidelines now recognize the role of professionals other than psychiatrists in the assessment and management of parasuicide patients (DHSS Circular 1984).

It may be that nurses can be used more appropriately than psychiatrists, as they are more adaptable (working in hospital, clinic and community settings), more available, and more likely to possess or have developed counselling skills. They are eclectic in their approach and can liaise effectively with both general and psychiatric medical and nursing colleagues as well as with other professionals within the hospital and community. This argument is strengthened by research findings which indicate that the large majority of parasuicide patients are not formally mentally ill but in a state of personal distress within the context of psychosocial difficulties. Research and experience does, however, emphasize the need for post-basic specialist training, and with such a vulnerable group of patients, clinical supervision and support are essential.

As all the research findings make clear, any parasuicide assessment should examine the patient's mental state, suicidal intent and psychosocial circumstances. The kind of treatment to be offered depends on the assessment, but those patients who are not actively suicidal or mentally ill can be offered crisis counselling (for an excellent presentation of care options for parasuicide patients, see Hawton & Catalan 1987). Crisis counselling can be described as a short-term focused therapy, offering immediate help in a time of crisis. It is important to note that 'the patient is not being treated as a sick or dependent person but as an adult with problems who is asking for help' (Bancroft, 1979, p. 93). Bancroft suggests that an explicit contract should be made with the patient, specifying the nature of the patient–therapist relationship, the time span involved and the objectives of the counselling. He points out that it is important to be aware not only of the therapeutic options but also of their limitations, and he emphasizes the need to be flexible.

With parasuicide patients the risk of further deliberate self-harm is always present; up to a quarter will repeat within a year (Hawton & Catalan 1987). This is an important fact to remember; firstly, in order to remain vigilant and to look for recurring suicidal feelings, and secondly, to be reassured that further parasuicide does not necessarily imply a failure on the part of the therapist. If a patient does repeat the act, it is worth discussing the event with the team and, of course, with the patient.

Finally, it is very probable that sooner or later a depressed patient in your care or a parasuicide patient you have assessed and counselled, will commit suicide. Such a tragedy will have many implications for all concerned: distressed and angry relatives, possible court appearances, psychiatric 'postmortems', attribution and re-attribution of blame and guilt may all have to be confronted. It is important to consider such a situation as *a crisis for the staff* as well as relatives, and that as such nurses need to support and help each other through this experience, encourage ventilation of feelings, facilitate communication, and show concern and empathy for each other. The family may also value this kind of support.

REFERENCES

Altschul A, McGovern M 1985 Psychiatric nursing, 6th ed. Baillière Tindall, London

Bancroft J, Skrimshire A, Casson J, Harvard-Watts O, Reynolds F 1977 People who deliberately poison or injure themselves: their problems and their contact with helping agencies. Psychological Medicine 7: 289–303

Bancroft J 1979 Crisis intervention. In: Bloch S (ed) An introduction to the psychotherapies. Oxford University Press, Oxford

Barraclough B, Bunch J, Nelson B, Sainsbury P 1974 A hundred cases of suicide; clinical aspects. British Journal of Psychiatry 125: 355–373

Bebbington P, Brugha T, MacCarthy B, Potter J, Sturt E, Wykes T, Katz R 1988 The Camberwell Collaborative Depression Study: I. Depressed probands: adversity and the form of depression. British Journal of Psychiatry 152: 754–765

Beck A T 1967 Depression: clinical, experimental & theoretical aspects. Staples Press, London

Beck A T 1976 Cognitive therapy and the emotional disorders. International University Press, New York

Beck A T, Rush A J, Shaw B F, Emery G 1980 Cognitive therapy of depression. J Wiley, London

Beck A T, Schuyler D, Herman J 1974 Development of suicidal intent scales in the prediction of suicide. In: Beck A T, Resnick H L P, Lettieri D J (eds). Charles Press, Maryland

Birtchnell J, Masters N, Deahl M 1988 Depression and the physical environment: a study of young married women on a London housing estate. British Journal of Psychiatry 153: 56–64

Bowlby J 1961 Processes of mourning. International Journal of Psychoanalysis XLII: 317–339

Brooking J I, Minghella E L 1987 Parasuicide. Nursing Times 83: 21, 40–43

Brown G, Harris T 1978 Social origins of depression. Tavistock, London

Buglass D, McCullough J W 1970 Further suicidal behaviour: the development and validation of predictive scales. British Journal of Psychiatry 116: 483–491

Catalan J, Marsack P, Hawton K E, Whitwell D, Fagg J, Bancroft J 1980 Comparison of doctors and nurses in the assessment of deliberate self-poisoning patients. Psychological Medicine 10: 483–491

Checkley S 1985 Biological markers in depression. In: Granville-Grossman K (ed) Recent advances in clinical psychiatry No 5. Churchill Livingstone, Edinburgh

Clare A 1979 Psychosurgery and electroconvulsive therapy. In: Hill P, Murray R, Thorley A (eds) Essentials of postgraduate psychiatry. Academic Press, London

Department of Health and Social Security Circular 1984 The management of deliberate self-harm (CMHN(84)25/LASL(84)5). HMSO, London

Freud S 1917 Mourning and melancholia. The standard edition of the complete psychological works, vol 14. Hogarth Press, London

Gelder M 1985 Cognitive therapy. In:Granville-Grossman K (eds) Recent Advances in Clinical Psychiatry No 5. Churchill Livingstone, Edinburgh

George L, Blazer G B, Hughes D C, Fowler N 1989 Social support and the outcome of major depression. British Journal of Psychiatry 154: 478–485

Goh S E, Salmons P H, Whittington R M 1989 Hospital suicides: are there preventable factors? British Journal of Psychiatry 154: 247–249

Goldberg D 1983 Depressive reactions in adults. In: Russell G F M, Henson L (eds) Neuroses and personality disorders. Handbook of psychiatry, vol 4. Cambridge University Press, Cambridge

Gordon V 1986 Reducing depression in women: research in the USA and Britain. In: Brooking J I (eds) Psychiatric nursing research. Wiley, Chichester

Greer H S 1981 Self-poisoning and suicide. Hospital Update: 667–677

Hawton K, Rose N 1986 Unemployment and attempted suicide among men in Oxford. Health Trends 18: 29–32

Hawton K, Catalan J 1987 Attempted suicide, 2nd edn. Oxford University Press, Oxford

Kennedy P, Kreitman N 1973 Epidemiological survey of parasuicide in general practice. British Journal of Psychiatry 123: 23–24

Kreitman N, Dyer J A T 1980 Suicide in relation to parasuicide. Medical Education: 1827–1830

Lawson A 1978 Book review. Psychological Medicine 8: 717–740

Linford Rees W L 1976 A short textbook of psychiatry, 2nd edn. Hodder & Stoughton, London

McClure G M G 1984 Trends in suicide rate for England and Wales 1975–80. British Journal of Psychiatry 144: 119–126

Maslow A H 1970 Motivation and personality, 2nd edn. Harper & Row, New York

Michel K 1987 Suicide risk factors: a comparison of suicide attempters with suicide completers. British Journal of Psychiatry 150: 78–82

Ministry of Health 1968 Hospital treatment of acute poisoning (Hill Report). HMSO, London

Morgan H G, Priest P 1984 Assessment of suicide risk in psychiatric in-patients. British Journal of Psychiatry 145: 467–469

Nelson-Jones R 1983 Practical counselling skills. Holt, Rinehart & Winston, London

Newson-Smith J G B, Hirsch S R 1979 Psychiatric symptoms in self-poisoning patients. Psychological Medicine 9: 493–500

Office of Health Economics 1981 Suicide and deliberate self-harm. HMSO, London

Ovenstone I M K, Kreitman N 1974 Two syndromes of suicide. British Journal of Psychiatry 124: 336–345

Pallis D J, Gibbons J S, Pierce D W 1984 Estimating suicide risk among attempted suicides: I. The development of new clinical scales. British Journal of Psychiatry 144: 139–148

Pedder J 1982 Failure to mourn and melancholia. British Journal of Psychiatry 141: 329–337

Peplau H 1987 Tomorrows world. Nursing Times, Jan 7: 29–32

Pierce P W 1981 Predictive validation of a suicide intent scale. British Journal of Psychiatry 139: 391–396

Pratt S, Kreitman N 1984 Trends in parasuicide and unemployment among men in Edinburgh 1968–1982. British Medical Journal 289: 1029–1032

Slater E, Cowie V 1971 The genetics of mental disorder. Oxford University Press, London

Stengel E 1964 Suicide and attempted suicide. Penguin, Harmondsworth

Storr A 1983 A psychotherapist looks at depression. British Journal of Psychiatry 143: 431–435

Tennant C 1985 Female vulnerability to depression. Psychological Medicine 15: 733–737

Trethowan W Sir, Sims A C P 1983 Psychiatry, 5th edn. Baillière Tindall, London

30

Anxiety

J. Wilson-Barnett

Most people have experienced the emotion of anxiety at some time in particular situations. For those who are ill, anxiety is common, as feeling unwell, receiving treatments and becoming a patient tend to increase feelings of vulnerability, both physically and emotionally. It is therefore essential for those providing care to recognize when people are anxious, to assess and understand the reasons for this and to become knowledgeable and skilled in providing relevant help.

ANXIETY — ORIGINS AND MEANINGS

Throughout the history of medicine emotions and 'sensitivity' have been recognized and studied for their influence on physical health. Sims (1985) quotes the inscription in Box 30.1 from a tombstone. He traces the history of the term anxiety and explains how ideas influenced treatments for anxiety.

Although mechanisms by which persistent or strong anxiety cause physical symptoms and illness were poorly understood (and to some extent still are), this relationship was documented and studied in the days of Hippocrates and Aristotle. The origin of the term is even earlier, the Latin derivation being '*anxietas*' meaning 'troubled in mind'.

Box 30.1 Inscription from a tombstone in Dorchester Abbey

READER!

If thou hast a Heart fam'd for
Tenderness and Pity, Contemplate
this Spot
In which are deposited the Remains
of a Young Lady, whose artless Beauty
innocence of Mind, and gentle Manners
once obtain'd her the Love and
Esteem of all who knew her. But when
Nerves were too delicately spun to
bear the rude Shakes and Jostlings
which we meet with in this transitory
World. Nature gave way: She sunk
and died a Martyr to Excessive
Sensibility.

MRS SARAH FLETCHER

Wife of Captain FLETCHER
departed this Life at the Village
of Clifton, on the 7 of June 1799.
In the 29th Year of her Age.
May her Soul meet that Peace in
Heaven which this Earth denied her.

Speilberger (1972 p. 24) defines anxiety as 'a palpable but transitory emotional state or condition characterized by feelings of tension and apprehension and heightened autonomic nervous system activity'. This is obviously closely related to the derivation from '*anxietas*' and '*angor*' meaning a sense of constriction. A threat of the unknown is often said to be the cause of anxiety. For example, Lazarus & Averill (1972) explain that this feeling results from an insufficient understanding of an event, and Rycroft (1968) also points to a vague threat in the future against which there is no action. May's (1950 p. 191) definition integrates most of these elements as he describes anxiety as 'a diffuse apprehension which is unspecific, vague and objectless. It is associated with feelings of uncertainty and helplessness resulting from a threat to the core or essence of the personality'.

When differentiating anxiety from fear, Hoch & Zubin (1950) point to the disproportionate reactions; whereas in fear they are related to directive

action, in anxiety the subject lacks power to act and the threat assumes disproportionate dimensions. Failure to be able to ward off a threat results in the complex emotion of anxiety which Rycroft (1968) recognizes as a combination of hope, fear, despondency and despair. Izard (1972) endorses this idea of a complex and ranked the components as follows: interest, fear, distress, disgust, guilt, surprise, shyness, fatigue, anger, contempt, enjoyment. Similarly Cattell's (1972 p. 288) sub-factors included guilt, ergic tension, poor ego strength, suspiciousness and a poorly developed self-sentiment.

In order to gauge how people experienced anxiety Davitz (1969 p. 36) found the following phrases to be most used when describing this emotion. 'I'm wound up inside; my whole body is tense; I'm jumpy, jittery; I want to do something, anything, to change the situation and relieve the tension; there is a tight knotted feeling in my stomach. There is a sense that I have no control over the situation, a sense of being gripped by the situation; there's a sense of uncertainty about the future. I have no appetite; I can't eat; there is an intense concern for what will happen next, a sense of anticipation, waiting for something to happen . . . .'

Anxiety as a personality factor

Characteristic forms of anxiety or anxiety traits are discussed by Levitt (1971). He suggests that describing people as anxious either means they are anxious at the moment or that they are often prone to anxiety. He considers that the term 'chronic' anxiety is not applicable to people who are prone to anxiety as this infers it is continuous and of low intensity. They are more likely to suffer from periods of anxiety but these are not necessarily of low intensity. Speilberger (1972) reiterates this when he says there is no evidence that a strong anxiety 'trait' is related to more or less intense experiences. He emphasizes that people's perception and defence mechanisms are essential to how they react to a threat. Arousal depends on a set of ordered events from perception, cognition and experience.

One personality factor that has been shown to

be strongly linked with anxiety-proneness is the level of self-esteem that a person holds. Research by Rosenberg (1962) showed that anxiety was associated with a low self-esteem, defined as the degree to which the subject holds attitudes of acceptance or rejection towards himself. A person with low self-esteem is likely to be sensitive to any evidence in the experience of daily life which testified to his inadequacy, incompetence or worthlessness. This was seen to be related to feelings of isolation and lack of social support. Speilberger (1972) endorses these findings by the observation that people with fear of failure (an obvious threat to the self-esteem) are also characterized by a high anxiety trait score. Sullivan (1956) also concurs with this view when he explains the origins of anxiety which rest in fear of losing social approval.

Guinn & Hill (1964) showed how a lowered self-acceptance and high level of anxiety were also associated with a lowered acceptance of others. Their interpretations were that:

- anxiety may disturb the person's capacity to relate positively to himself and others
- anxiety may stem from the subject's inability to relate to others
- anxiety is a symptom representing problems in relating to the self and others.

Causes of anxiety

Stimuli for emotional reactions vary between individuals as does their characteristic propensity to feeling anxious. Endler et al (1962) realized that stimuli varied with individual experience and they designed a stimulus–response inventory which gave many examples of events which would be relevant to a wide sample of the general population, such as going for an interview for a job, being ignored in a shop, waiting for a dental appointment, or walking into a crowded room full of strangers and making an announcement. The Fear Survey schedule, an instrument developed by Geer (1965) also lists specific fear or anxiety situations such as 'looking foolish', 'being alone', 'blood', 'driving a car' and 'snakes'.

Positive interpretations of anxiety exist, and al-though it is reviewed as an uncomfortable feeling, many people seek situations which evoke anxiety and seem to function better with the heightened awareness and energy it provides. Yerkes & Dodson's (1908) 'U-shaped curve' has had an immense effect on psychological thinking in that a low or moderate level of anxiety is found to be associated with improved performance in some situations but increased levels tend to result in disorganized behaviour. Related to this, Ray & Fitzgibbon (1982) consider that arousal rather than anxiety may be a more accurate description and constructive drive. In particular, when information processing is required by individuals in a particularly stressful situation (awaiting surgery), arousal rather than anxiety is desirable.

The uncomfortable nature of anxiety itself may spur people on to resolve these feelings by actions to reduce the threat of future events. For example, revising for examinations, visiting the doctor or asking questions to gain information, may all be seen as positive actions spurred on by anxiety leading to constructive behaviour. However, it is obviously the situations themselves, and the level and frequency of the anxious feelings they generate, which determine their effect and long-term influences on the physical state of the individual.

Anxiety — normal and pathological

The question of whether neurotic anxiety differs in quality or quantity from 'normal' everyday anxiety has been discussed by May (1950) who argues for a clear differentiation between normal and neurotic anxiety. Normal anxiety is seen to be proportional to the threat and subsides when the threat is removed, while neurotic anxiety is enduring and disproportionate and involves developing defence mechanisms. Freud (1936) and the neo-Freudians also differentiate between neurotic anxiety as pathological and normal anxiety resulting from threats or interpersonal relationships and conflicts.

More recent views by Hamilton (1969) and Lader (1975) disagree with this distinction. Hamilton claims that his research shows that the difference in anxiety felt by dermatology and

Box 30.2 Classification of anxiety terms (Lader 1975)

	Normal	Pathological
Trait	Anxiousness	Anxious personality
State	Feeling anxious	Anxiety state

Box 30.3 Effects of anxiety (modified from Aitken & Zealley 1970 p. 216)

Changes in thinking	Worry, dread and apprehension Reduced concentration and field of attention Distractibility and forgetfulness Irritability and depression Insomnia and nightmares Perceptual disturbance, such as depersonalization
Changes in physiological activity	
a. Motor activity	Muscular tension and trembling Restlessness and fidgeting Incoordination and impaired performance Startled reaction: 'Freezing'
b. Other somatic functions	Flushing and sweating (S) Dry mouth and anorexia (S) Choking feeling as if lump in throat (S) Rapid breathing and sometimes hyperventilation (S) Palpitations, fatigue, weakness and fainting (S) Dyspepsia and diarrhoea (P) Urgency and frequency of micturition (P) Impotence (P) Menstrual disturbance (P)

Key: P = parasympathetic S = sympathetic

psychiatric patients is only quantitative, not qualitative. He designed a test for anxiety in which neurotics scored much higher than dermatology patients. Psychiatric anxiety states are explained as a lowering of a threshold so that environmental stress which would not affect a normal person evokes anxiety in a neurotic. Lader (1975) talks in terms of a cut-off point on a continuum of anxiety beyond which levels are considered abnormal (Box 30.2). Pathological anxiety is more frequent, more severe and more persistent than is usual in terms of the individual.

Lader & Marks (1971) found that 3.2% of the British urban population suffer from anxiety states whereas only 2% of the rural population do so. This condition is found more frequently in females. In a transcultural study Lynn (1971) found that a thin build, alcoholism, accident proneness, high suicide rates and a low calorific intake were correlated with higher levels of anxiety.

Physical effects of anxiety

Both sympathetic and parasympathetic autonomic systems are stimulated in anxiety and produce the variety of symptoms listed in Box 30.3. Rises in catecholamine production, higher proportions of adrenaline to noradrenaline, occur in acute anxiety. Resulting physical sensations have a feedback mechanism and may cause a heightened awareness of these, which are then experienced as greater anxiety. Breggin (1964) discusses this as a self-perpetuating feedback loop. Recurrent attacks of anxiety may strengthen the conditioned association between anxiety and its sympatheticomimetic symptoms, thereby increasing the intensity of further anxiety reactions.

Coping with anxiety

It is well known that both Sigmund and Anna Freud contributed to current thought on how people defend themselves against the discomfort of anxiety. Displacement, sublimation, reaction formation, regression, rationalization and projection are discussed at length, and psychoanalysts have refined many of these early ideas. Normal functioning or coping depends on the subject using defences appropriately, without relying on one strategy to the exclusion of others.

Relief from anxiety symptoms, manifest as

somatic as well as psychic malaise, can also be reduced when such conditioned responses are weakened. New response patterns have to be learned which are considered appropriate to the situation and enviromental constraints. Recently, greater emphasis has been put on this relearning capacity as a cognitive activity within the control of the subject rather than as a result of understanding subconscious dynamics. However, this activity depends on the motivation and understanding of the individual. Adjustment to potentially anxiety-evoking events is the overall aim in order to reduce wasteful energy and uncoordinated responses. This aim of adjustment is even more essential for those who are more vulnerable through physical weaknesses and illness.

MEASUREMENT OF ANXIETY

Psychological measures

The importance of the time dimension when measuring emotions has been stressed by Speilberger (1966). 'Trait' tests measure the persistent level of any emotion or the personality 'proneness', whereas 'state' measurements measure the level of an emotion at one time such as 'at the moment' or 'today'. He suggests that tests should be chosen carefully, and the suitability of any test for a particular purpose will determine its usefulness.

Observer rating of subjects has been classically used in the psychiatric field and the format for rating scales can be structured in the same way as self-report scales. However, recognition of different moods from facial expression has been shown to be fairly difficult. A study reported by Rachman (1974) demonstrated that observers could not differentiate between fear, pain, hunger and surprise as so many things such as age and cultural background influence facial expression.

Training and standardization of raters is essential for obtaining useful assessments of others' emotions. Scales such as the Hamilton Anxiety Scale (1969) have been designed for professionals to rate those suffering from neurotic anxiety states. Another method by Gelder & Marks (1966) can be used to rate any symptom of anxiety, as shown in Figure 30.1.

In all these tests the rater must always establish the time dimension of the emotion, whether it is a long-term symptom or, as in the case of the linear scale in Figure 30.1, only for 3 days. The same applies when requesting subjects to report their own feelings. Personality tests of how anxious or depressed a person is, generally ask questions in terms of 'usually' or 'often'.

Self-report instruments

Trait scales. The trait of emotionality included in Cattell's (1954) 16 Personality Factors Test and Eysenck's Personality Inventory (EPI) (Eysenck & Eysenck 1964) is said to measure the characteristic proneness to anxiety and depression for each subject. The Cattell instrument is a lengthy self-report scale designed to provide a broad personality profile. The EPI provides scores on three scales measuring extroversion, neuroticism (or liability to feelings of anxiety and depression) and a lie scale. These two main dimensions of neuroticism 'N' and extroversion 'E' each have 24 component questions. A high 'N' scorer and low 'E' scorer would be known as an unstable introvert or 'dysthymic', likely to feel a high degree of negative emotions,

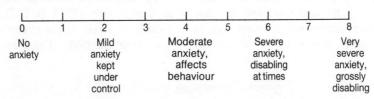

Fig. 30.1 Free-floating anxiety scale for observer rating anxious mood (from Lader & Marks 1971, p. 96). Rater: take note of persistent anxious mood, subjective tension, physical manifestation, poor concentration and motor restlessness. Base your assessment on the patient's state during the previous three days.

whereas a low 'N' score and high 'E' score of a stable extrovert would infer few of these emotional experiences.

Tests for measuring anxiety proneness, specifically, also exist. The Taylor Manifest Anxiety Scale (1953) is possibly the most widely used self-assessment personality test of anxiety. It consists of 50 questions requiring a 'true' or 'false' answer and is easy to score. It was originally devised as an index of drive but is found to be like an 'emotionality' trait test.

The Stimulus–Response (S–R) Inventory by Endler et al (1962), another attempt to measure anxiety proneness, presents 11 situations likely to evoke anxiety and requires checking 14 response tendencies, which are mainly physical. Situations can be adapted for the respondent as Hayward (1975) showed. The format appears lengthy and the maximum score is 770, as each of the 14 response tendencies are graded out of 5 points.

State scales are usually either linear or adjective check-lists, although Speilberger's (1983) popular State-Trait measure consists of 24 items which have to be rated on a 4-point scale. This scale is perhaps more appropriate for research uses. Clinical assessment monitoring needs a brief, easily completed instrument such as a linear scale.

Linear scales can be graduated and labelled quantitatively with such labels as 'none', 'a little', 'a moderate amount' or 'extremely', or they can extend from 'none at all' to 'maximum'. The subject merely crosses the line at the appropriate spot and the score equals the length along the line from 0, as shown in Figure 30.2. The scale is easy to mark and quantify and subjects are not distracted by a description of the amount of anxiety.

A mood adjective check-list, such as that used by Lishman (1972) containing 24 adjectives, each rated on a 4-point scale and covering the five dimensions of anxiety, depression, hostility, vigour and fatigue, has been shown to be useful for psychiatric patients as well as for general patients, as described by the author (Wilson-Barnett & Carrigy 1978). These adjectives provide a choice of terms used to describe feelings. Anxiety words are 'tense', 'on edge', 'shaky', 'nervous'. While 'unhappy', 'hopeless', 'discouraged', and 'miserable', 'worthless', 'depressed', 'helpless' and 'guilty' are included in Lishman's instrument to measure the degree of depression. The rationale for adjective check-lists is based on respondents' individual preference for an inferred meaning given to different words. They are an attempt to include a variety of words to enable the respondent to express his own feelings in familiar terms.

Physiological measures

Lader (1975) discusses the use of physiological indices of anxiety. He explains the poor correlation of these measurements to psychological test scores as a reflection of the two different systems which are being measured. Blood pressure, galvanic skin response (the measure of resistance to electrical current) and the electroencephalogram are linked to a system which primarily controls physiological function. Psychological tests are based on feelings which take only a small account of physical factors.

Several physiological indices have been used in the measurement of anxiety. Kelly (1967) has used forearm blood flow in the clinical situation and Munday (1973) used a fingertip count of sweat glands to assess the degree of anxiety. Boore (1976) used indices including temperature and urinary hydroxycorticosteroids. All these measures may be seen as indices of arousal rather than anxiety, and may be influenced by physical illness, drugs and idiopathic instability. They also require, as Lader says (1975 p. 207), special equipment (which in itself might evoke anxiety) and timely 'counting' methods. These methods are also often

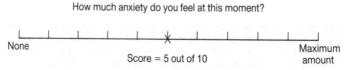

How much anxiety do you feel at this moment?

None   Maximum
                                        amount
Score = 5 out of 10

Fig. 30.2 A 10 centimetre line used as a linear scale.

not relevant to assessment of anxiety in psychiatric contexts.

ANXIETY AND ILLNESS

Anxiety as the cause of illness

Prolonged or excessive anxiety with accompanying physical responses is associated with an increased metabolic rate, reduced immunity and resistance to increased demand. It is not therefore, surprising that anxious people feel unwell and complain of physical symptoms. Many somatic complaints have been misinterpreted by medical staff as indicators of an organic pathological process which should be carefully investigated and treated. Many patients in turn explain this reaction to what they deem to be a physical disorder.

Relevant to this issue was a study (Wilson-Barnett & Trimble 1984) comparing a group with neurological conditions and another group with psychiatric disorders with those referred for assessment of 'hysterical' complaints. Patients in this last category had suffered fits, paralysis, disturbance of sensation or motor function. However, extensive investigations had been carried out without detecting abnormalities. When measuring affective components or emotions and personality dimensions we found those in the 'hysterical' group were highly anxious and/or depressed; in some cases severity was similar to the 'psychiatric' group. Most understood that their problems could have been psychological but tended to have an unrealistic view of their capabilities and life problems. Masked anxiety or depression resulting in physical or somatic problems such as these can be detected in many other specialties.

This area of care is frequently mismanaged, 'psychosomatic' or 'hysterical' being used by staff as a perjorative term which does not deserve medical and nursing time. It is this ignorance that tends to be associated with unsupportive reactions from staff and a worsening of the sufferers' condition.

It is sad that the fascinating mechanisms by which psychological factors affect physical health are not studied more, as they affect every person and patient. Holistic understanding has been deemed one of the unique perspectives for nursing

(Wilson-Barnett 1985) and these mechanisms may well hold the key to new ways in which nurses might have a positive influence on the overall health of their patients.

A very anxious patient, in whatever situation, will find it difficult to rest, sleep, concentrate and recover. Alleviation of this distressing emotion has therefore to be seen as vital for humanitarian and physically therapeutic reasons.

Those who are vulnerable to the effects of sympathetic stimulation, which increase the demands on the cardiovascular, digestive and immune systems, may of course fare worse under conditions of increased stress or anxiety. Angina, seen as a response to emotional excitement, is in fact named from the German 'angst' inferring constriction. It is a classic symptom associated with anxiety, and ischaemic heart disease is thought to be more prevalent in those of an anxious disposition (Olmsted & Kennedy 1975). Those with diabetes may also be unable to respond to the increased metabolism of cells, inadequate available insulin inhibiting the uptake of glucose. Alternatively, muscle wasting may occur through catabolic processes in response to other systems' need for energy and nutrients. Likewise, with reduced resistance consequent on protracted anxiety (Bartrop et al 1977), many patients would be vulnerable, particularly in hospital where pathogens abound.

It is now established that high anxiety is associated with both physical morbidity and a reduced ability to tolerate further discomfort. Both in a temporary situation postoperatively, and more persistently as a personality dimension, increased pain and anxiety correlate (Hayward 1975) and neuroticism is associated with more complicated and prolonged recovery (Mathew & Ridgeway 1981).

Anxiety as a response to illness

A feedback or circular relationship tends to exist between illness and anxiety — increased anxiety leading to illness, and illness being associated with greater emotional reactions of anxiety and often depression. Deep-seated fears of death and mutilation were discussed as the fundamental root of anxiety by Freud (see Jones 1955). Feelings of deep malaise or great pain and immobility tend to lead to morbid thoughts and feelings of dependence on others and vulnerability. Even influenza can produce such unpleasant symptoms which may evoke fears of death. 'I felt like death' is not a totally 'light-hearted' description.

Other reasons for anxiety during illness exist. In any situation the causes are individualistic or idiosyncratic, differing aspects of life seeming challenging or threatening to different people. Leaving the family, fearing disfigurement, being unable to cope with usual responsibilities and fearing the withdrawal of those one cares for, may all evoke anxiety (Lipowski 1975).

Seeking medical aid and advice from others may be encouraged through anxious feelings, but may in turn cause further concerns. In contrast, delays in seeking such help may be due to the fear of disclosing some dreaded condition, as Aitken et al (1955) found in their famous study of cancer patients.

Hospitalization

It is now well established that a majority of patients feel anxious about being hospitalized. Our own studies of those on medical wards (Wilson-Barnett & Carrigy 1978) demonstrate that emotional responses are greater than those normally experienced. At specific times, anxiety levels peak during the hospital stay. Almost without exception, they are higher than average on admission. Prior to adjusting to the patient role and making friends with others, patients are uncertain about forthcoming events or apprehensive about those they are expecting. Unfamiliar sights and sounds, particularly observing others who are very ill, listening to strange machines and being forced to perform daily living activities in the company of others may all cause distress (Robinson 1972, Wilson-Barnett 1976).

Particular groups of patients in general hospitals are consistently found to be vulnerable to emotional disturbance. This includes those with certain conditions such as viral infections, neurological or cardiac problems and those with cancer. Once more it is easy to explain why this should be so for some but not others. Long-term, chronic or fatal disorders may cause severe anxieties early on and at the time of diagnosis and early treatment, but later may give rise to depression. Viral conditions, even if short lived, such as influenza or chicken pox, may alter neuronal function and disturb mood, but this is still hypothetical.

Younger patients and females tend to be more emotionally reactive to hospitalization, often worrying about their children or partner and being more susceptible to feelings of embarrassment at the lack of privacy.

Lastly those patients in general wards who are being investigated, but do not have a specific diagnosis, are particularly prone to anxiety. Not only do the repeated tests cause this, but also the feeling that a grave diagnosis could be made, or alternatively that ultimately nothing is revealed and that others will label them a fraud.

Thus, so many patients may fall within a vulnerable group that nurses must be attentive to causes of anxiety and understand the type of care that is appropriate and effective.

NURSING THOSE WHO ARE ANXIOUS

By providing a sympathetic and understanding presence, a nurse can do a great deal to help those who may be feeling alone and anxious. Recognizing this need through being aware of cues and providing open communication is essential, but apparently not automatic from staff (Macleod Clark 1983). Asking patients open questions about their feelings and the reasons for these is clearly necessary to establish sensible strategies for care. In defining anxiety as fear of the unknown the reasons may be more or less specific or focused, realistic or not, temporary or long-standing. Feeling supported or cared for is said to be a fundamental buffer to stress and anxiety (Cassel 1974).

Research evaluating specific interventions to reduce anxiety and its unwanted consequences, has contributed greatly to recommendations for care. Many nursing studies have tested the effect of information-giving prior to stressful events such as surgery, special treatments or tests. Providing a realistic impression of what the patient will experience is thought to reduce 'the element of the unknown' (Johnson 1983). Benefits for patients have been shown in both recovery from surgery and reduced anxiety during specific procedures (for a review see Wilson-Barnett 1984).

Types of information and methods for providing this usefully have been devised. Guidance on physical exercises or coping with discomfort is seen to be very helpful for an investigation such as barium X-rays or cardiac catheterization (Finesilver 1979). However, information on the sensations (sensory information) of touch, sight, sound and smell is also found to be particularly helpful for major tests or surgical procedures such as gastroscopy or abdominal surgery (Johnson 1983). Such information has to be systematically based on accounts from patients who have experienced such events in order not only to provide accurate accounts but also to use a vocabulary that is accessible and meaningful to patients.

Although the majority of these studies have tested the effect of information given by interview, some patients may like to study a written account in their own time. In fact, on assessing preference for written or spoken information it tends to be roughly equally divided (Wild & Evans 1968).

Other studies of a similar nature using different interventions are also very useful. One example by Ridgeway & Mathew (1982) found that by focusing on major concerns about surgery rather than the whole pre- and postoperative experience, patients felt significant benefits. Common concerns such as the anaesthetic or pain were selected and discussed in a little booklet using the technique of positive reappraisal. Patients were encouraged to concentrate on the benefits of the surgery, and reduce the imagined disadvantage. This and other studies using this coping technique have found that patients can learn to employ positive reappraisal, and benefit more than those who are given a more comprehensive account with sensory information. This may of course be explained by the potency of an individualized approach as well as the effect of the positive reappraisal.

Providing a sense of support and some measure of self-control is therefore seen as important in alleviating anxiety. In longer-term situations, where people need to cope with chronic illness or recovery at home, similar resources should be provided by nurses. Allied to information-giving is the teaching of understanding and skills to enable patients to manage when they return home from hospital. Benefits from such help were found from a great majority of studies evaluating teaching (Wilson-Barnett & Oborne 1983). Not only understanding of the condition and treatments, but information which promotes independence and coping were found significantly to affect patients and their relatives. Psychological and physical welfare were influenced as those who did not receive such support frequently reported fear and apprehension when they experienced unexpected symptoms or practical problems.

These and other interventions should become part of every nurse's repertoire of care. Given that nurses have most opportunity for continuous communication with patients they are in a position to assess needs and plan such intervention. Explicit planning and scheduling for such care is the only way to reflect its importance (Bird 1955).

Careful discussion focused on people's feelings or problems may take on the character of counselling. Such interviews tend to use the same principles of open communication, active listening as well as the provision of information (Stewart 1983). Counselling skills are certainly built from those of facilitative communication and may well be employed for those with long-standing or serious psychosocial problems.

Appropriate interventions must be reviewed and chosen sensitively as those which do not rely on giving information may be indicated when patients are extremely anxious, or in a situation where there is, for example, news of loss (which may be initially greeted with anxiety rather than depression).

Physical coping strategies may be very useful for those who are suffering from the acute discomforts associated with sympathetic over-stimulation. Relaxation exercises or deep breathing and alternate contraction and relaxation of certain muscle groups can be learned and employed at times of need. It is obviously more helpful if individuals can master these techniques before they are really needed. Nurses themselves may benefit from a daily session of relaxation. This can provide 'rest' within a short period and refreshes the mind and body.

Although desensitization is discussed in other chapters the principles should be understood by all nurses. Experiences which are accompanied by anxiety are likely to be associated with the same or greater levels of anxiety in the future. Preventing feelings of anxiety through nurses anticipating and providing coping resources may reduce associations of fear in the future. Those which are already associated may be relearned through mastery of the event and new coping strategies. Reinforcement of poor coping should not be fostered in a situation where nurses could help and should be skilful and motivated to do so.

Referral

At times anxiety may be so great and protracted that a patient will not respond to nursing interventions. Referral to a specialist liaison psychologist or psychiatrist may be necessary. He should of course, work as part of a team learning relevant information from other staff as well as the patient and significant others. His recommendations should then be discussed and planned so that they can be speedily implemented. Strategies may include psychotherapy, relaxation or medication. These should not replace all the usual support and care previously tried by nurses. When patients recover they often find it is this continued presence rather than specific treatments which helped them to overcome their distress (Chastko et al 1971).

CONCLUSION

An understanding of how and why people become anxious is fundamental to nursing because of particular adverse effects on future mental and physical health. Assessment of pertinent personality factors and mood profiles may become more important in the future, as psychosomatic disorders become better understood and mind–body dualism no longer gains credibility.

Establishing a supportive relationship with anxious patients is fundamental to the role of the nurse. No other professional has such an explicit responsibility for the psychological welfare of patients or such opportunities and (potential) skills.

REFERENCES

Aitken R C B, Zealley A K 1970 Measurement of mood. British Journal of Hospital Medicine 8: 215–224

Aitken Swan J, Paterson R 1955 The cancer patient's delay in seeking advice. British Medical Journal 1: 623

Bartrop R W, Lazarus L, Luckhurst E, Kiloh L G, Penny R 1977 Depressed lymphocyte function after bereavement. Lancet 1: 834–6

Bird B 1955 Psychological aspects of preoperative and postoperative care. American Journal of Nursing 55(6): 685–687

Boore J 1976 Unpublished PhD Thesis. An investigation into the effects of some aspects of pre-operative preparation of patients on post-operative stress and recovery. May. University of Manchester

Breggin P B 1964 The psychophysiology of anxiety with a review of the literature concerning adrenaline. Journal of Nervous and Mental Diseases 139: 558–568

Cassel J 1974 Psychosocial processes and 'stress': theoretical formulation. International Journal of Health Services 4(3): 471–482

Cattell R B 1954 Sixteen personality factors. National Foundation for Educational Research, Bucks, England and Institute for Personality and Ability Testing, Illinois, USA

Cattell R B 1972 Current trends in theory and research. In: Speilberger C D (ed) Anxiety Vol 2. Academic Press, London

Chastko H E, Glick I D, Gould E, Hargreaves W A 1971 Patients' post-hospital evaluations of psychiatric nursing treatment. Nursing Research 20 (4): 333–338

Davitz J R 1969 The language of emotions. Academic Press, New York and London

Endler N S, Hunt Mc V J, Rosenstein A J 1962 An S-R Inventory of Anxiousness. Psychological monographs 76(17), (536)

Eysenck H J, Eysenck S B G 1964 Manual of the Eysenck Personality Inventory. University of London Press, London

Finesilver C 1979 Preparation of adult patients for cardiac catheterization and coronary cine-angiocardiography. International Journal of Nursing Studies 16: 211–221

Freud A 1936 The ego and mechanisms of defence. International University Press, New York

Geer J H 1965 The development of a scale to measure fear. Behaviour Research and Therapy 3: 5–53

Gelder M G, Marks I M 1966 Severe agoraphobia: a controlled prospective therapeutic trial. British Journal of Psychiatry 112: 309–319

Guinn R M, Hill H 1964 Influence of anxiety on the relationship between self-acceptance and acceptance of others. Journal of Consulting Psychology 28: 116–119

Hamilton M 1969 Diagnosis and rating of anxiety. In: Lader M (ed) Studies in anxiety. Headley Brothers Ltd, Ashford, Kent, pp 76–79

Hayward J C 1975 Information — a prescription against pain. Royal College of Nursing, London

Hoch P H, Zubin H 1950 Anxiety. Grune & Stratton Inc, New York

Izard C 1972 Patterns of emotions. Academic Press, New York and London

Johnson J 1983 Preparing patients to cope with stress while hospitalized. In: Wilson-Barnett J (ed) Patient teaching. Churchill Livingstone, Edinburgh

Jones E 1955 Sigmund Freud: life and work. Hogarth Press, London, vols 1 and 2

Kelly D H W 1967 The technique of forearm plethysmography for assessing anxiety. Journal of Psychomatic Research 10: 373–382

Lader M, Marks I 1971 Clinical anxiety. William Heineman Medical Books Ltd, London

Lader M 1975 In: Levi L (ed) Emotions, their parameters and measurement. Raven Press, New York (in discussion) p 341–367

Lazarus R S, Averill J R 1972 Emotion and cognition. In: Speilberger C D (ed) Anxiety: current trends in theory and research, vol 1. Academic Press, London

Levitt E E 1971 The psychology of anxiety. Granada Publishing Ltd, Paladin, London

Lipowski Z J 1975 Physical illness, the patient and his environment: psychosocial foundations of medicine. American Handbook of Psychiatry 4: 1–42

Lishman W A 1972 Selective factors in memory. Part 2 Affective Disorders. Psychological Medicine 2: 248–253

Lynn R 1971 National differences in anxiety. The Economic and Social Research Institute

Macleod Clark J 1983 Nurse-patient communication — an analysis of conversations from surgical wards. In: Wilson-Barnett J (ed) Nursing research: ten studies in patient care. John Wiley and Son, Chichester

Mathew A, Ridgeway V 1981 Personality and surgical recovery: a review. British Journal of Clinical Psychology 20: 243–260

May R 1950 The meaning of anxiety. Ronald Press, New York

Munday A 1973 Physiological measures of anxiety in hospital patients. Royal College of Nursing Study of Nursing Care, London

Olmsted R W, Kennedy D A 1975 In: Milton T (ed) Medical Behavioural Science. Saunders, London, pp 200–206

Rachman S 1974 The meaning of fear. Penguin, London

Ray C, Fitzgibbon G 1982 Stress arousal and coping with surgery. Psychological Medicine 11: 741–746

Ridgeway V, Mathew A 1982 Psychological preparation for surgery — a comparison of methods. British Journal of Clinical Psychology 21: 271–280

Robinson L 1972 Psychological aspects of the care of hospital patients. Davis Co, New York

Rosenberg M 1962 The association between self-esteem and anxiety. Journal of Psychiatric Research 1: 135–151

Rycroft C 1968 Anxiety and neurosis. Pelican, London

Sims A C P 1985 Anxiety in historical perspective. British Journal of Clinical Practice. Supplements 38, 39: 4–9

Speilberger C D 1966 Anxiety and behaviour. Academic Press, London

Speilberger C D 1972 (ed) Anxiety: Current trends in theory and research, Vol 1. Academic Press, London

Speilberger C D, Gorsuch R L, Lushene R, Vagol P R, Jacobs G A 1983 Manual for State Trait Anxiety Inventory (Form 4) 'Self evaluation questionnaire'. Consuttius Psychology Press, California

Sullivan H S 1956 Clinical studies in psychiatry. Norton, New York

Stewart W 1983 Counselling in nursing: a problem-solving approach. Harper & Row, London

Taylor J A 1953 A personality scale of manifest anxiety. Journal of Abnormal and Social Psychology 48: 285–295

Wild A A, Evans J 1968 The patient and the X-ray department. British Medical Journal 3: 107–109

Wilson-Barnett J 1976 Patients' emotional reactions to hospitalization: an exploratory study. Journal of Advanced Nursing 1: 351–358

Wilson-Barnett J, Carrigy A 1978 Factors influencing patients' emotional reactions to hospital. Journal of Advanced Nursing 3: 221–229

Wilson-Barnett J, Osborne J 1983 Studies evaluating patient teaching: implications for practice. International Journal of Nursing Studies 20(1): 33–44

Wilson-Barnett J 1984 Interventions to alleviate patients' stress: a review. Journal of Psychosomatic Research 28(1): 63–72

Wilson-Barnett J 1985 Key functions in nursing. Lampada 2: 35–39

Wilson-Barnett J, Trimble M 1984 Abnormal illness behaviour: the nursing contribution. International Journal of Nursing Studies 21(4): 267–278

Yerkes R M, Dodson J D 1908 The relation of strength of stimulus to rapidity of habit formation. Journal of Comparative Neurology and Psychology 18: 459–482

31

Phobic and obsessional disorders

K. Gournay

Twenty years ago nursing phobic and obsessional patients would have meant looking after those patients in custodial settings, perhaps even after a leucotomy had been performed, in an attempt to alleviate distress. More commonly, nurses provided very basic support in day-care settings or admission wards. In these situations doctors administered various drug therapies, modified insulin treatment or undertook psychoanalytic psychotherapy — all treatments in which the nurse played only a minor role.

Because of the behavioural revolution in psychiatry, the setting up of nurse therapy training programmes and a change of emphasis to treating patients in the community, phobic and obsessional patients are now nursed very differently. Treatment involves the provision of diagnosis, assessment, treatment and evaluation by the nurse, with no other professional involvement apart from the initial referral by a general practitioner or psychiatrist. This is not to say that all phobic and obsessional people are nursed in this way. Unfortunately some patients are still to be found in day hospitals or under the supervision of a community psychiatric nurse who may visit for 10 minutes every few weeks to check their tranquillizers. This chapter is concerned with nursing phobics and obsessionals in the former active fashion and will not attempt to discuss the latter.

Phobias and obsessive compulsive states are now eminently treatable conditions. There are many reviews (e.g. Rachman & Wilson 1980) showing that several years after relatively brief behavioural treatment, patients have significantly reduced symptomatology. In many other respects these patients show an improved quality of life as measured by such general indicators as increased social interaction and improved marital satisfaction (e.g. Lelliott et al 1986).

The advent of specialist training in behaviour therapy for Registered Mental Nurses in the early 1970s was contemporaneous with the dramatic developments in behavioural procedures for obsessions and phobias. (This landmark in the development of the nursing profession is described in Marks et al (1977) and discussed in Chapter 43 of this book.) In many health districts much of the treatment of phobic and obsessional states is now carried out by community nurses and nurse therapists. There is also encouraging evidence that routine behavioural treatment may be administered effectively in primary care settings by nurse therapists working in an even more autonomous fashion than the nurse therapists working in traditional settings (Marks 1985).

THE NATURE OF PHOBIAS AND OBSESSIONS

Phobias and obsessions can best be viewed as varieties of anxiety and as such are exaggerations of 'normal' behaviour. Behaviourists take the view that there is little evidence to treat these problems other than at face value.

As phobic and obsessional behaviour is present in everyone at some time during life, perhaps the greatest service nurses can give to patients when treating them is to keep this fact to the forefront, rather than viewing the patient as an abnormal object who suffers esoteric psychopathology. In this regard there is a rapidly growing amount of evidence (e.g. Buglass et al 1977, Chambless & Mason 1986, Gournay 1989) that on several measures of personality and function, even severe phobics are not different from matched normal controls other than with respect to their phobias.

An American psychologist, Dr Peter Lang, has described a model which has great utility when discussing anxiety (Lang 1971). He sees anxiety as being composed of three loosely correlated systems: the physiological, the cognitive and the behavioural. Thus, for example, typical 'exam nerves' would be a predominantly physiological phenomenon, with frequency of micturition, palpitations and other autonomic symptoms, while anxiety about the future of children in the nuclear age is predominantly cognitive (i.e. thinking and worrying). Thirdly, anxiety about meeting a lion on a country walk would be predominantly behavioural, with rapid escape and avoidance! These examples are perhaps overly simplistic but serve to illustrate that in Lang's words 'anxiety is not a lump'. Most anxiety states seen in clinical practice have symptoms in all three systems and the interrelationship of these symptoms changes subtly over time.

Using Lang's concept, a working model of phobias and obsessions can be developed. Phobias are anxiety states with a variety of physiological and cognitive symptoms and partial or total avoidance. In the case of the agoraphobic (see below) there are many situations which are completely avoided, while the aeroplane phobic may avoid cognitively by getting drunk before boarding the plane to Majorca for the yearly holiday! The obsessional ritualizer takes avoidance one stage further. For example, the obsessional patient with a phobia of germs not only avoids possible contact with germs but also takes many active measures (i.e. obsessional rituals) in the form of handwashing and cleaning to ensure that avoidance is total.

Alternative models of agoraphobia

Psychoanalytic models of agoraphobia have developed from Freud's original description of 'Little Hans' (Freud 1909). Freud stated that phobic states arise through a process of displacement and repression. While Freudian theory has been modified over the years and other schools of psychoanalytic theory have evolved, all psychoanalytic models stress that unconscious conflict underpins the whole syndrome. Analysts would therefore argue that the conflict needs to be resolved before recovery can take place.

Psychoanalytic treatment is therefore based on a protracted process of insight. For an up-to-date account of analytic theories and treatments the reader is referred to Freidman & Goldstein (1974).

While in most ways psychoanalytic models are diametrically opposed to the behavioural position, there are one or two points of agreement. For example, Mathews et al (1981) point out that Freud was most perceptive when he noted that what the patient actually fears is a repetition of panic. This notion of 'fear of fear' is of course central to the current cognitive-behavioural views of agoraphobia.

Recently, there have been some interesting alternative (non-psychoanalytical) psychological theories which are based on experimental data and which seem to be promising in providing a more comprehensive understanding of the syndrome. The current cognitive approach is based on experimental cognitive psychology rather than psychoanalytic theory. This initiative largely belongs to Dr Aaron Beck, who with others (Beck et al 1974) described anxiety and phobic anxiety states as a basic malfunction of cognitive processing. Beck argues that the phobic overestimates the possibility of personal risk and uses avoidance as a tactic. This hypothesis was tested experimentally by the author (Gournay 1985, 1989) in a controlled study. The data from this study seem to suggest prima-facie evidence that phobics differ from normal people in how they estimate the risk arising from everyday situations. More recently, Hallam (1986) has reviewed some very interesting work on information-processing theory and this seems to offer some fairly precise indicators about some of the cognitive mechanisms involved. In a somewhat looser sense, these cognitive approaches to agoraphobia have been used in the Personal Construct Model of George Kelly and have latterly been empirically tested on agoraphobic populations. (For a review, see Winter & Gournay 1987.) Briefly, the personal construct view would be that phobic patients construe the world and their position in the world vis-à-vis others in a very different way from non-phobic populations. However, as Winter & Gournay (1987) demonstrate, on the measure of the repertory grid, phobics clearly perceive themselves and the world in a significantly different way to 'normal' populations.

Outcome of non-behavioural treatments

While all the above theories are interesting, there is very little controlled research to test the utility of such approaches to treatment. With regard to psychoanalytic approaches, it should be pointed out that even Freud (1919), while stressing the importance of analysis, stated: 'One can hardly master a phobia if one waits until the patient lets the analysis influence him to give it up . . . . Analysis succeeds only when one can induce them to go through the influence of the analysis . . . . that is to go out alone and to struggle with their anxiety while they are making the attempt'. In reviewing current approaches, Freidman & Goldstein (1974) have also indicated that there needs to be active intervention to help the patient face the previously avoided situations. Although psychoanalytic psychotherapy is widely carried out in order to help patients with agoraphobia, there are few controlled studies to evaluate the effectiveness of such methods. In one classic enquiry by Gelder et al (1967), desensitization and psychodynamic psychotherapy were compared in a group of agoraphobics. The evidence from this study was that psychotherapy was no more effective than a placebo treatment. The major problem in evaluating psychoanalytic approaches is that psychotherapists seem to have their own idiosyncratic ways of carrying out treatment programmes. To compound the problem further, psychotherapists will often encourage exposure, and because of this, it is difficult to tease out the differential effects of psychoanalytic or psychodynamic psychotherapy and exposure treatment. Certainly, additions of cognitive approaches (of a non-analytic/dynamic variety) to behaviour therapy have shown little evidence of additional effectiveness. There are, however, many problems with the methodology of such enquiries, although one or two studies have overcome them. For an example of one of these excellent studies, the reader is referred to Mavissakalian et al (1983).

With regard to psychiatric nursing, the training in behaviour therapy (ENB 650) for nurse therapists is the only standardized and evaluated training for nurses in the treatment of agoraphobia. There is now a wealth of evidence which suggests that nurse therapists produce very significant and lasting change with agoraphobic patients, not only on agoraphobic avoidance, but on measures of life adjustment (e.g. Marks 1985).

If one looks to findings from various sciences, it is possible to compose a picture of how phobias and obsessions develop. Marks (1981) discusses such theories in detail and provides one of the several formulations currently available. The reader is referred to this work for more detail. In brief, the key features of Marks' formulation are as follows.

Certain objects and situations are more likely to become the source of phobias than others because of an innate survival mechanism. Thus, phobias of spiders or flying around the universe in aeroplanes are more likely to develop than, say, phobias of wooden chairs or musical instruments. The former are potentially more dangerous and thus man is biologically pre-programmed more readily to become phobic of these objects/situations. Furthermore, there is evidence that some people have a greater biological conditionality than others. Among other factors which may then contribute to the development of phobias are:

1. the learning of avoidance (by modelling) from parents
2. the possibility that specific frightening events act as a triggering mechanism
3. the subjection of the individual to the experience of several simultaneous stressful life events, which raises physiological arousal and therefore increases vulnerability to being phobically conditioned
4. physical illnesses of one kind or another (also raising arousal)
5. interpersonal 'stresses' such as severe marital conflict which raises general anxiety and hence arousal levels.

Most comprehensive theories of phobias and obsessions (e.g. Mathews et al 1981) suggest that it is a combination of many factors (some of which are listed above) which leads to the development of a phobia rather than one event. The trigger for the reaction may, for example, be the death of a spouse who previously acted as a source of safety or it may be the impact of childbirth. However, it should be pointed out that detective work in the form of insight-oriented therapy to search for the cause of the problem universally ends in failure. Most patients are intelligent and accepting enough, that the therapist can give an explanation based on the above factors, but at the same time point out to them that this explanation is probably incomplete. Comprehensive nursing assessment may, of course, reveal other problems which may be treated in separate (non-behavioural) programmes.

TREATMENT

Simple phobias

Phobias are so common that it is not practical to offer treatment to all sufferers. Treatment is reserved for people whose problem seriously upsets and/or interferes with normal activities.

In the great majority of cases, simple graduated exposure is the treatment of choice. The theory of exposure treatment is very simple. If the phobic faces the situation or object he fears for long enough, the anxiety normally experienced will diminish. The patient will experience a subjective feeling of coping and mastery. Together with this, adrenal output will fall and the patient will report feeling a reduction in autonomic arousal (e.g. rapid heart beat, sweating, etc.). In summary, the patient learns to cope with the evoked anxiety rather than escaping, and if the exercise is repeated often enough the anxiety reduces and eventually disappears.

To cite a simple example, a spider phobic can be exposed gradually to spiders over a couple of sessions of 2 to 3 hours each. At first the therapist exposes the patient to small live spiders in a closed container several feet away. The therapist encourages the patient to continue with this exposure and gradually the patient's anxiety level falls. At a pace which is acceptable to the patient, the therapist then continues, with the patient's exposure to spiders in open containers until finally the patient is handling large, live spiders. In very long sessions of several hours, the patient will get used to anxiety (habituate) and will probably be able to get over the problem more easily than he would in shorter sessions (of say one hour). Exposure is much facilitated by the therapist modelling each behaviour to be accomplished.

The patient is encouraged to practise exposure as homework, using a friend or relative as co-therapist. The therapist will, at assessment, have established what other avoidance measures the patient adopts: for example, a spider phobic may avoid going into the garage in case a spider is encountered. An exercise to deal will this will thus be incorporated into 'homework' tasks. The therapist asks the patient to record homework in the form of a written diary, getting the co-therapist to countersign when the exercise has been completed.

Some phobias are not so straightforward. One common problem is a phobia of becoming incontinent of urine. This leads the sufferer to reduce fluid intake and to restrict the length of journeys away from home. Patients with this phobia usually ensure that all toilets are carefully mapped out before they take a trip away from home. Exposure remains the central treatment approach for such cases. Treatment usually consists of a programme of gradually increasing fluid intake, and at the same time increasing the time the patient spends away from toilets and reducing the frequency of urination. The therapist is therefore principally involved with helping set up the programme and then meeting regularly with the patient to monitor progress. A simple behavioural diary is kept by the patient to aid this process. This diary is filled in daily and includes data on the amount of fluid consumed, number of urinations and places visited, together with a rating of anxiety for each task undertaken. This simple treatment has a very good outcome, with the large majority of patients achieving a very significant reduction in symptoms.

For some phobias it is difficult to arrange real life exposure. One example is thunder and lightening phobia. Sufferers often experience terror during thunderstorms and engage in avoidance behaviour such as putting cotton wool in their ears or hiding in soundproofed rooms. One patient actually spent several thousand pounds sound-proofing a room where he would retreat. Others resort to alcohol or drugs or avoid going out if thunder threatens. Patients will often take elaborate precautions to avoid being struck by lightening. For example, they might remove all metal objects from window sills or they may become preoccupied with checking weather forecasts or ringing the meteorological office incessantly. Conversely, they may avoid weather forecasts to the extent of not reading newspapers or watching the television news.

Exposure in these cases usually involves getting the patient to imagine terrible thunderstorms, perhaps using taped thunder noises or films to facilitate exposure. The therapist will also use the detailed assessment information to ask the patient to stop rituals, e.g. she might ask the patient to put a row of metal objects on the window sill during storms rather than remove them. If patients continually ring the meteorological office, they will be asked to refrain, or if they avoid weather forecasts they will be asked to read them regularly. The therapist will probably involve a spouse or friend as a co-therapist to help with these tasks. The therapist will then plan strategies for helping the patient to expose himself to the next thunderstorm. This may involve getting patient and co-therapist to stand out in the rain for a long period! As with simple phobias, prolonged exposure will lead to a reduction in anxiety. There is good evidence (e.g. Liddell & Lyons 1978) that behavioural treatment is very effective for this particular phobia.

Agoraphobia

This is one of the commonest disorders referred to behaviour therapists and community psychiatric nurses working with neurotic patients. In its classical form it involves multiple avoidance of public places, travelling and generally going far from a secure base. In such situations the phobic develops panic attacks with wide-ranging cognitive and physiological symptoms (for a comprehensive account of the syndrome the reader is reffered to Thorpe & Burns (1983) and Marks (1969)). The problem is often complicated by more generalized anxiety and depression, and also by addiction to benzodiazepine tranquillizers and alcohol. Fully developed agoraphobia probably occurs in 0.6% of the population, but recent research (Costello 1982) indicates that as many as one in six of the population experience some significant agoraphobic symptoms. This indicates that only a minority of agoraphobic patients actually receive treatment. Given that the syndrome has a low spontaneous remission rate (Agras et al 1969), it would be of great interest to know the fate of those who do not receive treatment.

The marital problems often seen in agoraphobia are often mistakenly seen as causative, but as with problems such as poor self-esteem, a vigorous approach to the phobic avoidance *per se* will often result in an enormous improvement in marital happiness and self-perception. It is common that cases referred to behaviour therapists have previously been managed by many hours of family therapy, marital therapy and insight-oriented treatment: all of these therapies have probably been to no avail. Then such cases have subsequently responded dramatically to 4 to 6 hours of behavioural intervention. Certainly there is much research evidence (e.g. Cobb et al 1980) which would suggest that an approach of changing avoidance behaviour should be the first strategy, rather than an attempt to treat apparent interpersonal problems. In Cobb's study, a group of agoraphobics who also had severe marital difficulties were randomly allocated to either exposure therapy for agoraphobia followed by marital therapy, or to marital therapy followed by exposure therapy. The results indicated clearly that successful treatment for agoraphobia leads to an improvement in marital satisfaction. However, marital therapy on its own does not change agoraphobic avoidance, nor does it seem to produce a lasting or significant change in the marital relationship.

Alcohol and tranquillizers

Before starting any exposure programme for agoraphobic avoidance, it is vital to ensure that the use of drugs and alcohol is not complicating the problem. Gournay's (1985) findings are in accord with several other studies which show that these factors are of crucial importance. Up to 20% of agoraphobics presenting for treatment may have a significant alcohol problem. Although these

patients may have begun using alcohol to reduce anxiety, it is fallacious to assume that successful treatment for the phobic state will lead to a reduction in alcohol intake. Very often the alcohol problem has developed its own momentum and arguably may produce its own anxiety symptoms. Thus, a carefully recorded drinking history with substantiation from a reliable witness is essential. If an alcohol problem is evident, then referral to an appropriate specialist is desirable. Certainly, any exposure programme with such individuals should only be conducted if they are totally abstinent and have been so for at least three months.

Tranquillizer-taking among agoraphobics is very common, and probably at least half of the agoraphobics presenting for treatment have been taking a regular benzodiazepine tranquillizer (e.g. Ativan, Valium, Tranxene) for at least one year (Gournay 1985). The same research showed that taking tranquillizers leads to poor outcome with treatment, a higher incidence of drop-out from treatment and a greater frequency of post-treatment relapse. Apart from these findings there is ample evidence to suggest that long-term tranquillizer use is of little or no lasting benefit in anxiety states (Murray et al 1981). Therefore, the therapist needs to liaise very closely with the patient's general practitioner or psychiatrist to ensure that tranquillizers are carefully and gradually discontinued before treatment commences.

Exposure treatment in agoraphobia

Systematic desensitization (Wolpe 1954) and flooding (Stampfl & Levis 1967) as described in many textbooks are best viewed as interesting anachronisms. The most effective treatment approach is graduated exposure in real life to the avoided situations. Simply keeping the patient in the situation from which he would normally escape or would avoid completely is the essential component of exposure treatment. Eventually the initial high anxiety experienced will decline, and the role of the therapist is to help persuade the patient to remain in the situation until this happens. Exposure sessions need to be long (2 hours or more) for this to be most effective. Research evidence indicates that short exposure sessions are not as effective as long sessions (Stern & Marks 1973), and allowing the patient to leave the situation while still highly anxious may be damaging.

This simple treatment is carried out only after adequate assessment and preparation, and there are several other factors which will help maximize the effect of treatment.

A detailed assessment of the patient's problem, history and general circumstances should be followed by a detailed evaluation which will be repeated during treatment, after treatment and at follow-up intervals. This is usually effected by using rating scales to measure phobic problem severity (see Fig. 31.1), mood, fear and avoidance.

Furthermore, the therapist usually asks the patient to attempt a task which would normally evoke anxiety (e.g. visiting a shop, travelling by bus). This Behavioural Avoidance Test gives a measure of actual function and is repeated at the end of treatment to assess progress. The therapist will also use rating scales to assess the impact of the problem on work, social and family relationships and other general areas (for an example, see

Fig. 31.2). Thus using a battery of measures, the patient's programme can be evaluated effectively.

The therapist then negotiates a range of target behaviours with the patient which are then rated after treatment and at follow-up (an example is shown in Fig. 31.3).

Usually the therapist enlists the help of a family member or friend to give additional information and more importantly to help the patient as a co-therapist. This co-therapy involves helping the patient regularly repeat exposure exercises. There is ample evidence (e.g. Mathews et al 1981) to suggest that for many patients a therapist may need to give only one exposure session. This would involve demonstrating the exposure principle to patient and co-therapist. After that the bulk of therapy can be carried out using programmed practice manuals. The therapist then has a simple advisory/monitoring role.

For patients who require a full exposure programme, the most effective delivery is to use group exposure. This entails two therapists treating six to eight patients in four to eight exposure

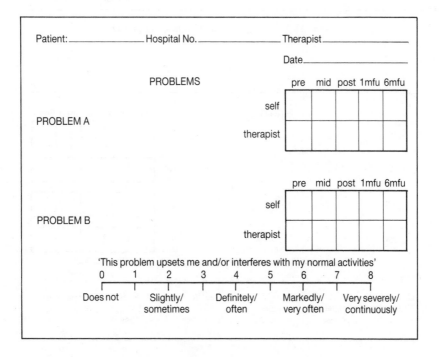

Fig. 31.1 Problem severity (Marks 1986).

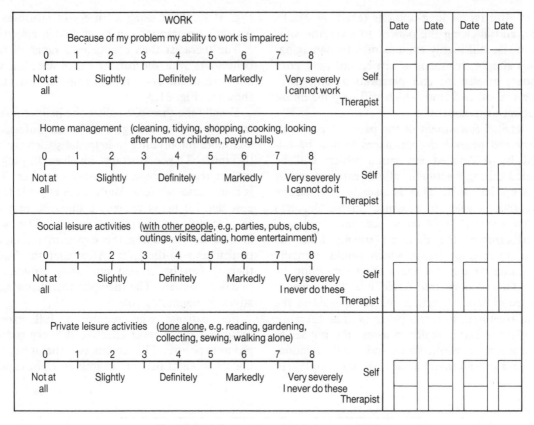

Fig. 31.2 Adjustment scale (Marks et al 1977).

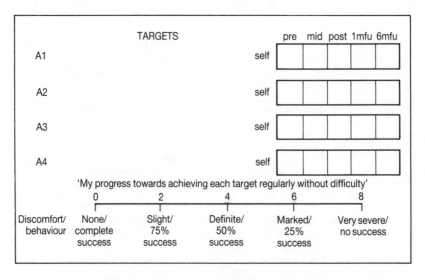

Fig. 31.3 Target behaviours (Marks et al 1977).

sessions of 2 hours plus. There is plentiful evidence that such group exposure is at least as effective as individual exposure (Hand et al 1974). The support that group members give each other seems to ensure the maintenance of treatment gains.

Following comprehensive individual assessment, members of the group meet for a preliminary session of about 1½ hours. The therapists introduce themselves and allow the patients to get to know each other. A verbal description of the programme with an explanation of treatment principles are given. A video used as a pre-therapy preparation showing exposure treatment taking place seems to be helpful in dispelling myths, and the observation of role models is obviously an important route to acquiring coping skills. Patients then ask questions, discuss the programme and explicitly commit themselves to a course of exposure treatment. After this first session, treatment proper begins with each exposure session being preceded by a brief session of anxiety management training concentrating on breathing control. Some recent work (Bonn et al 1984) has suggested that agoraphobics may chronically hyperventilate, thus increasing anxiety. Immediately following the anxiety management training, patients start 3 to 4 hours of exposure, adhering to the simple rule that they will tackle difficult, but just manageable tasks. A therapist may, for example, travel with two or three patients on the underground railway and over the session gradually 'fade out', encouraging patients gradually to attempt more tasks alone. For example, the therapist may sit at the opposite end of the carriage, then in the next compartment, then on the next train, and so on. Eventually, after 3 or 4 hours, most patients will be accomplishing significant tasks alone and be feeling relatively comfortable. The group then reconvenes for a brief discussion of the session and homework tasks will be negotiated. These tasks are attempted before the next session. The patient's co-therapist (spouse or friend) will be used to assist in this.

Over the sessions, patients travel by bus, train and tube; they visit various shopping centres; they eat and drink in public; drive along motorways; walk alone; travel in lifts and on escalators; cross bridges; and attempt the wide range of situations avoided by agoraphobics. This of course means that therapists must be flexible and at times visit strange and interesting places! In the author's treatment centre, psychology students and various nursing personnel are used as therapists, as well as, on occasion, having previously-treated patients act as therapists. A nurse therapist or community nurse would be the ideal person to direct and organize the group, and she could certainly delegate less qualified personnel to conduct exposure. The group director or leader needs to assume overall clinical responsibility and in doing so ensure detailed assessment and adequate evaluation, as well as writing comprehensive reports to the patient's doctor or referring agent. Apart from six sessions of exposure spread over 3 weeks, there is also a group where spouses or friends can be instructed as co-therapists. This provides a forum for questions and discussion. Amongst spouses, there is only a very small minority who choose not to attend this group.

When the programme is complete, individual evaluation is repeated for all patients. Most need no further treatment and attend a follow-up group which reassesses progress at 3 months, 6 months and yearly after treatment. Patients are encouraged to meet between sessions to continue exposure exercises. Occasionally, some patients need additional help and this is provided as required.

Before embarking on many hours of therapist-aided exposure, it is worth considering whether the patient can carry out his own exposure treatment with only minimal help. Mathews and his colleagues have described a programme (Mathews et al 1981) which is principally home based and involves:

1. Assessment by the therapist in the patient's home in the presence of a suitable co-therapist (e.g. spouse or friend)
2. A single session of exposure to demonstrate the principle of treatment (also involving the co-therapist)
3. The use of programmed practice manuals (one for the patient and one for the co-therapist)
4. Follow-up monitoring by the therapist. This could involve telephone contact.

Mathews' programme, which used only about 7½ hours in total of therapist time, achieved excellent results which were maintained long after active treatment ended. The results of this programme can be favourably compared to other more (time) costly programmes. This simple approach seems to be suitable for up to half of the agoraphobics referred to a district behaviour therapy service.

Other possibilities for self-directed treatment are the use of manuals alone, programmed practice directed by computer (Carr & Ghosh 1983) or the use of self-help groups. One promising possibility would be that primary-care-based community psychiatric nurses (CPNs) could set up neighbourhood groups and act as facilitators. This would ensure that the exposure experience remains central and is not replaced by symptom-swapping sessions where patients merely meet to discuss their problems without attempting behaviour change. The CPN could use ex-patients to help run exposure sessions and thus ensure the most efficient use of her time.

Failures in the treatment of agoraphobia

Gournay (1985) has carried out the first systematic enquiry of failures in the behavioural treatment of agoraphobia in British literature. Briefly, he investigated four groups of treatment failure. These were:

1. patients who did not respond to behavioural treatment
2. patients who initially responded and then relapsed
3. patients who dropped out from treatment
4. patients who refused treatment.

In all, 60 patients (of an initial cohort of 132) who entered a controlled treatment trial for agoraphobia were evaluated using multiple measures of change, including blind assessment, over a period of treatment and 2 years after. Several interesting findings emerged. People very often dropped out or refused treatment because they were frightened of the exposure treatment. This was somewhat surprising to the therapists, who felt that they had made considerable efforts to explain both treatment and rationale. Of the patients deemed to be treatment failures, their expectations of the treatment programme did not match those of the therapist. There were also several important factors associated with patients' own attributions of what would lead to recovery.

It seems very clear that many people do not see psychiatric treatment as a reasonable approach to their problems, believing instead that fears and phobias are the kind of problems that you have to get over on your own. This of course would confirm that a self-help approach is perhaps to be encouraged before offering a formal professional approach. It was also interesting that some patients who began a treatment programme and then dropped out, continued to improve during a follow-up period. This was presumably because they continued to use the principles of exposure taught to them. This would seem to confirm the view that one of the most important things about the behavioural treatment of agoraphobia is to persuade the patient to accept that the exposure principle must be paramount.

Of the patients who dropped out from treatment, many did so because professional treatment programmes did not fit with their needs. Furthermore, there was also some indication that fear of psychiatric stigma played an important part in some people refusing the offered treatment.

There are several mystifying problems concerned with the outcome of this study. For example, despite very thorough analyses there were no clear indications of what presenting features correlated with a good treatment outcome. Indeed, people with very marked and diverse symptomatology and handicap did just as well with treatment as people with milder, more circumscribed fears. However, there seem to be several factors which correlated with failure or drop out. The most important one was the concurrent use of benzodiazepine tranquillizers with exposure treatment. This factor was associated with twice as many people dropping out of treatment as those not taking benzodiazepine tranquillizers. The group taking tranquillizers also had a relapse rate twice that of those who took no medication. The other significant finding of the study was that nearly a fifth of the initial population of agoraphobics screened for the trial had a significant, if not abnormal, intake of alcohol. This points to the necessity of carefully screening for alcohol problems when making an initial assessment of a patient with agoraphobia.

Obsessional states

As with phobias, it can be argued that some obsessional thinking and behaviour may be viewed as a variant of normal behaviour. Marks (1981) pointed out that many children go through phases of obsessive rituals, perhaps avoiding stepping on cracks in the pavement or engaging in a nonsense rhyme or game. These rituals are carried out to stave off possible disaster. Most children of course 'grow out' of such patterns of behaviour. However, obsessional states of clinical proportions are relatively uncommon, accounting for perhaps only 0.05% of the general population (Beech 1974).

There are several definitions of obsessional disorders. However, there are some prominent features which are generally accepted as characteristic of obsessional states. Of most significance are the conscious ideas which the patient realizes are abnormal and are uncharacteristic of himself. The patient may attempt to resist and ward off these obsessional ideas either by adopting some form of ritualistic behaviour (rituals) or by using various mental devices (e.g. multiplication). For a consideration of the more complex theoretical issues, the reader is referred to Beech (1974).

Obsessional states can be divided into those with rituals and those with ruminations. In practice, however, most patients present with both rituals and ruminations, although one usually predominates. There may often be a focus for the ritual or rumination. This focus can be considered to be a phobic stimulus, and may be dirt, germs or some danger theme. These cues trigger the pattern of obsessive responses.

Assessment of the obsessional patient may be difficult for two main reasons. Firstly, the problem may be very complex with the patient engaging in extremely complex rituals; there may be extreme slowness and repetition and there may also be massive avoidance behaviour. Thus the therapist will need to be very patient and systematic.

Secondly, the patient may well be obsessional with regard to the information he gives. This may lead to the patient checking and reiterating and asking for reassurance. It is therefore wise to use standard assessment procedures and check-lists (see Fig. 31.4 for an example of an obsessional check-list). These procedures are detailed in Marks et al (1977).

For many patients, assessment is best carried out at home, as rituals may only be present in that environment. The patient can also demonstrate the problem in its natural setting and the therapist will be able to observe and record various activities. The therapist may also use rating scales (see Fig. 31.5) which specifically measure aspects of obsessional behaviour.

At the end of the assessment the therapist will negotiate a list of target behaviours using the same format described for agoraphobic patients (see Fig. 31.3).

A comprehensive treatment plan is formulated by the therapist and explained to the patient. Treatment rationale is discussed and again the emphasis is on the patient gradually facing the fear-evoking situations or objects or fear-evoking thoughts. This procedure may also be called cue exposure. Together with this exposure the therapist also concentrates on helping the patient to stop carrying out rituals or to practise alternative thoughts. This procedure is also called response prevention. Thus, for example, a patient with a contamination phobia will be asked to 'contaminate' himself. The therapist will demonstrate (model) the behaviour first. A patient with contamination fears may therefore need to touch dirt or waste bins. Patients would then be instructed that they should refrain from the normal ritual (e.g. cleaning or hand washing) and allow themselves to endure the anxiety. Eventually, anxiety levels fall (i.e. habituation occurs) and patients experience a feeling of coping and mastery. The prime role of the therapist is to help and encourage patients to continue facing anxiety and to model the appropriate behaviour.

Therapists should conduct sessions of several hours at a time to allow adequate exposure and hence anxiety reduction to take place. It is important that a co-therapist (in the form of a family

				ACTIVITY
Name_____		Hosp. No._____		Date_____ 19_____

INSTRUCTIONS: The following are a list of activities which people with your kind of problem sometimes have difficulty with. Please answer each question by putting a tick under the appropriate number

0 – I have no problems with activity – takes me about the same time as an average person. I do not need to repeat it or avoid it.

1 – This activity takes me about _twice_ as long as most people, or I have to repeat it _twice_ or _tend_ to avoid it.

2 – This activity takes me about _three_ times as long as most people, or I have to repeat it _three_ or more times, or I _usually_ avoid it.

3 – I am unable to complete or attempt activity.

				ACTIVITY
				Having a bath or shower
				Washing hands and face
				Care of hair (e.g. washing, combing, brushing)
				Brushing teeth
				Dressing and undressing
				Using toilet to urinate
				Using toilet to defaecate
				Touching people or being touched
				Handling waste or waste bins
				Washing clothes
				Washing dishes
				Handling or cooking food
				Cleaning the house
				Keeping things tidy
				Bed making
				Cleaning shoes
				Touching door handles
				Touching your genitals, petting or sexual intercourse
				Visiting a hospital
				Switching lights and taps on or off
				Locking or closing doors or windows
				Using electrical appliances (e.g. heaters)
				Doing arithmetic or accounts
				Getting to work
				Doing your work
				Writing
				Form filling
				Posting letters
				Reading
				Walking down the street
				Travelling by bus, train or car
				Looking after children
				Eating in restaurants
				Going to public toilets
				Keeping appointments
				Throwing things away
				Buying things in shops
TOTAL				
				Other (fill in)

Fig. 31.4 Compulsive check-list.

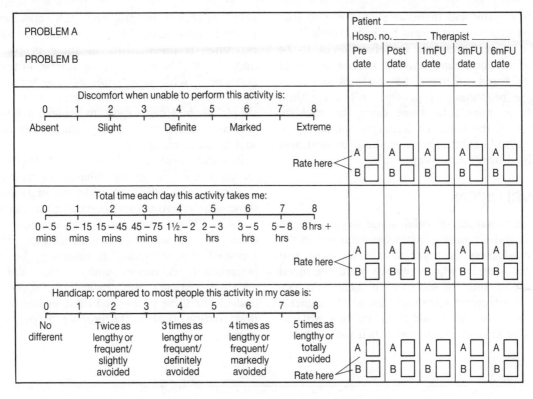

Fig. 31.5 Obsessive time and handicap (Marks et al 1977).

member or friend) is involved, and they should be present during the session. Even with severe obsessional states, two or three long exposure sessions may be sufficient to produce highly significant and lasting change. However, the therapist must be flexible and patient and be prepared to help the patient to perform many ordinary, mundane and sometimes intimate behaviours associated with daily living. This may involve bathing, dressing, cooking, laundering, putting out rubbish, feeding the baby etc. On occasion patients may require up to 50 hours of therapist-aided treatment, although the average is probably between 10 and 20 hours.

The therapist will also counsel the patient regarding developing a 'normal' behavioural repertoire to replace the time-consuming obsessions. If the patient has spent several years engaged in extensive rituals, discussing and negotiating 'normal' activity is a very important task. It will also be important to involve the co-therapist and to con-

duct family sessions to help prevent reassurance seeking. This may involve using role play with the therapist demonstrating appropriate responses to requests for reassurance. This should be done from the beginning of the programme, as reassurance seeking is very often centrally important in reinforcing obsessional behaviour.

For patients with obsessional thoughts, exposure sessions will involve getting the patient to face the distressing thought or ideas for long periods. This exposure may require the patient to use cues which normally evoke distress. Thus, for example, a patient who has obsessional ideas about death may be asked to read newspaper articles about death, visit cemeteries with the therapist, read accounts of life in a hospice for the dying, and generally attempt to evoke themes which are normally avoided. Other strategies which do not involve exposure are usually not very successful if used alone. Therefore, despite early promise, procedures such as thought stopping have not been very successful and therefore should not be considered as a main treatment for ruminations.

The current trend is for obsessionals to be treated at home, and only in rare cases should hospital-based treatment be used. Moreover, a sizeable proportion of patients will 'leave their rituals at home'. In these cases the problem centres on the home environment and does not transfer to hospital. Therefore, hospital treatment will be difficult if not impossible.

CONCLUSION

The development of behavioural approaches to phobic and obsessional states has been one of the major advances in psychiatry in the past two decades. Patients who previously were consigned to a life of suffering and were frequently the victims of iatrogenic (treatment-induced) problems such as tranquillizer addiction are now able to have a brief simple treatment which will consider-

ably reduce their problems. Of agoraphobic patients who undertake a reasonable trial of exposure treatment, 70% of these people will improve by 70% or more (on a number of reliable measures). With simple phobias the results are even more impressive. The great majority of simple phobics can expect to achieve a 90–95% reduction in symptomatology with perhaps only 3 to 4 hours of treatment.

Research evidence clearly demonstrates that nurses trained in giving behavioural treatments achieve results which are at least comparable to those of psychiatrists and psychologists (Marks et al 1977). These nurses work autonomously, and economic analyses demonstrate that they provide a cost-effective workforce. In summary, the use of behavioural techniques with phobic and obsessional patients has radically changed the outlook for these people and these procedures are now routine tools in the practice of psychiatric nursing.

REFERENCES

Agras W, Sylvester D, Oliveau D 1969 The epidemiology of common fears and phobias. Comprehensive Psychiatry 10: 2

Beck A T, Laude R, Bomhert M 1974 Ideational components of anxiety neurosis. Archives of General Psychiatry 31: 319–325

Beech H R 1974 (ed) Obsessional states. Methuen, London

Bonn J A, Readhead C P A, Timmons B H 1984 Enhanced adaptive behavioural response in agoraphobic patients pretreated with breathing retraining. Lancet 8404: 665–669

Buglass D, Clarke J, Henderson A S, Kreitman, N 1977 A study of agoraphobic housewives. Psychological Medicine 7: 73–86

Carr A C, Ghosh A 1983 Response of phobic patients to direct computer assessment. British Journal of Psychiatry 142: 60–65

Chambless D L, Mason J 1986 Sex, sex-role stereotyping and agoraphobia. Behaviour Research and Therapy 24(2): 231–285

Cobb J P, McDonald D R, Marks I M, Stern R S 1980 Marital versus exposure therapy: psychological treatment of co-existing marital and phobic-obsessive problems. Behaviour Analysis and Modification 4: 3–16

Costello, C G 1982 Fears and phobias in women. A community study. Journal of Abnormal Psychology 91: 280–286

Freud S 1909 Analysis of a phobia in a 5 year old boy. In: Collected papers, Vol 3. Hogarth Press, London, 1925

Freud S 1919 Obsessions and phobias. Reprinted as Chapter 7 in collected papers. Hogarth Press, London, 1924

Friedman P, Goldstein J 1974 Phobic reactions. In Arieti S, Brodie E G (eds). American handbook of psychiatry. Basic Books, New York

Gelder M G, Marks, I M, Wolff H H 1967 Desensitisation and psychotherapy in the treatment of phobic states. A controlled enquiry. British Journal of Psychiatry 113: 53–73

Gournay K J M 1985 Agoraphobia: a study of the syndrome and its treatment. PhD thesis, University of Leicester

Gournay K J M 1989 Agoraphobia: Current perspectives on theory and treatment. Routledge, London

Hallam R S 1986 Failures in the behavioural treatment of agoraphobia. Academic Press, London

Hand I, Lamontagne Y, Marks I M 1974 Group exposure (flooding) in vivo for agoraphobics. British Journal of Psychiatry 124: 588–602

Lang P 1971 In application of psychophysiological methods. In: Bergine A E, Garfield S (eds) Handbook of psychotherapy and behaviour change. Wiley, New York

Lelliott P T, Marks I M, Monteiro W O, Psakiris F, Noshirvani H F 1986 Agoraphobia five years after imipramine and exposure: outcome and predictors. Paper to European Association for Behaviour Therapy. Lausanne, Switzerland.

Liddell A, Lyons M 1978 Thunderstorm phobias. Behaviour Research and Therapy 16(4): 306–308

Marks I M 1969 Fears and phobias. Heinemann, London

Marks I M 1981 Care and cure of neurosis. Wiley, New York

Marks I M 1985 Psychiatric nurse therapists in primary care. Royal College of Nursing Research Series, London

Marks I M, Connolly J, Hallam R, Philpott R 1977 Nursing in behavioural psychotherapy. Royal College of Nursing Research Series, London

Mathews A, Gelder M G, Johnston D W 1981 Agoraphobia: nature and treatment. Tavistock, London

Mavissakalian M, Michaelson L, Greenwald D, Cornblith S, Greenwald M 1983 Cognitive behavioural treatment of agoraphobia. Paradoxical intention versus self-statement training. Behavioural Research and Therapy 21(1): 75–76

Murray R, Ghodse H, Harris C, Williams D, Williams P (eds) 1981 The misuse of psychotropic drugs. Gaskell, Royal College of Psychiatrists, London

Rachman S J, Wilson G T 1980 The effects of psychological therapy. Pergamon, Oxford

Stampfl T C, Levis D J 1967 Essentials of implosive therapy. Journal of Abnormal Psychology 72(4): 96–503

Stern R S, Marks I M 1973 Brief and prolonged flooding: A comparison in a agoraphobic patients. Archives of General Psychiatry 28: 270–276

Thorpe G L, Burns L E 1983 The agoraphobic syndrome. Wiley, London

Winter D, Gournay K J M 1987 Constriction and construction of agoraphobia. British Journal of Medical Psychology 60: 233–244.

Wolpe J 1954 Reciprocal inhibition as the main basis of psychotherapeutic effects. Archives of Neurology and Psychiatry 72: 205–226

32

Schizophrenia

J. I. Brooking and S. A. H. Ritter

AETIOLOGY OF SCHIZOPHRENIA

Cerebral pathology

The location and nature of cerebral pathology in schizophrenia are not easy to identify and describe. The debate about cognitive impairment, cerebral pathogenesis and schizophrenia has proved difficult to resolve, despite evidence which has accumulated since Johnstone et al (1976) demonstrated ventricular enlargement in a small group of hospitalized patients with chronic schizophrenia.

Perinatal complications

Beard & Slater (1962) noted a number of epileptic patients with schizophrenic-like psychoses who had had complicated deliveries. Hill (1962), in a commentary on their paper, suggested that more attention should be paid to 'the history of birth and to the history of infantile convulsions and febrile convulsions in early childhood' (p. 315). The associations between perinatal complications and later neurodevelopmental or psychosocial impairment require large and detailed studies to provide convincing explanations (Taylor & Rutter 1985).

Life expectancy

Lane & Albee (1966) investigated the comparative birth weights of schizophrenics and their siblings. Low birth weight predicts lifelong disadvantage, but it is also a measure of environmental variables during pregnancy, and these authors found that babies who were subsequently considered to be schizophrenic averaged lower birth weights than their siblings.

Gender

Flor-Henry's (1974) summary of the developmental and gender-related influences on psychosis, neurosis and epilepsy is also a summary of the directions for subsequent research into the causes of schizophrenia. Young men with a condition diagnosed as schizophrenic outnumber young women, who are more likely to be classified as manic-depressive. Boy infants are more likely than girl infants to develop lesions of the dominant hemisphere after febrile convulsions. Cerebral pathogenesis is most likely to be found in the dominant hemisphere of people with schizophrenia.

Season of birth

Hare (1975) observed that significantly more schizophrenics are born during the winter months.

Infection

Gualtieri & Hicks (1985) attempt to explain the observation that 'males are selectively afflicted with the neurodevelopmental and psychiatric disorders of childhood', including early-onset schizophrenia, by suggesting that the male fetus provokes a maternal immune reaction in utero. Selective male affliction may also be related to 'male vulnerability to environmental stressors, to the genetic endowment of the male, or to his complexity and relative immaturity', and these hypotheses require investigation (p. 436).

Investigations into a possibly viral aetiology of schizophrenia are based on the association between its incidence and the season of birth, as well as between its incidence and class and social differ-

ences (Fisman 1975). Currently, the questions of infection *in utero* and directly during the perinatal period are being investigated with a view to identifying possible neurodevelopmental defects.

Genetics

Twin studies of schizophrenia have not provided conclusive evidence about transmission nor about gender differences in concordance rates (the rate at which both twins will develop the disorder) (Samuels 1978). It is clear that, because concordance rates for monozygotic twins are at most 50%, genetic factors are not solely responsible for schizophrenia (Gottesman & Shields 1972). Nevertheless, the genetic factors responsible for the familial patterns of schizophrenia need to be identified in order to work out strategies for prevention, as well as mental health promotion.

Environment

Life events

Taylor & Rutter (1985) argue that because good psychosocial conditions in childhood and adolescence protect individuals from biological disadvantage, any investigation of the aetiology of schizophrenia must control for social and environmental factors. Conversely, any attempt to explain schizophrenia by hypotheses such as those involving family interaction must take into account the strong evidence of organic impairment. There is some evidence that first schizophrenic episodes are preceded for many people by significant life events. Link et al (1986) tackle one aspect of the question of whether the socio-economic status (SES) of schizophrenic people is the result of downward drift consequent upon the disorder, or whether SES is linked causally to the development of schizophrenia. They conclude that there is evidence that class-linked stress as defined by hazardous blue-collar work is associated with first schizophrenic episodes.

Experimental psychopathology

Experimental research methods have been extensively used to study the abnormal psychology of schizophrenia. In the absence of a theory that will satisfactorily explain the occurrence of mental events, it is difficult to come up with either an account or a classification of schizophrenic phenomena which clearly differentiates them from the mental processes occurring in other states such as mania or intoxication.

BEHAVIOUR AND LANGUAGE OF SCHIZOPHRENIC PEOPLE

Behaviour

Until recent developments in identifying the pathological mechanisms which appear to underlie schizophrenic disorders, diagnosis and treatment were based entirely on observations of patients' behaviour and language. Reasoning about the psychopathological process was worked back from observation and description of behaviour, and, depending on the point of view, explanation would be based on a range of theories from cerebral dysfunction to psychodynamics.

Patients' accounts of their hallucinations and their delusional beliefs have prompted observers to label their behaviour as bizarre, and thus not amenable to rational understanding. The resulting gulf between schizophrenic and non-schizophrenic people has led mental health workers to respond with anxiety to what is also labelled as crazy behaviour. This anxiety is discussed later in the chapter.

Because of the uncertainties about the causes of schizophrenia, it is still necessary to rely on observed behaviour to make a diagnosis, and treatment is necessarily symptomatic. Although a person's family, upbringing and personality have a pathoplastic influence on the underlying disease process, it is important to be clear about the reasoning which links them together. Otherwise it is all too easy for any unusual or deviant behaviour to be attributed to psychopathology which, because it is invisible to the observer, is not verifiable.

Language

People having an illness diagnosed as mental often find that other people do not readily comprehend what they say. There is a danger that someone may be classified as schizophrenic on the basis of assumptions which people who are not skilled in psycholinguistics are rarely competent to make. In his review of schizophrenic language, Schwartz (1982) argues that its oddities are the result of attentional dysfunction. Flor-Henry (1974) noted that if schizophrenics had a kind of sensory aphasia, they would appear to misinterpret words. Some schizophrenic people's ways of talking can be encouraged by staff who find them amusing or endearing, so that peculiarities of language are reinforced by smiling and friendly responses.

People who have difficulty in making themselves understood also encounter a lack of empathy on the part of others. This lack of empathy can be misinterpreted by the schizophrenic person, who may in turn appear hostile, thus diminishing further the possibility of empathic interaction. These interaction difficulties can be tackled at different levels, requiring a repertoire of skills in order, for example, to maximize cooperation between patients and staff.

Positive and negative symptoms

In order to try to understand schizophrenic processes, Strauss et al (1974) used Jackson's (1887) theories to distinguish between 'positive symptoms' which result from various causes including organic ones, and 'negative symptoms' which result from 'societal responses' to positive symptoms. Positive symptoms include hallucinations, delusions, complaints of interference with thoughts, language disorder and motor disorders such as excitement or catatonia. Negative symptoms include blunted or incongruent affect, withdrawal and apathy. A third category of symptoms can be grouped under disordered social relationships, which, according to Strauss et al (1974), are associated with a poor prognosis for both positive and negative symptoms. Wing & Brown (1970) had used the concept of 'florid' and 'negative' symptoms to distinguish between the primary evidence for schizophrenia (such as delusions and language disorder) and the secondary results of institutionalization ('social withdrawal, blunting of affect and poverty of speech' (p. 181)).

THE ROLE OF THE PSYCHIATRIC NURSE

In order to intervene effectively in such a complex disorder as schizophrenia, the psychiatric nurse must both deploy a range of skills and focus attention on specific aspects of the behaviour of schizophrenic people. Given the weight of evidence for organic pathology, the cognitive impairment of many schizophrenic people requires that the nurse carefully negotiates a clearly understandable, rational and focused plan so that the patient can collaborate in managing the disorder. The difficulties in establishing and maintaining an empathic relationship have been touched upon. The nurse will find much that is helpful in the work of Sullivan (1953), Searles (1965) and Arieti (1974), but a major problem for individuals and institutions is working with people who are unpredictable, sometimes accusatory and hostile, and whose reasoning and talk is difficult to understand. It may take a long time for a nurse to build a trusting relationship with a schizophrenic patient, who may be solitary, withdrawn and suspicious and may shun the nurse's attempts to be friendly. Many of the conventional communication skills taught to nurses may not be applicable in relationships with schizophrenics, who may feel threatened by physical closeness, touch, eye contact and attempts to talk.

Management of anxiety

S. J. Davidson (personal communication) describes the ward management of psychotic patients as coterminous with the management of institutional anxiety. The concept derives from human relations theories of management, and a number of strategies can be used so that patients are not over-medicated, locked up or, paradoxically, put at risk, as has been noted when schizophrenic patients close to discharge have killed themselves. Some of these strategies are described by Ritter in Chapters 24 and 37 of this book.

Assessment

The psychiatric nurse works, above all, within the context of the multi-disciplinary clinical team. The psychiatric nursing assessment of schizophrenic patients is a multi-modal one, on the principles described by Thomas (Ch. 18). Responsibility for aspects of the biological assessment is shared with medical staff, for aspects of the social assessment with the social worker and occupational therapist, and for aspects of the psychological assessment with the psychologist and occupational therapist.

Cognitive processes represent a particular challenge for accurate assessment because of the difficulties involved in remembering and recording apparent disturbances of language and speech.

Typically, goals of care will include the following items.

Short-term goals of care:

- The patient will feel safe and secure in the ward environment
- The patient will maintain good physical health and carry out all activities of daily living
- The patient will have a trusting relationship with his/her key nurses
- The patient will engage in structured purposeful activity and will participate in the ward community
- Psychotic symptoms, such as delusions, hallucinations and thought disorder, will be reduced
- Abnormal behaviour such as aggressiveness and extreme withdrawal will be reduced.

Long-term goals of care:

- The patient will understand and accept and deal effectively with the disorder
- The patient will maintain his/her self-esteem and strengths and will function at the maximum possible level of independence
- The patient will have an understanding of the importance of drug treatment and will comply with the treatment prescribed
- The patient will maintain relationships with family and/or friends.

Implementation of care

Some would argue that the use of coercion to

change behaviour is unethical, and that nurses should not attempt to change pre-morbid behaviour patterns. However, much of the abnormal behaviour displayed by schizophrenic patients is a direct result of the pathological process; and the nurse is responsible for protecting the patient by setting limits on aggressiveness, exaggerated withdrawal and clearly bizarre behaviour. Schizophrenics may withdraw from normal social contact for many reasons: they may lack the social skills necessary to make friends and may have a history of being rejected; they may suffer low esteem and believe that others dislike them; they may be suspicious and paranoid; they may be preoccupied with their fantasy world; or they may suffer delusions which would prohibit social contact, such as beliefs about smelling obnoxious or being contaminated.

Depending on the causes of withdrawal, nurses can attempt to engage with the patient by showing acceptance and recognition, without unduly pressuring him or her. They can sit near the patient and exchange a few words; they can invite the patient to help with certain activities, such as setting a meal table; they can encourage the patient to engage in favourite activities or to discuss hobbies and areas of expertise; they can help him or her to make friends with other patients and to attend social functions. It is important to remember that this may be a long process with patchy progress and frequent set-backs.

IN THE COMMUNITY
Family assessment

The presence of one member of the family with schizophrenia has a profound impact on the family as a whole, and with increasing care of patients in the community the degree of burden on the family has increased. Families report two main problems: extreme withdrawal of the schizophrenic and failure to interact with the family; and disturbed and embarrassing behaviour such as violence and sexual disinhibition. Not surprisingly, the effects on their lives are severe and relatives are often anxious, depressed and bewildered. They do not

know how to deal with odd and difficult behaviour, and they receive little sympathy and understanding from friends and neighbours. Relatives are sometimes aware of aetiological theories which implicate the family in the causation of schizophrenia; this may increase their feelings of guilt and responsibility.

In hospital, it is generally beneficial for patients to maintain close relationships with family and friends, although there may be circumstances in which this would be intolerably stressful for one or other. Normally, visitors will be encouraged to come, will be warmly welcomed by nurses, offered hospitality if possible, and given a quiet, private and comfortable place to sit and talk.

Families need information about the disorder, its cause and response to treatment, to help them to know what to expect, to give them control and help them to promote medication compliance. Hospital staff are typically evasive with families, avoid giving information and avoid using the term schizophrenia. It may be helpful for the families of several schizophrenic patients to meet as a group for the exchange of basic information, to learn skills to help the schizophrenic family member and to support each other. These groups could be led by nurses.

Expressed emotion

A series of influential studies on the relationship between family factors and the course of recovery after discharge have shown that relapse during the nine months after discharge is significantly associated with high levels of 'expressed emotion' in the family, exemplified by critical comments, hostility and over-involvement.

Patients living in 'high emotion' families were significantly more likely to relapse than those living in 'low emotion' families. Schizophrenics who lived in 'high emotion' families, had a high degree of contact with the family and took no phenothiazine medication, had a 90% chance of relapse. If only two out of these three factors was present, they had a 40% to 50% chance of relapse. These important research findings have obvious implications for family education (Goldstein et al

1978, Falloon et al 1982, Leff et al 1982).

Various forms of family therapy or meetings or both have been advocated to involve the family more effectively in after-care. In all these programmes, the focus was on helping the family to help the patient to develop coping skills. All the programmes had clear aims, structure and duration and adopted an approach which was gentle, supportive and concrete, focusing on current transactions rather than the past, and respecting the help given by family members.

UNDERSTANDING AND ACCEPTING THE LONG-TERM ILLNESS

The long-term course of schizophrenia is variable. It has been suggested that of all the patients suffering from schizophrenia about: 25% recover fully; 65% have acute relapses and develop mild to moderate impairment; 10% become severely disabled.

Many patients communicate little or no insight into the nature of the disorder and the problems associated with it. Some appear to have grossly unrealistic expectations of their future lives. In recognizing the variability of the prognosis, patients need help to accept the limitations the illness will impose on their future lives — socially, emotionally, domestically, financially and occupationally — and to make the necessary adjustments. They must be made aware of the possibility of further relapses, the early signs of relapse and come to terms with the likelihood of long-term contact with the mental health service. Patients need to learn to modify their life-style in order to protect themselves from the social stresses that can contribute to further breakdown.

Maintaining self-esteem, strengths and independence

Sufferers from severe mental illnesses occupy a particularly vulnerable place in society. Shunned, feared, denigrated or patronized by the general public, it is difficult for them to maintain self-esteem. Their strengths and independence are often subtly undermined by nurses who focus on deficits rather than abilities, who treat them like children and, however well intentioned, often deprive them of the respect and everyday freedoms normally afforded to adults. Nurses must be constantly vigilant against any tendencies they may have to assume that they should make decisions for rather than with patients, and to deprive patients of control over everyday activities and participation in decision-making. Nurses are frequently attracted into the profession because of a strong desire to care for sick and dependent people as a means of satisfying their own emotional needs, but to allow as much independence as possible to schizophrenic patients this desire must be overcome.

In preparing patients for discharge, nurses often underestimate or ignore the amount of discrimination faced by ex-mental patients. Goffman (1961) described the importance of ex-patients learning 'stigma management', which includes strategies such as concealing the illness from friends and colleagues. This is a major source of stress and should be considered realistically. Relationships with mental health professionals are no substitute for ordinary social contacts; patients should be informed about, and put in contact with, self-help groups, lay and voluntary organizations and befriending schemes.

THERAPEUTIC MILIEU

The nursing of schizophrenic patients is not easy. The importance of 'social treatments' is well recognized in the psychiatric literature and is clearly a major nursing responsibility, but research on how this can be provided most effectively has reached conflicting conclusions. Building a relationship with a schizophrenic patient is likely to be a slow process, and fragile relationships can easily be damaged. It is initially helpful to attempt contact by the odd friendly word and by sitting with the patient, but he or she must be allowed to set the pace for the relationship, so that the nurse should not be deterred by occasional rebuffs.

Safety

In the acute stages of illness, the patient must be supervised in order to protect him or her from harm. The risk of self-injury, either deliberate or from self-neglect, should be assessed. Attention should be given to ensuring that the physical environment of the ward is safe for an acutely disturbed patient and that the ward atmosphere is friendly, relaxed and homely. Other patients may need help to tolerate and understand the patient's psychotic behaviour. In order to protect other patients, it may be necessary to remove an acutely disturbed patient from a crowded room. Careful assessment is needed before including an acutely psychotic patient in ward group meetings (Yalom 1983).

Primary nursing

An organizational system of nursing which affords individualized care of patients is one which allows careful assessment, truly collaborative care-planning, and case presentation skills which give the nurse a voice in the multiprofessional team. Primary nursing is stressful and can only be implemented in a setting where anxiety management, safety and supervisory systems are effective.

Supervision

An essential component of the therapeutic milieu is a system of supervision of all staff. The first-line manager of a ward is in a supervisory grade, and is responsible for ensuring that all staff carry out their work to agreed standards and in an atmosphere of psychological and well as physical safety. A paranoid patient is often a very frightened person whose fear is expressed in hostility, thus generating fear and anxiety among nurses. Supervision will include anticipation of and rehearsal for difficult situations, as well as techniques such as critical incident debriefing after untoward events. A cycle of increasing fear and hostility develops when nurses feel unprotected. Once it is entrenched, and once it is expressed in violence by patients and in absenteeism and sickness by nurses, it is difficult to regain control other than

by scapegoating individuals. Nurses must be able to talk about their anxieties without fear of being thought inadequate, and in the context of continuing professional development which encourages learning new as well as refining existing skills.

Physical health

An acutely ill patient may be unable or unwilling to deal normally with the activities of daily living, and the nurse will assist with these as needed. The patient may need help with hygiene, grooming, clothes and laundry, with food and fluid intake, with elimination, and with rest and exercise. Smoking may need to be supervised because of the risk of fire. As far as possible, patients should retain choice and control over activities of daily living, but safety and dignity must be protected if the patient is unable to make rational decisions. If the patient is unable to attend to his or her own general physical health, this becomes a nursing responsibility and any indications of illness or pain must be taken seriously.

Purposeful activity

Wing & Brown (1970) found that the strongest predictor of institutionalism and thus 'negative' symptoms in schizophrenic patients was idleness. A simple structure or routine will help the patient to engage in purposeful activity and promote feelings of security and self-esteem. As far as possible, the patient participates in planning a daily programme which is tailored to meet individual needs and allows adequate private time for reflection, relaxation and the pursuit of personal interests. Patients can be offered a wide variety of social, recreational, creative and work-related activities, some of which can be planned with the occupational therapy department. These activities have an important therapeutic value and are discussed further in Chapter 44. In planning activities, it is necessary to achieve a balance between overstimulating an already disturbed patient who may find social contact and group activities stressful, and allowing the patient to become passive, apathetic and withdrawn, with the attendant risks of isolation and institutionalization.

A structured predictable environment with appropriate activities can promote a sense of reality. Ambiguous stimuli, such as whispered conversation or a television in the next room, can precipitate hallucinations and delusional thoughts. In getting to know patients, nurses become aware of clues that they may be hallucinating. Some schizophrenics are able to control these symptoms to some extent by deliberately distracting themselves, thinking about or doing other things, or shouting 'shut up' to imaginary voices. Conversations should be kept simple, direct and specific, avoiding theoretical and ideological topics. Paranoid patients can be suspicious, highly sensitive and easily offended. Because paranoia is so often associated with real sensory deficits, the nurse will include these in the assessment, and ensure that deafness and poor eyesight are dealt with. It is important not to provoke suspicion by prying into the patient's affairs or whispering in his or her presence, but to be as open and honest as possible. In doing so, it will become easier firstly to assess the nature of any hallucinations and secondly to discuss with the patient strategies for coping with them.

Medication

It is generally agreed that drug treatment controls symptoms, but does not actually cure schizophrenia. As well as administering drugs and monitoring their effects, nurses also have the major responsibility for observing and reporting unwanted side-effects, some of which can be eliminated or reduced, although tardive dyskinesia is irreversible unless detected early. For this reason, nurses must have a thorough understanding of drug side-effects.

The administration of neuroleptic drugs to mentally disordered people originated with the observation of their sedating effects on patients being prepared for surgery, when they were being used for their antihistamine action. All the drugs which appear to reduce schizophrenic symptoms also reduce dopamine, a catecholamine neuro-

transmitter found in the mesolimbic system, the corpus striatum and the hypothalamus–pituitary system. The theory that dopamine over-activity in these areas is associated with the development of schizophrenic symptoms depends on observations of the effects of neuroleptic drugs and of the psychoses associated with dopaminergic drugs such as amphetamine (Davis & Gierl 1984, Snyder 1986). Dopamine receptors are blockaded by neuroleptic drugs, but because some receptors have excitatory and others have inhibitory mechanisms, it is not clear exactly how dopamine is involved in biological processes as well as psychomotor behaviour. Moreover, it is not clear which receptors are blockaded by which drugs (Alpert & Friedhoff 1980). The evidence that neuroleptics are specifically antischizophrenic is debatable. Research into the antipsychotic effects of neuroleptics has followed the lines of that which identified the activities of opiate receptors, especially in the limbic system, where their effects on mood and emotion have been studied (Snyder 1986).

Nevertheless, neuroleptic drugs appear especially effective in reducing symptoms of language disorder, hallucinations and resistiveness, and so there is a clinical rationale for their use (Davis & Gierl 1984). The problem has been that the more powerful the antipsychotic action of a drug the more troublesome its other effects have tended to be. The most visibly problematic effects of neuroleptics arise from their interference with dopamine receptors in the corpus striatum, thus causing extrapyramidal or Parkinsonian symptoms of tremor, muscular hypertonia, festinant gait and hypokinesia which interfere significantly with activities such as writing and walking. A common and, for the patient, frightening extrapyramidal effect is acute dystonia, where the head and neck twist uncontrollably, while the tongue protrudes. It is a psychiatric emergency which requires immediate attention from a doctor, who will usually administer a benzodiazepine or an antiparkinsonian drug intravenously. Another effect of blocking dopamine receptors in the pituitary area is to increase serum prolactin levels, since prolactin release is no longer prevented by dopamine. The results for women may be amenorrhoea and galactorrhoea, and for men may be gynaecomastia, impotence and diminished libido. It seems that weight gain results from interference with serotonin receptors in the hypothalamic–pituitary area. Finally, it appears that with long-term use of neuroleptics, dopamine receptors in the corpus striatum increase in number. The patient develops involuntary movements such as writhing tongue and mouth, and jerking limbs. Stopping the drug tends to make no difference to the condition, which is known as tardive dyskinesia (Snyder 1986), However, in examining nineteenth century case records of severely mentally ill patients, Turner (1987) found descriptions of similar phenomena, which led him to speculate that the syndrome may be, at least partly, a late stage in the natural history of schizophrenia.

As well as acting on the central nervous system, neuroleptics affect the autonomic nervous system, interfering with the action of acetylcholine, a neurotransmitter for nerves in voluntary muscles and the endocrine system. Their anticholinergic effects include dry mouth, constipation and blurred vision. Epinephrine is synthethized in the same chain as dopamine, so that some neuroleptics block its receptors along with dopamine receptors, resulting in postural hypotension and tachycardia (Lader 1980).

Neuroleptic drugs affect other organ systems. For instance, up to three-quarters of oral chlorpromazine is partly metabolized by the liver before it reaches the brain, and jaundice can develop. Agranulocytosis can occur. Trifluoperazine and thioridazine can cause pigmentation of the retina, with a resulting impairment of sight. Increased photosensitivity leads to sunburn, even in spring and autumn. Thioridazine can be toxic to the myocardium, leading to ventricular tachycardia, which may account for some unexplained sudden deaths (Lader 1980, British National Formulary).

Long-established neuroleptics include the phenothiazines: chlorpromazine, thioridazine, prochlorperazine, fluphenazine and trifluoperazine; the butyrophenones: haloperidol and droperidol; the thioxanthenes: flupenthixol; and the diphenylbutylpiperidines: pimozide. As work progresses on identifying different types of dopamine and other receptors, so different types of neuroleptic medication are now available, developed, according to their manufacturers, specifically to target psychotic symptoms without producing the distressing effects of existing drugs. Nurses who are well informed about the actions of the different neuroleptics and who record meticulously their observations and patients' accounts of the effects of prescribed medication are in a position to contribute constructively to discussions about which drugs are desirable for which individuals.

Antiparkinsonian drugs

Antiparkinsonian drugs are anticholinergic, and so will exacerbate the anticholinergic effects of neuroleptics. They induce or stimulate liver enzymes to metabolize them more rapidly, interacting with the induction effects of drugs such as chlorpromazine and decreasing the antipsychotic effects. They are not now used routinely with antipsychotic medication (Lader 1980).

Treatment compliance

In hospital, nurses have the major responsibility for administering prescribed drugs, monitoring their effects, observing for side-effects and reporting these to the medical staff. Patients may refuse medication for numerous reasons: they may not know what the drug is or why it has been prescribed; they may have no confidence in the drug or may be troubled by side-effects; they may fear they are being poisoned or in some way harmed by the drug; they may be asserting their independence in one of the few ways possible; or they may be reacting against an authoritarian regimen. Rather than simply trying to insist the patient takes the drugs, the nurse must find out the reasons for the patient's refusal. Patients can only be expected to cooperate if they trust the staff and have confidence in them, and they need clear information about the reasons for the treatment, the effects and possible side-effects of the drug. Other misconceptions can usually be resolved once the reasons for non-compliance are understood. Some patients may be more willing to receive medication in elixir form or as long-acting depot injections, rather than as tablets and vice versa. If patients are to give informed consent to treatment, it is essential that all these issues are openly and clearly discussed with them.

In the long-term, schizophrenic patients need to understand the importance of continuing to take prescribed medication, even when acute symptoms have abated. Failure to take prescribed neuroleptic drugs is thought to be the biggest cause of subsequent relapse, and this fact must be made absolutely explicit. The patient's family members may be helpful in promoting long-term medication compliance if they are also fully informed.

Maintenance therapy

Given the evidence that apparently mentally healthy people often fail to complete short courses of antibiotics for troublesome ailments, it is not surprising that schizophrenic people are unreliable in taking oral medication over long periods of time. Suspension of neuroleptic medication in oil for deep intramuscular injection is designed to relieve patients of the responsibility for taking their pills, to minimize unwanted effects and maximize antipsychotic effects by a predictable absorption rate of a known quantity of a drug. Two provisos are important. Firstly, if the person who administers the depot injection uses a faulty technique, the medication can be rendered partly ineffective and, by producing tissue necrosis and abscesses, make the patient disinclined to accept further injections. Secondly, maintenance therapy appears to be less effective if it consists merely of an injection. Supportive interpersonal interaction, whether in the form of individual counselling or family meetings, not only intervenes in the disordered social relationships that characterize schizophrenia, but provides opportunities for monitoring a person's mental state and for offering help at times of stress.

REFERENCES

Alpert M, Friedhoff A J 1980 An un-dopamine hypothesis of schizophrenia. Schizophrenia Bulletin 6(3): 387–390

Arieti S 1974 Interpretation of schizophrenia. Crosby Lockwood Staples, London

Beard A W, Slater E 1962 The schizophrenic-like psychoses of epilepsy. Proceedings of the Royal Society of Medicine 55: 311–314

British National Formulary (published annually) Pharmaceutical Society and British Medical Association, London

Davis J M, Gierl B 1984 Pharmacological treatment in the care of schizophrenic patients. In: A S Bellack (ed) Schizophrenia. Grune & Stratton, Orlando, Fla

Falloon I R H, Boyd J L, McGill C W et al 1982 Family management in the prevention of exacerbations of schizophrenia: a controlled study. New England Journal of Medicine 306(24): 1437–1440

Fisman M 1975 The brain stem in psychosis. British Journal of Psychiatry 126: 414–422

Flor-Henry P 1974 Psychosis, neurosis and epilepsy. British Journal of Psychiatry 124: 144–150

Goffman E 1961 Asylums: essays on the social situation of mental patients and other inmates. Penguin, Harmondsworth

Goldstein M J, Rodnick E H, Evans J R et al 1978 Drug and family therapy in the aftercare of acute schizophrenics. Archives of General Psychiatry 35: 1169–1177

Gottesman I I, Shields J 1972 Schizophrenia and genetics. Academic Press, New York

Gualtieri T, Hicks R E 1985 An immunoreactive theory of selective male affliction. Behavioural and Brain Sciences 8: 427–441

Hare E 1975 Season of birth in schizophrenia and neurosis. American Journal of Psychiatry 132: 1168–1171

Hill D 1962 Commentary. Proceedings of the Royal Society of Medicine 55: 315–316

Jackson H 1887 Remarks on evolution and dissolution of the nervous system. Journal of Mental Science 33: 25–48

Johnstone E C, Crow T J, Frith C D, Husband J, Kreel L 1976 Cerebral ventricular size and cognitive impairment in chronic schizophrenia. Lancet ii (7992): 924–926

Lader M 1980 Introduction to psychopharmacology. Upjohn, Kalamazoo, Mich

Lane E A, Albee G W 1966 Comparative birth weights of schizophrenics and their siblings. Journal of Psychology 64: 227–231

Leff J P, Kuipers L, Berkowtiz R et al 1982 A controlled trial of social intervention in the families of schizophrenic patients. British Journal of Psychiatry 141: 121–134

Link B G, Dohrenwend B P, Skodol A E 1986 Socio-economic status and schizophrenia: noisome occupational characteristics as a risk factor. American Sociological Review 51: 242–258

Samuels L 1978 Sex differences in concordance rates for schizophrenia: finding or artefact? Schizophrenia Bulletin 4(1): 14–15

Schwartz S 1982 Is there a schizophrenic language? Behavioural and Brain Sciences 5: 579–626

Searles H 1965 Collected papers on schizophrenia and related subjects. Hogarth Press, London

Snyder S 1986 Drugs and the brain. Scientific American Library, New York

Strauss J S, Carpenter W T, Bartko J J 1974 Speculations on the processes that underlie schizophrenic symptoms and signs. Schizophrenia Bulletin 1(11): 61–75

Sullivan H S 1953 The interpersonal theory of psychiatry. Norton, New York

Taylor E, Rutter M 1985 Sex differences in neurodevelopmental and psychiatric disorders: one explanation or many? Behavioural and Brain Sciences 8: 460

Turner T 1987 Rich and mad in Victorian England. In: Murray R M, Turner T H (eds) 1990 Lectures on the history of psychiatry: the Squibb series. Gaskell, London

Wing J K, Brown G W 1970 Institutionalism and schizophrenia. Oxford University Press

Yalom I D 1983 Inpatient group psychotherapy. Basic Books, New York

33

Eating disorders

J. I. Brooking

Changes in body weight, appetite and eating patterns are common features of numerous physical and mental disorders. For example, some people overeat when depressed or anxious because food may be comforting, whereas others lose their appetite. Conversely, obesity can contribute to reduced self-esteem and morale and may be implicated in the development of depression or anxiety. Patients with psychotic and organic disorders may be too confused to prepare food, may forget to eat, refuse food which is believed to be poisoned, and may develop chaotic patterns of eating or preferences for bizarre foods. Manic patients may be too preoccupied or distractible to sit down for a complete meal. Drug and alcohol abusers are likely to develop severe nutritional deficiencies. Weight gain may also be a side-effect of neuroleptic drugs such as antidepressants and lithium. Although abnormal eating may be associated with many psychiatric problems, this chapter is specifically concerned with two major eating disorders, anorexia nervosa and a more recently identified related condition, bulimia nervosa.

ANOREXIA NERVOSA

The nature of the disorder

The term anorexia nervosa was first used by William Gull in 1874 to label a condition described

413

nearly 200 years earlier by Richard Morton in 1689. However, there was little interest in anorexia nervosa as a specific clinical entity until the 1960s, and some psychiatrists still do not consider it to be a distinct illness (Hsu 1980). Anorexia nervosa occurs predominantly in middle class females (Crisp et al 1976) in developed countries and originates mainly in adolescence, the commonest age for weight loss to begin being about 15 years (Crisp & Stonehill 1971). It is difficult to assess the incidence of the disorder because of concealment, under-reporting and misdiagnosis, but it is believed that the number of cases may be increasing (Palmer 1980) and there are estimated to be about 10 000 severely affected sufferers in Britain at any one time (Crisp 1983).

Russell (1970) has outlined three essential features: behaviour leading to a marked loss of body weight, mainly limiting food intake, but also excessive exercise, self-induced vomiting and purgation; an endocrine disorder shown by amenorrhoea in females; and a morbid fear of becoming fat.

Characteristic patterns of eating behaviour have been identified in anorexia nervosa: there is a restriction of food intake, with feelings of bloatedness after eating even small amounts, and this often begins with social pressures to diet. Studies have indicated that many sufferers are overweight prior to the onset of the disorder (Crisp 1980). The patient is usually secretive and defensive about her eating and greatly overestimates how much she consumes. She is preoccupied with food, knowledgeable about it and may prepare lavish meals for others, constantly testing her will power in a struggle against extreme hunger. The anorexic has a great fear of becoming fat and thinness is symbolic of perfection and freedom from anxiety: it desexualizes her and reduces the anxiety associated with libido. Bodily perception is distorted, so that the sufferer perceives herself as fat, although she appears emaciated to others (Crisp 1980). Psychologically the typical patient is mistrustful and will reject offers of help. She shows rigidity in her daily routines of eating, suggesting obsessionality, and she seems poorly equipped to cope with newly emerging sexuality and separation from her parents.

Physiological consequences of self-induced starvation include obvious emaciation, oedematous ankles, cold extremities, rough, dry and inelastic skin, bradycardia, amenorrhoea, lowered metabolic rate, increase in body hair, constipation and electrolyte imbalance which can be life threatening.

Causes of anorexia nervosa

In common with many other psychiatric disorders, there is little consensus about the aetiology of anorexia nervosa. Many theories have been proposed and each has some evidence to support it. The main causative theories are summarized below.

Sociocultural theory

Research cited by Hsu (1980) found that about half of the schoolgirls studied were weight conscious and engaged in some form of dieting. Hsu (1980) considers that the social emphasis on slimness has a share in producing illness. However, this idea fails to explain why only some girls who diet to lose weight go on to develop anorexia nervosa.

Psychoanalytic theory

Traditional psychoanalytic theory focused on the sexual symbolism of food for the anorexic, emphasizing fears of oral impregnation. Modern psychoanalytic thinking concentrates on the parent–child interaction. Bruch (1973, 1977) considers that some families fail to transmit an adequate sense of competence and self-value to the child, thus leaving the child without inward control and awareness. Bruch maintains that the main issues in anorexia are the struggles for control, identity, competence and effectiveness.

Some evidence in support of Bruch's theory is provided by research into early parent–child interactions (e.g. Dally et al 1979, Crisp 1965, Kay & Leigh 1954). These studies of anorexics have found increased separations from parents and above average levels of infant feeding difficulties with maternal over-concern about the child's eating.

Hypothalamic dysfunction theory

One of the functions of the anterior pituitary is impaired in anorexia nervosa, that is the release of gonadotrophins. Russell (1970) found that restoration to normal body weight was not sufficient to return gonadotrophin levels back to normal, therefore suggesting that the rhythmic control of gonadotrophins may not be a consequence of anorexia nervosa, but a more central feature of it. Since the hypothalamus also influences, among other functions, appetite, eating and sexual behaviour, it was proposed that hypothalamic impairment may be a causative factor (Russell 1970). According to Hsu (1980) animal studies have linked hypothalamic lesions with feeding disorders and menstrual irregularities, and a few reports have indicated that tumours in or near the hypothalamus can give rise to an anorexia nervosa-like syndrome in humans.

Family interaction theory

It is widely believed that parental personality and patterns of interaction within the family can influence the development and continuation of anorexia nervosa. Dally et al (1979) reported that at least one parent of 24% of patients in their study had been treated for a psychiatric disorder, although no consistent parental personality was found. Crisp (1973) also believes that family pathology often underlies anorexia nervosa and can serve to stabilize an insecure marriage and protect parents from anxiety and depression.

Minuchin et al (1975, 1978) postulate that certain types of family transactions are closely related to the development and maintenance of the disorder and that the symptoms in turn play an important part in maintaining the family homeostasis. The family characteristics identified include: enmeshment, extreme intensity and proximity in relationships; overprotectiveness and rigidity, which inhibit the development of autonomy; and a characteristic avoidance of conflict.

Psychobiological theory

Palmer (1980) proposes a psychobiological regression hypothesis. He suggests that weight loss starts following a decision to slim, possibly in response to social pressure, and in vulnerable individuals this may develop into anorexia nervosa. Vulnerability to the condition is thought to be associated with difficulties in coping with the transition through adolescence. Declining weight is accompanied by regression of the neuroendocrine system to its pre-pubertal state, demonstrated by hormonal changes and amenorrhoea. Palmer (1980) claims that neuroendocrine regression brings with it psychological changes which facilitate avoidance of the conflicts and turmoil of adolescence. Once established, in this 'switched off' avoidance state the individual fears weight gain with the implications of 'switching on' again, and hence a phobic avoidance of normal weight develops.

Crisp (1980) supports this hypothesis, stressing that once the pubertal process has been reversed, the individual has succeeded in avoiding the maturational challenge of puberty. He sees anorexia nervosa as part of the repertoire of possible morbid responses to maturational problems.

Treatment and care

There is little general agreement about the treatment of anorexia nervosa as its aetiology is not well understood. Approaches to treatment reflect the theoretical orientation of the practitioner and may include medically-oriented approaches such as tube feeding, high calorie diets, insulin and hormone preparations, psychotropic drugs and ECT, as well as psychologically-oriented approaches such as behaviour therapy, and more psychodynamic individual, family and group psychotherapy.

It is widely agreed that for treatment to be effective, the cooperation of the patient must be obtained (Crisp 1980, Russell 1973). Cooperation is often difficult to secure as the fear of change may far outweigh the miseries of starvation. Compulsory admission under the 1983 Mental Health Act is rarely required except in the most life-threatening states of malnutrition.

The aims of treatment vary according to the theoretical orientation of the clinician, but most authors agree that weight restoration and correction of abnormal eating patterns are central.

Treatment also attempts to alter the psychological state of the patient with eventual loss of the weight phobia (Palmer 1980, Russell 1981). Bruch (1978) sees the primary objective of treatment as maturing the 'undifferentiated slave-like self-concept' of the sufferer, and secondary to this is the clarification and unlocking of the stagnating patterns of family interaction. Similarly, Minuchin et al (1978) see the goal of therapy as 'not only a changed individual but a functional family system, one that can meet all of its members' needs for both autonomy and support'.

Restoration of normal weight, behavioural and physical treatments

If the patient has reached a life-threatening condition, compulsory inpatient treatment may be necessary with complete bedrest and refeeding, which may take the form of naso-gastric or intravenous feeding if the patient is unable or unwilling to take food orally. Crisp (1983) prefers tube feeding to intravenous infusions since 'the exact metabolic deficit and need for replacement electrolytes, fluid and energy are almost impossible to calculate'.

In less critically-ill sufferers, a near to normal oral diet is recommended. Palmer (1980) stresses that a mixed balanced diet should be eaten at conventional meal-times. The use of calorie-rich liquid supplements was recommended by Russell (1960) who believed they could be useful for patients who feel apprehensive at the sight of a bulky meal. Views differ concerning the best daily calorie intake. Dally et al (1979) suggested that very emaciated patients should initially receive food every 2 hours, to prevent paralytic ileus and gastric dilation, gradually increasing intake to 4000–5000 calories a day after 2 weeks. However Crisp (1967a) advocated a steady intake of 3000 calories a day to control the impulse to overeat. Minuchin et al (1978) do not specify a particular intake, believing that patients should control their own eating within certain limits, that is that meals should be well balanced and eaten in an allocated time.

Target weights are usually established at the beginning of treatment, although criteria for defining the target weight vary. Crisp (1980) recommends that the target should be the mean population weight for the patient's sex and height at the age of onset, whereas Dally et al (1979) believe the figure should be based upon 90% of the mean weight for the patient's present age, sex and height.

Most authors recommend initial bedrest with a gradual increase in activity as weight is restored (Palmer 1980, Minuchin et al 1978, Dally et al 1979, Russell 1973, Crisp 1980), although Bruch (1978) considers that bedrest may increase the patient's sense of helplessness. The patient should be weighed at regular intervals and Dally et al (1979) suggest that a weight chart by the bed may provide the patient with further incentive and diminish the fear of weight gain.

Behavioural principles are commonly used to enhance the effectiveness of refeeding (Garfinkel et al 1977, Dally et al 1979). The basic idea is to make contingent upon weight gain certain privileges such as telephone calls, visitors, bathing, television and weekend leave. The contract negotiated with the patient specifies the exact nature of the rewards given or withheld depending on an agreed daily or weekly weight gain. While acknowledging that behaviour therapy produces weight gain during treatment, Bruch (1974) argues that this method may be damaging in the longer term. She claims that behaviour therapy forces patients to relinquish control over their bodies and lives and thus undermines self-esteem, reducing the hope of achieving autonomy.

Occasionally, refeeding and general nursing may be effective without formal psychiatric help in patients who are only mildly ill or close to spontaneous recovery (Crisp 1980), although Dally et al (1979) consider that such treatment may provide only temporary benefit, and Bruch (1978) emphasizes that it may be harmful or even fatal.

The use of drugs and other physical treatments was widespread in the past and continues in some centres. Chlorpromazine may be given to decrease the anxiety associated with eating and therefore enhance cooperation with treatment; however Crisp et al (1985) believe that only about 10% will benefit from its use. Appetite-stimulating drugs and insulin have been recommended (e.g.

Goldberg et al 1979). However, many writers argue that anorexic patients have not lost their appetite, but are in constant struggle against the desire to eat (Palmer 1980, Crisp et al 1985). Moreover these drugs carry the risk of converting abstainers to bingers (Crisp 1980). Antidepressant drugs and electroconvulsive therapy are sometimes used, on the assumption that the disorder is a form of depressive illness. Current opinion is divided. Crisp et al (1985) pointed out that 'ECT is in our experience never helpful and often harmful', whereas Russell (1973) suggests that it has a place in the treatment of anorexia accompanied by severe depression if attempts at increasing weight fail.

Psychotherapeutic approaches

Psychotherapy is generally thought to be beneficial, although Hsu (1980) pointed out that there is little evidence of its efficacy in the treatment of anorexia nervosa. Individual, group, marital and family therapy may all be used and vary according to the theoretical orientation of the clinicians.

On the basis of the regression hypothesis, Palmer (1980) considers that weight restoration exposes the patient to emotional experiences from which she was previously protected and thus psychotherapy involves mobilization of alternative ways of coping with the emotional aspects of her rekindled biological maturity. He believes that emotional support should come from all members of the team to supplement formal non-directive psychotherapy sessions in which the patient is encouraged to explore and discover thoughts and feelings previously unspoken, poorly understood or denied. Palmer feels that this therapeutic relationship should begin early in the process of weight restoration so that it is established when the patient is nearing normal weight and is experiencing heightened turmoil. He adds that counselling should continue for 1 or 2 years after discharge.

Palmer proposes that individual psychotherapy should be supplemented by family or marital therapy in which past and present family difficulties are explored in an attempt to modify the environment to which the anorexic will return. The view that family therapy is a useful adjunct

to individual work is supported by Dally et al (1979).

Crisp (1973) also emphasizes that need for intensive emotional support as the anxieties of puberty are rekindled by weight gain, and he stresses the value of individual psychotherapy in assisting personal growth and independence from old relationships. This is supplemented at a later stage by small group therapy. Psychotherapy for the patient's parents is deemed essential to help them cope with changes resulting from treatment, and family therapy is considered appropriate to examine patterns of development in the family and allow sharing of feelings and experiences (Crisp 1980).

Bruch (1978) stresses that successful treatment must always involve resolution of underlying family problems. In fairly young patients who are relatively healthy emotionally Bruch sees family therapy as the mainstay of treatment; however in those with severe emotional and developmental disturbances individual psychotherapy is of ultimate importance. She sees the therapist's task as helping to liberate the patient from the influence of early experiences and to realize her own worth in an attempt to aid the patient in her search for autonomy and identity. In contrast to traditional psychoanalysts Bruch feels that giving interpretations of the unconscious meanings of, for example, fantasies and dreams is harmful as it reinforces the patient's view that she is incompetent since she is led to believe that she does not even understand her own thoughts. Bruch believes that meaningful therapeutic work cannot be done until a certain degree of weight restoration has taken place.

In contrast to other authors, Minuchin et al (1978) believe there is little place for individual psychotherapy in the treatment of anorexia. Their systems theory hypothesizes that the condition is caused and supported by various patterns of family interaction and hence therapy aims to identify and challenge these patterns and help the family to find alternative ways of interacting. Therapy begins with a lunch session during which the therapist observes family patterns and decides on strategies to challenge them. Minuchin et al (1978) describe methods by which enmeshment, over-protection, rigidity and conflict avoidance may be challenged in the therapeutic setting. For example, conflict avoidance may be reduced by insisting that family members discuss any disagreement fully.

Occupational therapy is often used to supplement psychotherapy. Projective art and psychodrama can help the patient to express herself as well as enhancing the therapist's understanding of relationships within the family (Crisp 1980, Dally et al 1979). Assertion, communication and discussion groups may help the patient to learn new ways of relating to people and increase her confidence in expressing her own views. Crisp (1980) suggests that occupational therapy sessions may also be utilized in helping the patient cook for herself in a normal way and grow accustomed to her new shape by making clothes. Examples of patients' behaviour and feelings during these activities can be taken to psychotherapeutic settings for further examination.

Finally, there are a number of lay organizations which are concerned with self-help. Examples in Britain include Anorexia Aid and the Women's Therapy Centre, which uses feminist principles. These organizations provide opportunities for sufferers to make contact with others with similar problems, and they provide support, guidance and counselling for sufferers, families and friends. Crisp (1980) considers that such groups can be helpful if competently run and if they have professional services to which sufferers can be referred for more specialist help.

Outcome of treatment

Assessment of the effectiveness of treatment is hindered by a number of difficulties. Firstly, assessment requires knowledge of the progress of the untreated condition which can only be estimated since the majority of untreated cases are not brought to the attention of researchers. Crisp (1980) estimates that 40% of severely ill anorexics can expect to have recovered naturally or be very much improved after 6 years. Criteria for assessing the success of therapy are also ill defined, and the time interval following treatment before its outcome can be properly assessed is debatable. Dally

et al (1979) consider that at least 4 years are necessary.

Comparison of the results of different outcome studies is difficult because of differences in diagnostic criteria, recovery criteria and severity of the disorder as well as the therapist's lack of control over the environment to which the patient returns after discharge. Treatment regimes consist of a variety of elements which change over time, thus making comparisons impossible. At the moment, there is little consensus about which types of treatment are most effective.

There is general agreement that hospital treatment involving refeeding, behavioural and psychotherapeutic elements is almost always effective in the short term in saving life and restoring weight, but relapse is common even after long periods of recovery. Numerous studies have been carried out, some of which followed up sufferers for many years, e.g. Hsu et al (1979), Burns & Crisp (1984), Russell (1977) Crisp (1977), Minuchin et al (1979), Bruch (1974). Studies have produced widely differing results, but generally more than half the subjects appear to be well about 2 years after treatment and about two-thirds after 5 years. In the long term Hsu (1980) considers that more than half remain preoccupied with weight, shape and food and have chaotic eating habits. Anxiety, social phobia, obsessive–compulsive symptoms and relationship problems are common in the long term. Studies show about 5% mortality in the long term.

Crisp (1980) considers that poor outcome is commonly associated with older age of onset, longer duration of illness, more severe weight loss, poor social adjustment in childhood, underlying neurotic disorders, such as anxiety, depression and obsessionality, and neurotic disorders, rigidity and hostility in the parents. Working class and male patients also seem to have poorer outcomes.

Description of the treatment regime in a specialist unit

The anorexia unit at Atkinson Morley's Hospital, London, is part of a busy acute psychiatric unit employing some therapeutic community principles. The treatment regime is described in more detail elsewhere (e.g. Crisp 1980, 1983, Crisp et al 1985).

The treatment approach combines psycho-analytic, behavioural and biological elements. Crisp considers that inpatient treatment is essential for success, because of the enormous magnitude of the task confronting patients and therapists. The patient must have some willingness to change in order to be treated successfully, and cooperation from the family is also important. The main psychological tasks of treatment are to enlarge the patient's experience of herself and to provide opportunities for personal growth. But psychological development is not possible without weight gain to a normal adult level.

Prior to admission the prospective patient is assessed and her cooperation enlisted: she is shown around the unit by a nurse and the regime explained in detail; she is given a pamphlet about the unit and introduced to another anorexic patient; she is shown a videotape on the unit's view of the disorder and is given a list of recommended books on anorexia. Thus the prospective patient is fully informed about all aspects of the regime before she decides whether or not to commit herself to treatment.

On admission the patient is given a target weight, which is the mean weight for height and sex at the age of onset of the illness, i.e. a 19-year-old with a 3-year history of anorexia would have as a target the average weight of a 16-year-old of her height.

The patient is expected to hand over control of her food intake and weight to the staff. The high carbohydrate diet is about 3000 calories a day on which a weight gain of $1\frac{1}{2}$ kg (4 lb) a week is expected. Everything must be eaten and no other food is allowed. No visitors are allowed while eating, but a nurse may sit with the patient to encourage her and to ensure that all food is eaten and not thrown away, hidden or vomited.

Activity is severely restricted until target weight is achieved, usually in about 8 to 12 weeks. The patient is nursed in a single cubicle on complete bedrest and is taken to the bathroom in a wheelchair by a nurse.

The patient has individual psychotherapy throughout the period of admission and small group and family or marital psychotherapy begins after the first month. Areas of psychopathology addressed in treatment include the meaning of shape, family relations, sense of self — social and sexual — anxiety, conflict, depression, helping others, relationships to authority and impulse control. Gradually the patient begins to attend community meetings and other forms of therapy such as projective art, relaxation groups, communication and trust groups, movement and exercise groups, social skills and assertion training, cookery and dressmaking.

The patient maintains a 'log book' throughout treatment, which remains her property. This includes personal diary space and sections for rating particular problems each week. The contents of the log book are discussed regularly with the 'individual assessor', usually an experienced nurse, who also relates to the patient over management issues.

From the time of achieving target weight, the patient leaves her cubicle and has a bed in the main ward. She is allowed to get up and get dressed and to leave the ward for gradually increasing periods, culminating in overnight or weekend leave at home about 4 or 5 weeks after attaining target weight. Flexibility in eating arrangements is gradually introduced, so that the patient begins to choose her own menu and eventually eats out in a restaurant.

Outpatient support continues for about 2 years and may include individual, group and family therapy. Some ex-patients are referred to self-help groups such as Anorexia Aid.

Role of the nurse

Literature on the role of the nurse in caring for anorexic patients was reviewed by Abell (1986) who found no research studies and a dearth of prescriptive literature. The predominant theme in the nursing literature was the importance of good relationships with patients and the notion that recovery hinged, at least partially, on the nurse's interpersonal skills. Misik (1981) claimed that nurses were valuable to the treatment of anorexics because of their similarity in age to the patients and McNamara (1982) considered that nurses are central to treatment because of the amount of contact they have with patients.

The importance of the nursing contribution is recognized in the psychiatric literature. For example, Dally et al (1979) wrote that 'no doctor can manage any but the mildest case of anorexia nervosa without devoted cooperation from the whole of his team'. Nevertheless, a review of 20 British and American psychiatric nursing textbooks published between 1976 and 1985 (Abell 1986) revealed little information about nursing anorexic patients. Only 11 texts referred to anorexia nervosa and none contained more than 500 words. Abell (1986) also found little input on eating disorders in British psychiatric nursing education.

It is clear that the treatment of anorexia nervosa varies according to the psychiatrist's theoretical orientation, and the role of the nurse will be largely determined by the treatment regime and will be influenced by the setting of care and other treatment resources available. In Crisp's regime (Crisp et al 1985) the nursing responsibilities are clearly prescribed. Nurses are expected: to be familiar with the details of the programme and to explain treatment to the patient; to be consistent with the whole team and to refer information back to the team; to manage the diet, to encourage and persuade the patient to eat, to ensure that meals are eaten, not disposed of or hidden, if necessary sitting with patients during meals; to monitor weight and to provide all necessary physical care; to support the formal psychotherapy by friendship, sharing experiences and discussion of fears and anxieties; and to be friend, mother substitute and confidant.

Observation and good physical care are crucial for critically ill patients, who may have all the symptoms of starvation. Patients may have a low blood pressure, temperature and pulse as the body tries to conserve energy; there may be poor peripheral circulation with peripheral cyanosis; amenorrhoea may result from the shutdown of reproductive functions; and dehydration, electrolyte imbalance and potassium depletion may occur, especially if the patient vomits and uses laxatives.

Nursing anorexics can be particularly stressful because of the risks of close identification with patients who may be very similar in age, social and educational background to their carers. Crisp (1980) considers that about half of the nurses in his team have worries over their own weight and therefore risk colluding with patients against other members of the team. As members of a high risk group many nurses suffer from eating disorders, although Lacey, cited in Chudley (1986), doubts whether they have any particular susceptibility. Despite personal worries over weight, Crisp (1980) acknowledges that if nurses have successfully adjusted to adult life and are functioning in society, it can be helpful for them to share personal experiences with patients.

In interviews with nurses and patients in two specialist anorexia units, Abell (1986) found that nurses had received little information from others about their role, but both nurses and patients rated the nurses' contribution to care highly. Nurses claimed that members of other disciplines did not always recognize the value of nursing care.

BULIMIA NERVOSA

In recent years psychiatrists in Britain and America have observed the emergence of an eating disorder which had not previously been described. This 'ominous variant of anorexia nervosa' was termed bulimia nervosa by Russell (1979) who proposed three diagnostic criteria:

- powerful and intractable urges to overeat
- an attempt to avoid the fattening effects of food by induced vomiting, purging or both
- a morbid fear of becoming fat.

Various definitions and names for this disorder have been suggested, but Fairburn (1982) considers that bulimarexia, binge-eating syndrome, dietary chaos syndrome, bulimia, bulimic syndrome and bulimia nervosa all describe a similar clinical phenomenon.

Clinical features

Features of the disorder have been described by several writers based on a series of patients seen in their clinics (e.g. Russell 1979, Lacey 1984). Some have used standardized assessment procedures (e.g. Fairburn & Cooper 1984). These patients are almost all women, almost invariably with a history of dieting and previous weight disturbance, and most have normal or near normal weight at the time of referral. Between a quarter and a third have a history of anorexia nervosa, although most writers argue that bulimia is distinct from anorexia nervosa. Lacey (1984) considers that bulimics have more clinical similarity to the massively obese than to anorexics. Patients typically present in their 20s and 30s, somewhat older than anorexics. Fairburn & Cooper (1984) found that three-quarters of their sample came from social classes one and two. In a survey of young adult women Cooper & Fairburn (1983) found an estimated prevalence of between 1 and 2%.

These patients have grossly disturbed eating habits, accompanied by morbid beliefs concerning their shape and weight. Secret binge-eating is typical, with an average daily intake about three times greater than normal. Lacey (1984) found that his patients binged on average three times a day, but some binged 15 to 20 times a day, completely disrupting normal life. Episodes of binging leave the sufferer feeling guilt ridden and degraded and are usually followed by vomiting and/or purging. Two-thirds of Lacey's (1984) patients used purgatives, often in massive doses.

Binge-eating, vomiting and purging can produce serious physical complications, described by Fairburn (1982) and Lacey (1984). These include metabolic disturbances, especially hypokalaemia, which can lead to cardiac arrhythmias, renal damage, dehydration, tetany and peripheral paraesthesia, and epileptic seizures. Other physical complications can include swelling of the parotid glands, erosion of dental enamel, chronic hoarseness of the voice, gastrointestinal reflux, steatorrhoea, recurrent abdominal pain and gastric dilation, finger clubbing and rebound water retention. This list of physical complications illustrates the grave dangers of binge-eating accompanied by vomiting and purging.

Lacey (1984) described three categories of patients seen in his clinic. The smallest group had bulimia secondary to a physical illness such as epilepsy or diabetes. What he termed a neurotic group comprised about 80% of his patients. These women were typically hard working and ambitious with high ethical standards. They superficially appeared to be stable, competent and resourceful, but deeper examination revealed low self-esteem and fear of failure, especially in relationships. Many doubted their femininity and attractiveness and had poor peer relationships. Depressive symptoms were common and often masked anger revealed later in treatment. Lacey (1984) considers that the neurotic group generally do well in outpatient treatment if well motivated. The third group of patients Lacey (1984) described as personality disordered. This 20% of patients were thought to be most difficult to treat. Many of these women also abuse alcohol and drugs and may be sexually disinhibited. They present as emotionally shallow or histrionic, with overdosing and superficial wrist cutting common. Lacey (1984) acknowledged that in the context of these neurotic or personality problems, bulimia could be precipitated by threatening events such as loss of a loved one, change in occupation or geographical location, or a sexual conflict.

Treatment and care

There is considerable uncertainty over treatment as these patients have very different problems and differing treatment needs. Some writers are pessimistic about the possibilities of successful treatment (e.g. Russell 1979, Stunkard 1980), but some successes have been reported.

This section describes three approaches to treatment developed over a number of years by Dr Hubert Lacey and his colleagues at St George's Hospital Medical School, London. The regimes are described fully in Lacey (1984). These treatment programmes are eclectic in orientation, using behaviour therapy and counselling to deal with abnormal eating patterns and 'insight-directed therapy' to deal with emotional conflicts which emerge as eating is brought under control. Drug treatment is rarely used. The treatments aim to be cost-effective, in that they are time limited and conducted by non-medical psychiatric professionals. In a controlled study Lacey (1983) found that all 30 severely-affected bulimics in his sample reduced symptoms during treatment. In follow-up over 2 years, 20 demonstrated no dietary abuse and eight reduced bingeing episodes to an average of three a year.

Outpatient programme involving individual and group sessions

This programme was designed for the 'neurotic' group, within a normal weight range, who are usually working and for whom inpatient or lengthy treatment would be unsuitable or inconvenient. Bulimics with personality disorders are considered to need more intensive and prolonged treatment than this programme provides. Groups of five patients attend for half a day a week over 10 weeks. These sessions are run by two therapists, preferably women. Lacey found no differences in patient outcome in patients treated by therapists from different professional groups. Lacey described working with social workers and occupational therapists, but no reference was found in his writing to working with nurses as therapists. During the half day, each patient first meets for half an hour with her individual therapist, and later the five patients and two therapists meet for a one and a half hour group session.

This programme involves a number of therapeutic processes. Firstly, it involves the imposition of control on a disorder marked by behavioural chaos. Lacey (1984) claims that these patients crave control, but too much external control can produce anger and avoidance of treatment. In this programme, control includes the rigid structure of the programme itself, the structured relationship with the therapist, the ritual of weekly weighing, the diet sheet with outlines of the prescribed diet and the dietary diary. The diary is thought to be a central component of the therapy. In it the patient records all intake, vomiting and laxative abuse, as well as thoughts and feelings. The diary is discussed with the therapist each week and goals for the following week are agreed and recorded. The group meeting is another important part of the treatment. It provides mutual support to enable members to change eating habits and examine the difficulties and consequences of giving up symptoms. The group also provides a safe place to explore problems and feelings and to experiment with new ways of dealing with them. The final component of the treatment is the contract agreed with the patient before treatment begins. This includes a commitment to attend all sessions, to maintain the same weight and to eat the prescribed diet of three meals a day at set times. Patients are encouraged to stop bingeing and vomiting and most achieve this between the 3rd and 6th week of treatment.

Patients continue to be followed up at 3-monthly intervals, and about 5% need to be considered for inpatient treatment. Poor outcome seems to be associated with alcohol abuse, previous anorexia nervosa, and chronicity and severity of bulimia nervosa. Marriage problems sometimes result from changes brought about by treatment, especially if the marriage took place in the context of the illness. Marital or family therapy is offered if necessary.

Individual outpatient programme

There are some sufferers for whom group work is unsuitable or whose other commitments prevent regular attendance at a group. Such patients can be offered a time-limited individual programme consisting of weekly one hour meetings with a therapist (not necessarily a psychiatrist) over 12 weeks. Lacey (1984) considers that this approach is generally less successful than the combination of group and individual work and the drop-out rate is higher. The self-help component and mutual support of fellow group members is missing in this approach.

Inpatient treatment programme

Inpatient treatment is necessary only for the minority of patients suffering from personality disorders or who are suicidal. Patients must genuinely desire to change if good results are to be achieved. Patients are not admitted to deal with disordered eating itself, which should be controlled through an individual outpatient programme before admission. Binge-eating, vomiting and purgative use are prohibited on the unit and the patient is expected to maintain a consistent weight. Transgressions may result in discharge, on the assumption that the patient is not yet willing or able to change.

The aim of admission is to deal with underlying emotional difficulties by intensive individual, small group and large group psychotherapy in a structured ward setting. A variety of occupational therapy and creative art activities such as art therapy, psychodrama, dance and movement and trust groups, are used to supplement formal psychotherapy. Family or marital therapy is offered when appropriate. Although depression commonly arises during treatment, antidepressant drugs are avoided.

Relationships with nurses and other staff provide opportunities for discussion of feelings and exploration of problems. Lacey (1984) considers that nurses need to respond thoughtfully and non-judgementally and with care and firmness when appropriate. He believes that transference problems are common with these patients, who may become over-involved with their nurses. Patients may need to be reminded that the relationship is a professional one and that they should be wary of investing it with feelings more appropriate to their private relationships.

REFERENCES

Abell C 1986 The role of the psychiatric nurse in the care of patients with anorexia nervosa. Unpublished dissertation for BSc(Hons) Nursing Studies, King's College, University of London

Bruch H 1973 Eating disorders: obesity, anorexia and the person within. Basic Books, New York

Bruch H 1974 Perils of behaviour modification in treatment of anorexia nervosa. Journal of the America Medical Association 230: 1419–1422

Bruch H 1977 Antecedents of anorexia nervosa. In: Vigersky R A (ed) Anorexia nervosa. Raven Press, New York.

Bruch H 1978 The golden cage. Open Books, Harvard

Burns T, Crisp A H, 1984 Outcome of anorexia nervosa in males. British Journal of Psychiatry 145: 319–325

Chudley P 1986 An unhealthy obsession. Nursing Times, March 26, 50–52

Cooper P J, Fairburn C G 1983 Binge-eating and self-induced vomiting in the community: a preliminary study. British Journal of Psychiatry 142: 139–44

Crisp A H 1965 Some aspects of the evolution, presentation and follow-up of anorexia nervosa. Proceedings of the Royal Society of Medicine 58: 814–820

Crisp A H 1967a Anorexia nervosa. Hospital Medicine 5: 713–718

Crisp A H 1967b The nature of primary anorexia nervosa. In: Symposium — Anorexia nervosa and obesity, May 1972. Royal College of Physicians of Edinburgh. Publication No. 42: 18–30

Crisp A H 1977 Diagnosis and outcome of anorexia nercosa: the St George's view. Proceedings of the Royal Society of Medicine 70: 464–470

Crisp A H 1980 Anorexia nervosa: let me be. Academic Press, London

Crisp A H 1983 Anorexia nervosa. British Medical Journal 287: 855–858

Crisp A H, Stonehill E 1971 Relation between aspects of nutritional disturbance and menstrual activity in primary anorexia nervosa. British Medical Journal 3: 149–151

Crisp A H, Palmer R L, Kalucy R S 1976 How common is anorexia nervosa? a prevalence study. British Journal of Psychiatry 128: 549–554

Crisp A H, Norton K R S, Jurczak S, Bowyer C, Duncan S 1985 A treatment approach to anorexia nervosa — 25 years on. Journal of Psychiatric Research 19: 393–404

Dally P, Gomez J, Isaacs I J 1979 Anorexia nervosa. Heinemann, London

Fairburn C G 1982 Binge-eating and bulimia nervosa. Smith, Kline and French Laboratories, London

Fairburn C G, Cooper P J 1984 The clinical features of bulimia nervosa. British Journal of Psychiatry 144: 238–246

Garfinkel P E, Moldofsky H, Garnier M 1977 The outcome of anorexia nervosa: significance of clinical features, body image and behaviour modification. In: Vigersky R A (ed) Anorexia nervosa. Raven Press, New York

Goldberg S C, Halmi K A, Eckert E D, Casper R C, Davis J M 1979 Cyproheptadine in anorexia nervosa. British Journal of Psychiatry 134: 67–70

Hsu L K G 1980 Anorexia nervosa. Smith, Kline and French Laboratories, London

Hsu L K G, Crisp A H, Harding B 1979 Outcome of anorexia nervosa. Lancet: 62–65

Kay D W K, Leigh D 1954 The natural history, treatment and prognosis of anorexia nervosa. Journal of Mental Science 100: 411–428

Lacey J H 1983 Bulimia nervosa, binge eating and psychogenic vomiting: a controlled treatment study and long-term outcome. British Medical Journal 268: 1597–1678

Lacey J H 1984 The bulimic syndrome. In: Ferguson A (ed) Advanced Medicine — 20.

McNamara R J 1982 The challenge of treating eating disorders. Canadian Nurse 78 (10): 35–45

Minuchin S, Rosman B L, Baker L 1978 Psychosomatic families: anorexia nervosa in context. Harvard Press, Cambridge

Minuchin S, Baker L, Rosman B L, Liebman R, Milman L, Thomas C T 1975 A conceptual model of psychosomatic illness in children. Archives of General Psychiatry 32: 1031–1038

Minuchin S, Rosman B L, Liebman R, Baker B L 1977 Input and outcome of family therapy in anorexia nervosa.

In: Fernstein S C, Giovacchini D L (eds) Adolescent
psychiatry, 5th edn. Jason Aronson, New York

Misik I M 1981 When the anorexic patient challenges you.
Nursing 11 (12): 46–49

Palmer P L 1980 Anorexia nervosa. Penguin,
Harmondsworth

Russell G F M 1970 Anorexia nervosa, its identity as an
illness and its treatment. In: Price J H (ed) Modern
trends in psychological medicine, 2nd edn. Butterworth,
London

Russell G F M 1973 The management of anorexia nervosa.
In: Symposium — Anorexia nervosa and obesity, May
1972. Royal College of Physicians of Edinburgh.
Publication No. 42

Russell G F M 1977 The present status of anorexia nervosa.
Psychological Medicine 7: 363–367

Russell G F M 1981 The current treatment of anorexia
nervosa. British Journal of Psychiatry 138: 164–166

Stunkard A J 1980 Psychoanalysis and psychotherapy. In:
Stunkard A J (ed) Obesity. W B Saunders, Philadelphia

34

Personality disorders

C. A. Barnes and R. Frisby

In the classification of psychiatric conditions, personality disorders have been somewhat tangential in the past, but are now viewed by many as major clinical entities (Millon 1981). The frequency of the diagnosis 'personality disorder', together with the implications for the person so labelled necessitate a careful and critical overview. As Campbell & Russell (1984) observe:

. . . attributions of personality disorder tend to carry with them negative connotations of chronicity and unresponsiveness to treatment. There is a temptation to see the patient in terms of unfavourable stereotypes.

Words such as 'abnormality' and 'disorder' are in themselves powerfully suggestive. They imply a medical model: a notion of some morbid process (Howells 1982). Yet there is often inadequate exploration in psychiatric nursing texts of the extent of subjectivity involved in a diagnosis of abnormal personality. An assumption that personality disorder exists as an identifiable psychiatric problem is implicit in much of the available literature. While it is true that nurses are asked to care for patients whose behaviour causes problems, yet who display no obvious psychiatric symptomatology, it seems inappropriate to discuss nursing intervention in terms of an assumed 'group'.

The primary aim of this chapter is to assist the reader in a personal consideration of 'abnormal personality': its definition, acceptability as a 'psychiatric problem' and the implications for nursing practice. Attention is initially given to matters of definition and classification, illustrated by reference to psychopathy. Aspects of treatment and the environment in which it occurs will follow. The final sections of the chapter consider the nursing response to individuals with personality and behavioural problems who have entered the psychiatric system: their assessment, some difficulties associated with their management, and ideas about the planning of their care.

ABNORMAL PERSONALITY: ISSUES OF DEFINITION AND CLASSIFICATION

When considering the labelling of certain individuals as abnormal personalities or personality disordered, it is helpful to remember that the words 'normal' and 'abnormal' can be used in different ways and with different connotations (Hamilton 1985). The commonest meaning is a statistical one, where 'normal' equates with 'common' and 'abnormal' with 'uncommon'. In the development of definitive criteria for distinguishing psychological abnormality from normality, the most frequent attempts have been statistical, involving the identification of behaviours within social groups (Millon 1981). However, as Orme (1984) comments, there are difficulties in defining abnormal personality types statistically. Such an approach may be attractive in its notional simplicity but is complicated by factors such as social desirability and acceptability. What is considered abnormal may change with social and moral values. Whether behaviour that is statistically 'deviant' is of concern reflects the degree of associated cultural approval or unease at any particular time (Barker 1985).

It should also be remembered that the situation is further complicated by personality itself having a multitude of definitions and a 'long and controversial history within psychology' (Turner & Hersen 1981). Definitions typically emphasize the existence of attributes or characteristics by which individuals are distinguished from one another, with specific reference to the importance of traits

(see Harré & Lamb 1983, Hamilton 1985).

In the final analysis, normality and abnormality of personality are relative concepts;

. . . they represent arbitrary points on a continuum or gradient, since no sharp line divides normal from pathological behaviour.

(Millon 1981)

It could be argued that if normal and abnormal personality merely form a continuum, then there can be no true system of classification. However, such schema exist, the best known of which appear in the International Classification of Diseases (World Health Organization 1978) and DSM-III-R (American Psychiatric Association 1987). As Millon (1981) notes, current personality classification is the result of 'a long and continuing history'. Jenkins (1960) views the history of classification of personality disorders as 'a reluctant fumbling toward working definitions'. He draws attention to the fact that whilst a diagnosis of schizophrenia can be made from *qualitative* differences from normal experience (such as delusions), one of personality disorder is made purely from difficulties in adjustment and an absence of qualitatively abnormal symptoms. Their determination relies on *quantitative* measures and a subjective evaluation of individuals by diagnosticians. Weller (1986) observes:

We all have personality deficiencies and when these become disorders, and when disorders become illnesses, if they ever do so, are issues which are difficult to resolve.

Classification attempts have been regarded at best as artificial and unhelpful, and at worst, serving to medicalize problems for purposes of social control and convenience.

However, Turner & Hersen (1981) probably best reflect the consensus view that personality disorders do exist despite being 'one of the least understood and researched of all the psychiatric disorders'. Pichot comments on the clinical consensus (despite considerable conceptual confusion) of there being . . .

. . . a set of states, distinct from psychoses and neuroses, and characterized by relatively permanent quantitative deviations of personality which are considered pathological on the basis of a criterion of 'suffering' (of the individual or society).

(Pichot 1978)

Pathological personalities, according to Millon (1981), are characterized by: an inability to adapt effectively to life events ('adaptive inflexibility'); a tendency to foster vicious, self-defeating circles by the perpetuation and intensification of pre-existing difficulties; and fragility and instability under stress.

PSYCHOPATHIC PERSONALITY DISORDER

Issues of definition and classification can perhaps best be illustrated by reference to the diagnosis of psychopathic personality disorder (here used synonymously with psychopathy, and also referred to as sociopathy and antisocial personality). This is just one of a collection of terms used since the early 19th century to denote a condition characterized, according to Lewis (1974), by a 'life-long propensity to behaviour which falls mid-way between normality and psychosis'. Reviews of the concept's history are provided by a number of authors (Walker & McCabe 1973, Lewis 1974, Pichot 1978). It is difficult to do justice to the great volume of literature on, and the controversy which surrounds, the use of the term without reference to historical and medico-legal considerations, such as the inclusion of psychopathic disorder in successive Mental Health Acts. However, it is important to be aware of the ways in which such a diagnosis may be reached, the evidence for and arguments against the existence of such a condition and the possible implications for a person so labelled.

Definitions

A review of the literature reveals numerous definitions of psychopathic personality. Blackburn (1974) found that the number of identifying criteria used in definitions of psychopathy varied between two and 14. He makes the important point that the criteria themselves are 'essentially negative social value judgements' rather than signs and symptoms of disease, distress or dysfunction. This is illustrated only too well by Cleckley's (1982) clinical profile of the psychopath which includes characteristics such as superficial charm and good intelligence, unreliability, lack of remorse and inadequately motivated antisocial behaviour. Apart from an obvious focus on its antisocial aspects (which have been reflected in the definitions of psychopathic disorder in the Mental Health Acts), there is still no real agreement on what such a disorder is (if it exists at all) or how it should be classified. As Orme (1984) comments 'the term psychopath is often criticized as being an ill-defined "rag-bag" one rather than one that defines a really homogeneous group of people'. Treves-Brown (1977) notes that there are really only two areas of near consensus between authors, that psychopathy is 'a bad thing to have' and is 'manifested by misbehaviour'.

It is clear from the literature that the production of a working definition of psychopathic personality has been the subject of intense speculation and fierce debate. However, it may be helpful to refer to Whiteley's (1970) general description of the psychopath, abstracted from different definitions to bring together some of their common features. Basically, a psychopath:

- persistently acts against current social norms
- is apparently unaware of the seriously deviant nature of his behaviour
- is neither totally 'bad' nor totally 'mad' as those terms are commonly understood.

The lure of label

In spite of its controversial nature, the concept of psychopathy has, as Howells (1982) notes, remained 'entrenched in psychiatric and legal thinking'. It is therefore unsurprising that many commentators have turned their attentions to possible hidden functions of a label which, observe Walker & McCabe (1973), seems 'likely to obliterate more information than it conveys'. Mental health workers are often faced with patients who are generally unrewarding — like the 'not nice' patients described by Scott: those who . . .

. . . habitually appear to be well able to look after themselves but don't . . . reject attempts to help them . . . break the institutional rules . . . get drunk . . . upset other patients . . . quietly go to the devil in their own way quite heedless of nurse and doctor.

(Scott 1975)

It is in coping with such clients that a label may be of use. Howells (1982) suggests that the notion of the 'untreatable psychopath' may serve to justify an unwillingness and failure to help aggressive, uncooperative patients. It may also function as a 'pseudo-diagnosis' (Walker & McCabe 1973). The current legal system asks the psychiatrist to distinguish between mentally normal and abnormal offenders, providing him with the label 'psychopathic disorder' to use if it is felt that the offender is abnormal but not mentally ill. On a more general level, society may need the psychopath in order to explain 'evil' —

. . . it may be reassuring in some way for society to localize the world's wickedness in a fantasized 'sick' abnormal group of deviants.

(Howells 1982)

Szasz's notion of 'semantic conversion and reconversion' also provides an insight into a possible function. He considers that certain types of behaviour were initially 'converted' to, or renamed as, mental disorders in order to justify 'therapeutic' intervention and control, until such time as it became necessary to reconvert them (perhaps as a result of therapeutic failure or policy convenience). To quote Szasz (1968):

. . . modern medical and psychiatric customs and opinions have removed the 'mentally ill' from among the class of fully respectable patients and returned them to the class of social deviants and troublemakers, which they formerly occupied. This is particularly evident in the present-day psychiatric posture towards patients who are stuck with labels such as . . . psychopathic or sociopathic personality.

Aetiology

Despite the critical nature of the above arguments against the existence of psychopathic personality disorder as a distinct clinical entity, the current professional consensus is that it exists . . .

. . . not [as] a single clinical disorder but a convenient label to describe a severe personality disorder which may show itself in a variety of attitudinal, emotional and inter-personal behaviour problems.
(Department of Health and Social Security/Home Office 1986)

Widespread professional acceptance accom-

panies what is now a vast literature on research into the disorder. In general, there is agreement that psychopathic disorder is the result of arrested emotional development which impedes normal social learning, but the aetiology of the abnormality remains obscure. As Prins (1980) points out 'as with many other aspects of mental disorder, the "nature" versus "nurture" debate has raged for many years in relation to psychopathy'.

Sutker et al (1981) remark that the subjection of clinical hypotheses about psychopathy to controlled investigation is only comparatively recent. Research has been criticized (Feldman 1977, Widom & Newman 1985) for an overwhelming emphasis on the study of criminal populations. This has resulted in biased subject selection. Critics (Feldman 1977, Howells 1982) have also noted that studies have used different measures and definitions of psychopathic disorder, making comparability of results difficult. Inevitably, a seemingly infinite number of organic and environmental factors have been implicated and the validity and reliability of findings have then been questioned and often dismissed. In a recent review, Weller (1986) concludes that 'several lines of evidence converge to suggest that at least some psychopaths, particularly violent psychopaths, are victims of abnormal brain functioning'. Claims that psychopathic behaviour may to some extent have an organic basis have emerged from neurophysiological, biochemical and genetic studies. 'Arousal theory' has been influential: several researchers have claimed, on the basis of abnormal electroencephalogram (EEG) patterns and electrodermal and cardiovascular responses, that psychopathy is related to cortical and autonomic under-arousal. Findings have been used to explain why the psychopath characteristically feels little guilt or anxiety and may actively need to seek stimulation by engaging in antisocial activities. According to Weller (1986) the claim that brain malfunction underlies psychopathy is further supported by the fact that such behaviour can result from brain damage, particularly to the frontal and temporal lobes. Weller (1986) also provides a useful reference to recent biochemical abnormalities which have been described, particularly in relation to violent behaviour.

Other studies (for example Eysenck & Eysenck 1978) have investigated genetic influences on psychopathic behaviour. Learning theory has also received considerable attention: the notion that psychopathy is the result of learned patterns of antisocial behaviour. Feldman (1977) reviews the evidence which links antisocial criminal behaviour to emotional separation, deprivation and disturbance in childhood, but makes the point that such studies have mostly been retrospective, with the result that the researcher who submits to socialization theory would more than likely *interpret* the childhood of a psychopath as 'disturbed'. Robins (1978) agrees that such retrospective studies 'are not likely to provide trustworthy results' because of the necessarily selective recall of the subjects and the difficulties in identifying appropriate control groups. However, an adverse home background and parental behaviour have been cited as key factors in the development of antisocial personalities (West & Farrington 1973).

Readers interested in more substantial reviews of relevant research in these areas should consult, for example, Hare & Schalling (1978) and Sutker et al (1981). In conclusion, the aetiology of psychopathic disorder is elusive. Research findings have been contested on methodological grounds and Cloninger et al (1978) comment that researchers have tended to introduce their own biases by emphasizing 'either genetic, physiological, sociological or behavioural learning factors to the exclusion of others'. Indeed, Blackburn's (1974) view that definitive conclusions cannot be drawn from research until the concept of psychopathy is itself more clearly defined seems as pertinent now as when he wrote.

ABNORMAL PERSONALITY: TREATMENT AND THERAPEUTIC ENVIRONMENTS

Before considering the nursing implications of abnormal personality, it is necessary to locate persons with such a diagnosis within the health care system, and to look briefly at treatment approaches.

Turner & Hersen (1981) comment on three traditional approaches. Firstly, personality disorder has customarily been a primary diagnosis amongst patients treated by a psychodynamic approach, with much of psychodynamic theory being based on the treatment of hysterical disorders. Psychodynamic therapy is essentially concerned with underlying psychopathology and internal conflict which 'often give rise to profound and personally unmanageable distress' (Swift 1984). The therapist aims to help the patient 'use the [therapist–patient] relationship to resolve the patient's interpersonal difficulties' (Turner & Hersen 1981), and explore both conscious and unconscious reasons for these. Swift (1984) notes the tendency to equate dynamic psychotherapy with psychotherapy in its general sense. She points out that many types of psychotherapy exist, but uses the primary distinction between dynamic and directive therapies. The latter, unlike the former, are not concerned with the patient's personality or psychopathology, but essentially focus on the relief of symptoms. Many mental health workers, including nurses, offer supportive therapy and counselling that would fall under the wide umbrella of the non-dynamic approach. In turn, many patients diagnosed as personality disordered are managed by supportive approaches. Any psychotherapeutic approach to treatment is difficult to evaluate systematically, which probably explains the lack of literature in this area. However, there is a general scepticism surrounding psychotherapy with the 'personality disordered'. This appears to be based on clinical experience: many patients so diagnosed have long-standing relationship difficulties and appear unable to make use of the one-to-one contact with the therapist. Especially in the case of psychopathic disorder, such a relatively intense relationship is avoided by 'discontinuing treatment, acting out or manipulating the therapist' (Whiteley 1970). Swift (1984) points out the dangers of dynamic treatment but feels that it is easier to select patients for other psychotherapeutic approaches.

The second traditional treatment approach is that of the therapeutic community. The principle of such an approach is to use the structure of the milieu, and the experience of the interactions within, to increase patients' awareness of their antisocial behaviour. This promotes the learning of more acceptable ways of relating. Problems of individual therapist–patient contact as described above can be avoided as 'a pool of people are available for interacting with the patient' (Turner & Hersen 1981). Clinical experience and research at the Henderson Hospital (Whiteley 1970, Copas & Whiteley 1976, Gudjonsson & Roberts 1985) suggest that certain psychopathic patients respond well to such an environment, although careful selection of patients is a prerequisite. Success has also been reported for therapeutic community principles in penal settings (Stürup 1968, Home Office 1985). Also, as Walton (1984) observes, there has been growing interest in applying these principles to various outpatient settings. Examples of both inpatient and outpatient approaches are provided in Hinshelwood & Manning (1979).

Thirdly, pharmacological treatment in personality disorder is sometimes used, but only in a palliative way. Many practitioners are opposed to the use of medication because of the risk of creating dependency or addiction; also patients may have a pre-existing history of drug abuse. The use of drugs is therefore largely incidental to the diagnosis, but may be given to certain patients to help combat anxiety or aggressiveness.

Turner & Hersen (1981) focus primarily on the behavioural approach. They conclude that behaviour therapy has produced some positive results in the social adjustment of some personality-disordered individuals, but warn that certain patients with severe disorders who are prone to suicidal or aggressive behaviour should be treated in structured, residential environments.

The above approaches, along with other relevant treatment principles and settings, are more thoroughly outlined in Russell & Hersov (1984). As patients diagnosed as personality disordered cover such a broad spectrum of referrals to psychiatric services, and as they present with such wide-ranging problems and histories, it is unsurprising that such a plethora of treatment approaches have been used.

A brief note about psychopathic disorder seems appropriate here, as it may serve to illustrate the wider position vis-à-vis personality disorder and its treatment. Psychopathy has classically been regarded as untreatable: little could be done until the condition 'burned out' with maturation.

However, certain practitioners (for example, Prins 1980) stress that management is generally more effective if different 'types' of psychopath are selected for different treatments. Suedfield & Landon (1978) and Sutker et al (1981) review treatment approaches specific to psychopathic disorder, pointing out that research in this area is again generally inadequate. Treatments have been very diverse with no clear demonstration that any one method is more effective than another (Gostin 1986). However, in the light of the uncertainty about the definition and aetiology of psychopathy and, indeed, 'personality disorder' itself, it seems inevitable that treatment methods and their evaluation have been based more on trial and error than on clinical, research-based knowledge.

ABNORMAL PERSONALITY: THE NURSING RESPONSE

Patient assessment and care planning

Barker (1985) recalls from his student days that the assessment of patients by psychiatric nurses was little more than . . .

. . . a scaled-down version of psychiatric diagnosis . . . [with] scant attention to studying the person who was sheltered by his towering label.

The ways in which psychiatric nurses have identified what should be done in the name of nursing care have in Barker's view been haphazard and 'rule-of-thumb'. His work offers an invaluable introduction to the principles and practice of a system of assessment which is based on problems of living arising from psychiatric disorders themselves. In this way, harmful stereotyping can be minimized and nurses have a more standardized tool with which they can work:

The rules, guidelines and specific procedures which are established in a formal system may help us to study different patients in more or less the same way. As a result, our own prejudices and idiosyncracies are reduced, if not cancelled out entirely.

(Barker 1985)

Essentially, assessment involves collecting information in such a way that will enable a judgement to be made about the kind of help the patient requires. Whenever possible, the process should involve cooperation by, and negotiation with, the patient. For many reasons this may be difficult when the patient has a disordered personality. These include problems in engaging the patient in therapeutic relationships and the effects of manipulative and/or antisocial behaviour. Such difficulties are highlighted by authors such as Stuart & Sundeen (1983) and Schultz & Dark (1986). These texts offer some useful directions in planning care. Firstly, there is the concept of the 'nursing diagnosis'. This appears to emerge logically from a process of nursing assessment and is couched in terms of patient problem and its underlying factors. Examples of such diagnoses could be 'unsatisfactory interpersonal relationships related to feelings of inadequacy and mistrust' or 'inability to express feelings of loneliness related to marital break-up'. Usually patients have multiple problems which need to be reflected in any care planning as separate diagnoses. In this way, nurses can work towards a comprehensive plan of appropriate and realistic interventions for each individual. Secondly, the above authors consider the care planning process as a response to some commonly experienced difficulties in personality disorder. Of these, three in particular merit attention here:

1. relating to patients with personality and behavioural difficulties
2. managing manipulative behaviour
3. managing antisocial behaviour.

Relating to patients with personality and behavioural difficulties

As the psychiatric ward is a community 'whose therapeutic potential is vitally influenced by the nursing staff' (Gillies & Russell 1984) the realization of such potential depends to a large extent on the management of nurse–patient relationships. These are generally accepted as the core of psychiatric nursing. With patients who have personality and behavioural problems, obstacles to the formation and continuation of therapeutic alliances can potentially lie in the feelings, attitudes and behaviour of both patients and nurses. It is unlikely

that nursing staff can be at all effective unless they try and remain aware of the interactive nature of their work with patients.

Schultz & Dark (1986) consider trust to be the foundation of a therapeutic relationship. They describe four phases of a 'trust relationship': introductory, testing, working and termination. The particular characteristics of each phase are considered with associated nursing objectives and interventions. For example, in the testing phase . . .

The client may say or do things to shock the nurse to see if he or she will reject the client. During this time the client may become manipulative in an attempt to discover the limits of the relationship or test the nurse's sincerity and dependability. The client's attitude may vary a great deal, from pleasant and eager to please to uncooperative or angry. This phase can be extremely trying and frustrating for the nurse.

(Schultz & Dark 1986)

Many nurses who have worked with patients with a 'personality disorder' label will recognize such testing. The underlying mistrust is often mutual; patients may present with a history of antisocial behaviour, a criminal record and a stigmatizing diagnosis, all of which can ensure that nurses are immediately 'on guard'. In turn, patients can be forgiven for regarding nurses as yet more institutional authoritarian figures, to try rather than to trust.

Gillies & Russell (1984) observe other obstacles to therapeutic relationships related to the institutional structure of the hospital and its implications for the nurse's role. Nurses, especially students, are not given full control of the maintenance and conclusion of such relationships. Reasons for this include: being moved between different wards; receiving inadequate supervision for the interpersonal aspects of their work; and having to share themselves as 'ward nurses' among patients making simultaneous demands.

The interpersonal process between nurse and patient is the focus of what has become an influential model in psychiatric nursing: the developmental model of Peplau (1952). Limitations of space prevent an in-depth consideration of Peplau's work, but the nurse seeking to explore this further is well served by other texts (see, for example, Pearson & Vaughan 1986, Collister 1986). In essence, four phases are identified which are reminiscent of Schultz & Dark above. After an 'orientation' phase during which the patient's problems are identified and initial contact developed, the patient passes through a phase of 'identification' in which he recognizes the relationship he is forming with the nurse who is offering help and formulating a plan of intervention. There follows an 'exploitation' phase when there is a response to what is on offer and a move towards goals which have been mutually agreed. Finally comes 'resolution' in which the patient regains independence. Undoubtedly, the realities of trying to help patients with personality and behavioural difficulties may cause some practitioners to dismiss such a model as Utopian. As Pearson & Vaughan (1986) acknowledge, Peplau's approach has been thought of as inappropriate in the many clinical settings which are not totally based on the client's ability to develop substantial insight into the cause of his difficulties. The nurse and patient may also be unable to negotiate mutually acceptable aims, or these may be repeatedly sabotaged by the patient. In other words,

. . . it may not be possible to progress beyond orientation or identification . . . [and] the nature of a particular patient's problem may be such that complete resolution is not possible.

(Collister 1986)

Nonetheless, a model which aims to make sense of nurse–patient contact and its vast potential should not be dismissed purely because of apparent difficulties in implementation. As Pearson & Vaughan (1986) claim, 'there is much to be learned from a model which lays emphasis on helping people to explore why they are facing difficulties'.

Managing manipulative behaviour

Manipulative behaviour is frequently viewed as a major problem in nursing patients with personality difficulties. It can be destructive to the therapeutic progress of patients and their peers and can generate extreme feelings of anger and hostility within staff. In essence, manipulation involves the use of one's control and influence to attempt to meet one's own goals, through a process whereby others are rendered powerless and their freedom of action curtailed. However, it is helpful to remember that manipulation can be (and often is) used by staff as well as by patients; the latter group may have their choices needlessly restricted by staff who want to exercise their power and authority. It could also be suggested that the frequent labelling and dismissal of patients as 'manipulative' possibly says as much about the labeller as the labelled!

Manipulation of nurses by patients leaves the former separated or split off from colleagues and deeply hostile towards the coercive patients. One invaluable account of manipulative behaviour and its effects within a psychotherapeutic relationship is provided by Murphy & Guze (1960). They emphasize that such behaviour 'retains the initiative for the patient, in a self-defeating way, and stands in the path of therapeutic progress'. The authors offer ways of understanding and managing such behaviour, based upon the setting of limits; these must be clear with both parties certain of what will and will not be tolerated. In this way, limit-setting can have what Murphy and Guze describe as a 'training function'. The patient learns the disadvantages of manipulation and more satisfying, rewarding ways of relating. They consider the patient's manipulative behaviour will only be abandoned if other ways of handling interpersonal situations are learned. Stuart & Sundeen (1983) tend to reinforce this point with their observation that manipulation is used by those who tolerate emotional closeness poorly, to keep others at arm's length.

Owing to the tendency of manipulative behaviour to cause or exacerbate splits between staff, it is vital that *multi-disciplinary* (not merely nursing) teamwork is of a high calibre, with each team member knowing the limits set for any particular patient. Working together in this way minimizes gaps in communication and enables colleagues to support each other in enforcing the limits. Once these have been agreed, staff should not 'debate, argue, rationalize or bargain' with the patient (Schultz & Dark 1986). Consistency and confrontation over infringements are also important, with patients being held responsible for their own actions. For the nurse in particular, the stress and general emotional cost involved in such confrontation should not be forgotten. As McCune (1987) remarks,

... the skilful handling of confrontation is potentially very helpful for patients but emotionally stressful for staff ... In general, doctors do not experience the stress of constant exposure to patients because they can more easily get 'time out' from particular patients.

Managing antisocial behaviour

Problems are also posed by those patients who exhibit 'socially deviant or antisocial behaviour [which] varies in intensity from mild to severe' (Turner & Hersen 1981), and which seems intrinsically related to their personality problems. Such behaviour may include verbal aggression, physical violence, substance abuse, self-mutilation or parasuicide. In such cases, a detailed knowledge of patients' personal and psychiatric histories can be a double-edged sword. Importantly, it may aid the assessment of a patient's level of dangerousness and enable nurses to take sensible precautions regarding safety. However, an over-emphasis on a patient's past can make staff excessively cautious and hence impede therapeutic progress.

Certain types of antisocial behaviour may be managed by behaviour modification techniques. Nurses can play an important role in this by limit-setting and developing specific consequences for unacceptable behaviour, as part of a planned behavioural approach. Individualized behavioural programmes may be designed in collaboration with clinical psychologists. Other methods are based on psychotherapeutic insights. Patients with personality problems may consider their world to be permanently full of antagonists; the problem lies within everyone else, not within them or their behaviour. Additionally, patients may 'split-off' or disown parts of themselves and their past actions which are too difficult to face (Grounds et al 1987). A nurse who engages with a patient is likely to become the subject of the latter's 'transference', a concept which in a general sense refers to a response to a new relationship based on feelings and attitudes developed in the past (Brown & Pedder 1979). The patient may therefore repeat previous patterns of antisocial behaviour which become targeted at the helper.

The extent to which nurses can work with patients towards an insightful understanding of such phenomena depends on several factors; these include the extent of patients' defences, their levels of maturity and ability to cope with confrontation, together with the skills of nurses involved. Clinical experience suggests it is inadvisable to adopt a psychodynamic approach with patients who resort to antisocial behaviour which is persistent and dangerous. The importance of accurate assessment of the individual patient together with consultation with and supervision by colleagues cannot be overstressed.

In conclusion, Schultz & Dark (1986) remind us that working in a hospital setting with patients who behave antisocially can be extremely frustrating due to difficulties in facilitating long-term change. It is important therefore to set realistic short-term goals, rather than aiming to transform patients' personalities and behaviours. Main (1957) observed that:

Only the most mature of therapists are able to encounter frustration of their hopes without some ambivalence towards the patient, and with patients who do not get better, or who even get worse in spite of long devoted care, major strain may arise. The patient's attendants are then pleased neither with him or themselves and the quality of their concern for him alters accordingly with consequences that can be severe both for patients and attendants.

The contribution of a 'primary nursing' approach

One way of organizing patient care on psychiatric wards is through a 'primary nursing' system. Each patient is allocated a primary nurse whose duty it is to plan and assume responsibility for that patient's care. When the primary nurse is off duty, designated 'associate nurses' maintain care according to the primary nurse's plan. It is an attempt to provide the patient with continuity of care and to ensure that accountability for patient care is held by individual nurses rather than being disseminated or abdicated. Primary nursing has been most commonly described and evaluated in general hospitals but psychiatric nursing care has also been organized in this way (Green 1983, Ritter 1985).

Clearly, such a system of care could contribute to meeting some of the relationship and management difficulties discussed above. If care is negotiated and planned with a primary nurse as opposed to a team in which no one individual assumes responsibility for implementation and evaluation, then manipulation and splitting of staff can be minimized. However, the patient may perceive the relationship as a ready-made vehicle to exploit: in other words, such a system can *facilitate* the splitting of staff, unless the primary nurse continues to seek and receive supervision from colleagues.

CONCLUSION

Perhaps the central difficulty in addressing the task of this chapter — the production of a text on nursing patients with abnormal personalities — has been in deciding which individuals merit being described in this way. Issues surrounding this particular diagnosis have been considered and illustrated by reference to a range of academic and clinical sources; an attempt has been made to provide a fairly rigorous examination of abnormal personality as a concept and personality disorder as a diagnosis. Yet many nurses *are* confronted with problems in managing patients with personality and behavioural problems who are not mentally ill in the commonly accepted sense of the word. The very heterogeneity of such a patient 'group' mitigates against a neat package of nursing interventions, but it is hoped that what has been offered here may be of help in facilitating an increased awareness of possible approaches to difficult situations. Whilst consideration of some special aspects and facilities (for example, those of a forensic nature) fall outside the scope of this chapter, it is acknowledged that nurses working in secure environments with offenders designated as personality disordered may face a range of concerns not dealt with here.

A psychiatric diagnosis, especially one as ambiguous as 'abnormal personality', does not in itself facilitate nursing care. Indeed, it may, as has been discussed, be severely stigmatizing and disabling. With psychiatric nurses becoming less bound by the rigidity of traditional and custodial roles, new directions in patient assessment and care planning can be pursued: those based on the capitalization of the nurse's unique contact with the patient rather than the restrictive framework of a psychiatric label such as abnormal personality.

REFERENCES

American Psychiatric Association 1987 Diagnostic and statistical manual of mental disorders (DSM-III-R). American Psychiatric Association, Washington

Barker P J 1985 Patient assessment in psychiatric nursing. Croom Helm, Beckenham, p 4

Blackburn R 1974 Personality and the classification of psychopathic disorders. Special Hospitals Research Report No 10. Special Hospitals Research Unit, London, p 2

Brown D, Pedder J 1979 Introduction to Psychotherapy. Tavistock, London

Campbell P G, Russell G F M 1984 The assessment of neurotic and personality disorders in adults. In: Russell G F M, Hersov L A (eds) Handbook of psychiatry, Vol 4. The neuroses and personality disorders. Cambridge University Press, Cambridge, p 65

Cleckley H 1982 The mask of sanity, 6th edn. Mosby, St Louis

Cloninger C R, Reich T, Guze S B 1978 Genetic-environmental interactions and antisocial behaviour. In: Hare R D, Schalling D (eds) Psychopathic behaviour: approaches to research. Wiley, Chichester, p 226

Collister B 1986 Psychiatric nursing and a developmental model. In: Kershaw B, Salvage J (eds) Models for nursing. Wiley, Chichester, p 93

Copas J B, Whiteley J S 1976 Predicting success in the treatment of psychopaths. British Journal of Psychiatry 129: 388–392

Department of Health and Social Security/Home Office 1986 Offenders suffering from psychopathic disorder. Department of Health and Social Security/Home Office, London, p 4

Eysenck H J, Eysenck S B G 1978 Psychopathy, personality and genetics. In: Hare R D, Schalling D (eds) Psychopathic behaviour: approaches to research. Wiley, Chichester

Feldman M P 1977 Criminal Behaviour. A psychological analysis. Wiley, Chichester

Gillies C, Russell G F M 1984 Nursing treatment. In: Russell G F M, Hersov L A (eds) Handbook of psychiatry, Vol 4. The neuroses and personality disorders. Cambridge University Press, Cambridge, p 115

Gostin L 1986 Institutions observed. King Edward's Hospital Fund for London, London

Green B 1983 Primary nursing in psychiatry. Nursing Times 79(3) January 19: 24–28

Grounds A T, Quayle M T, France J, Brett T, Cox M, Hamilton J R 1987 A unit for 'psychopathic disorder' patients in Broadmoor Hospital. Medicine, Science and the Law 27(1): 21–31

Gudjonsson G H, Roberts J C 1985 Psychological and physiological characteristics of personality-disordered patients. In: Farrington D P, Gunn J (eds) Aggression and dangerousness. Wiley, Chichester

Hamilton M (ed) 1985 Fish's clinical psychopathology, 2nd edn. Wright, Bristol

Hare R D, Schalling D (eds) 1978 Psychopathic behaviour: approaches to research. Wiley, Chichester

Harré R, Lamb R (eds) 1983 The encyclopaedic dictionary of psychology. Blackwell, Oxford

Hinshelwood R D, Manning N (eds) 1979 Therapeutic communities. Routledge & Kegan Paul, London

Home Office 1985 First Report of the Advisory Committee on the Therapeutic Regime at Grendon. Home Office, London

Howells K 1982 Mental disorder and violent behaviour. In: Feldman P (ed) Developments in the study of criminal behaviour, Vol 2: Violence. Wiley, Chichester, p 181

Jenkins R L 1960 The psychopathic or antisocial personality. Journal of Nervous and Mental Disease 319: 318–334

Lewis A 1974 Psychopathic personality: a most elusive category. In: The Later Papers of Sir Aubrey Lewis 1979. Oxford University Press, Oxford, p 205

Main T F 1957 The ailment. The British Journal of Medical Psychology 30(3): 129–145

McCune N 1987 In someone else's shoes. Bulletin of the Royal College of Psychiatrists 11(6) June: 196

Millon T 1981 Disorders of personality. Wiley, Chichester, pp 8, 24

Murphy G E, Guze S B 1960 Setting limits: the management of the manipulative patient. American Journal of Psychotherapy 14(1): 30–47

Orme J E 1984 Abnormal and clinical psychology. Croom Helm, Beckenham, p 25

Pearson A, Vaughan B 1986 Nursing models for practice. Heinemann, London, p 147

Peplau H E 1952 Interpersonal relations in nursing. Putnam, New York

Pichot P 1978 Psychopathic behaviour: a historical overview. In: Hare R D, Schalling D (eds) Psychopathic behaviour: approaches to research. Wiley, Chichester, p 68

Prins H 1980 Offenders, deviants or patients? Tavistock, London, p 143

Robins L N 1978 Aetiological implications in studies of childhood histories relating to antisocial personality. In:

Hare R D, Schalling D (eds) Psychopathic behaviour: approaches to research. Wiley, Chichester, p 257

Ritter S 1985 Primary nursing in mental illness. Nursing Mirror 160(17) April 24: 16–17

Russell G F M, Hersov L A (eds) 1984 Handbook of psychiatry, Vol 4. Cambridge University Press, Cambridge

Schultz J M, Dark S L 1986 Manual of psychiatric nursing care plans, 2nd edn. Little & Brown, Canada, pp 19, 168

Scott P D 1975 Has psychiatry failed in the treatment of offenders? (The Fifth Denis Carroll Memorial Lecture). Institute for the Study and Treatment of Delinquency, London, p 8

Stuart G W, Sundeen S J 1983 Principles and practice of psychiatric nursing, 2nd edn. Mosby, St Louis

Stürup G K 1968 Treating the 'untreatable' chronic criminals at Herstedvester. John Hopkins, Baltimore

Suedfield P, Landon P B 1978 Approaches to treatment. In: Hare R D, Schalling D (eds) Psychopathic behaviour: approaches to research. Wiley, Chichester

Sutker P B, Archer R P, Kilpatrick D G 1981 Sociopathy and antisocial behavior: theory and treatment. In: Turner S M, Calhoun K S, Adams H E (eds) Handbook of clinical behaviour therapy. Wiley, Chichester

Swift N 1984 Psychotherapy. In: Russell G F M, Hersov L A (eds) Handbook of psychiatry, Vol 4. The neuroses and personality disorders. Cambridge University Press, Cambridge, p 77

Szasz T S 1968 Law, liberty and psychiatry. Collier, New York, p 23

Treves-Brown C 1977 Who is the psychopath? Medicine, Science and the Law 17: 56–63

Turner S M, Hersen M 1981 Disorders of social behaviour: a behavioural approach to personality disorders. In: Turner S M, Calhoun K S, Adams H E (eds) Handbook of clinical behavior therapy. Wiley, Chichester, pp 103, 107, 120

Walker N, McCabe S 1973 Crime and insanity in England, Vols I and II. Edinburgh University Press, Edinburgh, pp 234, 235

Walton H 1984 In-patient care and therapeutic communities. In: Russell G F M, Hersov L A (eds) Handbook of psychiatry, Vol 4. The neuroses and personality disorders. Cambridge University Press, Cambridge

Weller M P I 1986 Medical concepts in psychopathy and violence. Medicine, Science and the Law 26(2): 131–143

West D J, Farrington D P 1973 Who becomes delinquent? Heinemann, London

Whiteley J S 1970 The psychopath and his treatment. British Journal of Hospital Medicine 3: 263–270

Widom C P, Newman J P 1985 Characteristics of non-institutionalized psychopaths. In: Farrington D P, Gunn J (eds) Aggression and dangerousness. Wiley, Chichester

World Health Organization 1978 Mental disorders: glossary and guide to their classification in accordance with the Ninth Revision of the International Classification of Diseases. World Health Organization, Geneva

35

Aggression and violence

C. A. Barnes

In recent years, psychiatric nurses have been increasingly concerned about the prevention and management of aggressive and violent behaviour by patients. They realise that any acceptable policy must balance patient care against staff safety. Aggression and violence is an emotive issue among psychiatric staff, and it is sometimes difficult to convey a sense of proportion about the problem in a text such as this. Popular wisdom often depicts the mentally ill as unpredictable and violent. However, research into the incidence of violent behaviour by patients (e.g. Fottrell 1979) has demonstrated that incidents of serious violence are rare. Most patients with whom psychiatric nurses come into contact prove no physical threat; however, there have been several reports that violent assaults by patients have increased in number (Confederation of Health Service Employees 1977, Psychiatric Nurses Association 1985), although this may be due to an increase in the proportion of incidents reported. Several studies of violent incidents have shown that nurses are the members of staff most likely to be attacked in psychiatric hospitals (e.g. Fottrell 1979, Drinkwater & Feldman 1982, Hodgkinson et al 1984, Casseem, 1984). Violent behaviour has also become a matter of concern for health service personnel in non-psychiatric settings.

To date, comparatively little research has been undertaken into the incidence of disturbed and violent behaviour and its management by nurses, and even less into the educational preparation of nurses in this respect. This makes a truly research-based approach to the nursing care of patients who are aggressive and violent impossible. There is also little literature on 'theoretically derived preventive nursing interventions' (Boettcher 1983) in this area. Some useful literature on the causes, prevention and management of violent behaviour has been written by nurses and other health professionals. Unfortunately, most of this material fails to convey the uniqueness of every aggressive act, or to provide methods for the systematic evaluation of each incident.

This chapter begins with an outline of recent developments in the treatment and placement of patients who may exhibit aggressive behaviour. This is followed by an analysis both of the nature of aggression and of the possible relationship of mental illness, ward environment and staff behaviour to its incidence. Some suggested strategies for preventing and managing violent behaviour are then described and discussed. The chapter concludes by considering future directions for this aspect of patient care.

CHANGING PHILOSOPHIES OF PSYCHIATRIC CARE

Until the 1950s, psychiatric patients were traditionally managed in the custodial environment of locked wards in large mental hospitals. This situation began to change with the advent of psychotropic medication and more active programmes of treatment and rehabilitation. Patients were cared for in less and less restrictive surroundings, a change which has unquestionably benefited most psychiatric patients. Early reports on these developments (e.g. Bell 1955, Pattemore 1957, Mandelbrote 1958) suggest that there were consequent improvements in nurse–patient relationships and reduced levels of violence in the wards and hospitals. However, as hospitals gradually relinquished their locked wards, nurses were increasingly deprived of the customary facilities for managing disturbed behaviour. In 1976, a *Lancet* editorial, in considering the needs of patients who required treatment in a secure setting, either during the acute phases of their illnesses or as part of a graduated programme of treatment and rehabilitation, noted that 'few mental hospitals provide even marginally secure wards or have nursing or medical staff with skills to man them' and that the revival of locked wards needed to be given further thought (*The Lancet* 1976). Other mental health practitioners felt that the necessary security could be provided without a return to a locked-door philosophy (e.g. Whitehead 1976).

The placement of patients who require periods of care in more secure wards and hospitals has been, and remains, controversial. The complex policy implications of this issue are discussed by the Home Office and Department of Health and Social Security (1975), MacCulloch (1977) and Bluglass (1978). Aspects with more obvious implications for nurses will be mentioned here.

Concern has been expressed that disturbed behaviour is now less tolerated by nurses working in 'open' psychiatric wards and units (Bluglass 1978). This could be caused by lack of experience in this aspect of patient care, owing to the dismantling of secure facilities within the health service. Altschul (1981) claims that nursing staff are now less competent in controlling violent behaviour, being afraid both of personal injury and of being accused of assault after physically restraining a patient. If this is so, such fears may contribute to the problems, discussed by Dell (1980), that special hospitals face when attempting to transfer patients to less restrictive hospitals. Many interim and regional secure units have had difficulties in recruiting suitably trained nursing staff (*Nursing Times* 1984), perhaps as a result of a general reduction in the level of skill and confidence amongst nurses in the management of violent behaviour. Some practitioners believe that competence in preventing and managing violence can only be acquired by experience, and not by training. If they are right, and if violent behaviour is now increasingly concentrated in special hospitals and prisons, then clearly it will be more difficult for nurses to gain relevant experience in this area.

AGGRESSION AND VIOLENCE: PROBLEMS OF DEFINITION

In discussions with nurses, it becomes clear that 'aggression' and 'violence' are terms which can mean different things to different people. Verbal abuse, experienced as traumatic by one nurse, may be considered by another as a routine, harmless display of anger or frustration, an unremarkable part of the job. One central difficulty in collecting data on violence in hospitals is the lack of consensus about what constitutes a 'violent incident'.

'Aggression' may be defined as 'an action that inflicts pain, anxiety or distress on another, and is in the service of a hostile motive or of the emotion of anger' (New Encyclopaedia Britannica 1985). Definitions of 'violence' tend to refer to the use of a greater degree of force, resulting in physical injury to a victim. Siann (1985) argues that the terms 'aggression' and 'violence' represent a 'complex amalgam of analytical concepts and intuitive understandings' and that attempts by academics to produce tight, exact definitions have resulted in explorations of human aggression that are narrow and restrictive. Certainly, there is a large subjective element in the use of such abstract terms. Whether an action is labelled as aggressive or violent tends to depend on personal values and the extent to which the behaviour is considered to be justified. The label usually implies that the act is intentional and has some element of motivation. Some of those who have written about aggression and violence (e.g. Marsh & Campbell 1982) use the terms interchangeably.

The latter convention is used in this chapter, on the premise that aggression and violence are inextricable and emanate from similar emotional states, even though they tend to describe different levels of behaviour by patients.

THE 'VIOLENT PATIENT'

Many existing texts tend to speak of 'the violent patient' and the problems he poses. Although this term may be technically and grammatically convenient, it usually implies that violent behaviour is a manifestation of the individual's psychopathological or physiological state. To explain a patient's aggressiveness solely in terms of a psychiatric diagnostic category can oversimplify the problem. Reference has been made to the 'uselessness of thinking of violent people or traits' (Hodgkinson 1980) and to the adoption of a broader understanding of the concept of violence, with an emphasis on the precise analysis of each violent incident. Violent behaviour has important interpersonal aspects and should always be examined in the context in which it occurs.

THE NATURE OF AGGRESSION

Psychiatric nursing demands 'an increased awareness of the process of human behaviour as a fundamental pre-requisite of intelligent intervention' (General Nursing Council 1982). Gaining an understanding of the nature of aggression is therefore essential to effective nursing practice. Many traditional theories have been criticized for concentrating upon explanations of aggression which lie in an individual's innate constitutional or psychological attributes; such approaches tend to minimize the role of the environment and socialization processes.

Belief in the existence of an inborn aggressive 'instinct' is at the basis of the writings of ethologists such as Lorenz (1966), psychoanalysts such as Storr (1968) and Fromm (1977), and some anthropologists (e.g. Fox 1982). These 'drive' theorists portray people as innately aggressive beings who need to find channels for the expression of such instincts. Human aggression is considered by most instinct theories as having potentially beneficial effects. Problems arise for both the individual and society when its expression is either blocked or takes an inappropriately destructive path. Mental illness, according to Storr (1968), arises when individuals are 'unable to integrate their aggression in a positive way'.

Frustration-aggression theory has also been influential. Dollard et al (1939) postulated that aggression was a natural response to some environmental frustration, and numerous psychological experiments were designed to demonstrate this causal link. However, it is now widely accepted that frustration is only one of many experiences that can precipitate an aggressive response. Also, an individual's response to being frustrated in the achievement of his goals is not always one of aggression.

More recent experimental approaches have developed a social learning analysis of aggression. Psychologists such as Bandura (1973) consider that most aggressive behaviour is learned through modelling and reinforcement processes. Models for such behaviour are initially parental, with peer groups and the media subsequently becoming influential. Bandura concludes that aggressive behaviour will only be imitated by an individual if it is beneficial.

Motivational aspects of aggression have also been widely studied. The main distinction to have emerged is one between reactive (or 'angry') and operant (or 'instrumental') aggression. The former is essentially a spontaneous reaction to some aversive event (or events), whilst aggression is seen as instrumental if there is some incentive by which it is motivated. The latter is felt to account for premeditated acts of violence. Owens & Ashcroft (1985) consider such reactive and operant processes to be fundamental, and capable of producing aggression without any other influences.

Aggression and violence have been studied from many differing academic perspectives, perhaps reflecting both the complexity of the subject and a deep-seated public concern about its implications. Some attempts have recently been made to produce an integrated theory which cuts across the boundaries of individual disciplines to bring together data from a wide range of sources within a single model of aggression. Examples of such efforts may be found in Owens & Ashcroft (1985) and Siann (1985), who also provide concise, readable reviews of different theoretical approaches. Although major disagreements about the nature of aggression are apparent, it seems likely that there are 'both biological and experiential factors that demonstrably affect aggressive behaviour' (Megargee & Hokanson 1970).

The implications of different theories can readily be observed in an examination of popular nursing and medical practices in psychiatric care (Karshmer 1978). For example, patients are often encouraged to ventilate their aggressive feelings by talking about them, by expressing them towards an inanimate object (for example, by hitting a pillow) or by partaking in physical exercise (such as going for a walk or playing table tennis). The underlying belief is that individuals can learn to dissipate their aggressive drive in an appropriate and acceptable fashion. The practice of housing 'disturbed' patients together in a locked ward or unit would be challenged by a social learning theorist, who would consider that such a policy amounts to the continued modelling of aggressive behaviour. Although it is important that the psychiatric nurse should possess sufficient knowledge of the different influential theories of aggression to allow an understanding of the theoretical bases of intervention strategies, the assumptions behind many nursing approaches have been neither clearly articulated nor subjected to any real critical assessment by practitioners.

AGGRESSIVE AND VIOLENT BEHAVIOUR BY PATIENTS: SOME SUGGESTED CAUSES

It may be useful to examine some possible explanations of violent behaviour by patients within three broad areas: mental disorder, environmental conditions and staff attitudes and behaviour.

Mental disorder

A review of research into the relationship between violent behaviour and psychiatric disorder appears in Howells (1982), who notes that 'virtually every category of mental illness has, at some time, been seen as causing violent behaviour'. Most of the work in this area has been concerned with criminal offenders but as they are unrepresentative of the general population who commit aggressive acts, it is difficult to draw reliable conclusions.

In a study of violent incidents at Tooting Bec Hospital, Fottrell (1979) found that schizophrenia was the most common psychiatric diagnosis of patients involved in incidents. However, as Hodgkinson et al (1984) point out, if associations are to be made between psychiatric diagnosis and the frequency of violent incidents, studies need to be designed to take into account the proportion of each diagnostic category in patient populations.

Some studies have associated paranoid ideas and violence (Howells 1982). McArthur (1972) drew attention to the perceptual distortions that may lead to misinterpretation of situations by psychotic patients, and hence to assaultive behaviour. Affective disorders may also predispose a patient to behave aggressively. Hypomanic excitability can result in a violent response if the activities of the sufferer are impeded. Depressed patients may commit assaults, but the difficulty in establishing a link between violent behaviour and depression lies in deciding whether the depression preceded the violent incident or was a guilt reaction to it. Organic conditions associated with changing levels of awareness, such as temporal lobe epilepsy and hypoglycaemia, have also been linked with violent behaviour, as have the effects of withdrawal from certain drugs.

The connection between violence and psychopathy is almost mythological. Although it has been claimed that the diagnosis of this condition presents few problems to the trained eye (Hood 1985), there can be no doubt that the notion of psychopathy has been beset with 'confusion and controversy of a philosophical, moral and clinical nature' (Howells 1982). Unfortunately, some nursing texts (e.g. Snell 1977, Darcy 1984) have tended to minimize or ignore the issues involved in the use of this diagnostic label. The definition of psychopathic disorder as 'a persistent disorder or disability of mind . . . which results in abnormally aggressive or seriously irresponsible conduct' (Mental Health Act 1983) gives rise to a circular process. Psychopathy is used as an explanation of aggressive behaviour, but aggression forms part of the definition of the disorder. However, clinical practice appears to confirm the existence of a minority of patients who exhibit persistently aggressive behaviour as part of a severely disordered personality, and who may pose great problems for nursing intervention.

Environmental conditions

It has been suggested that violent behaviour is more often 'the symptom of a disturbance in the hospital itself, rather than a symptom of a patient's particular mental state' (Harrington 1972); for 'environmental factors may be as important an antecedent to disruptive behaviour as is the individual's personality or his illness' (Weaver et al 1978). Studies into violent behaviour by patients in psychiatric settings (Brailsford & Stevenson 1973, Weaver et al 1978, Drinkwater & Feldman 1982, Armond 1982) suggest several environmental factors which may be influential in the instigation or continuation of aggression. However, in the absence of any systematic exploration and comparison of different ward environments, their relative impact remains unclear. It is therefore only possible to list tentatively some environmental factors which have been implicated by studies and the importance of which has been reinforced by the views and experiences of practitioners.

Low patient–staff ratio

A low patient–staff ratio can result in reduced levels of interaction opportunities and impede the observation and anticipation of changes in patient behaviour. Also, as Frost (1972) observed, patients are often afraid of their own violence, and badly staffed wards can act to increase this fear. Many mental hospital enquiry reports have drawn attention to the effects of staff shortages on nursing morale, and to how such situations are reflected in patient care (e.g. Ely Hospital Report 1969, Farleigh Hospital Report 1971).

Overcrowded wards

Ward overcrowding can create tension for patients and staff alike. Privacy is reduced and aggressive responses are more likely.

Unstructured time

The maintenance of a full programme of therapy, rehabilitation and occupation has been considered one of the most important factors in the prevention of violence. Drinkwater & Feldman's (1982) study supported this view in that they found a high number of incidents occurring when there were no planned ward activities.

Changes in physical surroundings

Armond (1982), in a study of a semi-secure ward of one psychiatric hospital, found that moving patients to different wards, and the administrative changes which were associated with such moves, caused psychological insecurity and an increase in the frequency of violence.

It is neither controversial nor surprising that an individual's environment can play a substantial part in influencing his or her behaviour. Psychiatric units often have particular environmental features which may increase the likelihood of aggressive reactions amongst their occupants. Many of the official inquiries into the alleged abuse of patients in hospitals serve to substantiate this view (e.g. Ely Hospital Report 1969, Farleigh Hospital Report 1971, South Ockendon Hospital Inquiry 1974).

Attitudes and behaviour of staff

A review of the aforementioned studies into violent behaviour provides some insight into the potential role of nurses and other staff in the generation of aggression. However, little work has been done in the analysis of staff–patient interaction. Hodgkinson (1980) considers that staff and patient behaviour have reciprocal effects, with staff responding to the anxieties caused by the disturbed behaviour of patients by over-control, which in turn can worsen the disturbance. Authoritarian attitudes on the part of nurses have been noted by patients (Raphael 1977) and staff alike. Brailsford & Stevenson (1973) undertook a survey, in two psychiatric hospitals, of views held by nursing and medical staff concerning factors related to violent and unpredictable behaviour. Staff attitudes were described as authoritarian, offhand, superior, tactless, inhuman, harsh, rigid and disrespectful. Inadequate direction and motivation by senior staff was also noted. It may be that nurses succumb to frustration due to lack of ward policy and a lack of praise and recognition of their work. However, the reliability of the data cannot be assessed, as no information about response rates is provided in the published report.

In a review of the few research studies of staff–patient interaction (generalizations from which are problematic due to a lack of comparability), Drinkwater (1982) notes that their main concern has been the frequency, rather than the content, of interactions. Taking up the suggestion made in these studies that staff spend more time interacting with each other and in administrative work than in contact with patients, Drinkwater (1982) speculates that extreme behaviour such as violence may be the most effective way of gaining staff attention. Weaver et al (1978) have suggested that sedating or physically restraining a patient may result in the inadvertent reinforcement by the nurse of an aggressive act. Such management of an incident, although apparently unpleasant for the patient, may provide him with the attention, concern and physical contact of which he may otherwise be deprived. In this way, aggressive behaviour may have beneficial rewards, in accordance with social learning theory.

Poor communication between members of staff can also contribute to the eruption of violence. There may be a failure to transmit important information to colleagues about a patient's mental state or other relevant circumstances. Admission policies can reveal the lack of adequate liaison between different disciplines. Brailsford & Stevenson (1973) suggested that patients were admitted regardless of the level and experience of nursing staff, and that nurses had too little influence in decisions involving the admission of potentially violent patients. This may be more an issue of disparities in power between professional groups than a simple communication problem. Nonetheless, the importance of a multi-disciplinary approach in the prevention and management of violence is a frequent theme in national guidelines (Department of Health and Social Security 1976, Confederation of Health Service Employees 1977). The failure by staff to keep patients informed about key aspects of treatment and policy can cause their feelings of fear and vulnerability to worsen, which may result in a violent incident.

PREVENTING VIOLENT BEHAVIOUR: A NURSING MODEL

Clearly, aggressive behaviour by patients is a complex phenomenon and is likely to be a combination of both intra- and interpersonal experiences and perceptions. Some potentially influential factors have been considered above. Drinkwater (1982) has suggested that violent behaviour in psychiatric hospitals is learned and can be environmentally controlled, with effective intervention being reliant on ward management policy. This indicates that future research should aim to identify aspects of psychiatric ward management that directly influence patient behaviour, and it is recommended that further studies be concerned with the content of staff–patient interaction, the attitudes of staff to violence, and styles of ward organisation and leadership. Such research would undoubtedly contribute to the overall understanding of why, and in what contexts, psychiatric patients may resort to violence; these insights seem crucial to effective prevention.

Must of the current guidance available to nurses on the prevention of violence, although potentially very helpful and practical, tends to be presented in a rather general and broad-based manner, failing to provide a systematic way of organizing knowledge about the patient as an individual. What seems to be needed for comprehensive, patient-centred, preventive nursing interventions is a framework whereby relevant information about the patient as an individual can be methodically collected and organized.

One of the most useful approaches to devising a theoretical model to help nurses understand and prevent violent behaviour, is offered by Boettcher (1983). This model is built on the premise that a number of basic human needs must be fulfilled if an individual is to remain psychologically healthy. If any of these needs are either partially or totally unmet, the individual experiences (either consciously or unconsciously) a blocking or alteration of these needs, which causes anxiety and stress. How people respond to this process depends on their 'repertoire of coping behaviour' (Boettcher 1983), and this might include resorting to violence. According to this theory, nursing intervention involves the collection of data relevant to patients' altered needs and usual responses to such a state. Boettcher provides a needs-assessment tool related to violent behaviour, to assist in establishing nursing diagnoses. Nine basic human needs are indicated (see Table 35.1) with examples of typical

Table 35.1   A needs-assessment tool (Based on Boettcher 1983)

Territoriality	Need for personal space and privacy
Communication	Need to talk with another person
Self-esteem	Need to have respect from others, and freedom from stigma and humiliation
Safety/security	Need for protection from harm
Autonomy	Need to make one's own decisions and to have control over one's own life
Own time	Need to be able to move at one's own pace
Personal identity	Need to retain personal belongings
Comfort	Need to be free from pain, hunger, thirst, excessive heat/cold, etc.
Cognitive understanding	Need to be aware of one's surroundings and to be free from confusion

aggressive responses by patients to the alteration of each need.

Using this assessment tool, it is clear that such needs can be infringed by each, or a combination, of the factors already discussed.

Mental disorder

Cognitive functioning and perceptual processes are adversely affected in many psychotic illnesses, with implications for individual awareness and interpretation of the environment. Alcohol and drug abuse can similarly affect cognitive processes. Psychiatric disorders can also reduce a patient's ability to communicate, whilst the stigma of mental illness has implications for self-esteem.

Environmental conditions

The physical organization of facilities can lead to overcrowding and the virtual abolition of privacy; the very act of hospitalization, especially if compulsory, reduces autonomy. Hospital routine and institutional 'rules' often have little regard for an individual's 'own time' or personal identity. Visiting regulations may reduce communication with relatives and friends, whilst staff shortages have implications for nurse–patient contact.

Attitudes and behaviour of staff

A patient's self-esteem and autonomy can be further reduced by the attitudes and behaviour of members of staff. Some impingement on privacy may be justifiable for the therapeutic purposes of observation, but thoughtless actions such as failing to knock on the door to a patient's room before entry encroach on the patient's privacy unjustifiably. Dismissive, patronizing or authoritarian attitudes shown by members of staff may serve to compound communication difficulties, and injure an individual's self-esteem. Insensitivity to the powerlessness and low status of the patient within a controlling environment is also an affront to needs fulfillment.

Other factors within an individual's personal circumstances may contribute to altering needs. Each patient has a unique history of coping strategies and interpersonal events which will precede his contact with the nurse and which may be central to present circumstances. Each patient seems to require individual assessment, with special attention to any stressful events that can prevent fulfillment of basic human needs, before preventive nursing interventions are possible. Boettcher claims that the combined use of the nursing process and the theoretical model based on altered needs 'can provide the nurse with a methodology to reduce the incidence of violence in health care settings' (Boettcher 1983). Her model provides a useful method of structuring both nursing assessment and intervention, which can facilitate the understanding of aggressive behaviour and contribute to its prevention and management.

It could be argued that a theoretical model based on needs theory, in conjunction with patient-centred nursing strategies, presents an explanation of aggressive behaviour which essentially locates the problem within the patient. Existing guidelines on the prevention and management of violence have been subjected to similar criticism (Hodgkinson 1980). However, one of the basic premises of Boettcher's model is that such behaviour involves both intra- and interpersonal events. Such an approach offers a means by which a wide range of factors that have been implicated in causing aggressive behaviour can be integrated to provide a working hypothesis. It seems to increase awareness of what makes patients feel and act in a violent way, and to safeguard against traditional, simplistic explanations of patient behaviour.

PREDICTION OF A VIOLENT EPISODE

Another important question is whether there are common warning signs that the nurse can pick up and act upon before a violent act occurs. Moran (1984) refers to indications that tension, fear, hostility, frustration or stress are building up; he lists muscular tension, twitching, pacing, jerkiness, change in the voice pitch and increased respiration rate as possible signals of aggression. Harrington (1972) considers that signs are not always obvious, and tend to be unique to any particular individual. Thus, the key to predicting violence is knowledge of the patient, and experience in developing predictive skills. Harrington points out that it is common for patients to give a verbal warning of their violent intent, and it is unwise to dismiss this as a simple threat.

MANAGEMENT OF VIOLENT BEHAVIOUR

There is considerable agreement among practitioners that, no matter how skilful nurses may be in preventive intervention, there will remain a level of violence committed by patients that resists prediction and prevention. One Canadian study points to the apparent existence of 'a core of incidents which are not preventable because they are unprovoked, unpremeditated outbursts' (Phillips 1977). Other authors reach similar conclusions (Harrington 1972, Penningroth 1975). Many nurses would agree with McArthur (1972) who asserts that 'psychiatric nurses throughout the hospital service accept as an occupational hazard the possibility of being on the receiving end of a violent attack'. Such a belief has lead to an understandable emphasis, especially over the last fifteen years, on the need for practical guidance as to how incidents can be managed as well as prevented.

Most psychiatric units now have some form of written policy concerned with the prevention and management of violent behaviour by patients, some of which are based on the guidelines devised by national bodies (National Association for Mental Health 1971, Royal College of Psychiatrists and the Royal College of Nursing 1972, Department of Health and Social Security 1976, Confederation of Health Service Employees 1977).

Most documents emphasize that the decision to restrain a patient physically should only be made as a last resort. Although they vary widely in detail and emphasis, written guidelines attempt to describe techniques that are both effective and safe for patients and staff. The central difficulty, due to the uniqueness of every incident, is that no one formula exists that will be adequate for all incidents. The frequent reference to the need to use 'the minimum force necessary' has been criticized for its failure to provide sufficiently precise guidance to the many nurses who are not trained in physical restraint (Drinkwater 1982).

Some principles of incident management

The objective in the therapeutic control of violence is to help the violent patient effect self-control while at the same time protecting him, other patients, and staff from injury' (Penningroth 1975)

Whilst recognizing the futility of attempting to produce a definitive statement on 'the management of the violent incident', a number of principles can be derived from the available literature.

Many incidents can be averted by talking to the patient on the verge of aggressive behaviour. Lion et al (1972) and Anders (1977) offer helpful phrases which the nurse can use to acknowledge the patient's hostile feelings and offer him the chance to talk rather than act upon them, whilst reassuring the patient that he will not be allowed to lose control. For example, saying to a patient, 'I'm going to stop you from hitting anybody with that chair — put it down and let's talk it over — you seem really angry' (Lion et al 1972), can defuse a situation. If an attack appears inevitable, or is already in process, shouting loudly at the patient to stop can be effective.

No attempt should be made to deal alone with an incident, unless this is completely unavoidable. Assistance can be summoned in a number of ways: shouting for help, asking another patient to summon other members of staff, or using the appropriate alarm call or emergency procedure.

Other patients should be asked to leave the area, both to ensure their safety and to prevent a possible escalation of the incident.

Organization and cooperation are crucial when help arrives. A numerical 'show of force' can be effective in preventing the instigation or continuation of an attack (Rusk 1970, Packham 1978), but for some patients, such confrontation would provoke an incident. The nurse who knows the patient best should take charge of the situation and instruct the team to either stay, or be at hand but out of sight of the patient.

The discreet removal of any potentially dangerous item is advisable. This includes potential weapons (such as a pen) and anything worn by the nurse (for example, a watch) which could damage a patient during restraint.

If physical restraint is unavoidable, the nurse in charge should designate each nurse to gain control of a particular limb of the patient, with one team member responsible for controlling the head to protect the patient's airway. Clothing, in preference to limbs, should be held in restraint; when limbs are grasped, they should be held near a major joint to reduce leverage and the danger of the patient sustaining a fracture or dislocation.

It is dangerous to apply pressure to the patient's abdomen, chest, throat or neck.

Placing the patient face down on the floor reduces leverage and aids immobilization.

Whenever possible, another nurse should be designated to stay with and explain the situation to other patients, who may either be frightened or think that the patient is being assaulted by staff.

Once the patient is immobilized, a decision must be taken about immediate management. Staff should maintain their hold until the patient either voluntarily and convincingly ceases the attack, or is adequately sedated and/or secluded. Restraint applied rapidly and firmly can be comforting for a patient who feels frightened and out of control (Burrows 1984) and is a crucial psychiatric nursing skill.

More detailed techniques concerning the immobilization of patients in different situations are contained in many hospital procedure manuals, and readers should consult the policy relevant to the area in which they work. Some organizations, for example South East Thames Regional Health Authority, have produced films on the use of such techniques (*Nursing Times* 1977). Having a repertoire of basic skills in restraint can greatly increase the confidence of the psychiatric nurse. However, many nurses feel ill-prepared to deal with violent incidents, partly because of a lack of training opportunities to acquire and practise basic techniques of physical restraint.

Structured role play can be a particularly effective teaching method to enable nurses to obtain such skills (DiFabio & Ackerhalt 1978). Special hospital nurses have expressed concern about patient attacks and have called for more specific training in the techniques of control and restraint (*Nursing Times* 1985). The Ritchie Report (Department of Health and Social Security 1985) on the death of a patient at Broadmoor recommended that all special hospital staff should receive special training in the principles of safe restraint. Many nurses in secure hospitals have already completed the Home Office approved 'control and restraint' course.

Seclusion

Seclusion is the enforced isolation of a patient in a locked room and is another method of managing patients who are behaving in a violent manner. Many psychiatric units will have specifically-modified seclusion rooms devoid of anything with which the patient can either accidentally or intentionally harm himself. Seclusion is seen primarily as 'a means of dealing with severely disturbed behaviour where there is an immediate danger to the patient or others' (Royal College of Nursing Society of Psychiatric Nursing 1979). Normally, there are specific regulations governing the observation and retention of patients in seclusion, and nurses should familiarize themselves with the requirements of their particular hospital. The seclusion of a patient must be reviewed at regular and frequent intervals, and terminated as soon as the danger to himself or others has passed. Seclusion is a highly controversial technique (see e.g. Strutt et al 1980, Leopoldt 1985) and has been criticized on both moral and therapeutic grounds. There have been few studies of either the method employed or the rationale for the use of seclusion; at times its occurrence has doubtless been a reflection more of a poor patient–staff ratio than of therapeutic necessity.

Seclusion should be distinguished from 'time out' (an abbreviation of 'time out from positive reinforcement'), which is part of a behavioural programme whereby the patient is denied reinforcers following undesirable behaviour. As Thorpe (1980) notes, seclusion and time out may be confused, as social isolation is one of three possible procedures used in a time-out programme.

Post-incident procedures

The importance of post-incident procedures has also been frequently emphasized. Detailed recording and analysis should follow every incident, each of which can be a valuable learning experience for all involved; its management should be critically examined so that lessons may be learned in handling future situations.

DiFabio & Ackerhalt (1978) have suggested that staff avoid discussing the use of physical restraint, partly because of the emotiveness of the issue. In a later paper, DiFabio (1981) concluded, on the basis of interviewing a small group of nurses, that the use of restraint was a stressful experience. This was often because nurses failed to receive help in dealing with the intrapersonal conflicts involved. Post-incident meetings can be a valuable forum for staff support.

CONCLUSION

The role of the psychiatric nurse in the prevention and management of violent behaviour by patients appears to have developed greatly since the days when custodial care was considered an acceptable means of exercising control, and nurses were not expected to examine the factors related to violence or their own part in its generation. If psychiatric nursing is to distance itself from the use of 'ad hoc methods in an unplanned and unevaluated manner' (Altschul 1981), and from practices largely based on what Brooking (1985) has called 'ritual and routine', it needs to develop intervention strategies based on theoretical models. This

will involve the critical use of existing knowledge, and a research-based clarification and expansion of the nurse's role in a number of key areas, not the least of which is in the prevention and management of violence.

ACKNOWLEDGEMENTS

I wish to thank my former colleagues at the Nursing Research Unit, King's College, University of London for their comments and help in the preparation of this text.

REFERENCES

Altschul A T 1981 Issues in psychiatric nursing. In: Hockey L (ed) Current issues in nursing. Churchill Livingstone, Edinburgh, p 95–103

Anders R L 1977 When a patient becomes violent. American Journal of Nursing 77(7): 1144–1148

Armond A D 1982 Violence in the semi-secure ward of a psychiatric hospital. Medicine, Science and the Law 22(3): 203–209

Bandura A 1973 Aggression: a social learning analysis. Prentice-Hall, New Jersey

Bell G M 1955 A mental hospital with open doors. International Journal of Social Psychiatry 1: 42–48

Bluglass R 1978 Regional secure units and interim security for psychiatric patients. British Medical Journal 1: 489–493

Boettcher E G 1983 Preventing violent behaviour: an integrated theoretical model for nursing. Perspectives in Psychiatric Care 21(2): 54–58

Brailsford D S, Stevenson J 1973 Factors related to violent and unpredictable behaviour in psychiatric hospitals. Nursing Times 69(3) Jan 18: 9–11

Brooking J I 1985 Advanced psychiatric nursing education in Britain. Journal of Advanced Nursing 10: 455–468

Burrows R 1984 Nurses and violence. Nursing Times 80(4) January 25: 56–58

Casseem M 1984 Violence on the wards. Nursing Mirror 158 (21) May 23: 14–16

Confederation of Health Service Employees 1977 The management of violent or potentially violent patients. COHSE, Banstead

Darcy P T 1984 Theory and practice of psychiatric care. Hodder and Stoughton, London

Dell S 1980 Transfer of special hospital patients to the NHS. British Journal of Psychiatry 136: 222–234

Department of Health and Social Security 1976 The management of violent, or potentially violent, hospital patients, HC(76) 11. DHSS, London

Department of Health and Social Security 1985 Report to the Secretary of State for Social Services concerning the death of Mr Michael Martin at Broadmoor Hospital on 6th July 1984 (The Ritchie Report). DHSS, London

DiFabio S 1981 Nurses' reactions to restraining patients. American Journal of Nursing 81(5) May: 973–975

DiFabio S, Ackerhalt E J 1978 Teaching the use of restraint through role play. Perspectives in Psychiatric Care 16(5–6): 218–222

Dollard J, Doob L W, Miller N E, Mowrer O H, Sears R R 1939 Frustration and aggression. Yale University Press, New Haven

Drinkwater J 1982 Violence in psychiatric hospitals. In: Feldman P (ed) Developments in the study of criminal behaviour. Volume 2: Violence. Wiley, Chichester, pp 111–130

Drinkwater J M, Feldman M P 1982 Violent incidents in a British psychiatric hospital: a preliminary study. Unpublished manuscript. Department of Psychology, University of Birmingham. Quoted in: Drinkwater J 1982 Violence in psychiatric hospitals. In: Feldman P (ed) Developments in the study of criminal behaviour. Volume 2: Violence. Wiley, Chichester, pp 111–130

Ely Hospital Report: National Health Service 1969 Report of the Committee of Inquiry into allegations of ill-treatment of patients and other irregularities at the Ely Hospital, Cardiff, Cmnd 3975. HMSO, London

Farleigh Hospital Report: National Health Service 1971 Report of the Farleigh Hospital Committee of Inquiry, Cmnd 4557. HMSO, London

Fottrell E M 1979 A study of violent behaviour among psychiatric in-patients. Unpublished thesis submitted for degree of doctor of medicine of the National University of Ireland

Fox R 1982 The violent imagination. In: Marsh P, Campbell A (eds) Aggression and violence. Blackwell, Oxford, pp 6–26

Fromm E 1977 The anatomy of human destructiveness. Penguin, Harmondsworth

Frost M 1972 Violence in psychiatric patients. Nursing Times 68(24) June 15: 748–749

The General Nursing Council for England and Wales 1982 Training syllabus for the certificate of mental nursing. General Nursing Council, London

Harrington J A 1972 Hospital violence. Nursing Mirror 135(12) July 21: 12–13

Hodgkinson P E 1980 Psychological approaches to violence. Nursing Times 76(32) August 7: 1399–1401

Hodgkinson P, Hillis T, Russell D 1984 Assaults on staff in a psychiatric hospital. Nursing Times 80(16) April 18: 44–46

Home Office, Department of Health and Social Security 1975 Report of the Committee on Mentally Abnormal Offenders, Cmnd 6244. HMSO, London

Hood M 1985 New horizons. Mental Health Nursing Supplement. Nursing Times 81(12) March 20: 53–54

Howells K 1982 Mental disorder and violent behaviour. In: Feldman P (ed) Developments in the study of criminal behaviour. Volume 2: Violence. Wiley, Chichester, pp 163–200

Karshmer J F 1978 The application of social learning theory to aggression. Perspectives in Psychiatric Care 16(5/6): 223–227

Lancet Editorial 1976 Who's for the locked ward? Lancet 1: 461

Leopoldt H 1985 A secure and secluded spot. Nursing Times 81(6) Feb 6: 26–28

Lion J R, Levenberg L B, Strange R E 1972 Restraining the violent patient. Journal of Psychiatric Nursing and Mental Health Services 10(2): 9–11

Lorenz K 1966 On aggression. Methuen, London

McArthur C H 1972 Nursing violent patients under security restrictions. Nursing Times 68(28) July 13: 861–863

MacCulloch J 1977 Some problems of placing psychiatric patients. Health Trends 9: 59–62

Mandelbrote B 1958 An experiment in the rapid conversion of a closed mental hospital into an open-door hospital. Mental Hygiene 42: 3–16

Marsh P, Campbell A 1982 In: Marsh P, Campbell A (eds) Aggression and violence. Blackwell, Oxford, pp 1–5

Megargee E I, Hokanson J E 1970 The dynamics of aggression. Quoted in Boettcher E G 1978 Preventing violent behaviour: an integrated theoretical model for nursing. Perspectives in Psychiatric Care 21(2): 54–58

Mental Health Act 1983 HMSO, London

Moran J 1984 Response and responsibility. Nursing Times 80(14) April 4: 28–31

National Association for Mental Health (MIND) 1971 Guidelines for the care of patients who exhibit violent behaviour in mental and mental subnormality hospitals: a consultative document. MIND, London

New Encyclopaedia Britannica 1985 Macropaedia, 15th edn. 14: 715

Nursing Times 1977 News feature: Management of violence. Nursing Times 73(46) November 17: 1782–1783

Nursing Times 1984 RSUs face staffing problems (Report of Rcn Society of Psychiatric Nursing Conference). Nursing Times 80(23) June 6: 8

Nursing Times 1985 Assaults on staff prompt call for training (Report of Prison Officers Association Conference). Nursing Times 81(44) October 30: 8

Owens R G, Ashcroft J B 1985 Violence: a guide for the caring professions. Croom Helm, Beckenham

Packham H 1978 Managing the violent patient. Nursing Mirror 146(25) June 22: 17–20

Pattemore J C 1957 The development of a disturbed ward between 1937 and 1956. Nursing Times 53, January 18: 73–75

Penningroth P E 1975 Control of violence in a mental health setting. American Journal of Nursing 75(4) April: 606–609

Phillips M 1977 Aggression control in the psychiatric hospital. Dimensions in Health Service 54(3) March: 39–41

Psychiatric Nurses Association 1985 Editorial. Mental Health Nursing Supplement. Nursing Times 81(12) March 20: 50

Raphael W 1977 Psychiatric hospitals viewed by their patients, 2nd edn. King Edward's Hospital Fund, London

Royal College of Nursing Society of Psychiatric Nursing 1979 Seclusion and restraint in hospitals and units for the mentally disordered. Royal College of Nursing, London

Royal College of Psychiatrists and the Royal College of Nursing 1972 Joint report on the care of the violent patient

Rusk T N 1970 Psychiatric emergencies in medical practice. Survey of the literature and some proposals. Journal of Oklahoma State Medical Association 63, October: 483–494

Siann G 1985 Accounting for aggression. Allen and Unwin, London

Snell H 1977 Mental disorder: an introductory textbook for nurses. Allen & Unwin, London

South Ockendon Hospital Inquiry 1974 Report of the Committee of Inquiry into South Ockendon Hospital. HMSO, London

Storr A 1968 Human aggression. Penguin, Harmondsworth. Pelican Edition 1970

Strutt R, Bailey C, Peermohamed R, Forrest A J, Corton B 1980 Seclusion: can it be justified? Nursing Times 76(37) Sept 11: 1629–1633

Thorpe J G 1980 Time out or seclusion? Nursing Times 76(14) April 3: 604

Weaver S M, Broome A K, Kat B J B 1978 Some patterns of disturbed behaviour in a closed ward environment. Journal of Advanced Nursing 3: 251–263

Whitehead T 1976 Security and the locked ward. Health and Social Service Journal 86(4505) August 28: 1552

36

Substance abuse

K. Ferguson

INTRODUCTION

This chapter reviews the extent of substance abuse in the United Kingdom, some reasons why people take mood altering substances and why some of them develop problems. The nature of drug and alcohol abuse is examined, first by giving an overview of the broad classes of drugs and general problems of their abuse, and then looking more specifically at particular drugs. Treatment methods are discussed, moving from the initial stages of the client admitting there is a problem, and then motivating him towards goal setting, detoxification and rehabilitation. Controlled drinking is also discussed. In the third section, the variety of treatment settings for alcohol and drug abusers are described, including both statutory and non-statutory services, advice-giving agencies and residential establishments. Lastly, a number of special topics are covered, including drugs in pregnancy, child care and drug/alcohol abuse, and some of the issues surrounding prevention.

In many treatment settings and often in the literature, alcohol and drug abuse are dealt with separately. In practice, this division is often artificial — drugs may be substituted for alcohol and vice versa. Fundamentally, the use of either type of substance involves a search for an altered state, and many of the problems related to alcohol use, tobacco or even some prescribed drugs are the same as those experienced by users of 'hard' drugs. There are, however, additional problems with these drugs just by virtue of their illegality. For this reason, the subject of substance abuse is dealt with as a whole, and where 'drugs' is written, this usually applies to alcohol, unless specified.

PART 1 THE NATURE OF SUBSTANCE ABUSE — AN OVERVIEW

In almost every society through the ages, people have used substances which alter consciousness. In British culture a number of drugs are considered to be an integral part of society. They include alcohol, tobacco and caffeine. Huge numbers of mood-altering drugs are prescribed each year by doctors. There has been much concern recently about the increasing use of illegal drugs, particularly heroin.

People may use drugs at times of celebration and to intensify pleasure, or as a way of dealing with difficulties or painful emotions. Since drug use, then, is a central feature of society's way of coping, when is it that use of drugs becomes problematic? City Roads and Phoenix House Drug Resources Pack (1980) provides a helpful guide for work with clients . . .'When the individual's ability to function and handle living is handicapped by his drug use — in physical, social or psychological ways or a combination of these'.

However, the question of for whom the drug use is a problem can often cause dilemmas. It may be that it is the family, social workers, the law or society that considers there is primarily a problem. Society, too, may change its views towards different drugs and definitions of use and misuse over time.

CAUSES OF DRUG AND ALCOHOL ABUSE

There has been much research, mainly retrospective, into why some people develop drug and alcohol problems, and very little definite information has been found. Griffith Edwards, at the Addiction Research Unit, Institute of Psychiatry,

has studied this area. The important consideration is that the reasons for trying a drug and for continuing to use it may be very different (Edwards 1982). Although research so far cannot give us definite predictors for who is at risk of developing a drug problem, there are a number of possible factors to consider:

Personality factors

It may be difficult to distinguish cause from consequences of drug use. Initially, especially, curiosity and rebellion may play a part. People may take drugs to relieve shyness, boredom, stress, tension or frustration. There has been some research suggesting a genetic link for alcoholism (Cloniger et al 1981). Initial reasons for taking drugs may have 'burnt out', yet drug taking continues.

Social factors

Peer pressure seems to be important, especially early on. Inititation to illegal drugs, as to legal ones, is generally by sharing, contrary to media scare stories about 'pushers'. Use of the drug may be motivated by a feeling of wanting to be accepted or admired by the group. Social acceptability of drug taking within the individual's culture or ethnic group may be important, along with their attitudes to intoxication. People may voluntarily join certain subcultures where drug taking is common. Money and availability of drugs/alcohol affect consumption. Parental attitudes towards drink or drugs may 'shape' behaviour. Material factors, such as unemployment and poor housing, may lead to drug abuse.

The role of the agent

The pharmacological effects of the drug itself are important. The actual effect experienced depends on the individual, his past experience, mood, environment and expectations. Pleasant effects reinforce continued use.

There is, then, no typical misuser of drugs or alcohol, and no evidence of any uniform personality type who becomes an addict or who develops a drug or alcohol problem.

CLASSIFICATION

Drugs of misuse can broadly be divided into three categories:

1. central nervous system depressants, e.g. alcohol, barbiturates, benzodiazepines, opiates
2. central nervous system stimulants, e.g. amphetamines, cocaine, caffeine
3. drugs that alter perceptual function, e.g. cannabis and other hallucinogens.

Each group of drugs will be dealt with in more detail in a later section.

EXPLANATION OF TERMS

Drug dependence implies a compulsion to continue taking a drug, occurring after periodic or continued administration of the substance. It may consist of psychic and or physical elements; and it takes varying times to develop, depending on the individual, the drug, dosage and frequency of use.

Physical dependence occurs owing to the pharmacology of the drug. It is recognized by withdrawal symptoms on stopping the drug. The rate of development varies: for instance, opiates rapidly produce physical dependence. Some drugs are thought not to produce physical dependence e.g. amphetamines, cocaine, solvents.

Psychological dependence refers to the desire or compulsive need to continue taking the drug, either for its pleasant effects or to avoid unpleasant effects. This need may be very powerful, causing the individual to focus all his interest on future supplies, perhaps at the expense of family, food or work. It may lead to a dramatic change in life-style, and possible antisocial behaviour in order to obtain the drug. It is manifested by 'craving', i.e. an intense desire, only met by the substance.

Withdrawal effects are the body's reaction to sudden absence of a drug to which it has become adapted. They are a sign of physical dependence.

Tolerance refers to the ability of the body to deal with larger doses of the drug, so the individual requires higher doses to achieve the same effects. This may develop quickly or slowly. Tolerance may be rapidly lost after detoxification in hospital or prison, and resumption of use at the previous level of consumption may be fatal.

A 'problem drug taker' is any person who experiences social, psychological or physical problems as a result of drinking or drug taking to excess, or in inappropriate situations, or when the effect puts himself or others at risk or harm.

Polydrug abuse is abuse of more than one drug by an individual, and is relatively common. A person may abuse a variety of drugs from different groups, e.g. amphetamines, cocaine and cannabis; or a person may, in times of shortage of his main drug of abuse, substitute with another drug from the same group, which has similar properties, e.g. diazepam and alcohol, opiates and codeine linctus.

SOME GENERAL COMPLICATIONS OF DRUG OR ALCOHOL ABUSE

Many people who use drugs do not get into difficulties, experiencing instead feelings of well-being, increased alertness, relaxation. However, each drug carries its own risks, and it will become clear that, as nurses, we cannot only be guided by the legal restrictions. This section deals with some general problems of drug/alcohol abuse — physical, social and emotional. The individual drugs are dealt with in the next section.

Physical complications

Taking too much of a drug may be a problem, with the risk of overdose or accidents when intoxicated. With continued use and dependency, normal functioning may be impaired. The person may neglect himself, drugs becoming the main priority. Malnourishment and general deterioration in life-style may lead to secondary illness.

There are risks associated with injecting drugs, especially where dirty needles are shared, procedures are not sterile or tablets are crushed for injection. Risks include abcesses, gangrene, collapsed veins, hepatitis B, HIV infection, endocarditis, thrombophlebitis. The injection process itself may increase chances of dependency because of the immediate gratification of the experience, as the drug rapidly enters the body. With taking any illicit drug, there is the danger of adulteration. For example, heroin has been combined with brick dust. The identity of the drug can easily be mistaken, the strengths are unknown and the effects unpredictable, increasing the chances of accidental overdose. These dangers are particularly relevant where drugs are injected, and thus rapidly absorbed into the bloodstream.

Polydrug misuse is common, and the user may be unaware of the combined effects of various drugs. For example, a combination of diazepam and alcohol may be fatal at sufficient dosage. Most drugs affect motor control to some extent, and so decrease efficiency and make risk of accidents at work, on the road or in the home more likely. Individual reactions to drugs vary, depending on body weight, sex difference, physical and personality differences.

Psychological complications

People may experience psychological problems as a result of their drug taking or dependency, or drugs may be taken to mask psychological problems — 'self-medication'. Taking drugs may function to block out painful emotions such as sadness, anger, frustration. The drugs numb the pain and so the maladaptive way of coping is reinforced. Drug taking may alleviate feelings of severe anxiety, either generalized or specific, thus giving a false sense of security or confidence. Inability to cope with these feelings without drugs may precipitate relapse. Denial that there is a problem, both to oneself and to others, and rationalization are common psychological mechanisms manifested in addicted persons. Relatives of drug users may describe a 'change in personality' since addiction. Drugs now are the major preoccupation. The family may describe severe mood swings, such as extreme irritability, social withdrawal and possibly aggressive outbursts. Depressed mood is a relatively common feature among addicts, but may be related to the drinking/drug taking, or indeed a reason for starting. Depression is easier to assess after detoxification. Some stimulants and hallucinogens may cause an acute anxiety reaction in certain predisposed individuals or after heavy continued use. Conversely, certain individuals who suffer from psychosis may try to 'dampen down' their symptoms by using alcohol or drugs.

Social complications

It must be remembered that there are many addicts who lead relatively stable lives. However, there are a number of social problems which may arise from heavy alcohol or drug use, and these in turn may lead to stigmatization, lack of trust, loss of reputation, and so confirmation in the role of addict. Work troubles may be the first sign of a problem developing — sickness, inefficiency, indiscretion, poor judgement, unreliability. With time, the person may become unemployable owing to his poor work record, and so drift down the social scale. There may also be lack of educational qualifications or training if the problem starts early in life. Housing problems may occur owing to the strain of maintaining the addiction on a person's budget. Eventually, other addicts may be the only group he can identify with and membership of the subculture itself in turn reinforces dependency. Many addicts and their families suffer from financial problems. Bills and debts may accumulate, household items may be pawned. With a worsening habit, the addict may eventually be forced into illegal activities. A heroin habit requires a good deal of money to support it, so that crime and prostitution are common.

Drug use and crime

Possession of certain drugs is itself illegal. Many addicts will supply drugs in order to fund their own habit at the risk of quite severe sentences. Offences may be committed while the individual is in a state of intoxication, e.g. violent or sexual crimes, motoring offences. In some cases, however, crime may predate dependence. With increasing severity of addiction, a person tends to mix more with other drug takers or heavy drinkers, becoming alienated from the mainstream of society. Leaving behind the ties of the subculture and re-entering society can be among the most difficult elements of staying off drugs.

Effects on the family and relationships

Dependence on alcohol or drugs may have an intense effect on significant others. The family may suffer social isolation, unpredictable crises, practical problems, emotional strain, arguments and possible aggression and violence. Edwards (1982) describes a number of ways in which the family or friends may cope. They may try to hide the problem, becoming isolated and depressed. They may respond by fear or anger, punishing the person verbally or physically. The family may avoid contact with the addicted member; at the extreme, the partners may separate. Other possible ways of coping are attempts at manipulation, such as embarassing the person, making threats or imposing sanctions. The addict's family may 'mother' him, shielding the individual from the consequences of his behaviour. The partner may take on all the responsibilities of the household — working, paying bills, looking after the family. She may seek help from the general practitioner or from an agency such as Al Anon, a self-help group for relatives of alcoholics. She may attempt in a variety of ways to persuade the addict to seek help.

EFFECTS AND COMPLICATIONS OF SPECIFIC DRUGS

Alcohol

Over 90% of adults in the UK take alcohol. It is an integral part of our culture and customs. However, 6% of men and 1% of women are taking more than the medically safe limit, and there is evidence of the problem increasing (Wilson 1980). Alcoholic drinks are now more widely available and the price has dropped relatively over the past 30 years. There are believed to be at least 75 000 alcoholics in the UK and twice as many people with drink problems.

Alcohol is usually measured in 'units'.

Beverage	One unit
Fortified wine	one glass
Average beer	1/2 pint
Cider	1/2 pint
Spirits	1 measure
Table wine	1 glass

How much is too much?

1. More than 28 units for women and 40 units for men per week

2. Drinking every day
3. More than 5 units per hour.

Drinking may be orderly or chaotic, continuous or intermittent.

Immediate effects of alcohol

Increased heart rate, flushing, diminished control, decreased inhibitions, coordination, judgement, memory and performance. Alcohol may cause relaxation and joviality. Intoxication causes slurring, lability of emotion and possibly aggressiveness, staggering, blurred vision, loss of balance and eventual loss of consciousness. In very high doses, alcohol may cause coma and death.

Complications of heavy alcohol use

Dependence. Physical and psychological dependence may occur. The 'alcohol dependence syndrome' is characterized by:

1. narrowing of drinking repertoire — drinking only for the relief of withdrawals, difficulty in choosing to abstain.
2. preoccupation with alcohol — becomes a priority which increases with time.
3. increasing tolerance, cross tolerance with other CNS depressants. With liver damage, tolerance is eventually lost.
4. repeated withdrawals. Frequency and severity increases.
5. relief drinking to avoid withdrawals — an attempt to maintain steady blood alcohol level.
6. subjective awareness of a complusion to drink.
7. tendency for recurrence after abstinence (Royal College of Psychiatrists 1979).

Withdrawal effects

Mild or moderate symptoms may occur in the first two to three days. Symptoms range from tremor, sweatiness, tachycardia, nausea and vomiting to agitation, tremor, disorientation and hallucinations. If withdrawal is severe, the patient may experience convulsions or delirium tremens. Withdrawal fits may occur from 12 hours to several days after stopping drink. These are grand mal convulsions of which one third develop into delirium tremens. Detoxification as an inpatient is advisable after one episode of grand mal fit.

Delirium tremens can occur after abstinence following years of heavy drinking. It may be undiagnosed initially. This is a fluctuating condition, generally worsening at night, recognized by delirium and disorientation in time, place and person. Tremor may be mild or severe. The patient experiences vivid and bizarre hallucinations of any sense, e.g. smelling gas, seeing snakes. He may experience paranoid unsystematized delusions. The patient is restless and overactive, sweaty, with a fever and decreased appetite. There is a risk of dehydration and exhaustion. Between 1% and 5% of cases are fatal.

Liver disease

Twenty-five per cent of alcohol abusers of 20 years duration suffer from cirrhosis. Alcohol has a toxic effect, causing scarring and disorganization of tissue. There is diminished functioning of the liver, disturbance of metabolism and eventual liver failure. Oesophageal varices may occur owing to damming of liver blood vessels. Death may result from haemorrhage. Alcoholic hepatitis may develop, where the liver becomes inflamed. Symptoms are jaundice, nausea, anorexia, fever, swollen liver and ascites. Ten per cent of cases are fatal. 'Fatty liver' is a reversible condition arising from heavy alcohol use, where the liver becomes swollen and tender. Cancer of the liver may follow cirrhosis.

Malnutrition

This may result partly from general self-neglect and the drain of alcohol on finances. Alcohol abuse also causes anorexia, nausea, vomiting, malabsorption and diarrhoea. The alcohol abuser may be obese yet malnourished — alcohol is a source of empty calories.

Brain damage

Lack of thiamine in the diet may cause Wernicke's syndrome. It is recognized by weakness, tingling and pain in the legs, confusion, double vision, staggering, stupor and uncoordinated eye movements; 15–20% of cases are fatal. Korsakoff's syndrome is a residual defect in 5–10% of chronic alcoholics, manifested as loss of memory and confabulation. Alcoholic dementia may occur with chronic alcoholism. Onset is insidious. The person shows signs of personal deterioration and may be aggressive. There is no known cure.

Acute intoxication may lead to aggression and lack of coordination, drowsiness and increased chance of accidents. Death may occur from inhalation of vomit or respiratory depression. Head injuries are common. Amnesia or blackouts are often an indication of a serious drink problem. Transient hallucinations may occur during heavy drinking bouts or during withdrawal (alcoholic hallucinosis). These hallucinations may last weeks or months. Crimes may occasionally be committed during automatized behaviour while intoxicated. This is known as a 'fugue state'.

Alimentary disease. Gastrointestinal symptoms are common, from oesophagitis, gastritis, dyspepsia and ulcers. Pancreatitis is also relatively common, either acute, with sudden abdominal pain and vomiting which may be fatal, or chronic with repeated bouts of low grade pain. Complications are diabetes and malnutrition.

Cancer of the mouth, tongue and larynx are common. Heavy drinkers are often heavy smokers.

Chest conditions, e.g. pneumonia, tuberculosis, abcesses, also have a higher incidence in alcoholics.

Hypoglycaemia can occur. This may be fatal, often because not recognized, especially in the context of heavy drinking.

Peripheral neuropathy (neuritis). Because of vitamin B deficiency there may be degeneration of motor and sensory nerves of the limbs, causing tingling and numbness.

Impotence and subfertility. Heavy alcohol intake reduces secretion of testosterone, decreases libido and may cause impotence. Recovery is variable.

Potentiation of other drugs, e.g. antidepressants, other CNS depressants.

Cardiac abnormalities such as congestive cardiac failure and hypertension may result from alcoholism, as may haematological disorders such as anaemia and macrocytosis. Gout may develop where joints become painful and swollen intermittently owing to high blood uric acid levels.

Barbiturates

These drugs are now much less available on the illicit market, due to a reduction in the prescribing of barbiturates (Osselton et al 1984). The wide availability of these drugs in the 1960s caused many problems. Since January 1985, they have been controlled under the Misuse of Drugs Act. Barbiturates may be taken orally or intravenously.

Effects

Medically, these drugs are used in general anaesthesia and for epilepsy. They are also used as sedatives and hypnotics (for sleep). Effects are comparable to those of alcohol, and, similarly, they produce tolerance and physical and psychological dependence. Chronic barbiturate intoxication causes slurring of speech, aggression, fall in blood pressure, cyanosis and sleepiness. These drugs have a low fatal dose and in the 1960s, were responsible for many fatal accidental overdoses, due especially to the potentiation of their effects by other CNS depressants such as alcohol. Many of the problems of long-term barbiturates use are secondary to the often chaotic life-style of the user. There are also the risks associated with injection of drugs.

Withdrawal effects

These are similar to those of alcohol, and likewise there is a risk of grand mal convulsions if withdrawal is too rapid. With short-acting barbiturates, fits may occur in the first two days after withdrawal, and with the long-acting drugs anytime up to 10 days after stopping them.

Benzodiazepines (minor tranquillizers)

These are the most commonly prescribed drugs in the UK. They replaced barbiturates in the 1960s, in the belief that they were non-addictive. Many prescriptions are long-term 'repeats' (Haddon 1984). One in seven people take tranquillizers at some time through the year, and one in 40 people take them all year round. Women are twice as likely to be prescribed these drugs (Batt et al 1974). Benzodiazepines do have a street value on the black market, and are often abused by polydrug users.

At present, minor tranquillizers are not controlled under the Misuse of Drugs Act, so that it is not illegal to supply or possess them without a prescription.

Effects

This group of drugs sedate and relieve symptoms of anxiety. They cause relaxation of the muscles and are also used as anticonvulsants. Some benzodiazepines are used as sleeping tablets. Effects resemble those of alcohol, and the two drugs are interchangeable: 15 mg of diazepam is equivalent to approximately one quarter bottle of whisky (Haddon 1984).

Side-effects

Benzodiazepines cause diminished alertness and performance, affecting ability to drive and to operate machinery. Sleeping tablets may cause a hangover effect, and depression and double vision are common side-effects. Large doses may decrease inhibition, causing irritability and aggression. Sedation and death may result from overdose, especially if taken in combination with other CNS depressants. With regular use, there is tolerance and physical and psychological dependence. After only 2 weeks, benzodiazepines lose their effectiveness for insomnia, and after 4 months become ineffective for anxiety. It seems, therefore, that prescribing a low dose of benzodiazepines for a short period has maximum beneficial effect.

Withdrawal effects

These effects are similar to those of alcohol: anxiety, apprehension, weakness, tremor, irritability, craving, insomnia, vomiting, restlessness, breathlessness, sweating, dry mouth, raised heart rate and blood pressure. Withdrawal symptoms may be quite severe. These drugs must be tapered off slowly because of the risk of convulsions.

Solvents and gases

There is a huge range of possible substances of abuse in this group, most of which are common household products. There are no national and few local surveys on solvent abuse. Fieldwork reports suggest that it is common in local areas for short periods, especially among 13–15 year old boys mainly on an experimental level (Merrill 1985). The method of use depends on the substance. Glue may be put in a bag, fluids soaked in a rag, and the vapours of the solvent then breathed in. Solvent abuse is not subject to drugs legislation at present, although convictions may be made for disorderly behaviour or crimes committed while intoxicated.

Effects

In some respects the effects are similar to those to alcohol. The person experiences drunkenness, dizziness and blurred vision; he may stagger, be giggly, have glazed eyes or be drowsy. Solvent abusers describe 'dream-like visions', which may be unpleasant. The effect is rapid and may last from a few minutes to half an hour, depending on the chemical used. There may be a mild hangover afterwards.

Hazards of use

There is insufficient research in the UK to assess the extent of risk for the solvent user. Deaths do occur, however, some of which may be preventable. American research shows that aerosols are much more toxic to the individual than glues (Bass 1970) and that deaths often occur from suffocation, choking on vomit or accidents while intoxicated. Heart failure may occur, especially with aerosols and cleaning fluids. Long-term users may develop sores around the mouth, chest pain, breathlessness, chest infections, weight loss,

decreased concentration, depression and possibly kidney damage (Francis et al 1982). Tolerance develops with frequent use.

Dependence is mainly psychological, but can be quite severe. It seems that the majority of solvent abusers 'grow out of it', and that it is mainly a group activity of children and teenagers. A minority, however, persist in use and become 'lone sniffers' or move on to other drugs (Melville 1984).

Opiates

In the past few years there has been much concern about the rise in misuse of narcotics. Research has suggested that Home Office statistics are a fivefold underestimate of the problem (Drug Indicators Project 1984). There has been an increase in heroin seizures and in convictions for drug offences since the 1980s (Home Office 1985). Generally, it seems the drug is more widely available and is becoming increasingly 'normalized'. 'Chasing the dragon', or smoking heroin, has become more common and is aesthetically less of a problem to people than injecting.

The stronger opiates are controlled under the Misuse of Drugs Act 1971, class A. Other, milder analgesics such as dihydrocodeine tablets are only class B. Cough medicines and similar preparations may be on prescription only or have no controls at all.

Most of the different types of opiates are available on the black market. It is the responsibility of doctors to notify the Home Office if they see a patient whom they consider or suspect is dependent on certain drugs, including some opiates. Home Office records are used for statistical purposes and also to aid in the diagnosis of addiction. (DHSS 1984).

Effects

As well as their analgesic effect, opiates cause a sensation of drowsy euphoria, warmth and well-being. Libido and desire for food is decreased. The cough reflex is depressed, respirations and heart rate decreased, blood vessels dilated and the bowel slows down. In intoxication, pupils are pinpointed and, in withdrawal, dilated. There may be nausea and vomiting with initial use. Length of effect varies. Heroin lasts 2–3 hours. The effect of methadone which is a synthetic preparation and is available orally, lasts up to 12 hours.

With prolonged use, tolerance develops. Development of physical and psychological dependence is quite rapid, although people may use heroin relatively infrequently over quite long periods. Dependence is not inevitable. Along with dependence, there may be many physical, psychological and social problems. The drug itself does not do physical damage to the body, but complications are secondary and are usually due to injection practices and to the life-style of the addict. Ovulation is suppressed, but accidental pregnancies may occur during times of shortage of drugs. Dangers of intoxication are accidents, coma and death. Opiates potentiate the action of other CNS depressants.

Withdrawal effects

Opiates act on the synapses of the central nervous system, so that withdrawal causes overactivity of the sympathetic system. Heroin withdrawal starts 8–24 hours after the last dose. It is characterized by aches, tremor, sweating, chills, sneezing, yawning, muscle spasms, insomnia, gooseflesh, dilated pupils, anorexia, rhinorrhoea, abdominal cramps, possibly vomiting and diarrhoea, and intense craving for the drug.

Amphetamines

These drugs were commonly prescribed in the 1960s as slimming pills and antidepressants, and were widely available on the black market. They are now less widely prescribed, but there is evidence from fieldwork reports nationally of a rise in the illicit manufacture of amphetamine sulphate since the late 1970s, and misuse is prevalant among young people in some areas. Amphetamines are controlled under the Misuse of Drugs Act 1971, either in class B, or, if intravenous, in class A. Some of the milder amphetamine-type drugs are not controlled, but are available on prescription only. The drug may be sniffed, taken in tablet form or intravenously.

Short-term effects

Amphetamines cause arousal, increased heart rate and respirations, dilated pupils, decreased fatigue, increase in alertness, confidence and energy. Appetite is diminished and, with continued use, there is weight loss. The person is excitable, restless, talkative, possibly irritable and suffers from insomnia, dry mouth and sweating. Some general practitioners still prescribe appetite suppressants, which have similar effects but which would have to be taken in larger doses to achieve the same stimulation.

Hazards and long-term effects

Tolerance may develop, but is not inevitable. With regular use, there is psychological addiction, but no recognized physical withdrawal symptoms, although the person will feel lethargic, hungry, depressed and sleepy. Amphetamines may cause paranoia, hallucinations and delusions. This has been described as 'amphetamine psychosis', and it generally improves on stopping the drug. Long-term use may be quite debilitating owing to lack of food and sleep, causing general ill health. Complications may arise from injection practices and also from buying the drug on the black market. There may be skin effects such as picking of skin or nails.

Cocaine

This used to be a relatively rare and expensive drug, used mainly by a small rich sector. A rise in cocaine misuse happened in North America in the early 1980s, followed by increased use in the UK (Home Office 1985). Cocaine is controlled under the Misuse of Drugs Act, class A. Routes of ingestion are by sniffing, injecting or 'free-basing', i.e. heating and inhaling the fumes.

Effects

These include arousal, euphoria, decreased appetite and fatigue, feelings of increased physical strength and mental capacity. It is a local anaesthetic. In large doses, there may be agitation, anxiety and possibly hallucinations.

Hazards of use

There are complications due to illegality of the drug, and secondary to injection. There may be deterioration in life-style and self-care with continued heavy use. The individual may become restless, paranoid, hyperexcitable and anorexic with unpleasant skin sensations. Repeated sniffing damages the lining of the nose and the structure separating the nostrils. There are no significant physical withdrawal symptoms, although lethargy, hunger and depression (possibly severe) may be experienced. Cocaine, however, is psychologically reinforcing, causing severe craving and the tendency to increase the dose.

Caffeine

Tea and coffee drinking is pervasive throughout society. Caffeine is also available in soft drinks and in some analgesics. Caffeine allays drowsiness and fatigue, and increases performance and alertness. Large doses impair performance, causing anxiety, restlessness, insomnia, gastro-intestinal complaints, headaches and tremor. Dependence is mainly psychological, but drowsiness and irritability are likely on cessation of taking caffeine.

Tobacco

Forty-five per cent of men and 34% of women smoke cigarettes, one fifth of men and one tenth of women smoking more than 20 per day (General Household Survey 1982). There are some restrictions on the use of tobacco, such as age limits for sale, taxation and restricted advertising. Nicotine is a mild stimulant. Short-term effects are almost immediate and rapidly decline, contributing to the attraction and frequency of use. Nicotine causes arousal and maintains performance, but is also used to decrease stress and anxiety. Long-term effects include rapid and marked tolerance, physical and psychological dependence. Withdrawal is characterized by irritability, restlessness, hunger and strong craving. Cigarette smoking is correlated with lung infections, cardiovascular diseases, cancer of the lung, throat and mouth, and stomach ulcers. There are 100 000 premature deaths each year due to smoking, the likelihood increasing with number of cigarettes smoked, number of years of smoking and the earlier the person started. Ex-smokers can regain normal health and life expectancy if they stop smoking before there is irreparable damage.

Cannabis

This drug has the greatest non-medical use out of those controlled under the Misuse of Drugs Act. In 1982 a nationwide survey found that 5% of 16-year-olds and over had used cannabis, and large numbers of people use the drug on a regular basis, (Mott 1985). Cannabis accounts for 80–90% of all drug seizures. The psychoactive ingredient in cannabis is tetrahydro-cannabinol (THC). Cannabis may be eaten, or smoked by itself or with tobacco.

Effects

Short-term effects include hilarity, relaxation, talkativeness, increased appreciation of sound, colour and music. With intoxication, concentration, dexterity and intellectual functioning are decreased. There may be perceptual distortions, memory impairment, hunger and thirst. The effects last from one to several hours, depending on the dose taken and route of ingestion. There is no hangover as such, except possible tiredness. Inexperienced users may experience magnification of unpleasant feelings such as depression, anxiety, feelings of paranoia.

There is no conclusive evidence of any lasting physical or mental damage, but there have been few studies of users over long periods of time. It is likely that there is a risk of respiratory disorders as a result of smoking cannabis. There is no physical dependence, but there may be some psychological withdrawal symptoms such as irritability and poor sleep. Heavy and chronic use may lead to apathy and self-neglect, but there is no special 'amotivational' syndrome among recreational users. There are some anecdotal reports of 'cannabis psychosis', but this is rare in the majority of users, suggesting that perhaps heavy use in predisposed individuals may precipitate a temporarily psychotic state. Research is currently going on in this area.

Legalization of cannabis debate

The legalization of cannabis has been the subject of debate in the UK since the 1960s. Positions have been polarized, with differing interpretations of the available information on health risks.

Arguments against legalization include the following. Alcohol and tobacco cause damage already to the population, so why legalize another intoxicant? There is insufficient evidence on long-term damage. Legalization could be interpreted as a softening of governmental attitude to drug abuse. The 'escalation theory' argues that cannabis will lead to other drug use by increasing contacts with other drug users.

Arguments for legalization include the following. Nationwide surveys suggest that of those people who experiment with cannabis, only a small percentage will go on to use it regularly and of these only a small percentage will try, and then regularly use, other drugs. It does seem that cannabis users are more likely to use other drugs than those who have never used cannabis, but, equally, alcohol and tobacco users· are more likely to become hard-drug users. Those in favour of legalization argue that cannabis is less harmful and causes less disruption to society than alcohol. Some say that legalization would prevent users having to mix with hard-drug users. It is argued that the illegality of the drug, and consequent stigma, is the main problem for the majority of cannabis users.

Lysergic acid diethylamide (LSD)

Use of LSD became common in the l960s, before declining for some years, and is now thought to be increasing. It is illegally produced and is available in tablet form or in capsules, but is more often absorbed on paper squares or possibly on gelatin or sugar cubes. This is a class A drug (Misuse of Drugs Act 1971).

Effects

The 'trip' begins 0.5–1 hour after taking LSD, fading after about 12 hours. Intensified or distorted perceptions are reported — of shape, colour time and place. Emotions may be labile, with increased self-awareness and possible feelings of dissociation. There may be unpleasant feelings, e.g. panic, disorientation, depression — a 'bad trip'. There is no evidence of any lasting damage due to LSD. Brief psychotic reactions or anxiety states are possible, but generally manageable in a familiar environment and with reduced stimulation. Suicide and death due to false perceptions are rare. There is no evidence for dependence.

Hallucinogenic or 'magic' mushrooms

There are no statistics available on use, but it is reported as common. These mushrooms grow in the UK and are only illegal when prepared in any way. Effects are similar to those of LSD, with distorted perceptions and also euphoria, hilarity and arousal. At high doses there may be hallucinations and anxiety. Some nausea and mild stomach pains may be experienced. There are no known serious long-term effects, but there are no studies of extended frequent use.

PART 2 HELPING THOSE WITH DRUG AND ALCOHOL PROBLEMS

THE MULTI-DISCIPLINARY APPROACH

Drug and alcohol abuse is a multifactorial problem. No single treatment or discipline can deal with all the difficulties. There is a need for a co-ordinated multi-disciplinary approach. Inevitably, this leads to overlap of roles between disciplines. Nurses working in addiction may work in a number of settings and take on a variety of roles, including advice giver, coordinator, individual counsellor, group therapist.

It is important, when working with this type of client, for the nurse to examine her own attitudes towards drugs and drug taking, and her fears, prejudices and stereotypes. Ambivalence, denial, deceit, deviousness and the high relapse rate in addicts may cause negative feelings in the nurse. She needs to look behind the behaviour. Deceit and subterfuge may be learned responses to the pressures of being dependent on a substance. The nurse's approach should be non-judgemental, showing empathy and passing on a message of hope, while confronting the maladaptive behaviour and reinforcing more positive interactions.

PRECONTEMPLATION PHASE

This is the initial stage of admitting that there is a problem. This may be in the primary health care setting when the person presents with a complication of drug use. Nurses should include questions about drugs and alcohol in general assessments and be alert to signs of abuse. 'Early' intervention is an important but difficult field, as the nurse may be met with denial, shame, guilt, anger and rationalization. The nurse's approach may be one of supportive confrontation. Engagement is important because the person must recognize his drug or alcohol use as a problem if change is to occur. The nurse must convey the message that change is possible and that help is available whenever the person is ready for it.

ASSESSMENT

Thorough assessment is vital and may serve as an opportunity for a structured personal review by the client. Assessment is likely to take place over some time. There are a number of areas which need to be covered, as follows.

Drug history

A drug history will include levels and consistency of present use; length of use of alcohol and drugs and what types (including prescribed drugs); reasons for using drugs, benefits gained; progression of drug use and links with other factors such as mood, life events, periods of abstinence, circumstances and causes of relapse. The question of whether the patient is dependent involves detailed investigation of how much of the drug is used, how often, and whether there is experience of withdrawal. It may help to ask the client about a typical drug-taking day or to ask him to keep a daily drinking diary. Any complications of drug use, whether physical, psychological or social, are recorded. Client's interpretation of how and when drug use became a problem, the extent of the importance of drugs in his life-style, other interests, work, are elicited. The nurse will find out whether friends or partner are drug users, what level of control over use the client claims to have, history of contact with helping agencies and his perception of their value. Risk and protective factors as well as motivating factors must be identified. The nurse will ask what are the reasons for coming to treatment at this point, what does the client want from the agency?

The patient's personal life history is also obtained (see Ch. 18).

Objective signs

It is important to verify the history using objective signs, especially if drugs are to be prescribed.

Checking with Home Office records is one diagnostic aid. Confirmation of addiction is also made by regular urine screening for drugs. Drug screens are conducted on consecutive days, and the results compared with a record of objective signs of the patient's state of intoxication or withdrawal. If the patient shows no signs of intoxication and yet his urine is positive to morphine, drug dependence is likely. Prescribing for people not addicted to the drug may lead to diversion of supplies to the black market or may even be fatal. Recent intravenous track marks or injection sites are an indication of intravenous drug use.

For alcohol dependence, urine, blood or breath tests may be used. High blood alcohol in a sober person is an indication of dependence. A blood alcohol level of greater than 80 mg, especially in the morning, is highly suggestive of alcohol abuse; a blood alcohol level of greater then 150 mg is almost diagnostic. Other tests such as mean corpuscular volume, liver function tests and uric acid and lipid levels are an indication of extent of damage caused alcohol misuse.

Assessment with the spouse or partner

It may be helpful, with the agreement of the client, to take personal, family and drinking histories from the partner of the addict, and also to ask her views on development of the problem, current patterns and hardships. This may be an opportunity to assess the coping mechanisms of the partner. The interview is of dual value in assessing and planning how best the partner can help the patient, and also in planning how best their needs can be met.

MOTIVATING FOR CHANGE

Because change can be a frightening process, motivation will vary at different times during recovery of the addict, and often he may appear ambivalent. The trigger for deciding to change will vary among individuals. A court case or a partner leaving may initiate change. Alcoholics Anonymous describes everyone as having their own 'rock bottom', when things are so bad the person decides he must do something about his addiction. It is important that an agency responds quickly to this request for help.

Maintaining motivation, however, is an ongoing process and staff may become despondent. The skill is to be able to raise hope, to let the client see change is possible. Even though detoxification may ultimately end in relapse, at least he had a chance to experience a period of sobriety. Many units operate a 'revolving door' policy, so that if an individual drops out of treatment, he is accepted again fairly readily when he feels ready to have another try.

Guides to assisting motivation

1. Balance sheet. This can be filled in by the client, showing positive and negative consequences of taking the substance (a 'decision matrix'). It may help to separate long- and short-term reasons, to distinguish immediate gratification from the long-term rewards. It is important that the client puts down his own perceptions.

2. Education. 'Frighteners' have been proved to have no lasting effect (TACADE 1979). Instead, information should be factual and relevant to financial and health matters, as well as the social and performance effects of the substance. The Health Education Council produces some useful literature.

3. Exposure to former addicts who are now abstinent or who have controlled their drink or drug use, whether individually or in self-help groups, may give the client hope and help him to confront some of his defences.

4. Enhancement of efficacy feelings means reinforcing the belief of the client in his ability to carry things through. This may involve practising coping imagery (imagining oneself coping and being sober in certain situations), positive self talk, and focus on past successes rather than failures.

GOAL SETTING

Setting clear goals avoids confusion and drift and helps to maintain continuity of purpose, also giving the client an opportunity to see his progress. It is an area, however, where there may be conflict between nurse and client, and it is important for there to be discussion and negotiation so that some agreement on goals is reached. The nurse should not be too directive — it is important for the client to assume responsibility and to develop a sense of control. This teaches planning ahead and the setting of realistic goals. There is room later for evaluation and change for goals if necessary.

Goal setting may be difficult if the patient has been coerced into treatment, perhaps by his family or by the court. Goals should be short term and attainable, although there is a need for some risk to aid motivation and self-esteem. Long-term goals may need breaking down. They should be stated in terms of the client's own behaviour such as things he can take control of. Getting rehoused could be worded as, 'The client will approach the council regarding an application for rehousing.'

Goal should be measurable and specific to enable evaluation to take place. Time limits on goals also aid evaluation. Everything should be recorded. Using a balance sheet may help in planning areas to work on. Goal setting should include all areas of the client's life, not just the drug taking. At each session, nurse and patient can discuss achievements and failures, and, from this, set goals for the next week. Commitment to long-term goals needs to be continually reinforced.

DETOXIFICATION

The aim of detoxification is to withdraw the person from drugs or alcohol as quickly, safely and comfortably as possible. This period will probably involve some physical investigations and a general building up of physical health.

Contrary to the fears of the addict and the family, detoxification is usually relatively easy. Maintaining abstinence is the major problem. Giving the family and the client information on what to expect and how they can help to relieve withdrawal symptoms may help motivation and reduce the actual distress experienced (Hayward 1974). Family support and education on how to deal with crises is vital, as they may occasionally contribute to relapse because of their inability to watch the addict suffer withdrawal symptoms.

There is no fixed regimen for detoxification, which varies depending on the type of drug, dosage, previous complications and supports. Most detoxification programmes are managed in the community. Unnecessary admissions may promote a sense of hopelessness and invalidism. Planning the detoxification (where, when and how) is an important part of goal setting. Detoxification is rarely effective in isolation but must be planned with prior goals for staying off drugs or alcohol.

Detoxification from alcohol

Detoxification from alcohol usually takes place at home. Criteria for admission to hospital are long dependence and previous complications such as fits, delirium tremens, confusion, poor home circumstances and supports, and isolation.

Detoxification at home may take about five days from the time that the person is advised to stop drinking. Plenty of support is needed, including daily checks by the community nurse or general practitioner. The family should also be aware of danger signs and of the risks of drinking on top of any tranquillizers prescribed. A balanced diet and plenty of fluids should be encouraged. A short-term course of benzodiazepines or chlormethiazole may be given, but only if really necessary because of their addictive properties. The patient is stabilized first, according to the history and objective signs of withdrawal. The dose is then gradually reduced over 5 to 7 days. Daily checks involve taking pulse and temperature, and observing for signs of diminished consciousness or of severe withdrawal symptoms such as tremor, restlessness, hallucinations. The patient is 'breathalysed' daily, and, if he has been drinking, the dose of sedatives may need to be reduced or omitted. Excessive drowsiness or a fall in blood pressure may indicate too high a dose of sedatives or illicit drinking.

Detoxification in hospital is done in a similar way, again using an individual and flexible programme. Objective monitoring of withdrawal is done and a careful watch is kept, especially for convulsions. In the early stages patients are escorted when off the ward. Prophylactic treatment such as short-term anticonvulsants may be prescribed in case of fits or status epilepticus. Intravenous diazepam and resuscitation equipment should be available in case of grand mal fits or other emergency situations.

If delirium tremens develops, close observation and maintenance of a calm, safe, restful environment is necessary. Light which illuminates but does not cast shadows will help. A limited dose of tranquillizers may be needed. Intramuscular vitamin replacement is often given. The patient may be overactive and sweaty, requiring rehydration and restoration of electrolyte balance. Delirium tremens generally resolves after about 4 days. Alcoholic hallucinosis may continue after withdrawal and require further treatment with antipsychotic medication.

Detoxification from benzodiazepines and barbiturates

With these drugs there is a risk of convulsions, and similar precautions should be taken as with alcohol. Detoxification from therapeutic doses of these drugs is possible in the community over a period of a few weeks. Drawing up an individual contract and reducing schedule, and arranging for the client to collect tablets on a regular basis may help. Polydrug users may not admit to use of these drugs, hence the importance of careful history taking and urine checks, so that hospitalization can be arranged if necessary.

Detoxification from opiates

Withdrawal from opiates, although distressing and uncomfortable, can be safely managed both in or out of hospital, even on high doses. Hospitalization may occasionally be used so as to establish a baseline dose before withdrawal starts in the community. It is possible to withdraw from opiates without any medication, and this may happen in police cells or when supplies run low. This is called 'cold turkey' and can be very distressing, so that it is not desirable in most cases.

Substitute drugs

Symptomatic medication, in the form of non-addictive drugs, may be given, either alone or with an opiate substitution regimen. Thioridazine (a sedative which relaxes and assists sleep) and diphenoxylate hydrocholoride (a mild opiate, which acts as an anti-emetic and anti-diarrhoea drug and relieves cramps) are often used. Propanolol may be used for a limited period for high somatic anxiety. Benzodiazepines are occasionally prescribed, especially for insomnia, but their use should be avoided in view of their addictive properties and black market value. Clonidine may also be used to alleviate withdrawal symptoms, but close monitoring is required because of its strongly hypotensive effect. Ideally, as few drugs should be prescribed as possible to avoid substitution.

Opiate stabilization and withdrawal

The drug of choice for opiate stabilization and withdrawal is oral methadone (a synthetic opiate). Assessing the required dosage is often the re-

sponsibility of the nurse. The dose is titrated against observable symptoms of intoxication and withdrawal, the aim being to achieve a dose where the patient is comfortable and yet can function normally. Less methadone may be required when heroin has been smoked.

Methadone is itself an addictive drug, and withdrawal symptoms may be more protracted than with heroin. The more severe symptoms last usually about 7 to 10 days, although some addicts complain of a general feeling of malaise for several weeks. Methadone produces less euphoria than heroin; it is longer acting and so causes less disruption to normal life; it is in liquid form, so there are no complications from injecting and overdose is less likely. Reduction may take place over as little as three weeks to several months. Longer detoxification may be arranged for more established addicts, if it is felt necessary for them to have time to sort out areas of their life before the crisis of coming off drugs.

Aids to detoxification

A contract system is operated by many clinics which prescribe drugs, to ensure that the addicts are taking the drug themselves and that they are not misusing other drugs of addiction which could potentially be dangerous. It may also help to prevent substitution of one drug with another. The contract system provides some form of external control, where internal control is often weak. Regular or random urine tests may be taken. The addict may receive his drug in daily doses, either at the clinic or at a local chemist.

It is important to be aware of the increased chance of relapse towards the end of detoxification. Extra support may be helpful at this point.

Maintenance therapy

Maintenance therapy is defined as continuing prescription of drugs with no plan for withdrawal. This is less common now, but is still practised in some clinics. Use of other drugs is usually prohibited and there may be a requirement to attend some form of therapy. The theory behind maintenance was that it would minimize the use of illegal drugs, problems with the law and complications of injecting. A few individuals have benefited and managed to lead more stable lives. It was quite commonly practised by private doctors but there are now heavy restrictions on prescribing.

REHABILITATION

Rehabilitation is an ongoing process, beginning at the first assessment interview. It involves maintaining abstinence and developing a new life-style without drugs or alcohol. Some kind of follow-up after detoxification is important, as relapse in the early stages is very common, and there is an opportunity to intervene early if progress is being monitored.

Some of the possible problems faced by a person trying to maintain a drug/alcohol-free life-style include difficulty of leaving old drinking or drug-taking friends. There may be loss of the excitement of being involved in an illegal sub-culture, of the comradeship or of the sense of belonging; facing up to unpleasant emotions and problems without drugs; learning new coping mechanisms; learning to delay gratification; stigmatization; adjustment to a new role in the family or with significant others who may not be trusting. Lack of occupation may necessitate dealing with boredom without resorting to drugs. Financial and housing problems exacerbate any lack of confidence and self-esteem. The person may be irritable and labile or low in mood, with sleep disturbance.

Counselling skills

These may be used in individual or group work. Both directive and non-directive approaches may be useful.

Group work

Groups may be more or less structured; behaviourally or psychoanalytically oriented; open or closed; drug-free or aiming towards abstinence or greater self-control. The value of group work is that it gives the client practice at expressing feelings, and at dealing with emotions and interpersonal relations without drugs. The group may provide role models. Peer support is extremely valuable in terms of giving information and sharing ways of coping. Peer confrontation also may be valuable. Socially, group work may help to boost the client's confidence and encourage independence.

In facilitating these types of groups, the nurse may have to work to be non-directive and encourage peer group work. The group facilitator is responsible for maintaining safety and providing support during examination of painful emotions. She may have to take a confrontative role if the group appears to be 'stuck'. She may also have to set limits, such as not allowing in a member of the group who is drunk, but the members of the group should be encouraged to do this work too.

Drug therapy assisting maintenance of abstinence

Alcohol sensitizing drugs

The two main drugs used are calcium carbimide (Abstem) and disulfiram (Antabuse). They can be used to aid motivation and in coping with high-risk situations. They sensitize the person to alcohol, causing flushing, breathlessness, dizziness, palpitations and possibly collapse if drink is taken. This occurs due to inhibition of normal breakdown of alcohol, causing a rise in blood levels of acetaldehyde. They should not be taken until at least 24 hours after the last drink. The nurse should explain to the patient and the family the consequences of drinking. The patient should give informed consent to the treatment. The family may initially have to be enrolled to give the daily tablet. These drugs should only be seen as an adjunct to treatment, not a cure.

Narcotic antagonists

Narcotic antagonists are being used clinically in some parts of the USA. Narcotic antagonists act competitively on opiate receptors in the brain, having 150 times greater affinity than opiates, so that a large amount of narcotic would be required to displace it. This means that any narcotics used would be unlikely to cause a euphoric effect. Antagonists are especially useful for preventing relapse after detoxification either in hospitals, prisons or therapeutic communities. The individual must be narcotic-free before starting antagonist therapy. The drugs are believed to be relatively safe with few side-effects.

Family work

Work with members of the family may involve using them in monitoring and assisting in the progress of the addict. It provides support for the family themselves. Marital therapy may be needed (Stanton et al 1978).

The family can be taught ways of helping the addict to maintain abstinence, and also to plan in case of relapse, and how to help by avoiding blame and pessimism. Where the person is still drinking and unwilling to get help, the family can be helped to develop coping strategies including devising a definite policy and sticking to it, not 'enabling' the person's dependency by giving money. Encouraging a cohesive approach by the family and encouraging involvement in self-help groups may help to alleviate the anxiety and guilt in carrying out a 'tough love' policy.

Children in the family of an addict may need particular help. They will need close monitoring if there is a risk of violence or neglect. They, too, should be given information, the opportunity to talk and the offer of support outside the home.

Behavioural techniques

Aversion therapy. This is rarely used now as it is quite unpleasant. It may be done in vivo or in vitro. Techniques include electric shocks, emetics or unpleasant images which are associated with alcohol or drugs.

Contingency management. Contingency management is based on operant conditioning. Rewards are given contingent on abstinence or controlled drinking, thus helping to increase a sense of control. It may be used in residential settings. A 'pass system' is an example where increasing freedom is given with length of abstinence. A marital contract may be set up in which the partner gives reinforcement only when the other is not drunk.

Cue exposure. This involves gradual exposure to high-risk situations which trigger the compulsive behaviour. Internal and external cues are identified, then the client is gradually exposed to them and helped to resist using drugs. He is taught that the anxiety and craving will disappear with time. This treatment is still in the early stages, but individual case studies show some positive results in extinguishing craving.

Attitude change techniques are also a new area. Difficult situations such as refusing a drink are rehearsed in role plays.

Relapse prevention techniques

Considerable research has been done in the USA on relapse prevention methods (Marlatt 1979, Marlatt & Gordon 1984). They are practised in some areas with misusers of drug and alcohol. The aim of the technique is to help the addict anticipate and cope with relapse, and it can be used in all indulgent behaviours. It is a self-control programme, combining behavioural skill training techniques and cognitive skills. It poses an alternative view to the 'disease model' of dependency, where relapse is viewed as failure, lack of control, and where one violation of abstinence is expected to be followed by total relapse. Marlatt believes that use of the drug after abstinence can be viewed as a single mistake, a 'lapse' or reversible slip, rather than total failure. In learning any new behaviour, mistakes are to be expected, and can be an opportunity for further learning.

Causes of relapse

Marlatt & Gordon (1984) identified a number of 'high-risk situations' which may be determinants of relapse. These were:

1. interpersonal determinants such as negative emotional states, including frustration, anger, boredom, negative physical states, including tiredness, illness, withdrawal symptoms; positive emotional states, including celebrations and testing of personal control, urges and temptations

2. interpersonal determinants such as interpersonal conflicts, social pressure either direct or indirect, and positive emotional states.

Social pressure was found to be an important factor in relapse, particularly with heroin (36%) and nicotine addiction (32%) and also with alcohol (18%). Negative emotional states were likely to lead to relapse in 38% of alcoholics, 37% of smokers and in 19% of heroin addicts. Marlatt suggests that the addict may make 'apparently ir-relevant decisions', leading him into very high-risk situations where he finds it impossible to fight the overwhelming desire to take drugs. For example, an ex-smoker may sit in the smoking car of a train. This behaviour is motivated by craving and by denial and rationalization. It may be that the per-son still feels ambivalent about giving up drugs, or that he has not learnt sufficient new coping mechanisms or that sobriety is not rewarding enough. All these are areas which can be worked on.

Marlatt suggests that effective coping in high-risk situations will lead to an increased sense of mastery and decrease the likelihood of relapse. If the alcoholic succumbs to accepting a whisky in the pub, he feels helpless, passive and that he cannot cope. He may deal with the stress and guilt by having another drink. Expectancies are impor-tant determinants of relapse, too.

Helping addicts to deal with high-risk situations

Identifying them. Firstly, the theory must be explained to the patient. Each individual has his own cue to relapse, which can be identified by taking a full drug history with details of where and when drugs are taken, who they are taken with, and what feelings are experienced afterwards. A history of relapses focusing on both internal and external cues is also needed. A diary kept by the patient may help. The decision matrix may also be used to identify areas of work. A hierarchy of high-risk situations is then prepared in order that appropriate coping skills can be mobilized.

Dealing with craving. Education on craving may help. Failing to respond to craving with the

substance will eventually lead to extinction. Giving in to it increases the chance of relapse. The addict can be taught that there is a pathway from craving to drug or alcohol use, with time to intervene by changing the response. He can be taught to rec-ognize the feeling and the need to strengthen his protective 'armoury' at that point, to recog-nize denial and to avoid 'apparently irrelevant decisions'. Repeated use of the decision matrix may help when the addict feels ambivalent. The nurse encourages the addict to develop his own strategies for dealing with craving, increasing the sense of self-control.

Avoidance of high-risk situations. This strategy may be used particularly in the early stages of abstinence before coping strategies are developed. For example, in rehabilitation units new clients may not be allowed out for a period unless escorted. The therapist plans, together with the addict, which situations can and cannot be avoided. An alcoholic may have to avoid pubs early on, but this may not be possible as a long-term strategy.

Developing coping responses. Development of coping responses depends on the particular dif-ficulties of an individual and involves the teaching of new strategies as well as encouraging the addict to use existing ones. Involvement in sports, hobbies, work or training may help to alleviate boredom. The addict also has to learn to tolerate it to some extent too. Anger may be dealt with by assertiveness training, control strategies or role play. Anxiety management and relaxation tech-niques can be taught. Interpersonal conflicts may be worked on in marital therapy, group therapy, social skills training or living in a therapeutic community.

If a slip occurs

The lapse should be regarded as a moment of danger and opportunity. A personal contract may be arranged beforehand to minimize the extent of the slip, stressing that this is a 'single event', not a personal failure, with no need for loss of personal control. A reminder card can be given to use in these situations, and also the phone number of the helping agency. The nurse should teach the client to maximize the learning benefits from the lapse. It can be reviewed in detail for early warning signals, and responses for the future planned. After the lapse, there is a need for renewed commitment and a plan for recovery.

Programmed relapses

Rarely, programmed relapse may be used as a treatment method to aid motivation. Relapse is planned and carefully supervised to show the discrepancy between the client's actual experience and his expectations.

Global intervention techniques

It would be impossible to plan for every high-risk situation, so that preventing relapse also involves the teaching of general problem-solving skills and intervention in the client's overall life-style. The person's life-style may be unbalanced, with too many 'shoulds', leading to a feeling of need to indulge oneself. He may need to be helped to modify his life-style and increase positive self-gratification in activities such as reading, creative hobbies or sport. Again, the focus should be on what the individual enjoys. Sobriety must be a rewarding experience if it is to be sustained.

Teaching of specific skills

Rehabilitation may involve training of the person in new areas, or revitalization of old skills which have not been used for sometime such as job-related skills, literacy or numeracy, social skills, assertiveness training, development of new leisure time activities, budgeting and domestic skills, child care skills and alternative ways of dealing with stress.

Controlled drinking

Whether it is possible to achieve controlled drinking has been the subject of much debate. It refers to subjectively normal drinking with no anxiety or preoccupation. Aims need to be clearly defined, as there are wide variations as to what is considered normal.

Predictors of successful outcome

It is difficult to give definite rules. There is often room for some experimentation. Where there is a long drinking history and fully developed dependency, then abstinence is the only goal.

Factors to consider:

1. Degree of dependence. A person with no experience of withdrawal or drinking only for about six months may be suitable
2. Evidence of recent sustained normal drinking
3. Length of drinking history
4. Age: younger alcoholics are generally more successful
5. The person's wishes
6. If the person is drinking to relieve psychiatric symptoms, controlled drinking is not appropriate
7. Presence or absence of alcohol-related physical illness
8. Are the family supportive? If they have alcohol problems, too, then abstinence is in better goal
9. A good indicator of success is whether the client is in regular employment.

How to do it

An interval of sobriety may be helpful initially. Aims and methods should be thoroughly discussed, along with the risk of self-deception. The type of beverage, quantity of intake and frequency should be defined. Motivations should be considered: for instance, do not have a drink when you 'need' a drink. High-risk situations should be avoided initially. Gradual exposure and resistance lead to extinction of craving. The partner may be involved in monitoring and acting as a restraining influence. Patients keep a diary, thus monitoring their own behaviour and self-control.

When objectively and subjectively the patient is drinking normally, contact may be decreased, with check-ups every few months. Referral to Drinkwatchers may help. If the person is unsuccessful, another attempt at control may be made, using a different strategy, or abstinence may be considered a more suitable goal.

PART 3 TREATMENT SETTINGS

Legislation in the UK over the past few decades has tended to be based on the theory that alcohol and drug dependency are social and medical problems rather than crimes. However, a large number of addicts are dealt with in the penal system. There is no compulsory treatment in Britain for the treatment of alcohol or drug dependence under the 1983 Mental Health Act. Services are often piecemeal, with local variations. There are many different agencies which deal with the problem of dependency in some way or another. Although a range of responses is needed for the varying problems, there is a need for coordination, planning and liaison. Drugs and alcohol services may be separately or jointly organized. Some cooperation is necessary, as there are many overlaps. Recent moves are towards community work and increasing integration of generic and specialist services.

PRIMARY HEALTH/SOCIAL SERVICES

Primary health care and social services include general practitioners, hospital emergency department staff, occupational health service staff, social workers, clergy and police. These workers are often best placed for early diagnosis and intervention. Support for the 'generalists' is needed from specialist services in the form of education, support and encouragement. The general services have the advantage of lack of stigma. Improvement of early detection and intervention will be achieved by thorough history taking, heightened awareness of signs of drug or alcohol abuse and the ability to treat and advise, knowing when and whom to refer to if necessary.

TREATMENT IN THE WORK SETTING FOR ALCOHOL PROBLEMS

This innovation has taken off primarily in the USA, but there are moves to introduce it on a wider scale in the UK. Problems often first become apparent at work. Certain occupations, too, are particularly at risk for development of alcohol problems. This type of programme would benefit employers and employees, avoiding cover up, denial, dismissal and disciplining. Minimal elements are a policy on drink, agreed by the employer and the unions, including, for example, a contract on help with review after six months, sick leave, job security, reporting of deterioration at work and screening. Referral routes or help within the organization and confidentiality are agreed on. Reed (1986) has shown the programme to be cost effective.

Nurses seem to be especially at risk of alcohol and drug problems. Finley (1982) recommended 'employee assistance programmes' for nurses, with increased knowledge about effects of drugs and alternative strategies for dealing with stress.

HOSPITAL SERVICES

Hospital services vary widely. There are relatively few specialized units, which are often attached to a general psychiatric ward or outpatients department.

Outpatient care usually involves detoxification and follow-up. There may be group therapy, behaviour therapy and social work support available.

Inpatient units may vary from provision of primarily custodial care to intensive therapy such as group work, family work, education, social skills and individual counselling. There seems to be a move recently away from inpatient treatment towards community care and working within the client's environment. However, a period of time away from those pressures may, in certain circumstances, still be beneficial. Units may be specialized or it may be that those people with problems of addiction are treated in the same ward as general psychiatric patients. This situation may be seen as less desirable than treatment in a specialized unit. Staff may see addicted patients as disruptive, blameworthy and not so seriously ill as the other patients.

Most units provide detoxification and there may be facilities for rehabilitation on site or for referral on to other units. The unit may often have quite rigid rules and expectations. A firm structure and visible limits, provided there is a shared rationale for them, are invaluable in helping this type of patient. There will probably be a no-drinking policy, which may be enforced by breath or urine tests. The policy is seen as useful both for the individual and for the community in the unit, and support from the group for the rule is engendered. There may be general or individual treatment contracts with stated rewards or sanctions. Staff may have a difficult task maintaining a therapeutic atmosphere, and encouraging individuals and the group to take responsibility. There is often quite a high level of conflict. Some units admit people only for detoxification, while others admit for stabilization or controlled drinking as well. It seems that segregation is a preferable situation, where all are working towards the same goal.

OTHER COMMUNITY FACILITIES

Detoxification centres

Detoxification centres exist in a few areas for offenders. It was felt that the revolving door of fines and a night in a cell were ineffective and uneconomical, and that there was a need for somewhere midway between punishment and treatment. Centres, therefore, were set up jointly by the probation and alcohol services in order to make available supervised withdrawal and medical services.

Halfway houses and hostels

These may be funded by local authorities or the voluntary sector. They may provide a place between hospital and home, or accommodation for the homeless. Counselling and rehabilitation may be provided. Abstinence is generally a condition of residence.

'Drop in' centres

Voluntary bodies may provide counselling, advice, and referral for drinkers and their families. They may also be involved in education and in social activities for recovering drinkers. There are various voluntary agencies providing advice and counselling for drug addicts, either by phone or at 'drop in' centres. Often this will be the first contact the addict has with any helping agency, and some people prefer their often more informal atmosphere. Some of the agencies have outreach workers as well.

Non-residential day care

There are a few day care facilities for alcoholics and drug addicts, operated either by voluntary or professional bodies. These usually have a structured programme of individual and group work, family support, recreational therapy, specific training and practical help. The need for this type of services is great, especially among young mothers, for whom long-term residential rehabilitation is often impractical and provision of services inadequate.

Therapeutic communities

The majority of these are drug-free communities. Some are voluntary agencies, some are privately funded. The focus is on group work, interpersonal relations and self-development. There may be an opportunity to work. The house is usually run by the residents. Some communities will recommend a minimum length of stay. Integration into the community and provision of follow-up support varies, since members often come from different parts of the country. Ideally though, there would be some type of follow-up support once the addict returns to his community.

Self-help groups

There are a number of these throughout the country. Alcoholics Anonymous and Narcotics Anonymous are the best known of these, as they operate world-wide. Their aim is for total abstinence from drugs and alcohol. Dependence is seen as a disease, which can be managed by working through the 'Twelve Steps'. Meetings are anonymous and involve sharing of experiences. The fellowship of the organization can be helpful in development of new social contacts.

Families Anonymous is the sister organization for relatives of dependent people. They believe that there is a 'sickness' in the family and that they have needs in their own right. They have a policy of 'tough love' with the addict, so that he has to take responsibility for his own behaviour. This may motivate him to get help.

Community services

There is now a move towards community work with drug and alcohol abusers. Community nurses may be generic workers, but specialist posts in the field are increasing. Nurses may be involved at various stages of treatment, and their role is very much evolving at present. They may practise early intervention, working with people before their drug problems are too severe and with people who are misusing a wider range of drugs. Nurses may be involved in home detoxification programmes. However, one major area of their work is in relapse prevention work: following up those who have recently come off drugs or alcohol and intervening early when there are problems. Inevitably, the work involves the family of the addict.

The community nurse can act as a liaison person between agencies. She can act as a consultant to other professional workers, thereby increasing knowledge and awareness of addiction in the community. Some community nurses will be involved in particular local projects such as day centres, 'drop in' agencies, telephone advisory services and self-help groups.

EFFECTIVENESS OF TREATMENT

Research to evaluate effectiveness of different types of treatment for addiction problems is inadequate. The clients in this group are renowned as being difficult to trace in follow-up studies. Stimson & Oppenheimer (1982) found that 40% of opiate addicts were off drugs after 10 years, suggesting that the long-term view is often more optimistic than short-term outcome. Addiction, however, is recognized as a chronic relapsing disorder with no easy cure. In terms of evaluating treatment, we need to look not only at whether the

person is totally abstinent, but also at their general quality of life.

PART 4 SPECIAL ISSUES

WOMEN AND DRUG/ALCOHOL ABUSE

Evidence shows that the gap between men and women in terms of drug and alcohol abuse is narrowing. However, there are differences in female drug abuse due to differing biology, social position, and expectations of women.

Drugs in pregnancy

Ellis & Fidler (1982) discuss the different effects of drugs used at various stages of pregnancy.

Alcohol

Heavy alcohol use may cause problems even before conception, as it decreases fertility and there is a greater chance of spontaneous abortion. Alcohol crosses the placenta. At present, there is no safe level established, so women are recommended not to drink at all during pregnancy and even pre-conceptually (Royal College of Psychiatrists 1979). It seems, though, that more than 40 g of alcohol daily may put the fetus at serious risk, either of retarded intra-uterine growth or of actual damage, the latter ranging from minor damage to fetal alcohol syndrome. In fetal alcohol syndrome there is retarded pre- and postnatal growth. It is a disorder of the central nervous system. causing hypotonia, irritability, mental retardation and uncoordination. There may be craniofacial abnormalities, abnormal eyes, ears and mouth. The baby may suffer from alcohol withdrawal at birth (Jones et al 1973).

Sedatives and hypnotics

It seems that heavy doses of barbiturate-type drugs or benzodiazepines may increase the risk of congenital malformations. There is a risk of fetal and neonatal depression of respiration. Babies may experience withdrawal at birth, and may have feeding problems, tremor, poor sleep, hypotonia, and hypothermia, symptoms which may last from a few weeks to several months.

Tobacco

Smoking during pregnancy can cause decreased birth weight and increased perinatal mortality.

Narcotics

Narcotics may cause low birth weight and increase perinatal mortality, but part of the problem may be neglect of diet and chaotic life-style of the mother. Many addicts come late for antenatal care. Opiates cause a withdrawal syndrome in the neonate. Ideally, if an addict presents early enough during her pregnancy, she can be slowly withdrawn from opiates so that the baby can be born drug-free. Regular monitoring will be necessary. If she feels unable to come off drugs, or if it is late in the pregnancy, then she may be stabilized on a low dose of a long-acting opiate such as methadone in order to avoid subjecting the baby to peaks of intoxication and troughs of withdrawal. There is no legal requirement on pregnant women to have treatment for addiction.

The Committee on Drugs (1983) describes symptoms of narcotic withdrawal in the neonatal as wakefulness, irritability, tremors, temperature variations, hyperactivity, high-pitched cry, feeding problems, diarrhoea, respiratory distress, weight loss, yawning, rhinorrhoea, and sneezing. There is a risk of convulsions. Onset of symptoms may be in the first 10 days. Subacute symptoms may be present for as long as 4 months, though the baby usually seems comfortable after about 2 weeks. Treatment is primarily supportive. An Abstinence Scoring Method may be used to assess the need for drug therapy. Treatment may involve prescribing of very small doses of a narcotic, a benzodiazepine, chlorpromazine, or phenobarbitone. The dosage is stabilized over 3–5 days and slowly reduced over a few weeks. The infant is ready for discharge when drug free and showing no symptoms of withdrawal.

CHILD CARE AND DRUG/ALCOHOL ABUSE

Child care and drug abuse is an issue often picked up by the media. Not every child of a drug or alcohol abuser is at risk, so that individual assessment of each case is essential. Because there is little precise information about long-term risks, management often deals with 'potential risks'. Care must be taken to work with facts rather than sterotypes. A blanket policy may deter addicts from seeking help.

PREVENTION

Prevention is a complex problem, with little information reliably available on effective ways of doing it (DHSS 1971, Advisory Council on Misuse of Drugs 1984). Prevention and treatment overlap (Caplan 1964).

Factors to consider

Since there is no single cause of substance abuse, there cannot be a single strategy for prevention. Current opinion varies from stopping drug use to minimizing harm. There is no natural progression of increased knowledge causing a change in attitudes or behaviour. Results of American drug abuse prevention campaigns are not very promising (Hanson 1982).

What should a prevention policy include?

The Advisory Council on Misuse of Drugs (1984) stress the need for a comprehensive policy considering the individual, the social group, supply of drugs, how drug abuse spreads and how to influence these factors using education, the media, and statutory controls.

They recommend:

1. Improved broad social and economic policy on housing, employment, leisure, and education, as this may have an indirect effect on substance misuse. This tends to be a less popular option politically.

2. Improved control of the availability of drugs, including restriction of supply of illegal drugs, improved customs and policing, controls on irresponsible prescribing, and political intervention in the price of alcohol, licensing laws, and age threshold for purchasing alcohol. Apart from cutting down on advertising, there is a trend away from these measures in the UK.

3. Education may be aimed towards 'at risk' or 'receptive' groups: generally the young. Information on drugs may be included in a general package, focussing on healthy life-styles along with discussion and practice of decision-making skills. It is felt that the teachers should present this material, and thus will require some training by specialists. Individual education is easier, as the message can be tailored, questions can be dealt with, and an individual plan of action can be made out. There are, unfortunately, obvious logistical problems.

Woodcock (1982) cites research indicating that denying access to one substance may lead to a shift towards use of others. It seems that health education has had no impact on experimentation with solvents. Woodcock suggests instead a campaign which was successful in the USA. Education via the mass media must also be approached with caution (Flay & Sobel 1983). Its effectiveness has been questioned, but it is popular politically, as governments can be 'seen to be doing something' about the problem. In 1989 the Scottish Health Education Council put out a national campaign of television and press releases, warning of the risks of excessive alcohol consumption. Evaluation showed that more people came forward for treatment after the national campaign. Three quarters of the adult population were reached by the campaign, but there was no significant increase in public knowledge, and no change in alcohol consumption after 8 months.

Education about alcohol is more subtle than the anti-smoking campaign, as alcohol is not seen as harmful for most people, and is socially acceptable. Abstinence is not a sensible goal for most. There are problems in setting any 'safe limits', as a safe amount for some may be too much for others and dangerous to others.

SUMMARY AND CONCLUSIONS

This chapter has presented some of the problems which may arise from drug or alcohol abuse, and how nurses may help this type of client. Strang (1982) described the nurse as often being the 'key worker' in establishing the therapeutic alliance with addicts. She may be able to use the less formal role and flexible style of the nurse to her advantage in engaging this type of patient. The chapter illustrates the variety of roles which the nurse may take on in helping dependent clients, and the wide range of treatment methods which may be utilized in different settings. This variety and flexibility of style is important in an area where there is no one simple cure for all. However, research on what nurses do, and particularly research by nurses in this field, is lacking. Work needs to be done, particularly in the areas of: initiation to drugs and alcohol; evaluation of treatment methods; follow-up studies, identification of cue for, and preventing, relapse; and the area of prevention.

APPENDIX

DRUG LAWS

Medicines Act 1908

This controls medicinal products in three categories:

Prescription only medicines — must be prescribed by a doctor and sold by a pharmacist.

Pharmacy medicines — no prescription is required, but these are sold only by pharmacists.

General sales list — these medicines may be bought from any shop, no prescription is necessary.

Misuse of Drugs Act (1971)

This Act aims to prevent the non-medical use of

certain drugs known as controlled drugs. It prohibits unlawful possession, supply, import, export and production.

The categories are:

Class A — carries the highest penalties. Includes opiates, hallucinogens and cocaine.

Class B — lower penalties. Includes cannabis, milder opiates, strong synthetic stimulants and sedatives. Any class B drug used intravenously, is classed as A.

Class C — lowest penalties. Includes less potent stimulants and dextropropoxyphene (a mild opioid analgesic.

The Mental Health Act 1983

In the new Mental Health Act, it is stated that dependence on drugs or alcohol alone should not be construed as a mental disorder, so there is no compulsory treatment.

ACKNOWLEDGEMENTS

I am grateful to the staff of the Drug Dependency Units at Bethlem Royal Hospital and also at St George's Hospital, Tooting Bec, for the experience I gained there, which helped in compiling this chapter.

REFERENCES

Advisory Council on Misuse of Drugs 1982 Treatment and rehabilitation. HMSO, London

Bass M 1970 Sudden sniffing deaths. Journal of the American Medical Association 212: 2075–2079

Batt M B, Levine J, Manheimer D I 1974 Cross national study of anti-anxiety sedative drug use. New England Journal of Medicine 290: 769–774

British Medical Journal 1982 Alcohol problems — articles from the British Medical Journal. Leagrave Press

Caplan G 1964 Prevent psychiatry. Tavistock, London

City Roads and Phoenix House 1980 Drugs Resource Pack. Available from City Roads, 358 City Road, London EC1, Tel: 071-278-8671

Cloninger C, Bohman M, Sigvardson S 1981 Inheritance of alcohol abuse. Archives of General Psychiatry 38: 861–868.

Committee on Drugs 1983 Neonatal drug withdrawal. American Academy of Paediatrics. (ISSN 0031 4005).

Department of Health and Social Security 1981 Prevention and health — drinking sensibly. HMSO, London

Department of Health and Social Security 1984 Report of the Medical Working Group on Drug Dependence. Guidelines on good clinical practice in the treatment of drug misuse.

Drug Indicators Project (Hartnoll R, Daviaud D, Lewis R, Mitcheson M) 1984 Drug problems — assessing local needs. Institute for the Study of Drug Dependence (ISDD), London

Edwards G 1982 The treatment of drinking problems — a guide for the helping professions. Grant McIntyre

Ellis C, Fidler J 1982 Drugs in pregnancy — adverse reactions. British Journal of Hospital Medicine 28: 575–584

Finley B 1982 Primary and secondary prevention of substance abuse. Nursing 30 (1): 271–280

Flay B, Sobel J 1983 The role of mass media in preventing adolescent drug abuse — intervention strategies. NIDA Research Monograph 47, Rockville Survey, National Institute of Drug Abuse. Department of Health and Human Services

Francis J, Murray V S G, Ruprah M, Flanagan R J, Ramsay J D Suspected solvent abuse in cases referred to the Poisons Unit at Guy's Hospital, July 1980–June 1981. Human Toxicology 1: 271–280

General Household Survey 1982 HMSO London

Haddon C 1984 Women and tranquillizers. Sheldon Press SPCK, London

Hanson D J 1982 Effectiveness of alcohol and drug education. Journal of Alcohol and Drug Education 272: 1–5

Hayward J 1974 Information — a prescription against pain. Royal College of Nursing, London

Home Office 1985 Tackling drug misuse — a summary of the Government's strategy. HMSO, London

Jones K L, Smith D W, Ulleland G N 1973 Pattern of malformation in offspring of chronic alcoholic mothers. Lancet 1: 1267–71

Marlatt G A 1979 Relapse prevention — introduction and overview of the model. British Journal of Addiction 74: 261–275

Marlatt G A, Gordon G R 1984 Relapse prevention — maintenance strategies in addictive behaviour change. Guildford Press, New York

Melville J 1984 The tranquillizer trap. Fontana, London

Mental Health Act 1982 HMSO, London

Mott J 1985 Self reported cannabis use in 1981 — Findings of the British Crime Survey. British Journal of Addiction 80: 37–43

Osselton M D, Blackmore R C, King L/A, Moffat A C I 1984 Poisoning associated deaths for England and Wales between 1973–80. Human Toxicology 3: 201–221

Reed M T 1986 Descriptive study of chemically dependent nurses. In: Brooking J (ed) Psychiatric nursing research. Wiley, Chichester

Royal College of Psychiatrists 1979 Alcohol and alcoholism. Tavistock, London

Stanton et al 1978 Heroin addiction as a family phenomenon. Americal Journal of Drug and Alcohol Abuse 5 (2): 125–150

Stimson G, Oppenheimer E 1982 Heroin addiction — treatment and control in Britain. Tavistock, London

Strang J 1982 Psychotherapy by nurses — some special characteristics. Journal of Advanced Nursing 7: 1671

Wilson P 1980 Survey on drinking in England and Wales. Office of Population Censuses and Surveys. HMSO, London

Woodcock J 1982 Solvent abuse from a health education perspective. Human Toxicology I: 331–336.

FURTHER READING

Curran V, Golumbock S 1985 Bottling it up. Faber, London

Dorn N, South N 1985 Helping drug users. Gower, Aldershot

Estes N J, Smith Dijulio K, Heinmann N E 1980 Nursing diagnosis of the alcoholic person. Mosby, St Louis

Faugier J 1986 The changing concept of dependence in the drug and alcohol field. Nursing Practice 1: 253–6

Glatt M 1982 Alcoholism. Teach Yourself Books, Sevenoaks

Gossop M 1982 Living with drugs. Morris Temple Smith

Heller T, Gott M, Jeffrey C 1987 Drug use and misuse. A reader. The Open University Department of Health and Social Welfare in association with the Health Education Authority. Open University Press, Milton Keynes

Institute for the Study of Drug Dependence 1985 Drug abuse briefing. ISDD, London

Manson R, Ritson B 1984 Alcohol and health — a handbook for nurses, midwives and health visitors. Medical Council on Alcoholism, London

Marlatt G A, George W H 1984 Relapse prevention. British Journal of Addiction 79: 261–74

Pearson G 1987 The new heroin users: voices from the street. Blackwell, Oxford

Pearson G, Gilman M, McIver S 1986 Young people and heroin: an examination of heroin use in the North of England. Health Education Council and Gower, London

Royal College of Psychiatrists 1986 Alcohol: our favourite drug. Tavistock, London

Strang J 1983 Problem Drug Taking. Medical Education International Ltd

USEFUL ADDRESSES AND INFORMATION

Information on services

Alcohol Concern, Grosvenor Crescent, London SW1. Tel: 071 233 4182

Institute for the Study of Drug Dependence (ISDD), 1–4 Hatton Place, Hatton Gardens, London EC1. Tel: 071 430 1991. Library and information service. Provides directories of rehabilitation projects, hospital services and advice and information agencies.

Teachers' Advisory Council on Alcohol and Drug Education (TACADE), 2 Mount Street, Manchester M2 5NG. Provides teaching materials.

Standing Conference on Drug Abuse (SCODA), 1 Hatton Place, Hatton Garden, London EC1. Tel: 071 430 2341. Coordinating body for the voluntary agencies — information on services.

Teaching materials (and advice on presentation)

Available from:

- Institute for the Study of Drug Dependence (ISDD) — address as above.
- Teachers Advisory Council on Alcohol and Drug Education (TACADE), 2 Mount Street, Manchester M2 5NG
- Health Education Council (for England and Wales), 78 New Oxford Street, London EC1. Tel: 071 673 1881
- Scottish Health Education Group, Woodburn House, Canaan Lane, Edinburgh EH10 4SG. Tel: 031 447 8044
- Health Education Service (Northern Ireland), 16 College Street, Belfast. Tel: 0232 41771.

37

Liaison psychiatric nursing

S. A. H. Ritter

Five main issues emerge from an examination of the literature on the psychosocial role of the nurse in the general hospital. These are the question of psychological factors in physical illness; psychiatric morbidity in general hospital patients; illness behaviour of patients; the relationship of the nurse and patient; and the relationships of the nurse within the nursing and multi-disciplinary clinical teams.

'THE PSYCHOSOCIAL HYPOTHESIS'

Henry's (1979) review of the literature on psychological factors in physical disease demonstrates the range of evidence for defining emotions as neuroendocrine behaviour and for considering this behaviour as inextricably linked to the development of physical disorders ranging from cancer to hypertension. What he calls 'the psychosocial hypothesis' suggests that psychosocial events cause neuroendocrine changes which are significantly related to the development and progress of organic disease.

A range of psychosocial events have been identified: from maternal loss in infancy through disturbed/abnormal sleep patterns to emigration. Other less explicitly measurable events such as inner city residence, and the experience of racism and poverty have been implicated as factors contributing to the chain of neuroendocrine changes resulting in the development of disease.

Personality variables have been found which characterize individuals with diagnoses ranging from coronary heart disease to lung cancer to urinary tract infection. Such factors include the so-called type A personality (Friedman & Rosenman 1974), and the difficulties of people with lung or breast cancer in expressing their emotions verbally (Kissen & Eysenck 1962, Greer & Morris 1975). According to Henry (1979), 'It is not the life situation nor the life changes alone that are critical. It is necessary to consider the social support and the personality, in fact, the overall social assets of the individual.'

PSYCHIATRIC MORBIDITY IN GENERAL HOSPITAL PATIENTS

Epidemiological studies of the amount of mental disorder seen in primary care settings indicate that emotional and psychological disturbance affects at least 15% of people consulting general practitioners and that such disturbance is also significantly associated with long-standing physical illness. Primary health care practitioners deal without reference to psychiatrists with much of the ill-health for which no organic cause can be found (Shepherd 1980). When the proportion of patients who require extensive investigation of their complaints is combined with the number of patients who develop psychological and emotional problems in the course of treatment for physical illness, the population at risk in hospital has been estimated at about 45% of patients in general hospitals (Sensky 1986).

ILLNESS BEHAVIOUR OF PATIENTS

Stockwell's study (1972) of the unpopular patient, and Kelly & May's (1982) review of the literature on good and bad patients show that nurses find only a narrow range of illness behaviour acceptable. Parsons (1951) and Mechanic (1962) have been influential in discussions of the beliefs and attitudes of individuals and society concerning illness and health. Mechanic reviewed the concept in 1986, and defined illness behaviour as involving

'the manner in which individuals monitor their bodies, define and interpret their symptoms, take remedial action, and utilize sources of help as well as the more formal health care system' (p. 1).

Pilowsky (1975) studied the definitions of the sick role and illness behaviour in order to validate the concept of abnormal illness behaviour. He was able to identify 'seven dimensions of abnormal illness behaviour': namely a general, mainly hypochondriasis factor, a 'disease conviction with symptom preoccupation' factor, a 'somatic versus psychologic' factor, an 'inhibition of affect' factor, an 'affective disturbance' factor, a life problems factor and an irritability factor.

Pilowsky's conclusions identify what is for many nurses a central problem of a psychosocial approach to abnormal illness behaviour: of being faced with angry and distressing complaints from patients who resist attempts to explore the origins of their anger and distress.

RELATIONSHIP OF THE NURSE AND PATIENT

However, anger and distress are also components of normal illness behaviours. They are communicated in ways which range from non-verbal yet expressive silence through various verbal expressions to non-verbal and often loud expression. If, when thinking of communication, the analogy of signal-to-noise ratio is remembered, anger and distress may be conceived as the noise through which the signal of a desire to understand and to be understood has to penetrate. The noise and the signal are integral parts of communication. Forming a professional and therapeutic relationship is, for the nurse, a matter of monitoring his or her response to the noise in order to remain attentive to the signal.

Menzies (1970) argued that hospital organizations are designed to protect nurses from what they experience as patients' emotional demands in the course of their work, which is accordingly designed to minimize opportunities for individual nurses and patients to form relationships. According to this view, nurses in traditional organizational settings are likely to regard any emotional demand by patients as excessively demanding of time and expertise.

RELATIONSHIPS OF THE NURSE WITHIN THE NURSING AND MULTI-DISCIPLINARY CLINICAL TEAMS

Membership and leadership of the multi-disciplinary clinical team is not always clearly defined: a factor which can lead to less effective relationships between staff and patients as well as between staff members themselves (Firman & Kaplan 1978).

THE PSYCHOSOCIAL APPROACH: RESPONSIBILITY OF THE GENERAL NURSE OR OF THE PSYCHIATRIC NURSE SPECIALIST?

Ray et al (1984) explored nurses' perceptions of their role in giving support to women who had breast cancer and mastectomy. In their review of the literature they noted that patients' distress tended not to be detected, and if recognized, not dealt with by nurses. Their study found that nurses felt doubtful about their ability to intervene in psychological aspects of patients' illness, and that they wished for specialist nurses to carry out such nursing care. However, Ray et al conclude, 'Where there is no specialist nurse, [ward nurses] may, indeed, be the patient's only source of professional support' (p. 110).

It seems clear that if nearly half of the general hospital inpatient population is regarded as having some kind of psychological or emotional dysfunction, their assessment and care is beyond the capacity of the small number of specialist psychiatric nurses who may be attached to the general hospital. If this is the case, psychosocial assessment needs to be effectively carried out in order to discriminate between those interventions that can be carried out by general nurses, and those for which specialist help is needed, whether from a specialist nurse or another member of the multi-disciplinary psychiatric team. Engel (1986) noted that where psychiatric consultation services have been set up, psychosocial approaches tend to be limited to patients whose behaviour interferes with the running of the ward or who do not comply with treatment regimens.

PSYCHOSOCIAL ASSESSMENT OF THE GENERAL HOSPITAL INPATIENT

Preparation for assessment

Wilson-Barnett & Trimble (1984) stress the need to conduct assessments in the context of 'an understanding relationship' with a single nurse over a period of time. A number of studies have shown that primary nursing provides the context for such relationships, enhancing patient and nurse satisfaction and improving clinical outcomes (Marram et al 1976, Sellick Russell & Beckmann 1983, Kent & Larson 1983, Culpepper et al 1986). The first step in psychosocial assessment is, therefore, the allocation of a primary nurse to a patient.

The second step is to determine the model by which the nurse's relationship with the patient will be structured during the patient's admission. Models which account for a beginning, middle and end to the nurse–patient relationship include those of Peplau (1952) and Sundeen et al (1985).

The third step is to determine how the nurse will collaborate with the patient's family or key friends. Brooking (1989) cautions against pressurizing patients' relatives into participating in nursing care. Her research, however, provides evidence of the lack of involvement by nurses of patients' significant others in planning their care. Among her recommendations are the provision of information booklets, pre-admission visits, oral information giving and teaching of practical care skills to supplement patients' self-care.

The fourth step is to determine the primary nurse's psychosocial role in relation to other members of the nursing and multi-disciplinary clinical teams. The role of the charge (or head) nurse in coordinating this step and supervising the competence of primary nurses has been emphasized by Shukla (1981) and Bartels et al (1977).

Assessment

Wilson-Barnett & Trimble (1984) note that in practice the liaison psychiatrist tends to be asked to confirm mental illness only when physical disease has been ruled out, and that if no formal mental disorder is found the patient tends to be discharged without treatment of any kind. The timing and management of collaboration with the specialist member of staff, of whatever discipline, is greatly facilitated by careful assessment by the patient's nurse: assessment which includes records of direct observations; process recordings of conversations with the patient; graphic representation of somatic measurements such as pulse rate or duration of sleep; and completion of validated rating scales.

Wilson-Barnett & Trimble (1984) recommend that Pilowsky's (1975) illness behaviour questionnaire is studied and some of its questions adapted by nurses in order to assess patients. They suggest that general nurses are educated in the use of other validated rating scales such as the Beck depression inventory (Beck 1979). Folstein & Folstein (1975) provide a brief format for what they call a minimental state assessment. Barker's (1985) very full account of assessment procedures for psychiatric patients includes many methods which can be used by primary nurses in the general setting. Millar (1981) provides a framework for communicating with patients in order to derive information, reduce emotional distress and to agree step by step behavioural commitments. He recommends the following techniques.

- Start with general open questions
- Move to specific open questions
- Only use specific open questions when establishing detail
- Clarification.

He criticizes as unhelpful the following responses to patients' emotions:

- inappropriate probing
- excess reassurance
- evasion
- hostility/judgement.

EXAMPLE OF SPECIFIC PROBLEMS
Withdrawal from alcohol

Delirium tremens is preventable by careful nursing assessment, using a drinking history and care-fully monitoring any withdrawal symptoms. Such monitoring can be done if the nurse is sceptical of the patient's account of his or her drinking, and can be used to titrate accurately the administration of medication such as chlormethiazole against the severity of withdrawal symptoms. Although delirium tremens develops in only a small population of patients, alcohol intake which is higher than the recommended amounts is present in many patients admitted to hospital. Withdrawal leads to dysphoria, some craving and physical discomfort, all of which affect patient's tolerance of pain, frustration and anxiety.

Depression and grief

Cavanaugh & Wettstein (1983) confirmed Moffic & Paykel's (1975) finding of significant amounts of depression in medically ill inpatients. They note that a diagnosis of depression may be confounded by patients' transient stress reactions to hospitalization. Linked with this observation is the occurrence of grief reactions in patients after major surgery, particularly that which alters a person's physical appearance, such as mastectomy or amputation, or sense of gender identification, such as hysterectomy or testicular surgery. Kelly (1985) used a personal experience of ileostomy to observe the process of grieving in himself, and concluded that hospital organizations do not facilitate nurses' helping patients to come to terms with their grief.

Two issues are important here. One is that depressed medical patients do not always recover from their depression as their physical illness resolves. Psychological intervention is generally required in order to treat the depression itself. The risk of suicide, though said to be small in medical inpatients, is nonetheless a factor to be considered when managing nursing care (Cavanaugh & Wettstein 1983). Therefore an accurate assessment of depression and suicidal intent is mandatory. The second issue is that some grief reactions and other emotional responses to illness and treatment are either health-promoting (for instance 'fighting spirit') (Moorey & Greer 1989) or are responsive to specific psychological interventions. An accurate assessment is required in order for the nurse to plan which behaviours to reinforce, which to suggest to the patient might change, and which require specialist assessment and interventions.

Davis & Payne (1986) assessed how general nurses trained to use clinical rating scales compared with an experienced psychotherapist who carried out a diagnostic interview of 50 post-myocardial infarction patients. They did find inter-rate reliability, and recommend that such systematized assessment is generally carried out by nurses.

Minghella & Brooking (1987) discussed the results of a study where patients who had attempted suicide were assessed and treated by nurses rather than psychiatrists. Their results confirm work in Edinburgh and Oxford where the assessment of patients and clinical outcomes for patients treated by the nurses compared favourably with those for patients assessed and treated by psychiatrists.

Psychosis and organic brain reactions

The acutely disturbed patient can present a serious threat to his or her own safety as well as that of other patients and staff. Such disturbance may be a more or less transient response to, among other things, medication, surgical procedures, metabolic crisis or trauma. Irreversible impairment may follow, among others, infection, trauma, or idiopathic destruction of brain tissue. These emotional responses to deficits usually constitute the nursing management difficulties in general wards. Such responses include impulsiveness, aggressiveness, withdrawal, and chaotic and apparently aimless activity. The primary nurse's recorded observations of the development of deficits and disturbance are inestimably valuable in assisting diagnosis and starting treatment. A clear picture of the inception and process of any disturbance is likely to allow rapid intervention and treatment of transient organic or psychotic reactions. It will at the same time clarify whether a condition is likely to be irreversible, so that consultation with specialists, transfer to a specialist unit, discussion with relatives and planning of staffing requirements can be carried out before a crisis overtakes matters.

A number of nursing actions have been iden-

tified as counterproductive in the assessment and nursing management of acute disturbance. They include avoidance of the patient, coercion, and overprotectiveness. It is suggested that such actions are related to nurses' own emotional responses to patients, including fear, disgust and anger.

Examples of nursing actions based on fear are described by Shilts (1987) in his account of the development of the AIDS epidemic. Ingham & Fielding (1985) reviewed the literature on attitudes towards old people, observing that it tended not to answer the charges made by Robb (1967). However, they do note that in one study which examined the relationship between nursing attitudes and patient behaviour, it was the nursing assistants allocated to carry out cleaning tasks for incontinence behaviours who reported the most negative attitudes to patients. Further work is required to clarify the relationship between organization, nurses' attitudes and patient behaviours. Spielvogel & Wile (1986) describe the anger of staff caring for women who become psychotic during and after pregnancy and who appear incompetent to look after their babies.

Pain

Mayer (1985) discusses available literature on non-pharmacological management of pain in patients with cancer. She observes that although a wide range of methods are available (including relaxation, distraction, cutaneous stimulation, hypnosis), there is no consistent guidance for nurses wishing to fit a particular method to the needs of an individual patient. Choice tends to be based on a combination of trial, error, experience and careful assessment. Mayer provides a useful reference list for nurses requiring specific assessment tools and stresses the need for careful documentation of outcomes in individual cases.

Chronic and terminal illness

If the need for psychosocial nursing intervention is perceived to be a function of the psychiatric morbidity of the patient, general nurses need to develop the skills of evaluating the evidence for such morbidity, and of distinguishing it from the normal range of psychological responses. As with the other problems already described, there are a number of psychological symptoms which are normal by-products of being seriously ill or which may be caused by treatment itself. They include complaints of weakness; lethargy; reduced concentration, attention and memory; and difficulties of adjustment to disfigurement, whether temporary or permanent. Laffrey & Crabtree (1988) compared self-reports of their health by people with cardiovascular disease with self-reports by a healthy control group. The authors suggest that the results show that the so-called chronically ill group defined their state of health in ways that were largely similar to the control group's self-concept.

Laffrey & Crabtree (1988), argue that health professionals need to approach patients from a wider perspective than an illness-oriented one. Following this line of thought, psychosocial nursing interventions would profitably be directed to identifying and reinforcing existing self-directed health behaviours. Knowledge of life-styles and of cultural influences is essential for this aspect of nursing assessment.

PLANNING

Behavioural and cognitive strategies are receiving a good deal of research attention whose preliminary results indicate that these rather than psychodynamically based approaches are more effective in the short term. That is, in the inpatient setting, it is not realistic to aim for the kind of lasting character changes sought in formal or dynamic psychotherapy. So-called supportive psychotherapy risks fostering a dependent relationship whose termination causes extensive problems, as at discharge.

Watson (1983) reviewed the literature on psychosocial interventions with cancer patients. She noted that studies which used mood as their measure of change in patients showed apparent success. What she terms 'entrenched behavioural responses and disturbances' were found to be far less amenable to brief interventions. She em-

phasizes the need for careful assessment of patients' problems in order that specific interventions are carried out with specific aims. She questions the general concept of support, finding that there is often confusion about what is meant by it. It is not clear, for instance, whether information-giving is a form of support or whether it is an activity to be contrasted with so-called therapeutic interventions such as counselling, group work or relaxation.

Many of the studies reviewed by Watson (1983) do not clarify whether patients knew their diagnoses. Evaluation of the effectiveness of nursing actions is impeded by the difficulty of comparison between studies and even between patients. Moreover, if the relationship between patient and nurse is seen as the vehicle by which support is provided, termination at the time of discharge could be seen as increasing the stress on a person already distressed by life-threatening illness or disfiguring treatment or both. It is not known what discharge from treatment at a later stage means to a seriously ill patient: for instance, a cancer patient in remission who is discharged from follow-up.

Behavioural and cognitive strategies depend for their effectiveness on the willingness and ability of the patient and/or the family to carry out 'homework' and so contain the possibility of continuing self-directed therapy in the absence of extensive contact with a therapist. They provide an example of a role for the psychiatric liaison nurse, who can devise and implement a treatment programme. However, the general nurse is still responsible for understanding the principles behind such programmes and for ensuring, say, that appropriate reinforcement is provided for target behaviours by the patient when the specialist is not present.

Nursing measures informed by behavioural and cognitive techniques are a useful first step in establishing a working relationship or partnership with the patient within which responsibility for the promotion of health behaviours is negotiated (Artinian 1983, Teasdale 1987).

An example of part of a simple care plan follows:

CASE EXAMPLE

Problem

Harry becomes so angry when disturbed late at night by nurses carrying out drug therapy with post-operative patients that he is unable to get to sleep until the small hours of the morning.

Objective

Harry will practise his relaxation routine in bed with his curtains drawn for 10 minutes after a warm non-caffeine-containing drink and before settling for the night.

Patient actions

Harry will practise his relaxation routine with one of his nurses until he is confident of carrying it out on his own.
Harry will refrain from watching television and drinking coffee in the late evenings.

Harry will ask the charge nurse to request that the nurses make less noise at night.
Harry will refrain from sleeping during the day, even if he has been kept awake in the night.
Harry will keep a sleep chart to record when and for how long he sleeps.

Nursing interventions

Harry's nurses will arrange times when they can practise Harry's relaxation routine with him uninterrupted and in privacy.
Harry's nurses will ensure that decaffeinated coffee and malted drinks are available as alternatives to coffee and tea.
Harry's nurses will discuss with Harry each day whether the relaxation routine is helping him to sleep.
Harry's nurses will help him find activities during the day to stop him becoming bored.

IMPLEMENTATION

Nursing interventions are designed to meet objectives which are directed to meeting needs or solving problems. Observation and scrupulous record-keeping are required at this stage to ascertain the effects of the interventions and to confirm that the interventions are being carried out correctly (Mason 1984). Nurses are required to provide information to the patient in the form of teaching and direct interaction, but the psychosocial dimension requires them also to work more intensively with each other and with other members of the multi-disciplinary team. Such work is carried out in formal and informal group settings, ranging from ad hoc management discussions to case conferences and reports. Problems may arise because of nurses' different motivations for self-awareness and for discussing emotional responses to patients in front of other people (Kohle et al 1973). Engström (1986) describes the practical difficulties encountered in an attempt to change patterns of staff–patient and staff–staff communication in a neurological ward. Luker & Box (1986) describes the reluctance of nurses in a

dialysis unit to be involved in teaching difficult patients new techniques of dialysis.

It is often in the process of implementation that deficiencies in a care plan can be realized. It is hoped that recording and discussing the effects of implementation prevent nurses from persisting with ineffective interventions.

The implications of the studies quoted are that it is in the areas of carrying out interventions, organizing priorities and communication between staff that the specialist liaison psychiatric nurse has most to offer. He or she can provide consultation to general nurses in working groups where problems in organizing and delivering nursing care can be discussed in order for the group to take responsibility for generating solutions. To be effective, working groups require a defined membership, a consistent location, a commitment by members to attend all scheduled meetings, a commitment to start and to finish on time, and privacy. The specialist nurse who facilitates such groups provides for nurses a model for cooperation and collaboration in problem-solving. Facilitation of working groups ensures that nurses' personal problems remain distinct from relationship problems with other staff or with patients.

EVALUATION

A number of questions require investigation before firm recommendations about training and service programmes can be made.

Evaluation of the provision of psychosocial nursing care to the general hospital inpatient attends both to the individual patient and to the organization of which he or she is more or less a member (Luker & Box 1986). It is not clear what psychiatric problems are seen by general nurses as occurring in their domain and thus as being their responsibility to intervene in. It is questionable whether general nurses are willing and able to consult with specialists and to carry out their recommendations. It is not always clear who may make referrals to the specialist member of staff. If, as implied in the preceding section on assessment, the primary nurse's careful observations reveal a developing problem, it is counterproductive if he or she is then unable to take steps to deal with it. Where channels of communication are unclear or obstructed, potential problems can insidiously develop into crises, because the patient's nurse does not have the authority to elicit help from a specialist when it is needed.

Although this chapter has assumed that assessment is the responsibility of the general nurse regardless of the availability of the specialist nurse, it may be that general nurses do not see it in this way. It is not known whether it is more cost-effective to educate and employ dual-trained nurses, or to educate general nurses in the specific skills required, or to provide a liaison–consultation service of specialist nurses. Identification and measurement of the extent to which psychosocial morbidity has been treated may be in terms of outcomes such as employment, family, marital and sexual relationships, continuing medical or psychiatric treatment, or in less easily measured terms such as anxiety and mood.

Evaluation in the ward setting involves discussion with the patient, the nurse's colleagues and with the specialist liason nurse, if available. Each ward is responsible for determining its standards of psychosocial nursing care and for comparing nursing activities and outcomes with these standards. The specialist liason nurse will work with the rest of the nursing and multidisciplinary teams to agree the standards to be used for audit. It is essential that problems revealed by attention to the kinds of outcomes listed above are also evaluated by reference to the process of nursing care delivery to discover whether standards can in fact be absolute. In particular, the concepts of advice, support, counselling and information-giving need to be 'operationalized' into specific nursing interventions which are then measured against patient outcomes, using psychosocial factors as the criteria for judgement.

THE PSYCHIATRIC LIAISON NURSE

The role of the psychiatric liaison nurse comprises direct clinical care, consultation, supervision, training and research (Tunmore 1987).

Direct clinical care

Case management skills are not part of the usual repertoire of general nurses, who may have difficulties with liaison nurses similar to these experienced with other members of the multidisciplinary clinical team. Active participation in case conferences involving the team is necessary in order that responsibilities can be clearly understood, and so that nurses can reinforce each other's interventions. Intervention by the liaison nurse will be based on an assessment conducted with the patient. Sometimes a single meeting with the patient will be enough for the nurse to plan his or her liaison with the nursing team. At other times it will lead to a planned treatment programme implemented by the liaison nurse.

Consultation

When the liaison nurse acts as consultant, he or she aims to mobilize the skills and knowledge of the general nurses to care for the patient, by helping to clarify problems and generate alternative approaches. However, the liaison nurse is not in charge of the management of a given patient, and so must understand aspects of organizations which facilitate or hinder colleagues' ability to act on consultation.

The focus of consultation may be on the patient or the organization of work, or on the skills of the nurses doing the consulting (Caplan 1970, Steinberg & Yule 1985).

Supervision

Supervision by the liaison nurse is directed towards providing 'supervisees' with an objective appraisal of their problem-solving strategies and either an appropriate support for interventions by less experienced and less confident nurses, or a counterbalance for excessive confidence. Thus general nurses who already possess the necessary skills will plan and carry out psychosocial interventions under supervision.

Training

Where treatment programmes require skills and knowledge beyond those possessed by general nurses it is up to the senior nursing staff, either to provide the training necessary to carry them out, or to arrange for suitably qualified nurses to be available. This requires both honesty (to acknowledge gaps in experience) and a willingness to learn skills, or to collaborate with interventions by colleagues.

Research

The liaison nurse has a key role in evaluating the effectiveness of nursing interventions both in retrospective audit and in commitment to research, including making material available to nurses and guiding them into research-based practice.

The success of the liaison nurse will depend on the quality of his or her relationships with colleagues. Integral to the work of a superviser in human service delivery, is the notion that a by-product of supervision will be the acquisition of confidence by, in this case, the general nurse, which allows him or her to begin collaborating with patients as partners in developing strategies to cope with illness and to attain the best possible level of health (Searles 1965).

REFERENCES

Artinian B M 1983 Becoming a dialysis patient. In: Hamrin E (ed) Research: a challege for nursing practice. Swedish Nurses Association, Stockholm

Barker P 1985 Patient assessment in psychiatric nursing. Croom Helm, Beckenham

Bartels D, Good V, Lampe S 1977 The role of the head nurse: principles of primary nursing. Canadian Nurse 3(3): 27–30

Beck A et al 1978 Cognitive therapy of depression. Guilford Press, New York

Brooking J 1989 A scale to measure use of the nursing process. Nursing Times 85 (15): pp. 44–46

Caplan G 1970 The theory and practice of mental health consultation. Basic Books, New York

Cavanaugh S A, Wettstein R M 1983 The relationship and severity of depression, cognitive dysfunction, and age in medical in-patients. American Journal of Psychiatry 140(4): 495–496

Culpepper R C et al 1986 The effect of primary nursing on nursing quality assurance. Journal of Nursing Administration 16(11): 24–31

Davis T M, Payne L A 1986 Identifying depression in medical patients: opitimal methods of nursing assessment. In Stinson S M et al (eds) New frontiers in nursing:

research. Proceedings of An International Nursing Research Conference. University of Alberta, Edmonton

Engel E T 1986 Psychosomatic medicine, behavioural medicine, just plain medicine. Psychosomatic Medicine 48(7): 466–479

Engström B 1986 A study of changes in the information routines in a neurological ward. International Journal of Nursing Studies 23(3): 231–245

Firman G J, Kaplan M P 1978 Staff 'splitting' on medical–surgical wards. Psychiatry 41: 289–295

Folstein M F, Folstein S E 1975 'Mini-mental state — a practical method for grading the cognitive state of patients for the clinician. Journal of Psychiatric Research 12: 189–198

Friedman M, Rosenman R H 1974 Association of specific overt behaviour pattern with blood and cardiovascular findings. Journal of the American Medical Association 169(12): 1286–1296

Greer S, Morris T 1975 Psychological attributes of women who develop breast cancer: a controlled study. Journal of Psychosomatic Research 19: 147–153

Henry J P 1979 Psychological factors in physical disease. In: Van Praag H M et al (eds) The handbook of biological psychiatry. Part II: Psychophysiology. Marcel Dekker, New York

Ingham R, Fielding P 1985 A review of the literature on attitudes towards old people. International Journal of Nursing Studies 22(3): 171–181

Kelly M 1985 Loss and grief reactions as responses to surgery. Journal of Advanced Nursing 10: 517–525

Kelly M, May D 1982 Good and bad patients: a review of the literature and a theoretical critique. Journal of Advanced Nursing 7: 147–156

Kent L A, Larsen E 1983 Evaluating the effectiveness of primary nursing practice. Journal of Nursing Administration 13(1): 34–41

Kissen D M, Eysenck H J 1962 Personality in male lung cancer patients. Journal of Psychosomatic Research 6: 123–127

Kohle K et al 1973 The training of a nursing staff in psychosomatic medicine in a medical clinic. Psychosomatics 14: 336–340

Laffrey S C, Crabtree K M 1988 Health and health behaviour of persons with chronic cardiovascular disease. International Journal of Nursing Studies 25(1): 41–52

Luker K A, Box D 1986 The response of nurses towards the management and teaching of patients on continuous ambulatory peritoneal dialysis (CAPD). International Journal of Nursing Studies 23(1): 51–59

Marram G et al 1976 Cost effectiveness of primary and team nursing. Contemporary Publishing, Wakefield, Mass

Mason E J 1984 How to write meaningful nursing standards. Wiley, New York

Mayer D K 1985 Non-pharmacologic management of pain in the person with cancer. Journal of Advanced Nursing 10: 325–330

Mechanic D 1961 The concept of illness behaviour. Journal of Chronic Disease 15: 189–194

Mechanic D 1986 Concept of illness behaviour. Psychological Medicine 16: 1–7

Menzies I 1970 The functioning of social systems as a defence against anxiety. Tavistock, London

Millar E 1981 Learning to communicate. Nursing 1: 1197–1199

Minghella E, Brooking J 1987 Parasuicide. Nursing Times 83(21): 40–43

Moffic H S, Paykel E S 1975 Depression in medical in-patients. British Journal of Psychiatry 126: 346–353

Moorey S, Greer S 1989 Psychotherapy for patients with cancer: a new approach. Heinemann, London

Parsons T 1951 The social system. Glencoe Press, Riverside, New Jersey

Peplau H 1952 Interpersonal relations in nursing. Putnam, New York

Pilowsky I 1975 Dimensions of abnormal illness behaviour. Australian and New Zealand Journal of Psychiatry 9: 141–147

Ray C et al 1984 Nurses' perception of early breast cancer and mastectomy, and their psychological implications, and of the role of health professionals in providing support. International Journal of Nursing Studies 21(2): 101–111

Robb B 1967 Sans everything. Nelson, London

Searles H 1965 Collected papers on schizophrenia. Hogarth, London

Sellick K, Russell S, Beckmann 1983 Primary nursing: an evaluation of its effects on patient perception of care and staff satisfaction. International Journal of Nursing Studies 20(4): 265–273

Sensky T 1986 The general hospital psychiatrist: too many tasks and too few roles? British Journal of Psychiatry 148: 151–158

Shepherd M 1980 Mental health as an integrant of primary medical care. Journal of the Royal College of General Practitioners 30: 657–664

Shilts R 1987 And the band played on. Penguin, Harmondsworth

Shukla R 1981 Structure vs people in primary nursing: an inquiry. Nursing Research 30: 236–241

Spielvogel A, Wile J 1986 Treatment of the psychotic pregnant patient. Psychosomatics 27(7): 487–492

Steinberg D, Yule W 1985 Consultative work. In: Rutter M Hersov (eds) Child and adolescent psychiatry: modern approaches. Blackwell, Oxford

Stockwell F 1972 The unpopular patient. Royal College of Nursing, London

Sundeen S J et al 1985 Nurse–client interaction: implementing the nursing process. Mosby, St Louis, Mo

Teasdale K 1987 Partnership with patients? Professional Nurse 2(12): 397–399

Tunmore R 1987 Personal communication

Watson M 1983 Psychosocial intervention with cancer patients: a review. Psychological Medicine 13: 839–846

Wilson-Barnett J, Trimble M 1984 Abnormal illness behaviour: the nursing contribution. International Journal of Nursing Studies 21(4): 267–278

38

The elderly mentally infirm

J. I. Brooking

Elderly people can suffer from a wide range of mental disorder, both organic and functional. Some of these disorders occur most frequently in this age group, such as dementia; others may occur at any time during the life span, such as depression or anxiety. Information contained in other parts of this book is relevant to the elderly, but the manifestations of mental disorders and their care and treatment are profoundly influenced by the ageing process. Consideration of the meaning of old age and the psychological and physiological changes associated with ageing are beyond the scope of this chapter, but are important background information against which nursing should be planned. Care of the elderly mentally infirm takes place in the context of declining physical health, which must also be considered when planning care. Distinctions between physical and mental health in the elderly are entirely artificial, although this chapter necessarily focuses on mental health care.

This chapter aims to introduce readers to the nature, causes and treatment of the most common mental disorders of old age, including dementia, confusional states and depression. Nursing interventions are discussed in detail. The chapter also introduces readers to the range of services available for elderly mentally infirm people, both in hospital and community care, and critically examines the quality of institutional care. Other topics considered briefly include the needs of families, terminal care, legal aspects and preventive aspects.

EPIDEMIOLOGY OF MENTAL DISORDERS IN OLD AGE

There has been a great deal of research into the frequency of various psychiatric disorders in the elderly. Generally, the incidence and prevalence of dementia have been found to increase with age. In a comprehensive review of studies, Eastwood & Corbin (1985) found that prevalence rates for severe dementia are generally less than 3% in the 65 to 69 age group, increasing to more than 20% in the 85 and over age group. In Newcastle, Kay et al (1964) found dementia to be the main determinant of the need for institutional care. Eastwood & Corbin (1985) claimed that the prevalence of dementia was significantly higher among the institutionalized elderly (with estimates ranging from 12 to 65%), than among the general elderly population. In a review of transient cognitive disorders in the elderly, Lipowski (1983) noted that delirium (acute confusion) is a frequent consequence or concomitant of other medical conditions. A reported 10 to 15% of those aged over 65 develop delirium following surgery and 16 to 25% of those admitted to general medical wards are either delirious on admission or develop delirium in the first month of hospitalization. Rates for patients in geriatric units are even higher, with from 35% to 80% of patients delirious at some time during their stay.

Epidemiological research on depression in old age has shown that on average about 10% of those over 65 have a clinical syndrome of depression (Eastwood & Corbin 1985). About 2% to 5% were found to be suffering from depressive illness (Kay & Bergmann 1980), which is thought to be more frequent in women than men. In Western societies the incidence of suicide rises with increasing age, especially among men. About 25% to 30% of all suicides occur in the over 65 age group, although they represent only about 10% to 15% of the population (Shulman 1978). In elderly people, attempted suicide is very rare and usually represents

genuine failure rather than a bid for attention, which is common in the young. The vast majority of suicides and parasuicides in old age are associated with a depressive illness (Post & Shulman 1985). In a study in which men of all ages who had attempted suicide were followed up, Shulman (1978) reported that ultimately fatal acts occurred 20 times more frequently in old rather than young men.

The incidence of neuroses appears to drop with age (Kay & Bergmann 1980). Neugebauer (1980) reviewed European surveys and described a prevalence rate for neuroses in the over 60s as varying from 1% to 10% with a median of 5%. The range in reported prevalence of personality disorders from European surveys was from 3% to 13% with a median of 5%. Combined rates from studies reporting prevalence of both neuroses and personality disorders ranged from 7% to 18% with a median of 12.5%. Reported rates have tended to be appreciably higher in women than men for neuroses and higher in men for personality disorders (Eastwood & Corbin 1985).

Although the peak time for the onset of schizophrenia is young adulthood, there is a subsidiary peak in old age. Kay (1963) found that 4% of schizophrenia in men and 14% in women occurred after the age of 65. In a review of studies of both institutionalized and non-institutionalized people over the age of 60, Neugebauer (1980) described prevalence rates for schizophrenia as ranging from zero to 2.22% with a median rate of 0.32%.

DISTINCTIONS BETWEEN NORMAL AGEING, DEMENTIA AND CONFUSION

In old age many people suffer impairment of cognitive, emotional and social functioning. In mild form these are regarded as non-pathological age-related changes. There has been some debate about whether dementia could be distinguished from normal ageing. The current view according to Levy & Post (1982) is that dementia is quantitatively and probably qualitatively different from the normal ageing process.

Nurses sometimes incorrectly use the terms

Table 38.1 Main differences between dementia and confusional states (from Millard and Bennet 1982)

	Dementia	Confusional states
Precipitant	Brain pathology	Disorder of neuronal metabolism
Onset	Long and gradual	Short and rapid
Course	Chronic	Acute
Variability	Slow deterioration over months	Marked from hour to hour
Recovery	No	Yes — and memory for event vague
Consciousness	Clear	Clouded. Fluctutating brief lucid spells
Orientation	Absent ———————————→	
Memory	Impaired. No insight into deficit	Impaired. May recognise deficit
Cognitive deficits	Global and consistent	Global but variable
Hallucinations	Rare	Frequent
Behaviour	Disinhibited ———————→	
Affect	Often bland, but varies	Perplexed, fearful ? aggressive

dementia and confusion interchangeably. This difficulty arises because patients with dementia are invariably confused. It is hoped that this chapter will show that it is important to recognize the distinctions between the two conditions as the care required for each may be very different (see Table 38.1).

Dementia can be defined as a steady, progressive and usually irreversible decline in previously normal mental function, which is associated with detectable brain pathology. Confusion is an acute or subacute alteration in previously normal mental function, which is often temporary and reversible, associated with impaired brain function usually secondary to a pathological process outside the nervous system.

CLASSIFICATION OF DEMENTIAS

Dementias are termed senile or pre-senile, according to the age of onset — before or after 65. This

chapter is mainly concerned with senile dementia. However, pre-senile dementia must be mentioned as these patients may come into the psychogeriatric services, as few provisions exist for them elsewhere. Others may appear in psychogeriatric wards some years after diagnosis.

There has been uncertainty about appropriate terminology for two reasons. Firstly, scientific understanding of the nature of dementia has increased and some early diagnostic categories found to be inaccurate, e.g. evidence has accumulated that in the absence of infarcts, cerebral arteriosclerosis is unlikely to produce detectable dementia (Levy & Post 1982). Secondly, some believed that the term dementia carried a stigma. Many writers made cosmetic attempts to develop new names for the same disease, e.g. organic brain syndrome, brain failure and cerebral atrophy. These created endless misunderstandings.

The classification outlined below has the advantage of being simple, logical and based on research evidence.

Pre-senile dementias

Several rare diseases have been described as presenile dementias. These include Pick's disease, Huntington's chorea, Jakob Creutzfeldt disease, normal pressure hydrocephalus and neurosyphilis (Miller 1977). Alzheimer's disease is more common and has a bimodal distribution with peaks at ages 40 to 54 and 70 to 84 (Katzman et al 1978). Thus early-onset Alzheimer's disease accounts for many cases of pre-senile dementia.

Senile dementias

In the past many subdivisions of senile dementia were described, but recent evidence shows these to have doubtful validity (Levy & Post 1982). A workshop in the USA (Katzman et al 1978) concluded that Alzheimer's disease accounts for over half of all cases. Less than a fifth of patients have what is now termed multi-infarct dementia. This is a more accurate term for what used to be called arteriosclerotic dementia.

The aetiology and pathology of dementia

Some possible risk factors identified by Katzman et al (1978) include a genetic link, increased brain aluminium concentration, latent viral infections, immunological factors and neurotransmitters. There is thought to be no association with social class, previous intelligence or geographical distribution.

Some or all of the following pathological changes have been found in the brains of demented patients. The brain cells atrophy, mainly in the cerebral cortex. The ventricles enlarge and the gyri are flattened with widening of the sulci. There may be a deficiency of acetyl choline in the cortical and sub-cortical areas. Microscopically, senile plaques, neuro-fibrillary tangles and granulo-vacuolar degeneration occur (Miller 1977).

ASSESSING DEMENTED PATIENTS

Identification of patients' problems

Nursing assessment should focus on the following four areas of functioning within which demented patients experience problems.

Cognitive problems

Memory failure and global intellectual deterioration are central. Some patients may confabulate, i.e. unintentionally fill in memory gaps with fabrications. Patients experience disorientation of time, place, person and self. Disorientation means lack of awareness of one's position relative to the environment. There is impairment of abstract reasoning and judgement.

Emotional problems

There is emotional blunting and lability, i.e. instability with rapid and inappropriate emotional changes. Some sufferers become depressed, suspicious and irritable. There may be exaggeration of the previous personality or the personality may alter markedly.

Social problems

There is narrowing of interests, loss of motivation, regression and desocialization. In some cases, superficial social skills may be retained for a long time. Speech becomes anecdotal, repetitive and increasingly meaningless. Domestic skills decline.

Physical problems

There is general physical deterioration and eventually self-care capabilities are lost. Specific neurological features may occur.

Factors influencing the nature and severity of problems

Although the problems described above are all central to dementia, nurses will find that patients' problems vary in nature and severity. The following factors influence these variations and should be considered during the nursing assessment.

Stage of the dementia

Because dementia is progressive, nurses will meet patients at various stages of the disease. Initially, sufferers may exhibit only mild deterioration such as failure to cope with complex tasks or when under pressure. The condition gradually deteriorates until eventually the patient is totally helpless and dependent.

Underlying pathology

The general features already described apply to most dementias, particularly Alzheimer's disease. However, each type of pre-senile and senile dementia has a different pathology and consequently slightly different clinical features. This is not important as a determinant of nursing care, but accurate diagnosis may be essential for other reasons. For example, Huntington's chorea is transmitted by a single dominant gene, thus genetic counselling of the offspring of sufferers is crucial.

Extent of compensation

Grimley Evans (1982) described how dementia may remain concealed within families for long periods. Families may engage in collusion, may accept deterioration as normal, may fail to notice because their interactions are always concrete and shallow, or fail to notice because the sufferer restricts his life-style so that deficiencies are concealed. This delicate balance can be disrupted by any alteration to the familiar environment, e.g. death of spouse, moving house, a family holiday or admission to hospital. These events can lead to acute decompensation and the previously hidden dementia becomes obvious.

Self-fulfilling prophecy

Described by Merton (1957), this is a prophecy which is fulfilled solely because it was made. It may influence the behaviour or feelings of the person who made it, or the person about whom it was made. It was identified as relevant to dementia by MacDonald (1973) and Libow (1978). Nurses may increase dementia in several ways. They may expect senility and treat patients as senile, which then fosters it. Secondly, patients may be nursed in an environment which is so unstimulating and lacking in orientation cues that dementia is worsened. Thirdly, reversible confusional states may be assumed to reflect dementia and ignored, eventually resulting in permanent damage (LaPorte 1982).

CARE REQUIRED FOR DEMENTED PATIENTS

Participation of the nurse in medical treatment

There are currently no effective medical treatments to reverse or slow the degenerative process of dementia. Patients may be given tranquillizers, antidepressants or sedatives as symptomatic treatment. Cerebrovascular dilators such as cyclo-spasmol (cyclandelate) are occasionally used to increase cortical perfusion where cerebral arterio-sclerosis exists. Ribonucleic acid, alleged to be a substrate of memory, has been used experimentally, but without convincing results. Hyperbaric oxygen treatment has also been tried experimentally, but reviewers conclude that there is little evidence of efficacy (Katzman et al 1978).

Psychological methods of treatment

Stimulation and activity

Studies reviewed by Holden & Woods (1988) suggest that the elderly are often deprived of sensory stimulation, which can increase confusion. Mental stimulation can have beneficial effects on cognitive function. Reviewing studies, Miller (1977) concluded that increased social stimulation of institutionalized demented patients would enhance the quality and quantity of their social interactions. However, gains often disappear once the intervention is withdrawn. It is necessary to devise a permanently stimulating environment to maintain improvements. A range of interesting and engaging activities should be offered to patients, including discussions, music, films, games, outings, visitors, occasional parties etc. Powell (1974) and Diesfeldt & Diesfeldt–Groenendijk (1977) found that structured physical exercise produced improvements in cognitive functioning. Physical activity offered to demented patients should include walking, ball games, keep-fit exercises, skittles, dancing etc.

Changes to the physical environment

This can be as simple as rearranging furniture so as to encourage social interaction. Peterson et al (1977) rearranged chairs in a psychogeriatric ward from straight lines round the walls to small groups. This led to an increase in social interaction among patients. Similarly, if patients eat at small rather than large tables they are more likely to talk to each other. Most people are not used to interacting in large groups. Furniture arrangements which bring together about four to six patients parallel family and work groups. Environmental changes can be more drastic. Marston & Gupta (1977) suggested that large wards or old people's homes should be divided into small living units of eight to 12 people. Holden & Woods (1982) reported that these arrangements seem to reduce confusion and incontinence and residents became more vocal and active. When making changes it is important to remember patients' needs for privacy and personal territory.

Increasing patient participation and choice

There have been several experiments with the institutionalized elderly in which patient participation, control and predictability were manipulated. Unfortunately, the extent to which the subjects were demented is not indicated. Schultz (1976) in a well-controlled experiment found that predictable positive events had a powerful beneficial effect on indicators of physical and psychological status as well as level of activity. Langer & Rodin (1976) in a conceptually similar study gave an experimental group a communication emphasizing their responsibility for themselves. They were given several choices and responsibility for looking after a plant. In comparison with a control group, the experimental group showed significant improvements in alertness, active participation, happiness, level of activity and general sense of well-being.

Both experiments included follow-up studies, but these produced equivocal findings. Rodin & Langer (1977) found that differences between the two groups were maintained and they concluded that decline of the aged can be slowed or reversed by inducing an increased sense of personal control. In his follow-up, Schulz (1980) found that the effects of the intervention had been temporary. This suggests that in order to maintain improvements, increased patient participation and choice need to be continued indefinitely.

Research demonstrating the importance of personal control, participation and choice for elderly people was comprehensively reviewed in Garber & Seligman (1980).

Behavioural methods

These are based on the principles of operant conditioning and require that the subject is sufficiently cognitively intact to learn the association between behaviour and reward. Holden & Woods (1982) reviewed some evidence that demented patients could learn new information. Rewards or reinforcers may take many forms, such as smiles, praise, food, money, cigarettes and extra privileges. In the elderly, reward must be immediate as delayed feedback is not nearly so powerful in modifying behaviour.

Studies have been carried out with elderly patients demonstrating improvements in specific behaviours, such as eating, mobility, continence, participation in purposeful activities and social and verbal interaction. In a detailed review of studies Holden & Woods (1982) concluded that behaviour modification is an extremely promising approach, but there is insufficient evidence of its effectiveness with demented patients.

General programmes for all patients on a ward have been tried. For example, Mishara & Kastenbaum (1973) evaluated a token-economy programme with elderly psychiatric patients. Patients were given tokens as rewards for specified behaviour, which could be exchanged for privileges or cigarettes, wine, extra food etc. The programme was successful in that patients became more independent in performing self-care tasks.

Reality orientation (RO)

RO was originated in the USA by Folsom in about 1958 (Taulbee & Folsom 1966). The first published account of its use in Britain was by Brook et al (1975). It is one of the first therapeutic techniques of a psychological nature designed for use with demented patients. According to Murray et al (1980) RO is intended to maintain reality contact and to reverse or halt confusion, disorientation, social withdrawal and apathy. It enables the patient to relearn and then continually use a range of basic information relating to his or her orientation. RO consists of two main components — informal or 24 hour RO and formal or classroom RO.

Staff attitudes are an essential prerequisite, and a consistent approach, geared to the patients' needs and personality, must be maintained by all staff. Staff must allow patients individuality, dignity, choice and independence. In informal RO, orientation cues are provided in the environment, e.g. clocks, calendars, menus, name tags and names of rooms on doors. Wards can have orientation boards on which the name of the ward and hospital and daily events are displayed in large letters. Family photographs and significant personal items can be displayed on patients' lockers and their names can be displayed over their beds. Current newspapers and magazines should be available. Staff introduce themselves by name at each meeting and repeatedly present current information to the patient. Realistic responses are rewarded with smiles and supportive statements.

During formal or classroom RO, a small group of patients meet daily with a familiar staff member. This is to teach information related to orientation, establish group participation and develop interpersonal relationships. The content of the group work is adjusted to suit the level of cognitive functioning of the group.

Several reviews of evaluation studies have appeared, e.g. Burton (1982), Powell et al (1982), and Woods & Britton (1985). All have pointed out the difficulty of drawing conclusions about the effectiveness of RO because the evaluation studies tend not to be comparable and many are methodologically unsound. However, it is clear that RO brings about improvements in patients' verbal orientation. Whether RO produces change in other dimensions of behaviour is not certain. Powell et al (1982) concluded that RO needs to be continued indefinitely to maintain changes, is good general background, but no substitute for specific therapies geared to individual needs.

Several reviewers have examined the question of how the effects of RO are achieved. Several possible mechanisms have been suggested: reactivation of neural pathways, increased stimulation, behavioural re-education, increased staff attention, patient participation and overcoming depressive withdrawal.

Validation therapy

This was described by Jones (1985) as a companion to RO. It consists of accepting and acknowledging the reality of disoriented patients' feelings. It does not reinforce inaccurate beliefs, but it acknowledges the feelings associated with memories and encourages their expression in order to finish unfinished business. This is a psychotherapeutic approach which helps to resolve emotional conflicts, to relive past pleasures and to come to terms with feelings of loneliness and uselessness.

Group work

Various approaches have been described as suitable for psychogeriatric patients by Murray et al (1980). These include:

RO groups — already discussed.

Reminiscence and life review groups — to be discussed later.

Activity groups. These are notionally intended for the completion of a task such as making a collage. Other components, such as social participation, discussion of feelings and taking responsibility are equally important.

Support groups. These are designed to help patients cope with the changes associated with old age. Topics are chosen by the group for discussion and might include loss, death, depression, isolation etc. These discussions help the elderly realize the universality of their experiences and support one another.

Discharge groups. These are to help patients to plan for their discharge from hospital.

Remotivation groups. A topic of general interest is debated among the patients with a staff member as group leader. Such discussions are claimed to prevent disengagement, increase interest in reality and stimulate thinking. Gray & Stevenson (1980) included reinforcement for sensible utterances. They found that remotivation groups increased social interactions between group members.

Irrespective of the type of group, Murray et al (1980) suggest that the following general principles are helpful with psychogeriatric patients. Groups should have clear goals, explicit rules about confidentiality, timing, membership, turn-taking etc., a leader who provides structure, and a climate of acceptance and mutual appreciation.

Reminiscence and life-review

Butler (1963) first described the need to review one's life in old age, which may be responsible for the increased reminiscence of older people. He described life-review as a 'normal naturally-occurring universal mental process characterized by looking back over life lived and recalling either pleasurable memories or unresolved conflicts which can be surveyed and integrated'. Ideally, life-review should result in new wisdom and insights, so that the old person can retire from life with an acceptable image and dignity.

Reminiscence in groups may be facilitated by a variety of items from the past, photographs and films. For example, Help the Aged Education Department (1981) produced the Recall Package, which consists of tape slide programmes about working-class life in London from the beginning of this century. These are designed to stimulate recollections and encourage communications between patients and carers. There is still much work to be done in evaluating the effects of reminiscence on the mentally infirm elderly.

The nurse's role is to encourage life-review and reminiscence by active listening, accepting, being interested, acknowledging achievements and providing constructive feedback. It should, of course, be remembered that recalling long-repressed emotions may be painful and that some patients may prefer to forget their past experiences, which should be respected (Post 1982).

Hughston & Merriam (1982) reviewed the research literature on reminiscence and concluded that it appeared to result in successful adaptation to old age, improved life satisfaction and enhanced self-concept. Some studies claimed that it improved cognitive functioning. Coleman (1984) carried out a longitudinal study over 10 years and found great individual variations in old people's attitudes towards reminiscence. Some valued memories as a most treasured possession; others regarded the past as finished and unimportant. On the basis of interviews with cognitively intact old people, Coleman (1984) claimed that those who adapted best over the 10 years were those for whom memories offered significant support and those who had plenty of current interests to take the place of the past. Problems were more likely to arise in those people worried by disturbing thoughts about the past and those who could not find means of compensating for the past.

An overview of psychological methods of treatment

There is much overlap among the various treatments described and it is not intended that any one should be used in isolation from the rest. Most of the methods contain the following common elements, which are probably the most important to develop:

1. The patient's environment is enriched and compensates for gaps in functioning
2. Meaningful activities and stimulation are provided
3. Patients are encouraged to participate and make choices
4. Social interaction and mutual help are encouraged
5. Activities take place in small groups
6. Appropriate behaviour is reinforced
7. The ward staff are active and involved. The nurses' role changes from being custodial, emphasizing physical tasks, to being rehabilitative, initiating care to meet all the patients' needs. These changes in nurses' behaviour, and subsequently ward atmosphere, may be the most important factors in all the psychological treatments.

Meeting the basic human needs of demented patients

Bergman (1986) suggested that the most important component of nursing demented people is an attitude of 'humane concern'. She considered that 'the nurse must truly understand and believe that those she cares for are worthwhile individuals with needs and feelings, who deserve respect and love'. This basic value underpins all aspects of care and without it care is no more than maintaining body functions. It is important to remember that patients' problems will vary according to the stage and severity of dementia.

Nutrition

The diet should be adequate in quality and quantity, allowing the patient a choice of foods, which should be attractively presented and of manageable consistency. Modifications to china and cutlery may help the patient to feed him or herself. It is preferable to avoid bibs if possible as they look childish. The patient should wear dentures and attend to oral hygiene. The patient should maintain a reasonable weight. Adequate hydration can be ensured with a selection of drinks chosen by the patient. For more information about eating and drinking, see Thomas (1986).

Elimination

Incontinence is often regarded as an inevitable feature of dementia, but it can frequently be avoided. The causes and management of incontinence are discussed by Norton (1986). Incontinence may result from disorientation, especially in a strange environment. This can be helped by good signposting and lighting and appropriate reminders. Old people may retain high standards of modesty and may avoid asking for assistance due to embarrassment. Incontinence may be a response to the stress of hospitalization, related to loss of independence and self-esteem. It may be a form of regression or an expression of anger or frustration. In a socially impoverished, understaffed ward, incontinence may be rewarded as it is one of the few ways of obtaining attention from nurses. In advanced dementia incontinence aids such as pads and pants, penile sheaths and catheters may be used. Regular toileting coinciding with the most likely times, as revealed by an incontinence chart, may catch some urine. Constipation can be

a problem and should be avoided by a high fibre diet, plenty of fluids and exercise.

Movement and posture

Patients should be kept as mobile as possible with frequent exercise, including outdoor walks if possible. Clothes that allow mobility should be worn, including shoes rather than ill-fitting slippers. Regular chiropody may be needed. Bed- or chair-bound patients can be positioned to allow chest expansion, and active or passive limb movements should be carried out.

Cleanliness, skin care and grooming

The risk of pressure sores should be assessed and preventive measures taken. Patients can be assisted to look attractive and maintain self-esteem with regular hairdressing, removal of facial hair and cosmetics if desired.

Dressing and undressing

Patients should be encouraged to choose what to wear themselves, and clothes can be modified to make independent dressing and undressing easier. If possible, patients should be able to wear their own clothes. If hospital clothes must be worn, they should be attractive, well-matched and correctly fitting. Nightclothes should not be worn during the day.

Body temperature

Nurses should be aware of the risks of hypothermia, even for ambulant patients. The extremities should be kept warm, but movement should not be restrained with shawls and blankets over knees.

Sleep and rest

In many psychogeriatric wards patients doze in chairs all day and are in bed at night for about 12 hours. Understandably, they become restless and are then given unnecessary sedation which increases confusion and creates daytime drowsiness. If patients are busy and active during the day and go to bed for about 8 hours, night sedation is less likely to be needed. Many old people find an alcoholic drink is the best sedative. A short afternoon rest may be beneficial and restore energy for later activities.

Respiration

Bed rest and inactivity increase the risk of respiratory infections, and inactive patients should have deep breathing exercises several times a day. If patients smoke, they should be observed unobtrusively because of the risk of fire.

Avoiding dangers in the environment

Ambulant demented patients are particularly prone to accidents as they may wander away from the ward. Nurses are responsible for ensuring that the ward is a safe environment. Floors should be non-slip and there should be no frayed carpet edges. Dangerous items such as poisons and sharp knives should be locked away. Stairs and corridors should be well lit. Baths and lavatories should have handrails. Patients who tend to wander should be closely supervised and engaged in interesting activities.

The use of restraints. It is not uncommon for psychogeriatric patients to be restrained with the tacit approval of the institution, e.g. cot sides on beds, tables attached to tilting geriatric chairs, and sheets tying patients to beds or chairs. Miller (1975) reviewed the literature on the use of restraints and found a variety of adverse consequences: severe distress and regression; exacerbation of dementia; death wish; loss of ego strength; weight loss and incontinence. Miller cited several studies showing that the immobility resulting from the use of restraints produced muscle atrophy, osteoporosis, hypercalcaemia and other disorders. In addition to these medical and psychological reasons, there are also ethical objections to the use of restraints. They can rarely be justified.

Worship

Patients must be helped to continue practising their religion if they wish.

Communication

Nurses can help patients to overcome sensory deficits by arranging for spectacles and hearing aids to be provided as necessary. Excessive meaningless stimuli, such as background noise from unwatched televisions, should be avoided. Nurses should make use of touch and should remember the patient's needs for affection and friendship. Good relationships between patient, family and friends should be promoted. For a discussion of sexuality in old age see Webb (1986).

Work and accomplishment

The patient's skills should be used to maintain a sense of worth. If possible, the patient can be placed in an advisory or consultative role. Nurses should encourage creative expression, individuality, decision-making and participation in care. Assistance with financial affairs and official papers may be required.

Recreation

A wide range of recreational facilities should be available, e.g. games, cards, billiards, table tennis, books, newspapers, art and sewing materials, music and flower arranging.

Learning, discovery and curiosity

Demented patients need routine and order in their lives to increase predictability of events. The patient should establish the daily routine, then maintain a structured and dependable programme. Changes should be introduced slowly after careful preparation. If the patient is required to take part in activities and discussions which are too complex, frustration and disappointment may result.

CONFUSION

Classification and mechanisms of confusion

Confusional states are classified according to whether or not the onset is acute and the condition of short duration, or the onset sub-acute, with longer duration. The condition may also be classified according to its underlying cause. The mechanisms of confusion in the elderly are not fully understood. Grimley Evans (1982) hypothesized that they are more prone to delirium than younger adults because of increased neural noise and an impaired blood–brain barrier. Grimley Evans suggested that when neural noise is further increased by random neuro-transmitter activity, there is interference to perception, attention, memory etc.

A long-standing debate has existed as to the preferred diagnostic label for this syndrome. Terms used include reversible dementia, delirium, acute brain failure, pseudosenility, clouded states, acute brain syndrome and acute confusional states (Foreman 1986). All of these can be assumed to mean much the same as confusion.

Assessing confused patients

Identification of patients' problems

Nursing assessment should include the following four areas of functioning.

Cognitive problems. Patients are usually disorientated in time, place, person and self. They may experience perceptual problems such as illusions, i.e. misidentification of a real sensory stimulus, or visual hallucinations, i.e. a false perception occurring without any real sensory stimulus. Memory and learning will be affected and confabulation can occur. The patient cannot concentrate and is easily distracted. Thought processes are sluggish and confused. Information and events may be misunderstood.

Emotional problems. Patients may be anxious, apprehensive, fearful, agitated, perplexed or belligerent.

Social problems. Communication is inevitably disrupted by the cognitive deficits. Speech may become rambling, disorganized and verbose.

Physical problems. These are largely determined by the cause of the confusional state and some patients will be very ill. Confusion is often worse at night or in the dark, and sleep may be disturbed. Some patients exhibit stereotyped and

perseverating movements. Restlessness may be present.

Factors predisposing to confusion

Multiple factors may be responsible in the elderly. For example, Trimble (1981) described how mild electrolyte imbalance, mild anaemia and hypoxia, combined with a mild pyrexia, may be enough to precipitate the clinical illness. Furthermore, pre-existing mild dementia may lower the threshold for the appearance of an acute confusional state. Identification of the causes of a confusional state is an essential part of nursing assessment for three reasons: firstly, to enable nurses to understand and predict the pattern of problems experienced by patients; secondly, nurses can help to prevent confusion if they understand the predisposing conditions and try to reduce them at any early stage; thirdly, the main principle of treatment and care is to search for relevant causes and remove or reduce them. The main causes are discussed under nine headings.

Pharmacological causes. Drug-induced confusion may be a side-effect or a withdrawal effect, and even quite small dosages may induce toxicity in the elderly. Examples of drugs commonly associated with toxicity include L-dopa, steroids, diuretics, anti-hypertensives, insulin and oral hypoglycaemics, digitalis, barbiturates, benzodiazepines and other psychotropic drugs. The high incidence of drug-induced confusion points to the need for regular drug review and close monitoring.

Nutritional deficiencies. These may be general malnutrition or specific vitamin deficiencies.

General medical conditions. These include cardiac, hepatic and renal diseases. Other conditions which may precipitate acute confusional states are alcoholism, anaemia, hypotension and hypothermia.

Infections. Any systemic infection with high fever involving dehydration and electrolyte imbalance may cause confusion. Most commonly, this includes pneumonia, septicaemia and pyelitis.

Endocrine disorders. Any hormonal imbalance may be a causative factor. These include thyroid, pancreatic, pituitary or adrenal cortex disease.

Neurological conditions. These include trauma, neoplasms, anoxia, infections and haemorrhages involving the nervous system. Epilepsy, strokes and dementia also increase the risk of confusional states.

Surgical causes. Confusional states are sometimes precipitated by major surgery, especially to the heart, brain, eye and reproductive organs. Other causes associated with surgery include prolonged anaesthesia, shock, electrolyte imbalance, pain and anxiety.

Environmental causes. Patients may lack sensory supports such as spectacles and hearing aids to enable them to perceive their environment correctly. Hospital wards are often noisy and confusing, lacking familiar objects, clocks and calendars etc. The general disturbance of the ward may cause sleep disruption and the normal cycle of light and dark may be interrupted, e.g. intensive care unit lights on all the time. Armstrong-Esther & Hawkins (1982) argued that admission to hospital could eliminate the social cues which elderly people need to maintain synchronization of circadian rhythms. They argued that if desynchronization occurred this could lead to confusion, sleep disturbances and incontinence.

Psychological causes. The importance of the self-fulfilling prophecy has already been mentioned. Once a patient has been labelled as confused, the ward staff often sustain the confusion by their behaviour (Chisholm et al 1982). Other important psychological factors include depersonalization, loss of personal control over events and self, stress and anxiety, and social isolation.

Care required for confused patients

Prevention of confusion is of first importance. Given an understanding of the conditions prodromal to confusion, the nurse can attempt to reduce them. If a patient has developed a confusional state, then the main principles of treatment are to search for the cause, to treat or reduce all precipitating factors, and to provide supportive and symptomatic care (Foreman 1986).

Participation of the nurse in medical treatments

Hypnotics are rarely used as they cause dangerous sleepiness, make assessment difficult and increase confusion. Sometimes the patient may be so agitated that sedation is essential. Post (1982) then recommends the use of promazine (sparine), haloperidol or droperidol. Specific medical interventions will vary according to the cause of the condition.

Controlling the patient's environment

The environment should be kept constant to make it familiar and should be quiet and peaceful. These patients are best nursed in single rooms. The room should contain orientation cues such as clocks, calendars, windows and familiar objects. Background noise from radios, conversations etc. adds further to ambiguous and random stimuli, thus increasing confusion.

Dealing with psychological distress

Anxiety, hyperactivity, fear and screaming are not uncommon. A frightened patient should not be left alone and the nurse should be calm and supportive. If hallucinations and illusions occur, it is helpful to explain to the patient what is happening and reassure him or her. Realistic responses should be rewarded with appropriate reinforcement. The room should be well lit all the time to reduce confusion and fear.

Meeting the basic human needs of confused patients

The nursing interventions discussed here are required for most acutely confused patients, irrespective of the cause. However, other problems are likely to exist, depending on the cause of the confusional state. The need for other nursing actions should be assessed individually.

Nutrition. Hydration is often a problem and patients must be offered drinks constantly. Many patients are anorexic and may need help and encouragement to eat a light but nutritious diet.

Elimination. Incontinence can be reduced if the patient is taken to the lavatory or commode every hour or two. Constipation is common.

Movement and posture. The patient may wander restlessly, but it is preferable not to restrict movements too much.

Cleanliness, skin care and grooming. Patients can be helped to maintain their body image by wearing their own day clothes or night wear. Help may be required with grooming.

Dressing and undressing. The steps involved in dressing may be too complex for a confused patient who will become frustrated at his or her own incompetence. Patients should be helped with dressing. Clothes which are comfortable and easy to wear, such as night clothes, may be most appropriate.

Sleep and rest. Typically, confusion is worse at night and in the dark. The room should thus be adequately lit, even at night. Other measures which will help to avoid the 'sundown syndrome' include: avoiding fatigue and pain, ensuring that bladder and bowels are emptied, giving clear explanations of all occurrences, and keeping the environment constant.

Avoiding dangers in the environment. The safety of the patient is a major concern as he or she may be restless and wandering. These patients need careful constant observation within a safe and reasonably enclosed environment.

Communication. Ideally, the same nurses should care for the patient all the time. Any strangers should be introduced and the purpose of the visit explained. The patient should be informed of everything happening. Nurses should present a calm, concerned and understanding demeanour, speaking in a clear voice using simple statements. A quiet, soothing voice helps to reduce agitation. Touch can be used to calm and reassure the patient. Occasional lucid intervals should be used to establish rapport. The patient should be encouraged to wear his or her spectacles and hearing aid to support sensory reception.

DEPRESSION

According to Bergmann (1982) depression in the elderly is relatively common, but is often not recognized, and even when recognized, often not treated. Two inaccurate assumptions are commonly held: firstly, that depression is inevitable in old age and therefore not worth treating; secondly, that depression is a prodromal phase of senility and therefore not treatable.

Nurses will meet patients who have suffered from recurrent attacks of depression all their lives, and others who have developed a late-onset depression. Post (1982) suggested that depression in the elderly shows the influence of the ageing process, but is not essentially different from depression in other age groups. He considered that elderly depressives can appear anywhere in the classical spectrum from psychotic to neurotic manifestations with a large overlap in the middle. One important age-related difference is that elderly depressives have more hypochondriacal symptoms than younger depressives (Gurland 1976).

Factors causing depression in the elderly

The causes of depression in the elderly can be discussed under three main headings:

Social factors

Many stresses and losses occur in old age which may precipitate depression. Post (1972) reported the existence of precipitating events in more than 60% of the elderly depressives he studied. These social factors may include bereavement; retirement with its loss of status and income; reduced efficiency of the body and reduced mobility; awareness of one's own mortality; and overt or covert messages from the rest of society about reduced worth. Murphy (1982) found that elderly people lacking a confiding relationship were more vulnerable to depression. Often such people had never had a confidant, so this seemed related to life-long personality vulnerability.

Biological factors

Physical illness is known to be an important causative factor (Salzman & Shader 1979, Murphy

1982). A family history of depression is found in many patients. Other possible biological causes include changes in circadian rhythms, lower levels of biogenic amines and cerebral hypofunction. Many commonly prescribed drugs have been found to induce depression in the elderly (Davison 1978).

Personality factors

Learned helplessness, associated with perceived loss of control, was first identified as a major cause of depression by Seligman (1974) and shown relevant to the elderly by Schulz (1976). About half of elderly depressives have shown earlier neurotic tendencies with anxiety, depression or sexual maladjustment.

It is important for nurses to be aware of the causes of depression so that they are alert to the possible onset of depression. The two single most important antecedents are physical illness and bereavement, especially loss of spouse. Of course, old people vary in their reactions to bereavement, depending on their coping skills, other resources, personality and dependence on the lost spouse.

The relationship between depression and physical illness

Several possible relationships occur. Depression is a common reaction to serious illness of surgery, especially amputation, colostomy and chronic infections. Some physical illnesses, such as occult malignancies and giant-cell arteritis, may present initially as depression (Grimley Evans 1982). 'Masked depression' (Pfeiffer 1977) may present as vague physical symptoms against a background of anorexia, weight loss, loss of energy, sleep disturbance and constipation. Elderly people with functional psychiatric disorders show higher morbidity and mortality rates than average for their age (Kay et al 1966).

The relationship between depression and dementia

The two commonly co-exist and according to

Lader (1981) five forms of association can be found:

- They can co-exist by chance
- The same brain pathology, e.g. multiple infarcts, can cause both
- Incipient dementia may make the patient become depressed as he or she realizes that his or her mental capacity is decaying
- Incipient dementia may lead to self-neglect and social isolation, resulting in situational depression
- Depression may lead to self-neglect with malnutrition and vitamin deficiencies, which in turn result in confusion and mental deterioration.

Whatever form the relationship takes, any associated intellectual impairment makes the assessment of depression more difficult, as symptoms may be masked.

Clinical features of depression

In a study of elderly depressives admitted to a psychiatric unit, Post (1972) found that approximately a third exhibited severely psychotic symptoms. These patients experienced bizarre, paranoid and nihilistic delusions. Some had auditory hallucinations. Many were physically retarded with sleeplessness, anorexia and weight loss. Hypochondria, bodily complaints, self-deprecation, guilt and ideas of poverty were common. Many communicated great sadness, fear, dread, agitation and despair. Another third of the patients exhibited more neurotic than psychotic symptoms. Generally they conveyed less avert sadness than is typical in younger patients and more anxiety. These patients preserved the capacity to see that their feelings were due to their emotional state. They had many physical complaints and sought constant reassurance about their health. They experienced feelings of worthlessness and self-reproach.

Nursing assessment

Self-care capability should be considered and physical assessment should include level of activity, sleep pattern, appetite and bowel function. Physical complaints should be investigated. Psychological factors to be assessed include mood, self-esteem, level of anxiety, feelings of guilt and cognitive processes. The existence of psychotic symptoms such as hallucinations and delusions should be assessed and their content noted. It is important to examine the patient's social relationships with family and friends.

Care required for depressed patients

In general the techniques of therapy appropriate to younger adults are equally relevant to the elderly. Woods & Britton (1985) consider that the most significant special consideration is physical health. Deafness, for example, makes individual and group psychotherapy very difficult. It is difficult for a nurse to sound empathic when talking loudly to a very deaf patient.

Participation of the nurse in medical treatments

Drug treatment. Tricyclic antidepressants are used most frequently. These include amitriptyline, imipramine and doxepin. The elderly tend to be more sensitive than younger adults to smaller dosages and may experience serious side-effects. Anticholinergic effects, i.e. signs of sympathetic overactivity, are common and include dry mouth, blurred vision, tremor and palpitations. Dangerous side-effects such as glaucoma, prostate damage and cardiotoxicity can occur. These drugs may take about 2 weeks to exert their antidepressant effect and they may also cause undesirable sleepiness. The tetracyclic antidepressants are newer drugs with fewer anticholinergic effects. They include mianserin hydrochloride. Monoamine oxidase inhibitors (MAOIs), e.g. phenelzine and isocarboxazid, are now rarely used unless tricyclics are ineffective. They have very serious side-effects and special dietary restrictions are essential.

Electroconvulsive therapy (ECT). Old age is not a contraindication, although the risk of troublesome side-effects is somewhat increased. Reviewing the evidence on the use of ECT with the elderly, Fraser (1982) concluded that the treatment is very effective against a wide range of depressive symptoms. It is particularly useful when drug treatment has failed or with suicide risk or risk of serious self-neglect.

Participation of the nurse in psychotherapy and counselling

It was traditional psychiatric wisdom that psychotherapy was ineffective with the elderly. Eisdorfer & Stotsky (1977) reported that this view is now changing and psychotherapy is being used with success. Studies reviewed by Post (1982) suggest that psychotherapeutic approaches with the depressed elderly should be directive and combined with somatic treatments.

Bergmann (1978) summarized the major tasks facing elderly people which form the focus of psychotherapy. These included: accepting the closeness of death; adjusting to declining health and physical disabilities; achieving a rational dependence on medical, family and social support, while exercising available choices; and maintaining emotionally gratifying relationships with friends and family. Other important themes in psychotherapy with the elderly were identified by Butler & Lewis (1982). These included: the need for assertion to redress helplessness and reduced self-esteem; making reparations for guilt; adjusting to losses, both of loved ones and body function; enjoying the limited time left for life; coping with the fear of death; and restructuring social life and relationships. Woods & Britton (1985) claimed that the main differences between psychotherapy with old and young people are that no attempts should be made with the elderly to change long-standing personality patterns or to trace dynamics back to childhood.

Other therapeutic approaches which may be used with the depressed elderly include behavioural treatments such as anxiety reduction, cognitive therapy, activity programmes, problem-solving, increasing personal control and social skills training. Bereavement counselling may be particularly relevant as this is such a major cause of depression in old age. Life review and reminiscence may be used for depression and other neurotic disorders. Group work may include discussion groups, support and activity groups, and could be led by nurses with relatively little extra training. The extent of nurses' involvement in formal therapy depends on their expertise in using these techniques. With appropriate training, nurses can function as psychotherapists and counsellors.

Nursing actions to help patients overcome depression

This is the central part of nurses' work with depressed patients, yet surprisingly there is little literature about what nurses can do to relieve depression. The nurse's attitude and manner can be therapeutic. Nurses should convey to patients that they are accepted and appreciated as valuable. The nurse should attempt to be calm, caring, supportive and empathic, communicating these qualities verbally and non-verbally. The patient may be helped by information about the illness. It is important to convey that negative feelings are temporary and treatable. It is helpful to explain that physical symptoms may be a feature of the depression. Patients should be encouraged to ventilate their feelings and negative emotions including sadness, anger and guilt. Conflicts and feelings of loss may be resolved by rational discussion with a sympathetic nurse. Thus patients can be helped to see that a happy future is possible. The patient should also be encouraged to engage in a wide range of physical and mental activities. Positive responses and behaviour should be reinforced. At times of great adversity, many people turn to religion to seek meaning in their existence (Weber 1961). Attendance at church services and visits from a chaplain may be a great comfort to depressed patients.

Meeting the patient's physical needs

Elderly depressed patients, even if they have no associated physical illness, commonly experience many physical problems, each of which should be treated. Patients may need assistance and encouragement with basic hygiene and grooming. Loss of appetite, weight loss and constipation are common. Sleep disturbance may be associated with anxiety and inability to relax. Patients may become lethargic and unwilling to exercise.

SUICIDE

Suicide risk should be assessed in collaboration with the whole health care team so as to determine the intensity of precautions required. Any threat of suicide must be taken seriously. A patient's predisposition to suicide should be considered under the following three headings.

Psychiatric predisposition

In young people suicide attempts are associated more frequently with personality disorders than with depression. However, in the elderly, suicidal ideas and behaviour are almost always related to clinical depression. A small percentage of elderly suicides are those of alcoholics, patients with organic brain disease and the terminally ill.

Social predisposition

An important characteristic of suicide is social isolation and lack of integration into the community. Typically there are few important ties, whether familial, religious, occupational, cultural or social. Sainsbury (1968) found that 39% of elderly suicides lived alone. Men are more likely to kill themselves than women. Retirement, for men, may produce a social void as most friendships were with colleagues. For housewives, the domestic and social roles change little with increasing age and most friendships continue to be with neighbours.

Stressful events

Sainsbury (1968) found that 35% of elderly suicides suffered from a physical illness and 16% were recently bereaved. Any major crisis or interpersonal conflict can be seen as a risk factor.

Helping suicidal patients

Nurses' responsibilities to potentially suicidal patients include dealing with the factors precipitating suicide, developing a supportive relationship, close observation and providing a safe environment. The care of depressed patients has been discussed earlier and is relevant here. Nurses can help to reduce social isolation by encouraging visits from family and friends, helping patients to make new friends, encouraging involvement in community activities, clubs, churches, etc. Bereavement counselling may be helpful.

The nurse should try to develop a supportive relationship with the patient and should find out what and whom still matter to the patient. The sources of distress should be identified and discussed openly. The nurse should assure the patient that such feelings are not unusual. The nurse must be aware of his or her possible importance to the patient. If going off-duty or leaving the ward, this should be explained and the patient introduced to the replacement nurse.

During the crisis period the nurse should take all precautions necessary to prevent suicide or self-mutilation. The first principle is constant unobtrusive observation by a designated nurse in a tactful way which will not be stressful designs or offensive to the patient. This is best achieved by sharing the patient's activities rather than scrutiny without participation. It is preferable to explain these basic precautions to the patient, using an honest but kindly attitude. Dangerous objects such as razors, scissors, belts, drugs, matches, glass objects, etc. should be removed. Windows should be locked or blocked. The patient should be supervised when bathing, using a razor or knife and when smoking. Despite these precautions nurses should try to convey a feeling of empathic optimism that the patient will feel better. Staff should be aware of the dangers of the self-fulfilling prophecy if they feel hopeless about the patient.

OTHER EMOTIONAL DISORDERS

This section desribes some of those psychiatric disorders (often termed 'functional' disorders) in which there is no currently demonstrable organic pathology. The aetiology of many so-called functional disorders is not yet fully understood, but may include organic factors such as biochemical abnormalities. Thus the distinction between organic and functional disorders is not clear cut, especially in the psychiatry of old age, where the effects of the ageing process and of the deteriorating brain are relevant. There is no sharp demarcation between neurotic and psychotic disorders and it is preferable to view them as a continuum rather than a dichotomy. Personality disorders form another category. For a more detailed discussion see Post (1982).

Schizophrenia and paranoid states

There is a large population of schizophrenics who have been in psychiatric hospitals for decades and are now elderly. Although some classic symptoms such as delusions and hallucinations may remain, their main problem is severe institutionalization with flat affect, passivity and loss of capacity for autonomous action.

Paranoia is the attribution to other people of motivations which do not exist (Pfeiffer 1977). In young people it is usually indicative of schizophrenia, but in the elderly it is very common and less serious. It is typically associated with solitary living, insecurity, anxiety and encounters with ageism. Reduced sensory input can lead to misinterpretation of the environment and suspicion. It should be remembered that old people can genuinely be persecuted, discriminated against and rejected by their families and neighbours. In mild forms of paranoid psychosis there is a transitory delusionary state, often precipitated by stress. In more severe forms this becomes paraphrenia, a form of schizophrenia in which persecutory delusions and sometimes hallucinations occur, although the personality remains intact. This is most common in women and is often associated with social isolation and deafness.

Psychotropic drugs have greatly improved what used to be a poor prognosis. Nursing interventions should be aimed at reducing stress, reducing any genuine persecution, helping the patient to explore reality, increasing self-esteem, maximizing remaining cognitive capabilities, improving sensory input and developing a trusting relationship. It is pointless to contradict delusions, but nor should they be reinforced. It is best to admit puzzlement and gently suggest alternative explanations.

Affective psychoses

Depression, which may be neurotic or psychotic, has already been discussed. Mania, studied by Shulman & Post (1980), is much rarer than depression and typically occurs in women. Some cases are just mania, others are mixed manic-depressive. Shulman & Post (1980) argued that mania in old people rarely shows the classical 'flights of ideas'. A hostile, surly affect is more usual and depression is never very far away. The prognosis has been improved by drug treatment, such as lithium carbonate. Nursing interventions for manic patients should be aimed at ensuring that basic needs such as diet, elimination, hygiene, rest etc. are not neglected, providing a safe and calming environment and redirecting the patient's energies in purposeful activities.

Neuroses

Because elderly neurotic people are rarely referred to psychiatrists except after a suicide attempt, the study of neuroses in old age has been rather neglected (Kral 1982). Some people suffer from neuroses all their lives and, according to Müller (1969), neuroses tend to become less disabling in later life. As the personality becomes less extroverted, patterns of neurotic symptoms tend to shift from outward manifestations to more inwardly directed states. Post (1982) wrote that late-onset neurotics differ from life-long neurotics in that they are more often afflicted with real physical illness, have a higher mortality risk, are lonely and have low incomes.

Obsessive-compulsive neurosis is the only classical neurosis which appears for the first time in old age (Post 1982). Hypochondria is common, especially in women, due to increased concern with health and illness in old age. According to Vogel (1982) acute anxiety states are rare, but chronic anxious ruminations are common. Anxiety may arise from losses, changes and helplessness, and is likely to exacerbate physical problems. Drugs

should be used to treat neurotic symptoms, such as anxiety or depression. Distressing life circumstances should as far as possible be reduced. Individual and/or group psychotherapy may be helpful, unless denial is the patient's preferred coping strategy. It may be possible to work with relatives to improve family relationships.

Personality disorders

It is thought that 'deviant' personalities tend to become more normal with old age. Aggression reduces, but inadequacy worsens. Alcoholism is fairly common (Mishara & Kastenbaum 1980). Diogenes syndrome was described by Clark et al (1975), although Muir Gray (1985) suggested that 'this term is a reflection more of the desire of the medical profession to classify individuals than of the objective existence of any such condition'. These eccentrics have a history of being independent, quarrelsome and secretive. They reject social contact and live in squalor, although they are not poor. They tend to have at least average intelligence and are often middle or upper class. On the other hand, social isolation often occurs because of bereavement or rejection and can significantly reduce life satisfaction. That kind of isolation is remediable, whereas elderly eccentrics neither want nor need help.

SERVICES FOR THE ELDERLY MENTALLY INFIRM

The development of psychogeriatric medicine and nursing

Specialized psychiatric services for the elderly began during the 1960s (e.g. Robinson 1962); since then there has been increasing recognition and acceptance of the need for special services in each locality. The Royal College of Psychiatrists established a Specialist Section for the Psychiatry of Old Age which has been important in the development of ideas and has generated a series of policy statements and guidelines for practice (e.g. Royal College of Psychiatrists 1973). A Department of Health and Social Security (DHSS) Working Party also endorsed the trend towards special psychiatric services for the aged (DHSS 1981).

Factors which have contributed to the development of psychogeriatric services were described by Arie & Jolley (1982) as: the increase in the number of elderly people, especially the very old; developments in psychiatry leading to more effective treatments for the elderly; and acceptance that health services should be planned for defined populations. The purposes of psychogeriatric services were described by Arie & Jolley (1982) as maintaining mental health, preserving independence, and providing permanent or intermittent institutional care when necessary.

After years of neglect, psychogeriatric medicine has become a recognized specialty. Both psychiatrists and geriatricians have chosen to specialize in this subject. By 1984, at least 150 consultant psychiatrists described psychogeriatrics as their main activity, which was some 14% of consultants in general psychiatry (Arie et al 1985). The Royal College of Psychiatrists (1981) suggested that there should be at least two psychogeriatricians in each health district. The role should include the organization of facilities and staff in the district, representing the specialty in planning committees, clinical practice, education and research (Arie & Jolley 1982).

The care of the elderly mentally infirm has traditionally been regarded as an unattractive and low-prestige area of nursing. There is, however, evidence that attitudes are beginning to change. For example, in Scottish surveys Jones (1986) found very positive attitudes among nurses to psychogeriatric nursing.

General and psychiatric nursing students gain experience in the care of the elderly during training, although general nursing students may not work with psychogeriatric patients. As these patients may be cared for in general or psychiatric settings, their carers may be either general or psychiatric nurses. Possibly a combination of both kinds of nursing experience provides the best preparation for work in this specialized area. Post-basic clinical courses relevant to psychogeriatric nursing include Nursing Elderly People, Community Psychiatric Nursing and Advanced Psychiatric Nursing. There are no clinical courses which are specific to psychogeriatric nursing. The setting up of such a course would provide a major landmark in establishing the care of the elderly mentally infirm as a recognized branch of nursing.

Categories of psychogeriatric patients and services required

A DHSS document published in 1972 classified mentally ill old people into four groups, and defined the relative responsibilities of geriatric, psychiatric and medical units and social services departments in caring for this population. This classification inevitably creates a lack of integration in services. The four categories were as follows:

1. Patients who entered psychiatric hospitals before modern treatment was available, have grown old and are likely to live out their lives in hospitals. They are about 20% of the current psychiatric hospital population (Macdonald 1982). The fate of their successors, the middle-aged chronic schizophrenics, is uncertain, but it is likely that some will remain in psychiatric hospitals. These groups of patients are the responsibility of psychiatrists within the general psychiatric services.
2. The elderly with functional mental illnesses contribute more than half the referrals to most psychiatric services. They are also likely to remain within the spectrum of general psychiatry.
3. Patients with a mild degree of senile dementia but no physical disease can usually be cared for in their own home. Their social circumstances may require residential or day care under the social services department.
4. Severely demented ambulant patients could be cared for in psychogeriatric day hospitals or admitted to psychiatric care. Demented patients with an associated physical illness are mainly the responsibility of the geriatric medical services, whether as inpatients or day patients.

Services for sufferers living at home

Government policy in Britain emphasizes the importance of treatment and care in the community rather than in hospital (e.g. Department of Health and Social Security 1978). In European countries studies show that less than 10% of the elderly with psychiatric disorders receive institutional care (World Health Organization 1985). Hemsi (1982) described reasons for this community emphasis: the disorders are such that no hospital investigations may be required and little is gained by admission; old people are members of social networks which should be maintained; institutional resources are scarce and expensive; and there are well recognized disadvantages of hospital care. Therefore, Hemsi (1982) argued that it is better to support the patient (and his or her carers) in the community.

It is usual in psychogeriatric practice for initial assessment to take place in the patient's home (Arie & Jolley 1982). This is because functioning at home gives an accurate picture of the patient's capacities, whereas moving the patient can increase confusion. Hemsi (1982) argued that hospital assessment is only appropriate when special investigations are necessary.

Large numbers of people are involved in community care. These include families, friends and neighbours; statutory authorities such as social services and community health services; and a variety of charities and voluntary agencies such as church groups. In trying to achieve the goal of community care, obstacles arise because of the administrative separation of the health services, provided by central government, and the social services, provided by local authorities.

Many mentally infirm old people are cared for by relatives. According to Pasker et al (1976) families carry a formidable burden, yet rarely receive adequate support from the domiciliary services. Services which should be available include home-helps, meals-on-wheels, laundry services, telephones, emergency call systems, etc. Bergmann et al (1978) argued that if resources are limited, more domiciliary services should be directed to people living with their families than to those living alone. This is because the former

can often remain at home given adequate support, whereas many of the latter will inevitably require eventual admission. Woods & Britton (1985) argued that 'the task of all agencies is to attempt to support these supporters, who often experience considerable strain. This arises as much from the emotional demands of caring as the physical burden'. Support for families/home carers should include information in the form of 'a clear basic description of the problems of the patient, what is wrong and its likely implications, in simple straightforward language' (Woods & Britton 1985).

The World Health Organization has made efforts to stimulate the production of self-health care guides for the elderly and literature for family carers (World Health Organization 1984). In Britain, the Alzheimer's Disease Society provides literature for families on caring for a relative with dementia. Respite care ranges from a 'sitter' for a few hours to allow a shopping trip or an evening out, to holiday admissions of a fortnight or longer. Individual and/or group psychological support is also important, and Woods & Britton (1985) suggested that 'relatives' support groups can provide a focus for communication and sharing of problems and support, both practical and emotional'. The Alzheimer's Disease Society, founded in London in 1979, runs a counselling service and self-help groups, as well as providing literature on aids, services and other resources.

Elderly mentally infirm people living alone, without family support, pose considerable problems, and innovative patterns of community care are required to avoid hospitalization. One example is the Intensive Domiciliary Care Scheme started in Liverpool in 1981 and evaluated by Crosby et al (1984). This is a flexible and comprehensive package of home care for people suffering from dementia who would otherwise be dependent on hospital care. Sufferers receive care for up to 5 hours every day from specially trained aides working under the close supervision of a community psychiatric nurse. Training for the aides stresses the importance of stimulating the patients mentally and socially and maintaining independence. The aides meet their supervisor at least weekly and patients are monitored by the community psychiatric nurse.

In Britain general practitioners (family doctors) deal with most of the problems of the elderly mentally infirm without referring them to consultants. However, a study by Williamson et al (1964) found that general practitioners were unaware of many of the psychiatric disorders suffered by their elderly patients. It also appeared that patients did not always receive adequate long-term medical supervision. These problems may be due to the organization of general practice as a patient-initiated service.

Community psychiatric nurses are playing an increasing role in the care of mentally abnormal old people (Ainsworth & Jolley 1978), and many specialist posts have been created within general community psychiatric nursing teams. District nurses, health visitors and social workers are also likely to be involved in home care.

Day-care facilities

Day care is a natural link between institutional and home care, and may provide enough support for patients who would otherwise be unable to remain at home. Patients can benefit from social interaction, nursing care, medical treatment and stimulating activities. Day facilities are entirely dependent on the availability of transport. Discharge from day care is most often by death or admission to another form of care (Greene & Timbury 1979). Psychogeriatric day care may be an extension of the hospital service or it may consist of local authority day centres, social clubs or luncheon clubs. The work of one joint Social Services and Health Authority day centre in Birmingham was described by Keegan (1984). Studies of day centres (e.g. Gilliard et al 1984) have emphasized that one of their most important functions is to reduce the family strain associated with caring for a demented relative.

Residential homes

Part III of the National Assistance Act of 1948 gives local authorities responsibility for providing old people's homes and other sheltered accommodation. Britain has no significant nursing home

sector to fill the gap between old people's homes and hospitals. Indeed, nurses have very limited involvement in this type of care. In a comparison of New York and London, Gurland et al (1979) found that both cities provide residential care for about 4% of their elderly. In New York about two-thirds were in nurse-run nursing homes, whereas in London about two-thirds were in local authority homes staffed by wardens and domestic helpers.

Residential homes have a proportion of mentally infirm residents and this is likely to increase (Wilkin et al 1978). The question of whether mentally alert and mentally infirm residents should live in integrated homes or whether they should be separated has been debated. Those in favour of integrated homes argue that confused people are less likely to be subjected to 'infantilizing processes' in mixed homes (Meacher 1972) and that rational residents assist and encourage confused residents. Arguments in favour of segregated homes are that a safer environment can be created in which wandering can be contained without resort to restraint (Bergmann 1973). Staff in integrated homes are unlikely to have been adequately trained in the specialized management of old people with psychiatric disorders. A compromise may be integration, but with some separate facilities so that the needs of each group can be met. The work of one residential home in Birmingham, specifically for the elderly mentally infirm, was described by Pettitt (1984).

Hospital care

Elderly mentally infirm patients may be found in geriatric hospitals, psychiatric hospitals, general hospitals and in specialized assessment units.

Psychogeriatric assessment units

Studies in the 1960s, e.g. Kidd (1962), concluded that extensive misplacement of patients between geriatric and psychiatric hospitals led to poor treatment, prolonged stay and unnecessary mortality. Concern about misplacement led to an official policy of developing psychogeriatric short-stay assessment units, jointly directed by psychiatrists and geriatricians (DHSS 1970). Arie (1981) argued that they should be located in general hospitals because diagnosis, especially of acute confusional states, requires painstaking investigation. Some assessment units have worked well, but many have had difficulty functioning effectively because of the lack of places to which patients could be transferred following assessment.

Psychiatric hospitals

Fifty per cent of all mental illness beds are occupied by the over 65s and they account for 20% to 40% of psychiatric admissions (DHSS 1976). Describing the distribution of elderly patients in a typical large psychiatric hospital, Macdonald (1982) found 8% suffering from acute functional illness, 30% severely demented and 20% had 'graduated' from the long-stay wards and were mainly chronic psychotics. There was also another large group of middle-aged institutionalized schizophrenics who were likely to grow old in hospital.

General and geriatric hospitals

Elderly mentally infirm patients may be found in geriatric, medical, surgical and orthopaedic wards. They are also in geriatric hospitals. If patients are suffering from physical illness or disability, the medical geriatric services should provide care and should be able to cope with associated mental disturbance. It is understandable that geriatric services are often reluctant to take ambulant demented patients, as their wandering takes up much nursing time and they may disturb mentally alert patients.

The quality of institutional care

Many British studies have observed the care given to elderly mentally infirm people in various institutional settings. Several researchers have used the case study approach to examine the role of nurses in a psychogeriatric ward of a psychiatric hospital.

Towell (1975) found that the main concern of the ward was the 'routine servicing' of patients, and while patient-centred care was seen as an ideal, it was said to be impossible due to lack of resources. There was little verbal interaction between staff and patients, and patients were regarded as depersonalized objects. In a similar study Savage et al (1979) found that nurses spent more than half their time on physical care. Increasing staff numbers led to more physical care but no increase in psychological care. They discussed how the Warehousing Model (Miller & Gwynne 1974), implicit in the ward, reinforced dependency and reduced patient autonomy. Unwin (1981) studied a ward in which most patients were diagnosed as demented. She found that the nurse's day typically involved 'tremendous onslaughts' of physical care, followed by long periods away from patients, sitting relaxing. The ethic of the ward was 'to get the work done' quickly and then relax, which was one reason nurses said they liked working there. Unwin observed that nurses' conversations with patients occurred randomly and had no planned therapeutic content. Patients were forced into dependent roles irrespective of actual needs. Nurses perceived their problems to be (in rank order): shortage of staff; insufficient time for psychological care; lack of equipment; wandering patients; and lack of understanding by senior staff. Unwin argued that lack of systematic psychological care was not due to lack of time but to a lack of training in interpersonal skills and psychological aspects of care. She suggested that there was a need for more contact between ward nurses and managers and for involvement of nurses in decision-making if improvements were to be seen.

In a larger study Miller (1978) evaluated the care given to demented patients in six long-stay wards. She found that physical care was adequate, but there was a lack of clear goals, communication and overall policy, with no attempt to individualize care. The severely demented patients spent only a third of their time engaged in any activity. Miller recommended the introduction of individual care plans, written objectives and increased support from senior staff.

Another relevant study was carried out on general geriatric wards by Wells (1980). She found that trainee nurses and auxiliaries gave most of the physical care, while qualified nurses were engaged in administrative duties. Wells considered that nursing was focused not on the patients but on the routine. Periods of intense rushed nursing activity alternated with periods of relative inactivity away from the patients. Wells argued that the excuse of staff shortage was a rationalization to alleviate feelings of failure. The real problem was lack of organization, and a more individualized approach was needed. Armstrong-Esther & Browne (1986) also studied a general geriatric ward and found very low levels of staff–patient communication, with nurses interacting least with the most confused and demented patients. Patients were inactive most of the time, sitting dozing or staring into space.

Wilkin et al (1985) studied six residential homes for both lucid and demented residents. The standard of physical care varied between homes and between members of staff. In the worst cases residents received care which was 'utterly undignified and which paid scant concern to their physical comfort, let alone their rights as individuals and their personal feelings'. In general, levels of social interaction were low. The lack of importance given to communication was demonstrated by one officer-in-charge who said that care staff could talk to residents 'when they have finished their work'. The researchers commented that poor standards originated not solely from individual staff members, but from failures in policy making, management and training. Care staff responded to the lead provided by officers-in-charge.

Reviewing research on the quality of care Woods & Britton (1985) concluded that 'institutions for the elderly may then be characterized as places where inactivity is the norm, where there is little social interaction, where staff contact relates mainly to physical care and where dependence is likely to be positively encouraged'. They also noted that relationships were characterized by staff dominance and staff control over daily living activities, so that residents/patients lost their normal adult freedoms.

Characteristics of high quality inpatient care

It is sometimes argued that elderly patients with functional disorders should be placed alongside younger patients with similar disorders. However, there are also advantages in an age-related service, and it should be possible to care for patients with organic and functional disorders together, especially as there are often blurred boundaries between the two groups.

It may be preferable for assessment, acute and long-term treatment to take place in the same unit. This facilitates continuity of care as patients are cared for by the same staff throughout their stay in hospital. It also eliminates the stigma and problems of low status associated with long-stay wards and is likely to result in a more vigorous unit with enthusiastic staff. The psychogeriatric unit should be small and should accommodate men and women. It should be close to the catchment area to encourage visiting and family participation. Ideally, patients should have their own bedrooms or cubicles to allow privacy and personal space. Patients should be encouraged to have personal belongings in their bedrooms. There should be a sitting room and dining room, and ideally a separate room for noisy activities such as television.

It should be possible to deal with uncomplicated physical illness and disability within a psychogeriatric unit rather than having to transfer patients to geriatric medical wards. The unit should be able to offer vigorous, individually planned, psychiatric and physical treatments, but there should also be recognition when active treatment and rehabilitation are no longer appropriate. The unit should be able to provide skilled terminal care.

Irrespective of physical surroundings, the attitudes and behaviour of staff are the main determinants of the quality of care. Central principles of high quality care and strategies for changing institutions were discussed by Woods & Britton (1985). Care should be individually planned with the patient in order to meet that individual's needs. Elderly patients should retain normal adult freedoms, such as privacy and control over daily living activities. Staff should treat elderly people with the same respect and courtesy that they would give to younger adults. Independence should be encouraged and the daily routine should be sufficiently flexible to allow patients to carry out activities at their own pace. Staff–patient relationships are helped by a primary nursing (or key worker) system, so that each nurse works with the same small group of patients over a long period. Staff should remember that old people have the same needs for companionship and affection as younger adults.

Nursing the elderly mentally infirm requires particular motivation and specialized education. There are currently few educational opportunities, either at pre- or post-registration level, and an in-service educational programme is essential to a successful unit. The presence of students of all disciplines can be helpful in developing new ideas and maintaining enthusiasm.

Working with demented and depressed patients is emotionally draining. Staff can easily feel inadequate and discouraged when patients fail to improve. Support is essential if high calibre nurses and doctors are to be attracted into this area and stay. Clear communication among staff at all levels is a first essential. Frequent patient review by the multi-disciplinary team and nursing care planning meetings facilitate this. All staff must be fully informed about goals for their patients. Support groups can help staff to become aware of their own reactions and to ventilate their worries and frustrations, but they only work if the ward atmosphere encourages mutual respect and acceptance.

Helping the families of elderly mentally infirm patients

Families may experience distress, anxiety and guilt about the patient's illness. Many relatives express a desire for increased participation in decision-making about care and in giving care (Brooking 1982). This can be brought about by encouraging and welcoming visitors and providing a pleasant and private place for visits. With the patient's permission, relatives should be given information about all aspects of care and treatment. One geriatric hospital established a 'relatives' corner' in each ward, where relatives could make tea, arrange flowers, wash clothes, help the patients with hygiene, grooming, hairdressing, etc. (Callaghan & Silver 1974). Success depended on the attitude and encouragement of ward staff.

Relatives' groups, led by a staff member, can provide mutual support and discussion of problems common to all. Hayter (1982) established monthly support groups for the families of de-

mented patients. These allowed an outlet for expression of grief and guilt and tended to be cohesive and mutually supportive. Relatives can be involved in care at all stages of the nursing process. It may also be possible to invite relatives to multi-disciplinary meetings at which the patient's care is discussed (Leeming & Luke 1977). Working with demented patients' families, Hayter (1982) found a number of recurrent themes — topics about which families worried or needed information. These included: need for information about the disease process — cause, course, prognosis and treatment; fear that they would develop the disease; need for information about their role and responsibility; guilt about having negative feelings towards the patient; worries about the patient's physical appearance; desire for contact with other sufferers' families; and desire to contribute to research and education about dementia.

CARE OF THE DYING

Terminal care may seem a surprising subject for a textbook of psychiatric nursing. However, large numbers of elderly mentally infirm patients die in psychiatric care and few psychiatric nurses are knowledgeable about this complex and sensitive subject. A terminally ill patient is one in whom the advent of death is certain and not too far distant, and for whom treatment has changed from the curative to the palliative. Terminal care aims to improve the quality of daily life by alleviating unpleasant symptoms, preventing loneliness and fear, and promoting psychological well-being.

Communication, social and spiritual needs

As most deaths occur in hospital, many people have no experience of death or dying, so death remains a taboo subject. Kübler-Ross (1973) interviewed 200 dying patients and identified five stages which many went through in preparing for death. These were:

- denial and isolation, 'it can't be true'
- anger towards everyone, including family and carers

- bargaining, trying to negotiate with people and God to make sense of it
- depression and grief
- acceptance.

Open communication is essential to help patients to move towards acceptance. This requires the nurse to: respond honestly to patients' wishes for information; allow time for discussion; allow patients to express fears and feelings; encourage life review and reminiscence to make sense of life; and provide companionship and human warmth. Patients may be offered a range of activities to avoid boredom and give a sense of purpose. These might include television, radio, letter writing, reading materials, knitting and sewing, or any other hobbies or interests. Depending on the patients' wishes visitors should be encouraged, including pets. Many people turn to religion when facing death and patients' spiritual needs should be assessed. Visits from ministers can be arranged and patients can be taken to services.

Basic comfort measures

The main aims of physical care are to relieve pain, to promote comfort and to support the deteriorating body systems.

The causes of pain should be identified, remembering the importance of fear, anxiety and anticipation of pain. Analgesics should be used to prevent pain breakthrough. Oral analgesics are preferable to avoid the discomfort of injections. Typically, dying patients are given opiates too late and in too small dosages because of staff concern about addiction. Commonly-used opiates include morphine and diamorphine. Drug-induced constipation can be avoided with laxatives, fibre in the diet and adequate fluids.

Loss of appetite is common and patients should be offered favourite foods at whatever time they want them. Meals should be made to look attractive and the appetite may be stimulated by alcoholic drinks such as sherry. Fluids are more important than solid food and patients should be offered favourite drinks. Oral hygiene is essential and some patients find it soothing to suck a fresh ice cube. Nausea and vomiting can be reduced by emetics.

Good general hygiene is important for morale and includes regular changes of bed linen and clothes. Some patients enjoy soaking in a warm bath, but others find it too tiring. Hair and nails should be kept clean and well groomed and patients may enjoy scented talcum powder, perfume and cosmetics. Pressure areas should be treated as usual, but if turning is very painful, a rational decision should be taken about the frequency of pressure area care, depending on the patient's prognosis. Existing sores are unlikely to heal in the terminal phase of life, so should be treated with the aim of keeping the patient as comfortable as possible.

Intractable incontinence causes enormous distress, both physically and emotionally. Catheterization is usually necessary for women, but men can be kept dry with a penile sheath, such as Paul's tubing, or a urinary bottle in situ. Diarrhoea should be treated, bearing in mind that leakage of faecal fluid may indicate severe constipation.

Other general comfort measures include ensuring warmth, ensuring a well-supported position, frequent changes of position according to the patient's wishes, passive and active limb movements and gentle massage. Deep breathing and coughing exercises and upright posture may help to avoid chest infections. Observations, such as temperature, pulse, blood pressure, weight etc., should only be checked if the results are to be acted upon, as they may be uncomfortable or irritating to the patient.

Relatives' needs

Relatives need practical and emotional support from nurses, both before and after death. They need information about the patient's condition, care and prognosis, and they need practical information concerning arrangements for the patient's property, the funeral and the death certificate. They may need assistance with overnight accommodation and meals. Visitors should be welcomed at any reasonable time, but patients must be protected against being over-tired by too many visitors. Relatives should be given privacy during visits, and the use of touch and physical contact can be encouraged. Relatives may wish to participate in care-giving and can be encouraged to assist with feeding, giving drinks and washing. Nurses can offer emotional support to relatives, especially to elderly lonely spouses.

The needs of staff

It is sadly quite common for elderly people to die in hospital without the staff ever having acknowledged that the patient was dying. As palliative care is different from vigorous curative treatment it is important for the whole team to meet and agree on the patient's prognosis and future care. It is important for staff to be able to admit their own feelings of sadness and to feel supported by colleagues. Giving good physical and psychological care to dying patients and their families is emotionally draining. If nurses are not supported they will inevitably use blocking techniques to avoid hurt to themselves, e.g. they become too busy to answer patients' questions.

At the time of death

Patients should not be left to die alone. According to the wishes of the patient and family, the relatives and religious representative may be called as death approaches. After death, relatives should be allowed some time alone with the deceased person; then they should be allowed to sit in a private room or chapel until they feel ready to leave. The nurse who knew the patient and family best may be able to offer some comfort by sharing his or her own feelings of sadness with the family. The patient's personal belongings should be returned to the family, but it may be kinder to leave this for a few days. Follow-up support for an elderly spouse living alone may be required, such as bereavement counselling, or informing the local minister, general practitioner or district nurse. Relatives should be given information about collecting the death certificate. Last offices should be carried out according to the hospital procedure and observing any special requirements of the patient's religion. It is usually pointless to attempt to conceal a death from other patients and import-

ant to respond supportively to the feelings it evokes in them.

LEGAL ASPECTS OF PSYCHOGERIATRIC CARE

Hemsi (1982) considered that compulsory detention under the Mental Health Act is rarely justified in psychogeriatric medicine. He pointed out that basic care rather than treatment is required for dementia, and so the Act is irrelevant. A possible exception identified by Hemsi (1982) is the patient with an insight-impairing functional psychosis who may respond to physical treatment but refuses it, and can be detained in the interests of his or her own health and safety.

Section 47 of the National Assistance 1948, as amended in 1951, applies to the elderly who are living in unsanitary conditions and who are unable to give themselves, nor receive from others, proper care and attention. The Act enables such a person, under clearly defined procedures, to be taken to a hospital for 3 weeks. Muir Gray (1980) found that about 200 people a year were removed from their homes to hospitals or old people's homes each year under the provisions of Section 47.

If patients are lucid, financial decisions are entirely their own. If they are physically incapable or choose not to manage their own affairs, they can transfer that function by giving another person the 'power of attorney'. This can be revoked at any time and it lapses in law if the patient ceases to be lucid. The Court of Protection exists to protect and control the administration of the property of persons who become physically or mentally incapable of doing so themselves. The Court derives its statutory authority from Part VII of the Mental Health Act 1983. It is part of the Supreme Court and is staffed by judges nominated by the Lord Chancellor. A medical recommendation is required to place a patient under the jurisdiction of the Court and enquiries may be made by Officers of the Court. The Court can appoint a Receiver, often a family member, to administer the property under its direction. In 1983 about 23 000 people were under the jurisdiction of the Court of Protection (Bluglass 1983). Many are frail elderly people.

PREVENTION OF PSYCHIATRIC DISORDERS AND PROMOTION OF MENTAL WELL-BEING.

Pfeiffer (1977) viewed psychopathology in the elderly as a failure to adapt to this stage of life, and he identified three main adaptive tasks of old age:

- Adaptation to losses such as spouse, work and social roles, income and mobility. The task is replacement and learning to cope with loss
- Life review. The task is to mark out an identity which integrates the diverse elements of life and allows a positive view of one's life work
- The task of remaining active to retain physical, emotional, social and intellectual function.

Nurses have a role in helping elderly people to carry out these adaptive tasks and to reduce the likelihood of illness.

Ferguson Anderson (1978) considered that the two main causes of emotional disturbance in the elderly are physical disease and an adverse environment, including loneliness. Both have implications for nursing. Nurses can help to prevent physical disease by health education, patient teaching and health visiting. In order to improve the living environment of elderly people, nurses may need to broaden their perspectives beyond the individual to whole families and communities. Changing negative social attitudes to the elderly and campaigning on their behalf are legitimate nursing activities. In addition to the ideas outlined, it is also beneficial: to enhance family relationships; to change attitudes to retirement and educate people to use their extra leisure time productively; to change the negative attitudes of care-givers; and to facilitate elderly people's participation in former interests and activities, including the spiritual aspects of life.

CONCLUSION

This chapter began by considering the scope of the problem of mental disorder in elderly people. The nature, causes and treatment of dementia and confusional states were discussed. It is hoped that the many innovations in care and treatment will make readers realize that an optimistic approach to nursing demented and confused patients is entirely appropriate. The next section focused on the important problem of depression in the elderly. Nurses often feel incapable of helping these patients and consequently tend to ignore their problems. This chapter contains practical ideas which should facilitate effective care and treatment. The section on suicide in old age aimed to make the problem more understandable and to indicate what approaches to care will be most helpful. Other neurotic and psychotic disorders and personality disorders that are seen in elderly people were briefly considered. The next main section considered services for the elderly mentally infirm, including the development of specialized services and services required for specific categories of patients. Current provisions for the elderly mentally infirm were considered. These include community and day care, residential and hospital care. Problems concerning the quality of institutional care were considered, along with recommendations for improving the quality of care. The needs of patients' families were identified. As psychiatric nurses may care for elderly people who are dying, recommendations concerning terminal care were included. Some legal aspects of psychogeriatric practice were summarized and the chapter closed with a consideration of the prevention of mental disorders in the elderly.

REFERENCES

Ainsworth D, Jolley D 1978 The community nurse in a developing psychogeriatric service. Nursing Times 74: 873–874

Arie T 1981 Consideration for the future of psychogeriatric services. In: Kinniard J, Brotherston J, Williamson J (eds) The provision of care for the elderly. Churchill Livingstone, Edinburgh

Arie T, Jolley D 1982 Making services work: organization and style of psychogeriatric services. In: Levy R, Post F (eds) The psychiatry of late life. Blackwell, Oxford

Arie T, Jones R, Smith C 1985 The educational potential of old age psychiatry services. In: Arie T (ed) Recent advances in psychogeriatrics, vol 1. Churchill Livingstone, Edinburgh

Armstrong-Esther C A, Hawkins L H 1982 Day for night: circadian rhythms in the elderly. Nursing Times 78: 1263–1265

Armstrong-Esther C A, Browne K D 1986 The influence of elderly patients' mental impairment on nurse–patient interaction. Journal of Advanced Nursing 11: 379–387

Bergman R 1986 Nursing the aged with brain failure. Journal of Advanced Nursing 11: 361–367

Bergmann K 1973 Letter. New Society 22: 531

Bergmann K 1978 Neurosis and personality disorders in old age. In: Isaacs A D, Post F (eds) Studies in geriatric psychiatry. Wiley, New York

Bergmann K 1982 Depression in the elderly. In: Isaacs B (ed) Recent advances in geriatric medicine 2. Churchill Livingstone, Edinburgh

Bergmann K, Foster E M, Justice A W et al 1978 Management of the demented elderly patient in the community. British Journal of Psychiatry 132: 441–447

Bluglass R 1983 A guide to the mental health act 1983. Churchill Livingstone, Edinburgh

Brook P, Degun G, Mather M 1975 Reality orientation, a therapy for psychogeriatric patients: a controlled study. British Journal of Psychiatry 127: 42–45

Brooking J I 1982 Patient and family participation in nursing: a survey of opinions and current practices among patients, relatives and nurses. In: Hockey L, Keighly T C, Sisson A R (eds) Proceedings of the RCN Research Society 23rd Annual Conference, Royal College of Nursing, London

Burton M 1982 Reality orientation for the elderly: a critique. Journal of Advanced Nursing 7: 427–433

Butler R 1963 The life review: an interpretation of reminiscence in the aged. Psychiatry 26: 65–76

Butler R N, Lewis M I 1982 Ageing and mental health: positive psychosocial and biomedical approaches. Mosby, New York

Callaghan J, Silver C R 1974 Relatives' corner. Nursing Mirror 138: 76

Chisholm S E, Deniston O L, Igrisan R M, Barbus A J 1982 Prevalence of confusion in elderly hospitalized patients. Journal of Gerontological Nursing 8: 2, 87–96

Clark A N G, Mankikar G D, Gray I 1975 Diogenes syndrome. A clinical study of gross neglect in old age. Lancet i: 366–373

Coleman P G 1984 The value of reminiscence in adaptation to old age: longitudinal case studies over ten years. In:

Bromley D B (ed) Gerontology: social and behavioural perspectives. Croom Helm, London

Crosby C, Stevenson R C, Copeland J R M 1984 The evaluation of intensive domiciliary care for the elderly mentally ill. In: Bromley D B (ed) Gerontology: social and behavioural perspectives. Croom Helm, London

Davison W 1978 The hazards of drug treatment in old age. In: Brocklehurst J (ed) Textbook of geriatric medicine, 2nd edn. Churchill Livingstone, Edinburgh

Department of Health and Social Security 1970 Psychogeriatric assessment units. Circular H M (70)11. DHSS, London

Department of Health and Social Security 1976 Health and social services statistics for England 1975. HMSO, London

Department of Health and Social Security 1978 A happier old age: a discussion document on the elderly in our society. HMSO, London

Department of Health and Social Security 1981 Growing older. HMSO, London

Diesfeldt H F A, Diesfeldt-Groenendijk H 1977 Improving cognitive performance in psychogeriatric patients: the influence of physical exercise. Age and Ageing 6: 58–64

Eastwood R, Corbin S 1985 Epidemiology of mental disorders in old age. In: Arie T (ed) Recent advances in psychogeriatrics, vol 1. Churchill Livingstone, Edinburgh

Eisdorfer C, Stotsky B A 1977 Intervention, treatment and rehabilitation of psychiatric disorders. In: Birren J E, Schaie K W (eds) Handbook of the psychology of ageing. Van Nostrand, New York

Ferguson Anderson W 1978 Preventive medicine in old age. In: Brocklehurst J C (ed) Textbook of geriatric medicine and gerontology, 2nd edn. Churchill Livingstone, Edinburgh

Foreman M D 1986 Acute confusional states in hospitalized elderly: a research dilemma. Nursing Research 35: 34–38

Fraser M 1982 ECT: a clinical guide. Wiley, Chichester

Garber J, Seligman M E P 1980 (eds) Human helplessness: theory and applications. Academic, New York

Gilliard C J, Gilliard E, Whittick J E 1984 Impact of psychogeriatric day hospital care on the patient's family. British Journal of Psychiatry 145: 487–492

Gray P, Stevenson J S 1980 Changes in verbal interaction among members of resocialization groups. Journal of Gerontological Nursing 6: 86–90

Greene J G, Timbury G C 1979 A geriatric psychiatry day hospital service. Age and Ageing 8: 49–53

Grimley Evans J 1982 The psychiatric aspects of physical disease. In: Levy R, Post F (eds) The psychiatry of late life. Blackwell, Oxford

Gurland B J 1976 The comparative frequency of depression in various adult age groups. Journal of Gerontology 31: 283–292

Gurland B et al 1979 A cross-national comparison of the institutionalized elderly in the cities of New York and London. Psychological Medicine 9: 4, 781–788

Hayter J 1982 Helping families of patients with Alzheimer's disease. Journal of Gerontological Nursing 8: 81–86

Help the Aged Education Department 1981 Recall — a handbook. Help the Aged, London

Hemsi L 1982 Psychogeriatric care in the community. In:

Levy R, Post F (eds) The psychiatry of late life. Blackwell, Oxford

Holden V P, Woods R T 1988 Reality orientation, 2nd edn. Churchill Livingstone, Edinburgh

Hughston G A, Merriam S B 1982 Reminiscence: a non-formal technique for improving cognitive functioning in the aged. International Journal of Ageing and Human Development 15: 139–149

Jones G 1985 Validation therapy: a companion to reality orientation. The Canadian Nurse 81: 20–23

Jones R G 1986 Extended study to evaluate nurses' attitudes to geriatric psychiatry. In: Brooking J I (ed) Psychiatric nursing research. Wiley, Chichester

Katzman R, Terry R D, Bick K L (eds) 1978 Alzheimer's disease: senile dementia and related disorders. Raven Press, New York

Kay D W K 1963 Late paraphrenia and its bearing on the aetiology of schizophrenia. Acta Psychiatrica Scandinavica 39: 159–169

Kay D W K, Beamish P, Roth M 1964 Old age mental disorders in Newcastle upon Tyne. Part 1. A study of prevalence and Part 2 A study of possible social and medical causes. British Journal of Psychiatry 110: 146–158 and 668–682

Kay D W K, Bergmann K 1980 Epidemiology of mental disorders among the aged in the community. In: Birren J E, Sloane R B (eds) Handbook of mental health and ageing. Prentice-Hall, Englewood-Cliffs, New Jersey

Kay D W K, Bergmann K, Foster E M et al 1966 A four-year follow-up of a random sample of old people originally seen in their own homes. A physical, social and psychiatric enquiry. Excerpta Medica International Congress Series No 150, Proceedings of the Fourth World Congress of Psychiatry, pp 1668–1670

Keegan M 1984 A day centre for the elderly mentally infirm. In: Isaacs B, Evers H (eds) Innovations in the care of the elderly. Croom Helm, London

Kidd C D 1962 Misplacement of the elderly in hospital. British Medical Journal 2: 1491–1493

Kral V A 1982 Neuroses of the aged: a neglected area. Clinical Gerontologist 1: 29–35

Kübler-Ross E 1973 On death and dying. Tavistock, London

Lader M H 1981 Focus on depression. Bencard, Middlesex

Langer E J, Rodin J 1976 The effects of choice and enhanced personal responsibility for the aged: a field experiment in an institutional setting. Journal of Personality and Social Psychology 34: 191–198

LaPorte H J 1982 Reversible causes of dementia: a nursing challenge. Journal of Gerontological Nursing 8: 213–216

Leeming J T, Luke A 1977 Multidisciplinary meetings with relatives of elderly hospital patients in continuing care wards. Age and Ageing 6: 1–5

Levy R, Post F 1982 The dementias of old age. In: Levy R, Post F (eds) The psychiatry of late life. Blackwell, Oxford

Libow L S 1978 Senile dementias and pseudo-dementias, clinical diagnosis. In: Eisdorfer C, Friedal R O (eds) Cognitive and emotional disturbance in the elderly. Year Book Medical Publishers, Chicago

Lipowski Z J 1983 Transient cognitive disorders in the elderly. American Journal of Psychiatry 140(11): 1426–1436

Macdonald C 1982 A psychogeriatric rehabilitation programme. In: McCreadie R G (ed) Rehabilitation in psychiatric practice. Pitman, London

Macdonald M L 1973 The forgotten Americans: a sociopsychological analysis of ageing and nursing homes. American Journal of Community Psychology 3: 272–292

Marston N, Gupta H 1977 Interesting the old. Community Care, November 16: 26–28

Meacher M 1972 Taken for a ride. Longman, London

Merton R K 1957 Social theory and social structure (revised edn). Free Press, Illinois

Millard P H, Bennett G C J 1982 Geriatric medicine — a practical guide. St George's Hospital Medical School, Department of Geriatric Medicine

Miller A E 1978 Evaluation of the care provided for patients with dementia in six hospital wards. Unpublished MSc thesis, University of Manchester

Miller E 1977 Abnormal ageing: the psychology of senile and presenile dementia. Wiley, Chichester

Miller E, Gwynne G V 1974 A life apart: a pilot study of residential institutions for the physically handicapped and young chronic sick. Tavistock, London

Miller M 1975 Iatrogenic and nursigenic effects of prolonged immobilization of the ill aged. Journal of the American Geriatric Society 23: 360–369

Mishara B L, Kastenbaum R 1973 Self-injurious behaviour and environmental change in the institutionalized elderly. International Journal of Ageing and Human Development 4: 133–145

Mishara B L, Kastenbaum R 1980 Alcohol and old age. Grune and Stratton, New York

Muir Gray J A 1980 Section 47. Age and Ageing 9: 205–209

Muir Gray J A 1985 The ethics of compulsory removal. In: Lockwood M (ed) Moral dilemmas in modern medicine. Oxford University Press, Oxford

Müller C 1969 Manuel de geronto-psychiatrie. Masson et Cie, Paris

Murphy E 1982 Social origins of depression in old age. British Journal of Psychiatry 141: 135–142

Murray R, Huelskoetter M M, O'Driscoll D 1980 The Nursing process in later maturity. Prentice-Hall, New Jersey

Neugebauer R 1980 Formulation of hypotheses about the true prevalence of functional and organic psychiatric disorders among the elderly in the United States. In: Dohrenwend B P, Dohrenwend B S (eds) Mental illness in the United States: epidemiological estimates. Praeger, New York

Norton C 1986 Eliminating. In: Redfern S J (ed) Nursing elderly people. Churchill Livingstone, Edinburgh

Pasker P, Thomas J P R, Ashley J S A 1976 The elderly mentally ill — whose responsibility? British Medical Journal ii: 164–166

Peterson R F, Knapp T J, Rosen J C, Pither B F 1977 The effects of furniture arrangements on the behaviour of geriatric patients. Behaviour Therapy 8: 464–467

Pettitt D 1984 Residential home for the elderly mentally infirm. In: Isaacs B, Evers H (eds) Innovations in the care of the elderly. Croom Helm, London

Pfeiffer E 1977 Psychopathology and social pathology. In: Birren J E, Schaie K W (eds) Handbook of the psychology of ageing. Van Nostrand, New York

Post F 1972 The management and nature of depressive illness in late life: a follow-through study. British Journal of Psychiatry 121: 393–404

Post F 1982 Functional disorders. In: Levy R, Post F (eds)

The psychiatry of late life. Blackwell, Oxford

Post F, Shulman K 1985 New views on old age affective disorders. In: Arie T (ed) Recent advances in psychogeriatrics, vol 1. Churchill Livingstone, Edinburgh

Powell R R 1974 Psychological effects of exercise therapy upon institutionalized geriatric mental patients. Gerontologist 14: 157–161

Powell Proctor L, Miller E 1982 Reality orientation: a critical appraisal. British Journal of Psychiatry 140: 457–463

Robinson R A 1962 The Practice of a psychiatric geriatric unit. Gerontologia Clinica 1: 1–19

Rodin J, Langer E J 1977 Long-term effects of a control-relevant intervention with the institutionalized aged. Journal of Personality and Social Psychology 35: 897–902

Royal College of Psychiatrists 1973 News and Notes. August. Joint Report of the British Geriatrics Society and the Royal College Of Psychiatrists on matters relating to the care of psycho-geriatric patients. Royal College of Psychiatrists, London

Royal College of Psychiatrists 1981 Interim guidelines for regional advisers on consultant posts in psychiatry of old age. Bulletin, June

Sainsbury P 1968 Suicide and depression. In: Coppen A, Walk A (eds) British Journal of Psychiatry, Special Publication No 2

Salzman C, Shader R I 1979 Clinical evaluation of depression in the elderly. In: Raskin H, Jarvik L H (eds) Psychiatric symptoms and cognitive loss in the elderly. Wiley, New York

Savage B, Widdowson T, Wright T 1979 Improving the care of the elderly. In: Towell D, Harries C (eds) Innovation in patient care. Croom Helm, London

Schulz R 1976 Effects of control and predictability on the physical and psychological well-being of the institutionalized aged. Journal of Personality and Social Psychology 33: 563–573

Seligman M E P 1974 Depression and learned helplessness. In: Friedman R J, Katz M M (eds) The psychology of depression: contemporary theory and research. V H Winston, Washington

Shulman K 1978 Suicide and parasuicide in old age: a review. Age and Ageing 7:201–209

Shulman K, Post F 1980 Bipolar affective disorder in old age. British Journal of Psychiatry 136: 26–32

Taulbee L R, Folsom J C 1966 Reality orientation for geriatric patients. Hospital and Community Psychiatry 17: 133--135

Thomas S 1986 Eating and drinking. In: Redfern S J (ed) Nursing elderly people. Churchill Livingstone, Edinburgh

Towell D 1975 Understanding psychiatric nursing. London, Royal College of Nursing

Trimble M 1981 Neuropsychiatry. Wiley, Chichester.

Unwin K 1981 A case study to investigate problems faced by nurses on a psychogeriatric ward. Unpublished BSc dissertation, University of London, Chelsea College

Vogel C H 1982 Anxiety and depression among the elderly. Journal of Gerontological Nursing 8: 213–216

Wattis J, Wattis L, Arie T 1981 Psychogeriatrics: a national survey of a new branch of psychiatry. British Medical Journal 282: 1529–1533

Webb C 1986 Expressing sexuality. In: Redfern S J (ed) Nursing elderly people. Churchill Livingstone, Edinburgh

Weber M 1961 The social psychology of the world religions. In: Gerth H H, Mills C W (eds) From Max Weber: essays in sociology. Routledge and Kegan Paul, London

Weissman M M 1979 Environmental factors in affective disorders. Hospital Practice 14: 103–109

Wells T J 1980 Problems in geriatric nursing. Churchill Livingstone, Edinburgh

Wilkin D, Hughes B, Jolley D J 1985 Quality of care in institutions. In: Arie T (ed) Recent advances in psychogeriatrics, vol 1. Churchill Livingstone, Edinburgh

Wilkin D, Mashiah T, Jolley D 1978 Changes in behavioural characteristics of local authority homes and long-stay hospital wards, 1976–77. British Medical Journal ii: 1274–1276

Williamson J, Stokoe I H, Gray S et al 1964 Old people at home: their unreported needs. Lancet i: 1117–1120

Woods R T, Britton P G 1985 Clinical psychology with the elderly. Croom Helm, Beckenham, Kent

World Health Organization 1984 Self-health care and older people: a manual for public policy and programme development. Copenhagen

World Health Organization 1985 Senile dementia. Report of a scientific group, Geneva. Cited in Henderson J H, Macfadyen D M 1985 In: Arie T (ed) Recent advances in psychogeriatrics, vol 1. Churchill Livingstone, Edinburgh

FURTHER READING

Arie T 1985 (ed) Recent advances in psychogeriatrics, vol 1, Churchill Livingstone, Edinburgh — This edited textbook reviews current knowledge about various aspects of psychogeriatrics. Some of the chapters concern scientific and technical developments, but there are useful chapters on clinical topics, such as affective disorders, quality of care and epidemiology.

Butler R, Lewis M 1982 Ageing and mental health, 3rd edn. Mosby, London — Contains useful material on reminiscence and recall.

Cormack D F S (ed) 1985 Geriatric nursing: a conceptual approach. Blackwell Scientific, Oxford — Contains practical information on dealing with common problems such as disorientation, anxiety and depression.

Hanley I, Hodge J, 1984 (eds) Psychological approaches to the care of the elderly. Croom Helm, London – Contains extensive coverage on psychological interventions such as reality orientation, behavioural techniques and psychotherapy, including reviews of evaluative research on these techniques.

Holden U P, Woods R T 1988 Reality orientation: psychological approaches to the confused elderly, 2nd edn. Churchill Livingstone, Edinburgh — Discusses theory and research as well as the practical applications of reality orientation.

Levy R, Post F 1982 (eds) The psychiatry of late life. Blackwell Scientific, Oxford — This advanced psychiatric textbook contains clearly written, concise reviews of a range of clinical topics, written by well-known researchers and psychiatrists.

Redfern S J 1991 (ed) Nursing elderly people, 2nd edn. Churchill Livingstone, Edinburgh — This edited textbook contains research-based chapters on all aspects of caring for the elderly. Part 1 contains chapters on the meaning of old age and the psychology and physiology of ageing.

Part 2 contains chapters on a range of aspects of daily living, such as sight and hearing, mobility, sleep, pain etc. Part 3 concerns the organization of care in various settings and Part 4 contains a discussion of general issues concerning ageing and society and the nurse's role.

Schulz R 1980 Ageing and control. In: Garber J, Seligman M E P (eds) Human helplessness: theory and applications. Academic, New York — An excellent review on the importance of personal control to the psychological well-being of the elderly.

Woods R T, Britton P G 1985 Clinical psychology with the elderly. Croom Helm, London — Contains interesting chapters on patient assessment and quality of care in various settings as well as useful material on making changes in institutional practices.

Part 5

Methods of therapy in psychiatric nursing

39

Drug treatment

J. K. Davies

Over the last 30 years, there has been a progressive decline in the population of patients receiving treatment in psychiatric hospitals, matched by a corresponding increase in the population receiving treatment in outpatient clinics or from general practitioners. This trend began to appear around the time that a number of new drugs were discovered which appeared to be genuinely beneficial in the treatment of psychiatric illness. Notable amongst these were chlorpromazine, introduced for the treatment of schizophrenia in 1952, iproniazid and imipramine for depressive illness, in 1954 and 1958 respectively, and the benzodiazepine drugs chlordiazepoxide (1962) and diazepam (1964) for the treatment of anxious neurotic disorders. So-called 'psychotropic' drugs have been the subject of continuous development up to the present time, and the period of decline in the psychiatric hospital population has been one in which drugs have come to assume a pre-eminent position in the treatment of mental illness.

Undoubtedly the use of drugs has enabled many patients to resume life in the community who would formerly have required to be institutionalized, but it would be facile to attribute the overall demographic changes solely to the availability of new medicines. In the light of the recommendations of the 1959 and 1983 Mental Health Acts, and with the provision of resources to support psychiatric patients in the community, it is likely that the population of the mental hospitals would have declined even without the advent of the new drugs. The question therefore remains: what is the extent of the benefit that patients can expect to derive through the use of psychotropic drugs?

No new drug can be introduced into routine medical practice until reliable information as to its safety and efficacy has been obtained. Drug clinical trials are performed in order to furnish this type of information, and their results, published in the scientific literature, provide a basis for assessing the benefits and limitations of drug therapy.

Before discussing any conclusions which can be drawn from them, it may be of interest to describe the essential features of the design and conduct of clinical trials and in particular, the precautions which are required in order to obtain a reliable assessment of the therapeutic value of a drug.

CLINICAL TRIALS OF PSYCHOTROPIC DRUGS

Definition and characteristics

A clinical trial is an investigation, conducted in patients, with the object of ascertaining what beneficial or harmful effects a drug may have. It is a form of experiment, an extension, in fact, of the experiments conducted in laboratory animals which provide the first indication of the potential value of a new compound. The main risk associated with the use of previously untried drugs is of toxicity, and the Department of Health Committee on Safety of Medicines requires a satisfactory report of a drug in animal toxicity tests before issuing the necessary authorization for it to be tested in patients. Approval is also required from the Ethical Committee of the Health Authority in which the trial is to be conducted, and the informed consent of patients selected to participate is normally required. In the case of severely ill psychiatric patients this may be impractical to obtain, in which case the consent of a legally authorized representative must be sought.

Apart from the possible novelty of the drug employed, the conduct of clinical trials differs

from the routine practice of drug therapy in three other respects:

1. Patients are selected to participate in trials, i.e. certain patients may be excluded, on grounds of age or pregnancy for example, who might be eligible to receive standard drug medication.
2. The progress of patients is carefully monitored during the trial by means of regular observations and measurements made by medical and nursing personnel.
3. An effort is made to perform the trial under controlled conditions.

The methods used to assess drug effects in trials of psychotropic drugs and the measures which are employed to achieve a measure of control are described in the following sections.

The assessment of drug activity

Drug effects appear in clinical trials as alterations in the thought, mood and behaviour of patients. It is unlikely that such alterations will be sudden and dramatic; rather they tend to be gradual in onset and possibly imperceptible on a day-to-day basis. As a consequence, drug effects may only become apparent by examining the records obtained from patients at intervals over a lengthy trial period. To achieve a measure of uniformity in the method of assessment of different patients at different times, it has become common practice for observers to use standard rating scales of various types. Global Rating Scales, for example, record the clinician's overall assessment of the status of the patient, often on a seven-point scale. Symptom Rating Scales identify symptoms which are clinically relevant and their severity is recorded on a shorter integer scale, as in the example of an Anxiety Rating Scale shown in Figure 39.1 (Hamilton 1959). Similar scales have been devised for assessing the symptoms of schizophrenia (Hamilton et al 1960, Lorr 1963) and depression (Hamilton 1960). Patients who retain insight and can give a good account of themselves can record their subjective mood by means of Self-Rating Scales, and scales have also been devised to enable nurses to record the ward behaviour of patients

Item no.	Score range	Symptom	Comments
1	0 – 4	Anxious mood	
2	0 – 4	Tension	
3	0 – 4	Fears	
4	0 – 4	Insomnia	
5	0 – 4	Intellectual	
6	0 – 4	Depressed mood	
7	0 – 4	Gen. som. muscular	
8	0 – 4	Gen. som. sensory	
9	0 – 4	Cardiovascular	
10	0 – 4	Respiratory	
11	0 – 4	Gastrointestinal	
12	0 – 4	Genitourinary	
13	0 – 4	Autonomic	
14	0 – 4	Behaviour at interview	
		TOTAL	Further notes

0 Absent   1 Mild or trivial   2 Moderate   3 Severe

4 Very severe to grossly disabling

Fig. 39.1 The Hamilton Anxiety Rating Scale.

(Honigfeld et al 1976). In trials involving outpatients, information in a similar form relating to the social adaptation of patients can be provided by relatives or guardians.

Figure 39.2 (Hamilton et al 1960) summarizes the results of a trial in which a clinician's rating scale was employed to evaluate two antipsychotic drugs. Eighteen symptoms were graded in severity on a scale 0–3, and the aggregate rating score for 18 schizophrenic patients was calculated before and after a period of drug medication. The bars in the figure represent differences between scores recorded pre- and post-treatment, and indicate, at a glance, the relative size and direction of overall changes in the status of the patients in each group. Data expressed in this manner are convenient for statistical analysis, and the use of standard rating procedures enables the results of one trial to be compared with, or even pooled with, those of others using the same scoring system.

It must be recognized, however, that while rating scales enable a large amount of data relating to the clinical status of patients to be expressed in a highly condensed form, a figure on a numerical scale conveys a less than complete picture of a real clinical situation or of changes which a clinician

might regard as significant. For example, the scores shown in Figure 39.2 indicate an improvement in the overall condition of patients without indicating their status either at the beginning or at the end of the trial. In addition, it is not unknown for drugs to modify some symptoms more than others, nor, indeed, to improve some symptoms and aggravate others (Hamilton et al 1960), but this information is impossible to extricate from an aggregated symptom score. Finally, it is not immediately obvious whether the size of change indicated by the different scores in Figure 39.2 is of any particular clinical significance. An average improvement by one point of all 18 symptoms in all 18 patients would register an aggregate change in score of 324, considerably in excess of the largest change noted in any group in the trial.

It is unfortunate that much published clinical trial data is of only limited value in assessing the effectiveness of drugs because information of immediate clinical relevance is either sparse or lacking.

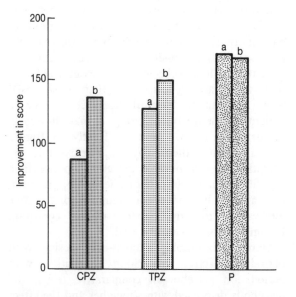

Fig. 39.2 Changes in aggregate rating score determined in a clinical trial of chlorpromazine and thiopropazate in schizophrenic patients. (See text for details.) CPZ: chlorpromazine; TPZ: thiopropazate; P: placebo. Duration of treatment — a: 2 weeks; b: 8 weeks. (From Hamilton et al 1960.)

The control of clinical trials

The importance of adequate control cannot be overemphasized if clinical trials are to provide reliable information about drug efficacy. This point is illustrated in the results of the trial shown in Figure 39.2. The improvement shown by drug-treated patients indicates a modest benefit derived from chlorpromazine and thiopropazate. Results obtained with a further group of patients, however, forces some reappraisal of this view. In these patients, active medication was substituted by a placebo, that is an inert substance formulated in an identical manner to the test substance. Comparing the results from the different groups suggests that neither drug was more efficacious than the placebo, i.e. than no drug at all. This verdict does not overlook the fact that the patients who took part in the trial seem to have derived some benefit from their treatment; rather, it recognizes that there is considerably more to the 'treatment' than the mere effect of the drug.

In a controlled trial, some attempt is made to assess the contribution made by non-drug factors to any observed changes in the condition of the patients. As in the example above, this may involve comparing the performance of a group of patients receiving active medication with that of a placebo group. Denial of active medication to patients in the placebo group raises ethical questions which are no less cogent than those raised when a potentially harmful substance is given to patients in the treatment group. It may, however, be justifiable on two grounds. Firstly, as Figure 39.2 illustrates, there may be a reasonable expectation of a favourable placebo response in a significant number of patients. Secondly, provision can always be made for administering active medication to any patient whose condition becomes worse during the trial.

Some trials employ a cross-over design with periods of active medication alternating with periods on placebo. In comparative trials, the placebo is dispensed with altogether and the effect of a new product is compared with that of a standard drug. Needless to say, the results of such trials are of little value unless it has been established that the reference drug is itself superior to placebo.

Efforts to control trials by the use of placebo are liable to be frustrated if patients are aware of whether or not they are receiving active medication. Similarly, observers who know which patients are on active medication may allow their expectation of its effect to bias their assessment. It is normal practice for trials to be conducted 'double-blind', i.e. under conditions where neither patient nor observer is aware of the nature of the treatment.

There is no doubt that failure to control clinical trials can create a quite misleading impression of the effectiveness of drugs. Reviewing the results of drug trials published over a 5-year period in British and American journals, Foulds (1958) noted that treatment was claimed as effective in 83% of trials in which no controls were used. By contrast, in only 25% of placebo-controlled trials was any significant effect claimed. It would be folly to represent pharmacotherapy as a panacea for mental illness in the face of evidence that controlled trials fail more often than they succeed. Admittedly, the drugs currently available may be superior to many which were in use 30 years ago, but even today it is not unusual to find conflicting reports of efficacy arising from clinical trials of the same drug. It seems safe to conclude only that drugs can be of some benefit under some conditions; a problem of some therapeutic importance is to identify the conditions under which drugs can be used to best advantage. A comparison of the methodology employed in different trials of the same drug, including both the successful and the failed, has brought to light certain variables, including the examples described in the following section, which appear to affect the results in a fairly systematic or predictable manner.

WHY DO TRIALS 'FAIL'?

Patient symptomatology

The organic disorders that give rise to the symptoms of psychiatric illness are far from clearly understood. The appearance of certain symptoms may enable patients to be placed within a particular broad diagnostic category ('schizophrenic', 'depressive'), but there is no reason to suppose that all patients within that category suffer from the same fundamental abnormality. Indeed, this seems unlikely in view of the variety of forms a disease can assume in different patients. Schizophrenia, for example, can be subclassified as simple, hebephrenic, catatonic or paranoid, and depression as unipolar or bipolar, endogenous or reactive. Since the action of psychotropic drugs tends to be localized to particular types of cell within the brain, it might be optimistic to expect a single drug to be uniformly effective in treating a disease in all its manifestations, and the experience of clinical trials appears to bear this out. Endogenous depressives, for example, appear to derive greater benefit from tricyclic drugs than do reactive cases (Kiloh & Garside 1963). Cases of depression with paranoid features appear to be particularly refractory to treatment with these drugs (Klerman & Cole 1965), while in cases of bipolar depression, tricyclic drugs have been known to precipitate manic episodes (Bunney 1978). It goes without saying that in psychiatry, as in any branch of medicine, the prospect of a successful outcome of treatment depends on the accuracy of the initial diagnosis.

Drug dosage

When clinical trials are designed, a decision has to be taken as to the daily dose of drug that each patient should receive. The dose must be set high enough to enable patients to derive the full benefit of the drug, yet not so high as to produce side-effects which are unacceptable to the patient and readily detected by a supposedly 'blind' observer. A comparison of the results of trials in which different doses of drugs have been used, e.g. of imipramine (Klerman & Cole 1965) and of chlorpromazine (Little 1958), indicates that better results have been obtained when higher doses have been used.

The notion of an optimal dose of drug which will benefit all patients to a similar extent is often fallacious. The size of dose determines the size of effect insofar as it determines the concentration of drug available to act at its target sites within the body. The relationship between dose and target site concentration is far from simple, particularly when drugs are given by mouth, and there is growing evidence that the relationship is not necessarily the same for all patients. For example, plasma levels of tricyclic antidepressants in patients taking the same dose have shown as much as a 20-fold variation (Kessler 1978). It follows that a standard dose may not suit all patients, and that some 'tailoring' of doses to suit the needs of individuals may be necessary. Some clinical trial protocols include a flexible dose-regimen. Since mild side-effects often accompany the therapeutic effect of psychotropic drugs, these can serve as an indicator that plasma concentrations are within the therapeutic range.

A not infrequent cause of treatment failure is a more prosaic one: patients simply fail to take their medication. Many psychiatric patients dislike taking drugs and become skilful at avoiding it. Nursing staff have an important role in clinical trials in ensuring that patients comply with the prescribed dose-regimen. Needless to say, problems with patient compliance become particularly troublesome when trials involve hospital outpatients.

Treatment duration

Clinical trials have to be of sufficient duration to allow the full effect of the drug to develop. In the case of tricyclic antidepressants, there may be a delay of up to 3 weeks before any therapeutic response is seen (Kessler 1978). In trials lasting several weeks, or even months, a failure to show drug effects can hardly be attributed to inadequate duration of treatment. Paradoxically, however, the effect of drugs may appear to diminish with the increased length of a trial. In acute depression and anxiety neurosis there is a good prognosis for spontaneous recovery, which is likely to occur with increasing frequency as time goes by. In one clinical trial of imipramine (Robin & Langley 1964), patients in the placebo group had improved sufficiently after 4 weeks to bring them more or less on a par with patients in the treatment group who had shown a more rapid improvement 2 weeks into the trial. If, as in this example, the effect of a drug is to accelerate a natural process of recovery without increasing the extent of any eventual improvement, the timing of observations becomes critical if the effect of the drug is to be detected.

Therapeutic environment

A natural process of recovery in psychiatric illness can be accelerated not only by drugs, but also by non-drug factors. In drug trials involving depressed patients it has been observed that the placebo response rate is considerably higher in patients treated in hospital than in outpatients (Klerman & Cole 1965). This gives an indication of the extent of the benefit that patients can derive from the care and attention they receive from nursing personnel, both in trials and in the normal hospital routine. As a corollary to this, if the therapeutic environment is one in which a significant recovery rate could be expected without medication, the additional benefit conferred by drugs appears to be diminished. Hordern & Hamilton (1963) offer this as a likely explanation for discrepant findings of clinical trials of chlorpromazine and other antipsychotic agents. They conclude: 'The best results have been obtained when neuroleptics have been given in situations in which patients were receiving a minimum of individual attention from nursing and medical staff. In other situations where, by contrast, the care of patients has been provided on an intensively organized individual or small group basis . . . the addition of neuroleptics to the therapeutic regime has conferred very little additional benefit.'

It does not detract from the value of neuroleptic drugs to suggest that intensive social therapy can be equally beneficial. Nevertheless, where alternative therapies can be just as effective, it is evident that the pre-eminent position of drugs in psychiatric medicine is not determined solely by therapeutic considerations.

STATISTICAL EVALUATION OF THE RESULTS OF DRUG TRIALS

Just as clinical trials of the same drug often give variable results, so variation is also likely to occur in the response of patients participating in any single drug trial. Some of this variation may be attributable to the influence of the type of systematic variable discussed in the previous section, but patients often fail to respond to a form of treatment for no accountable reason. The placebo response of patients is also subject to this type of random variation, and under certain circumstances this can create a spurious impression of efficacy in a compound which is actually inactive. Thus, if patients within a treatment group show a higher non-drug recovery rate than patients in a control group, a difference between the groups which, in reality, had occurred by chance might be wrongly attributed to the effect of the drug.

In general, an observed difference between treatment and control groups can be confidently attributed to the effect of a drug only if it can be shown to be too large, or too frequently observed, to have occurred by chance. In order to assess the possible influence of chance factors, it is accepted practice to design drug trials in such a way that the data can be evaluated by statistical means.

The requirement for statistical evaluation influences both the form and amount of data that clinical trials are designed to provide. Patient assessment by means of rating scales provides data in a form, and with the information content, required by the most powerful statistical tests. As far as the amount of data is concerned, no meaningful statistical analysis can be contemplated on data samples below a certain size. Unfortunately, if large numbers of patients are included in a trial, this may entail some loss of homogeneity in the patient sample, with a consequent increase in variability of the drug response.

It must be emphasized that the purpose of a clinical trial is to furnish information relating to the clinical value of a drug. Statistical tests can indicate whether a drug has had a genuine effect, but different criteria must be used to assess how useful it is likely to prove in a clinical context. A slight improvement might prove statistically significant if it occurred in a large number of patients, and yet be too small to be of any particular clinical significance. In many reports of clinical trials, a successful outcome is claimed if statistical tests show the drug to be significantly better than placebo. Without additional information as to the extent of the recovery the patients had made, this hardly constitutes a satisfactory basis on which to judge the effectiveness of the drug.

THE EFFECTIVENESS OF PSYCHOTROPIC DRUGS

Antipsychotic (neuroleptic) agents

Drugs currently available for the treatment of schizophrenia include the phenothiazine derivatives chlorpromazine, thioridazine and fluphenazine. Other chemical groups of antipsychotics include butyrophenones (e.g. haloperidol), diphenylbutylpiperidines (e.g. pimozide), thioxanthines (e.g. flupenthixol) and the substituted benzamide, sulpiride. There appears to be little to choose between these various agents in terms of their antipsychotic activity, although other considerations, notably the incidence of their sedative or extrapyramidal effects, may dictate the choice of a particular drug in practice (Davis & Casper 1978a).

The results of a 6-week collaborative study involving a large number of acute schizophrenic patients (Cole 1964) are probably typical of many trials in which a substantial effect of phenothiazine drugs has been demonstrated. Roughly three patients in four were judged to have improved markedly on drug treatment, although as many as one third of these might have improved to a similar extent on placebo. In the remaining patients, the improvement was minimal or nil, although there was an indication that in some cases drug treatment might have averted a further deterioration in the patient's condition. On average, patients on phenothiazines improved by two points on a seven-point global rating scale, from 'marked illness' to 'mildly ill' two points below 'normal'. The proportion of patients judged to be functioning at a normal level by the end of the trial was of the order of 16%, with around 30% judged 'borderline mentally-ill' (see Fig. 39.3).

When patients have successfully negotiated an episode of schizophrenia with the aid of drugs, the question arises when this support may safely be withdrawn. A conspectus of withdrawal studies

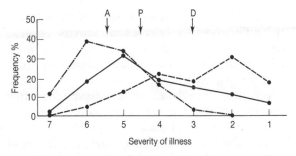

Fig. 39.3 Frequency distribution of global illness ratings in schizophrenic patients before and after treatment with phenothiazine drugs. (See text for details.) Illness rating grades are — 7: Extreme; 6: Severe; 5: Serious; 4: moderate; 3: Mild; 2: Borderline; 1: Normal. Dotted line shows the distribution of grades of illness in the total patient sample before treatment. The distributions of grades after treatment are for the drug group (dashed line) and the placebo group (solid line). Arrows denote median grades; A: before treatment; P: after placebo; D: after drug. (From Cole et al 1964.)

indicates that around 40% of patients relapse on withdrawal of medication (Gardos & Cole 1978). The majority of patients who relapse remit soon after pharmacotherapy is resumed, but may be considered a bad risk if discontinuation of treatment is considered at a later stage. Drug discontinuation is also contraindicated in patients for whom the consequences of relapse are potentially disastrous, e.g. patients with a history of assaultiveness or suicide attempts. Subject to these provisos, withdrawal of medication should be considered in any patient once a satisfactory response has been achieved, with a view to obviating the risk of long-term toxic effects of the drug.

Some studies have compared drug treatment with other therapies. Compared with social and psychotherapy, drugs are at least as, and often more, effective in both acute and chronic patients (reviews: Davis & Casper 1978b, Schooler 1978). A combination of drug with other forms of therapy often gives better results than does either form of treatment alone, particularly in the management of chronic hospitalized patients and in assisting the community rehabilitation of outpatients.

Antidepressant drugs

The term 'tricyclic' embraces a number of antidepressant drugs having a similar chemical structure, including imipramine, desipramine and amitryptiline. There is no evidence of any substantial difference in antidepressant activity between drugs of this type, nor between these and more recently-introduced compounds having one-, two- or four-ring structures. As in the case of antipsychotics, the choice of antidepressant often resides with the drug whose side-effects are likely to prove least troublesome to the patient.

Tricyclic and related compounds are the most widely-used drugs for the treatment of affective disorders. Surveys of numerous trials of tricyclic antidepressants (reviews: Kessler 1978, Klerman & Cole 1965) indicate that roughly two patients in three improve significantly while on medication. At the same time, a surprisingly large proportion of patients, perhaps one in three, improve by a similar amount on placebo. Acute depression has a good prognosis for spontaneous symptomatic recovery, and this probably contributes to the high placebo response rate in drug trials. Indeed, the indications are that almost as many patients as recover on drugs would do so without medication, albeit over a longer period of time than the 1 to 3 months encompassed by most drug trials (Alexander 1953). In many patients, therefore, the effect of drugs is to shorten what would otherwise be a protracted depressive episode. The therapeutic benefits that accrue are a reduction in the number of patients requiring to be admitted to hospital, a more rapid discharge of those who do, and a reduction in the mortality of patients through suicide or other disease-related causes.

Controlled long-term trials have shown a further effect of drugs of reducing the frequency of depressive episodes (review: Klerman 1978). Up to one half of patients who experience an acute depressive episode may never experience another; the remainder can expect at least one recurrence in their lives with the probability of further recurrences increasing with each successive episode. Continuation of treatment beyond the period required to achieve full remission of depressive symptoms, either with the original dose or with a reduced maintenance dose, can produce a marked reduction in both the likelihood and severity of further attacks. In a minority of patients, continuation or maintenance therapy may be indicated

for an indefinite period in order to prevent relapse (Ayd 1963).

As amongst schizophrenics, a sizeable proportion of depressive patients appear to derive little or no benefit from drugs. Inadequate dosage or lack of patient compliance in taking the prescribed medication may account for a proportion of these failures. In addition, cases of reactive or neurotic depression appear to be somewhat refractory to treatment with tricylic drugs (Kiloh & Garside 1963).

Tricyclic drugs are also of uncertain value in the treatment of bipolar depression — a form of endogenous depression in which depressive episodes are interspersed with periods of hypomania or mania. While the drugs may help to abate the depressive phase of the illness, there is some evidence that they may exacerbate the manic phase (Bunney 1978). In contrast, lithium salts have proved to be particularly effective in controlling manic symptoms and have become the drugs of choice for the maintenance therapy of patients with recurrent episodes of both mania and depression (Schou 1978).

The first effective pharmacotherapy in depression was with drugs of the mono-amine oxidase inhibitor (MAOI) type, examples of which are phenelzine and isocarboxazid. In terms of efficacy, there is probably little to choose between these and the tricyclic antidepressants (Robinson et al 1978), but the toxicity of MAOIs and, in particular, their adverse interactions with certain dietary constituents and with other drugs (Lasagna 1978), has led to a decline in their use in favour of tricyclic compounds. Nevertheless, some patients respond to MAOIs who have failed to do so to tricyclics, and there is some evidence for their superiority over tricyclics in the treatment of phobias (Lader & Petursson 1983).

It would be naive to suppose that drugs offer a complete treatment for affective disorders. Apart from the significant number of patients for whom, often unaccountably, drugs prove to be of no benefit, the beneficial effect they provide in other patients may fall well short of full social rehabilitation. On the other hand, drugs represent a form of therapy which is more readily accessible to patients than the alternatives of electroconvulsive therapy (ECT) and psychotherapy. ECT may be marginally more effective than tricyclics, and produces an effect with a more immediate onset, but requires to be administered by specialist staff in a hospital setting. A far greater number of patients can be treated with drugs by medical practitioners who do not necessarily have specialist psychiatric training.

Few, if any, studies of psychotherapy in depression have been conducted with the rigour of the best drug trials, and no meaningful comparison of the effects of drugs and alternative forms of treatment can be made at present.

Anxiolytic agents

Diazepam (Valium) and other benzodiazepine (BDZ) compounds are currently the drugs most frequently used for the treatment of anxiety. The drugs have remarkably similar pharmacological properties, but differ in potency and in duration of action. Anxiety is an emotional response to stress, and an all-too-frequent accompaniment to life in a modern industrialized society. Most of the adult population cope with the anxiety in their lives most of the time, but a surprisingly high proportion, of perhaps one in three, are likely to consult their family practitioner concerning anxiety or other stress-related problems (Lader & Petursson 1983). Drugs are frequently prescribed for these conditions, and, in the view of some, are prescribed more frequently than is medically justified (e.g. see Editorial, Lancet 1973). There can be no doubt, however, that when appropriately used, BDZs represent an effective treatment for psychoneurotic disorders in which anxiety is a prominent symptom.

Superiority of BDZs over placebo has been demonstrated in numerous clinical trials (review: Greenblatt & Shader 1978). The drugs are effective in relieving anxiety accompanied by insomnia and/or somatic symptoms, or attributable to somatic disorders. In contrast, they are of doubtful value in treating neurotic conditions characterized by phobias and depression, or by personality disturbances which affect work performance and interpersonal relationships (Rickels et al 1978).

BDZs appear to be of comparable benefit in cases of acute and chronic anxiety, although a case can be made for withholding them in acute anxiety of mild to moderate intensity, where recovery is likely to occur spontaneously or after adequate reassurance (Lader & Petursson 1983). Reassurance can also enhance the therapeutic effect of BDZ drugs (Rickels et al 1978).

As to the extent of the benefit obtained by patients, large-scale studies of BDZ in general practice (Rickels et al 1978) indicate an average improvement not exceeding one point on a four-point physician rating scale, or two points on a seven-point global rating scale, irrespective of the initial level of anxiety. This implies that the prospects of drug therapy achieving the full social rehabilitation of the patient diminishes with the increased severity of the patient's symptoms. In practice, the majority of patients studied in the trial continued to function below par even after 4 to 6 weeks of BDZ treatment, and as many as one in three derived no benefit at all.

Long-term use of BDZs is discouraged on the grounds that the drugs are liable to produce physical and psychological dependence (Lader 1983). There is no evidence that patients improve any more if a course of treatment is extended beyond 4 to 6 weeks, and in one follow-up study, very little change was found to have occurred in the condition of patients 6 months after treatment had been discontinued (Rickels et al 1978). The benefits of continued medication may outweigh the risk of dependence in patients suffering chronic, disabling anxiety whose symptoms are found to recur after withdrawal of medication.

Since the introduction of BDZs, the use of barbiturates for the treatment of anxiety, and also for insomnia, has declined drastically. BDZs are more effective, produce fewer side-effects and are far safer in overdose (Lader 1983). As an alternative to BDZs, patients who find the somatic symptoms of anxiety troublesome often find relief when beta-blocking drugs are prescribed (Greenblatt & Shader 1978). These drugs ameliorate the symptoms caused by overactivity of the sympathetic nervous system, for example on the cardiovascular and gastrointestinal systems.

SIDE-EFFECTS OF PSYCHOTROPIC DRUGS

Table 39.1 lists various undesirable effects which are encountered with the use of psychotropic drugs. Severe side-effects are, fortunately, rare and are often avoidable, for example, when they are a result of an interaction with other drugs or when predisposing factors like cardiovascular disease or renal or hepatic impairment are present. Nevertheless, even mild side-effects can add to the discomfort of patients whose health is already impaired, and are a cause for concern, not least because they may lead to non-compliance of the patient with the prescribed dose-regimen. Whether the benefit derived by the patient outweighs any actual or potential insult inflicted should be the subject of continuous appraisal. By judicious adjustment of dosage, it should be possible to strike an optimal balance between the desired and undesired aspects of a drug's action.

Most side-effects disappear once the drug is withdrawn; whether the symptoms return at the same time depends on the natural history of the disease and, in particular, on the likelihood of a natural remission having occurred during the period of drug administration. Clinical experience with antidepressant drugs, for example, suggests that the gradual reduction and eventual termination of dosage can be contemplated after 6 to 9 months of treatment (Kessler 1978). Unfortunately, there is no escaping the fact that chronic illness may require chronic treatment, and patients who suffer relapse on withdrawal of medication, or who have a history of recurrent episodes of disease, may require treatment for an indefinite period.

These patients are subject to additional adverse drug effects which appear in the long-term, and which protocols of maintenance drug therapy are designed to obviate or minimize. In general, maintenance doses are kept to a minimum and increased only if indicated by a deterioration in the patient's condition.

Long-term treatment with antipsychotic drugs is approached with particular care because of the risk of tardive dyskinesia, an irreversible disorder of motor function attributed to the long-term use of these agents (Baldessarini & Tarsy 1978). Chronic schizophrenics who derive only marginal benefit from antipsychotic drugs may be withdrawn from them altogether, while other patients may be withdrawn periodically for as long as they can continue to function satisfactorily, possibly for several months.

THE DEVELOPMENT OF PSYCHOTROPIC DRUGS

There is no doubt that drugs effect a speedy return to normal health for a significant proportion of patients who experience acute attacks of psychiatric illness. At the same time, large numbers of patients give rise to concern because drugs seem to offer them no relief, or because the cost of even modest relief is the burden of severe short- or long-term side-effects. The achievements of psychopharmacotherapy over the last 30 years have created a climate of optimism that successful forms of treatment for these recalcitrant cases will eventually be found. If progress towards this objective appears to have been slow, it is a reflection of the fact that the discovery of new types of drug requires an element of luck as well as scientific judgement.

If it appears that no existing class of drug holds the key to the treatment of a particular type of psychiatric disorder, the hope must be that drugs having an entirely novel mode of action may do so. The development of drugs in the pharmaceutical industry proceeds from the synthesis of a series of organic compounds through a sequence of testing procedures in animals designed to reveal which compounds, if any, have pharmacological properties relevant to the treatment of human disease. There is, unfortunately, little guidance to be offered as to the shape and form such compounds might take.

Restoring normal function to the diseased brain may well involve selectively augmenting or inhibiting the action of one of the many chemical messenger substances which regulate the activity of brain cells. There are many examples of drugs which produce this kind of effect by virtue of

Table 39.1 Typical side-effects produced by therapeutic doses of psychotropic drugs

	INCIDENCE	SEVERITY	LATENCY	REVERSIBILITY
Antipsychotics				
Anticholinergic:				
(dry mouth blurred vision constipation urinary retention impotence)	+	+	1	+
Cardiovascular:				
postural hypotension	++	+	1	+
CNS:				
extrapyramidal (dystonia, akathisia, parkinsonism)	++	++	1	+
tardive dyskinesia	++	++	2	−
sedation	++	+	1	+
Endocrine:				
(prolactinaemia galactorrhoea weight gain)	+	+	1	+
Hypersensitivity/idiosyncratic:				
blood dyscrasias	+	+++	1	+
skin reactions jaundice	+	+	1	+
Miscellaneous:				
(photosensitivity ocular deposits skin discolouration)	+	+	1	+
Antidepressants: tricyclics				
Anticholinergic:				
(dry mouth blurred vision constipation urinary retention)	++	++	1	+
Cardiovascular:				
postural hypotension	+	+	1	+
cardiac dysrhythmias	+	++	1	+
CNS:				
(hypomania confusion/delerium tremor)	++	+	1	+
sedation	++	+	1	+
Hypersensitivity/idiosyncratic:				
blood dyscrasias	+	+++	1	+
jaundice	+	+	1	+
Potentially hazardous interactions with: guanethidine MAOI				

Table 39.1 (cont'd)

	INCIDENCE	SEVERITY	LATENCY	REVERSIBILITY
Antidepressants: MAOI				
Autonomic:				
(dry mouth				
blurred vision				
constipation				
urinary retention	+	+	1	+
impotence)				
postural hypotension	++	++	1	+
CNS:				
hypomania				
confusion/delerium	+	++	1	+
Potentially hazardous interactions with:				
sympathomimetic amines in food and medicines ('cheese' reaction)				
tricyclic antidepressants				
opiates				
Antidepressants: Lithium salts				
Cardiovascular:				
cardiac dysrythmias	+	+++	1	+
Gastrointestinal:				
(nausea				
vomiting	+	+	1	+
abdominal pain				
diarrhoea)				
CNS:				
tremor				
seizures	+	+++	1	+
sedation				
coma				
Endocrine:				
hypothyroidism	+	++	1	+
Hypersensitivity/idiosyncratic:				
dermatitis	+	+	1	+
blood dyscrasias	+	+++	1	+
Anxiolytics				
CNS:				
drowsiness	++	+	1	+
disinhibition of emotional, aggressive or sexual behaviour	+	++	1	+
tolerance and dependence (abstinence syndrome as withdrawal)	+	++	2	+
Hazardous interaction with ethanol				

Table 39.1 (cont'd)

Key:

Incidence of effect:	++	in > 10% of cases
	+	in < 10% of cases
Severity of effect:	+++	discontinuation of treatment normally indicated
	++	reduction of dose or corrective medication normally indicated
	+	tolerable
Latency of onset of effect:	1	appearing within 0–3 months
	2	appearing after 3 months
Reversibility of effect:	+	disappears after withdrawal of medication
	−	normally persists after withdrawal of medication

Refs: Baldessarini (1985), Baldessarini & Tarsy (1978), Davis & Casper (1978), Klerman & Cole (1965), Lasagna (1978), Sovner & DiMascio (1978).

having a similar chemical structure to that of a particular messenger. Once the chemical messengers involved in particular aspects of brain function have been identified, it should be possible to produce new psychotropic drugs by suitably modifying their chemical structure. Much effort is being directed towards identifying central messengers, but the picture is still far from complete. Until it is, the search for new drugs relies heavily on inspired guesswork of the type which led to the discovery of the benzodiazepine anxiolytic drugs in 1957 (Sternbach 1983).

The difficulty of identifying the appropriate type of chemical to synthesize is compounded by the problem of recognizing the therapeutic potential of any newly-synthesized compound which, by luck or judgement, happened to possess the requisite chemical structure for the desired activity. The type of effect that gives the most reliable indication of the potential therapeutic value of a novel compound in the laboratory is the animal equivalent of the effect which is sought in man. In the case of psychotropic drugs, this would be an effect on specific aspects of thought, mood and behaviour in the experimental animal. No means exists of communicating with animals, and the interview technique which enables a clinician to assess the mental state of a patient has no counterpart in animal experiments. As Kornetsky (1977) has observed: 'No matter how often you ask the animal, he will not be able to tell you that other animals or people are plotting against him.'

In other words, the most characteristic and sought-after effects of psychotropic drugs, their effects on the subjective mental state, are not accessible for study in animal experiments.

The behaviour of animals, including the way they respond to changes in their environment, can be altered by psychotropic drugs, and, more importantly, can be readily observed. Behavioural tests can be used to differentiate between active and inactive compounds, and the nature of behavioural changes can often provide an indication of the type of therapeutic application a drug may have. This is not to say that behavioural tests necessarily attempt to reproduce the abnormal behaviour of psychiatric patients; rather, they are tests in which drugs of proven therapeutic worth produce prominent and characteristic effects. It is perhaps inevitable that novel drugs which produce similar behavioural effects to existing ones in animal experiments, normally prove to have a similar mode of action with all that this implies in terms of limited clinical effectiveness and a tendency to produce particular side-effects. It is relevant to observe that chlorpromazine and imipramine remain among the drugs of first choice for the treatment of schizophrenia and depression, respectively, in spite of the bewildering number of alternatives that have been introduced in the 30 years since their discovery.

Most of the pharmacological properties of a new drug will have been learned in the laboratory before it enters the stage of clinical testing, but it is not unusual for unexpected effects to appear during the first trials in patients. These effects may be undesirable, or even harmful, but occasionally they provide an unexpected bonus by suggesting a new application for the product. Examples of such unexpected effects are the 'tranquillizing' activity of chlorpromazine and the mood-elevating effect of imipramine, which were first noticed while other effects of the drugs were being evaluated in the clinic. Thanks to the astuteness of clinicians in recognizing the significance of these properties, the drugs were rapidly redeployed into fields of psychiatric medicine where they could be put to good effect.

Although a systematic approach towards drug development would seem to offer the best prospect for rapid progress, there is always a chance that serendipity may play a similar role in the discovery of future psychotropic drugs as it has in the past with chlorpromazine and imipramine.

CONCLUSION

There is little doubt that the prospect of psychiatric patients being able to resume normal life in the community has improved considerably since the advent of modern psychotropic drugs. At the same time, it is invidious to attempt to compare the effectiveness of drug and non-drug therapies, since the best results have normally been obtained by using a combination of different treatments. It is difficult to envisage how patients could become fully rehabilitated in society, with or without drugs, unless they were able to feel that other people had a genuine concern for their welfare.

A disturbing fact to emerge from the results of clinical trials is that a significant proportion of patients appear to derive little or no benefit from drugs. To avoid the situation where large numbers of patients are being prescribed powerful drugs to no good effect requires that some means be found of identifying probable refractory cases at the time their illness is diagnosed. In addition, there is an obvious need for new drugs to fill the void left by existing ones. A new chapter in psychiatric medicine opened 30 years ago with the discovery of the first effective psychotropic agents. Who can say what the next 30 years may bring?

REFERENCES

Alexander L 1953 Treatment of mental disorder. W B Saunders, Philadelphia

Ayd F J Jnr 1963 Five years of antidepressant therapy. Mind 1: 6–11

Baldessarini R J 1985 Drugs and the treatment of psychiatric disorders. In: Goodman A G, Goodman L S, Rall T W, Murad F (eds) The Pharmacological Basis of Therapeutics. Macmillan, NY, pp 385–445

Baldessarini R J, Tarsy D 1978 Tardive dyskinesia. In: Lipton M A, DiMascio A, Killam K F (eds) Psychopharmacology: a generation of progress. Raven Press, NY, pp 993–1004

Bunney W E 1978 Psychopharmacology of the switch process in affective illness. In: Lipton M A, DiMascio A, Killam K F (eds) Psychopharmacology: a generation of progress. Raven Press, NY, pp 1249–1259

Cole J O 1964 Phenothiazine treatment of acute schizophrenia. Archives of General Psychiatry 10: 246–261

Davis J M, Casper R C 1978a General principles of the clinical use of neuroleptics. In: Clark W G, del Guidice J (eds) Principles of Psychopharmacology. Academic Press, NY, pp 511–536

Davis J M, Casper R C 1978b Side-effects of psychotropic drugs and their management. In: Clark W G, del Guidice J (eds) Principles of Pharmacology. Academic Press, NY, pp 479–494

Editorial 1973 Benzodiazepines; overuse, misuse or abuse? Lancet, May: 1101–1102

Foulds G A 1958 Clinical research in psychiatry. Journal of Mental Science 104: 259–265

Gardos G, Cole J O 1978 Maintenance antipsychotic therapy: for whom and for how long? In: Lipton M A, DiMascio A, Killam K F (eds) Psychopharmacology: a generation of progress. Raven Press, NY, pp 1169–1178

Greenblatt D J, Shader R I 1978 Pharmacotherapy of anxiety with benzodiazepines and beta-adrenergic blockers. In: Lipton M A, DiMascio A, Killam K F (eds) Psychopharmacology: a generation of progress. Raven Press, NY, pp 1381–1390

Hamilton M 1959 The assessment of anxiety states by rating. British Journal of Medical Psychology 32: 50–55

Hamilton M 1960 A rating scale for depression. Journal of Neurology, Neurosurgery and Psychiatry 23: 56–61

Hamilton M, Smith A L G, Lapidus H E, Cadogan E P

1960 A contolled trial of thiopropazate dihydrochloride (Dartalan), chlorpromazine and occupational therapy in chronic schizophrenics. Journal of Mental Science 106: 40–55

Honigfeld G, Gillis R D, Klett C J 1976 NOSIE. Nurses' Observational Scale for Inpatient Evaluation. In: Guy W (ed) ECDEU assessment manual for psychopharmacology, rev. edn. Rockville, Maryland, pp 265–273

Hordern A, Hamilton M 1963 Drugs and moral treatment. British Journal of Psychiatry 109: 500–509

Kessler K A 1978 Tricyclic antidepressants: mode of action and clinical use. In: Lipton M A, DiMascio A, Killam K F (eds) Psychopharmacology: a generation of progress. Raven Press, NY, pp 1289–1302

Kiloh L G, Garside R F 1963 The independence of neurotic depression and endogenous depression. British Journal of Psychiatry 109: 451–463

Klerman G L 1978 Long-term treament of affective disorders. In: Lipton M A, DiMascio A, Killam K F (eds) Psychopharmacology: a generation of progress. Raven Press, NY, pp 1303–1311

Klerman G L, Cole J O 1965 Clinical Pharmacology of imipramine and related antidepressant compounds. Pharmacological Reviews 17: 101–141

Kornetsky C 1977 Animal models: promises and problems. In: Hanin I, Usdin E (eds) Animal models in psychiatry and neurology. Pergamon, Oxford, pp 1–7

Lader M 1983 Benzodiazepine withdrawal states. In: Trimble M R (ed) Benzodiazepines divided. John Wiley Chichester, pp 17–32

Lader M, Petursson H 1983 Rational use of anxiolytic/sedative drugs. Drugs 25: 514–528

Lasagna L 1978 Some adverse interactions with other drugs. In: Lipton M A, DiMascio A, Killam K F (eds)

Psychopharmacology: a generation of progress. Raven Press, NY, pp 1005–1020

Little J C 1958 A double-blind controlled comparison of the effects of chlorpromazine, barbiturate and a placebo in 142 chronic psychotic inpatients. Journal of Mental Science 104: 334–349

Lorr M 1963 Inpatient multidimensional psychiatric scale. Consulting Psychiatrists Press, Palo Alto, California

Rickels K, Downing R W, Winokur A 1978 Anti-anxiety drugs: clinical use in psychiatry. In: Iversen L L, Iversen D, Snyder S H (eds) Handbook of psychopharmacology, vol 13, Biology of mood and antianxiety drugs. Plenum Press, NY, pp 395–430

Robin A A, Langley G E 1964 A controlled trial of imipramine. Journal of Psychiatry 110: 419–422

Robinson D S, Nies A, Ravais C L, Ives J O, Bartlett D 1978 Clinical pharmacology of phenelzine. Archives of General Psychiatry 35: 629–635

Schooler N R 1978 Antipsychotic drugs and psychological treatment in schizophrenia. In: Lipton M A, DiMascio A, Killam K F (eds) Psychopharmacology: a generation of progress. Raven Press, NY, pp 1155–1168

Schou M 1978 Clinical use of lithium. In: Clark W G, del Guidice J (eds) Principles of psychopharmacology. Academic Press, New York, pp 553–560

Sovner R, DiMascio A 1978 Extrapyramidal syndromes and other neurological side-effects of psychotropic drugs. In: Lipton M A, DiMascio A, Killam K F (eds) Psychopharmacology: a generation of progress. Raven Press, NY, pp 1021–1032

Sternbach L H 1983 The discovery of CNS-active 1,4 benzodiazepines. In: Costa E (ed) The benzodiazepines: from molecular biology to clinical practice. Raven Press, NY, pp 1–6

40

Physical treatments

J. I. Brooking

Drugs are the most widely used physical treatment in psychiatry and are discussed in Chapters 15 and 39. This chapter introduces the other major physical treatments and considers the role of the nurse in relation to these treatments. Electro-convulsive therapy is frequently used and is discussed in detail. Psychosurgery, although very rare, is highly controversial and therefore justifies detailed consideration. A number of other unusual physical treatments are mentioned briefly.

To some extent, it is artificial to separate physical from other treatments as psychotherapeutic techniques and social support accompany physical treatments and contribute substantially to their success or failure. Irrespective of the therapeutic model used, psychiatric nurses talk with their patients, counsel them and whether formally or informally, help them to solve problems and provide social and emotional support. Patients' attitudes to their treatments and to their nurses and other carers will of course influence their responses to therapy.

ELECTROCONVULSIVE THERAPY

Electroconvulsive therapy (ECT) is the application of a controlled electrical current to the brain, resulting in a convulsion resembling a grand mal seizure. Prior to this the patient is anaesthetized and given a muscle relaxant. ECT is also known as electric shock therapy (EST), electrotherapy and electroplexy.

The history of ECT was described by Dally & Connolly (1981). In 1798 Weickhardt recommended giving camphor to the point of producing fits for mental disorder. In its present form ECT dates from 1937 when it was developed by Cerlitti and Bini. It was then believed that the correlation between schizophrenia and epilepsy was very low and that when they did occur together, the epileptic seizure modified the schizophrenic symptoms. Thus, ECT originally developed as a treatment for schizophrenia, although there was later found to be no biological antagonism between epilepsy and schizophrenia. In the late 1940s muscle relaxants were introduced to lessen the risk of fracture and short-acting anaesthetics began to be used. Dally & Connolly (1981) claimed that ECT was abused and over-used in the early days. It was not uncommon for schizophrenics to be given twice weekly ECT indefinitely as a means of controlling disturbed behaviour. This over-use came to an end in the 1950s with the introduction of more effective drug treatments.

ECT began to be criticized in the 1970s, so much so that many American psychiatrists have abandoned its use for fear of litigation. Crow (1979) claimed, however, that 'despite criticisms from a number of sources, most psychiatrists remain convinced that ECT has a unique place in the treatment of depression'. In 1981 Pippard and Ellam sent postal questionnaires to all members of the Royal College of Psychiatrists in Britain and obtained replies from 3045 psychiatrists, a response rate of 95%. They found that 87% of all their respondents and 97% of clinical consultants regarded ECT as at least occasionally justified. 78% of consultants had prescribed ECT in the previous 6 months. The researchers found that 200 000 ECT treatments were administered in 1979, in 390 NHS and private psychiatric establishments. Clearly, this is still a very widely-used treatment.

Indications and contraindications

The main indication for ECT today is severe endogenous depression. Reviewing the evidence for its effectiveness, Fraser (1982) concluded that there was nothing for which ECT could be recommended except depression. Its use in schizophrenia has now been largely abandoned, except occasionally when affective, catatonic or paranoid features predominate. It is sometimes used in the treatment of mania, but this has been largely superseded by drugs such as lithium.

Old age is not a contraindication; indeed many psychiatrists consider that elderly depressed patients respond particularly well to ECT. Fraser (1982) claimed that cardiac arrhythmias and memory damage are theoretically more likely to occur as side-effects in elderly rather than in young people. However, he considered that these risks are less severe than the hazards of suicide and self-neglect associated with untreated depression in the elderly. The use of ECT in children and adolescents is minimal, except in the most severe depressive illnesses, and is banned in some American states.

Fraser (1982) listed several contraindications to ECT. These include any organic brain disease such as cerebral tumour, haemorrhage or infarcts, cardiovascular disease and recent myocardial infarction, demyelinating disease such as multiple sclerosis, asthma, active bone disease because of the risk of fractures, anxiety states, pregnancy and any contraindications to a general anaesthetic.

Effectiveness of ECT

Much of the controversy surrounding ECT concerns the question of its effectiveness. Numerous studies have compared ECT with other treatments or with no treatment, but many studies fail to control for the powerful placebo effect of receiving a complex treatment involving much extra attention and care. Since 1978 there have been at least five methodologically rigorous studies in Britain using double-blind placebo-controlled designs. In this type of research, patients suffering from endogenous depression are randomly assigned to one of two groups. The experimental group receive a course of ECT and the control group receive the same number of simulated ECT treatments, that is all aspects of the procedure, including the anaesthetic and muscle relaxant, but not the electric shock. Neither the patients nor the assessors know to which condition individuals have been assigned. Patients are then assessed at fixed points during and after the treatment period using standard measures of depression and other symptoms. These studies have produced varying results.

Lambourn & Gill (1978) found that both groups of patients did well and they demonstrated no more than a trend in favour of ECT. Other studies showed greater improvement in patients given a full course of ECT compared with a simulated ECT group (Freeman et al 1978, Brandon et al 1984, Gregory et al 1985). In the Northwick Park trial Johnstone et al (1980) found a significantly superior effect for ECT but also a high placebo effect in the simulated ECT group, i.e. both groups recovered considerably, but the ECT group were significantly less depressed during the treatment period. A month and 6 months after treatment there were no differences between the two groups on patient' self-ratings and psychiatrists' ratings. From these studies it appears that ECT, which includes an electrically induced convulsion, has a more rapidly antidepressant effect than simulated ECT, but that the effect may be short-lived. Johnstone et al (1980) concluded that intensive medical and nursing care might prove an adequate alternative for depression as patients given simulated ECT eventually recovered as much as those given real ECT. Nevertheless, antidepressant drugs take 2 to 3 weeks to work and a rapidly acting treatment might reduce the risk of suicide, physical neglect and the other serious social consequences of depression in that time.

Mode of action

There are various theories about how ECT works, but none are clearly established. Psychoanalytic and other psychological explanations have been postulated, but, reviewing the evidence, Fraser (1982) concluded that biochemical explanations are the most plausible. He considered that the therapeutic effect depends on altered post-synaptic response to mono-amine and other neurotransmitters in the central nervous system. ECT stimulates synaptic remodelling and there is a temporary enhanced behavioural response to released neurotransmitters. Alterations are widespread in the brain, but relief of depression is more directly related to changes in the diencephalon part of the hypothalamus which affects appetite, sleep, weight etc. The strong placebo effect was demonstrated in the Northwick Park trial by patients who believed they received ECT and who actually received a simulated treatment, but nevertheless made substantial therapeutic gains.

ROLE OF THE NURSE IN RELATION TO ECT

Nursing interventions in relation to ECT can be divided into three periods: preparation of the patient, care during the procedure, and care after the procedure.

Preparation of the patient for ECT

ECT is usually prescribed by a consultant psychiatrist. Nurses can contribute to the selection of patients for ECT if they have assessed their patients thoroughly and have a good understanding of the patient's condition. Features of depression which are thought to be predictors of a good response include sudden onset, diurnal variation, retardation, weight loss, early waking, somatic delusions and guilt (Trimble 1981).

In order to give valid consent to treatment patients must be competent to understand the nature, purpose and likely effects of ECT, must be given full information, and consent must be voluntary. Pippard & Ellam (1981) found that it was usually doctors who explained ECT to patients and their families, although nurses were sometimes involved. Discussion was often brief and patients were rarely given written information. Both doctors and nurses are responsible for explaining the procedure to patients and their relatives. Information should be given in clear non-medical language, and should be repeated if necessary and ideally should be supplemented by a simple written summary. An example of a 'package' of information designed by a nurse (Wilby 1986) to be given to patients before ECT is shown in Figure 40.1.

Section 58 of the 1983 Mental Health Act deals with consent to ECT. Informal patients cannot be given any treatment without consent. If a detained

1. Verbal information to be given to patients before ECT

I understand that you are having the first in a course of ECT treatments on _____ , so what I'm hoping to be able to do in the next 20 minutes or so is to explain the procedure to you and answer any questions that you might have about your treatments. Is that OK with you?

ECT has been shown to have beneficial effects for many patients, and everyone who is looking after you feels that it will probably help lift your depression or feelings of sadness.

No one is absolutely sure how ECT works to reduce depression, although there are quite a lot of well-researched theories about it. But what they are sure about is how safe it is.

Before you actually have the treatment there are a few things that have to be done. The doctors will make sure that they have an X-ray of your chest, and if not, you will have one taken. You won't be able to eat or drink anything from midnight before, to make sure that your stomach is empty. On the actual morning of treatment you may be given a small injection to dry up the saliva in your mouth, and also to make you feel a little more relaxed. When you get into the ECT Clinic you will be asked to take out any dentures if you have them, and it is usual that you go to the toilet before going to the Clinic.

All of these things are done with any patient who is having an anaesthetic, even if they are only having an ingrowing toenail removed.

On the morning you are to have your treatment, you will go to the ECT Clinic, first to the waiting room with a nurse who you know from your ward. You will then be called through into a room with a few beds in it; there will be an anaesthetist who will put you to sleep, and another doctor who carries out the treatment. You'll lie on a bed with the curtains drawn round; the nurse from your ward will still be with you. The anaesthetist will give you an injection in the back of your hand that will send you to sleep quickly for just a few minutes.

While you are asleep the other doctor will place an electrode on your forehead, and give you a small shock, which you will not be able to feel.

Within a few minutes of it all being over you wake up; you may feel a bit muzzy and have a slight headache, but this will soon pass, and you will be able to take some Aspirin or Paradon for it, if you want. You might also find it difficult to remember little things, but again this will go away in a few hours, and once you have finished your course of treatments, these effects will not recur.

Once you feel like it, you will be given a cup of tea and biscuits, and then you can go back to the ward with the nurse, where you can lie down and relax.

You will have between 6 and 12 treatments depending on how quickly they begin to have some effect, and you will probably have them twice a week. I've told you quite a lot about what will happen when you have your ECT treatments in the last few minutes, but I don't know if there are any questions you'd like to ask me or if you would like anything repeated or made clearer because I am quite willing to do so. Is there anything about the treatment that worries you, that you would like to talk about?

2. Written information to be given to patients before ECT

ECT electroconvulsive therapy is a form of treatment which has been in use for many years now. It has been shown in research studies to be very effective in treating depression for many people. Although there is no absolute guarantee that every case of depression will be completely cured by ECT, your doctors think that it is likely to help you. There are many theories about how ECT actually works. One thing about which we are sure is that the treatment is very safe with no lasting side-effects.

1. Before the day you are to have your first ECT treatment, the doctors will make sure they have an X-ray of your chest.

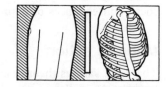

2. As with any anaesthetic you will not be able to eat or drink from midnight before you have your treatment.

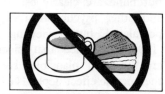

3. You may have an injection that morning which will make your mouth dry, and help you to relax.

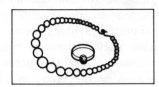

4. You will be asked to remove any dentures and jewellery when you are in the ECT Clinic.

5. Before you go to the Clinic with a nurse from your ward it might be a good idea to go to the toilet.

   All of these things are usual for any patient who is to have a general anaesthetic.

6. Once you are at the Clinic you will lie down and be put to sleep by an anaesthetist for a few minutes. Another doctor will give you a small shock which you will not be able to feel.

7. After a few minutes you will wake up. You may feel a bit muzzy and have a headache but these will soon pass.

8. After tea and biscuits you can go back to the ward with the nurse who will have stayed with you throughout.

   If you have any questions about your ECT treatments, which have not been answered do not hesitate to ask any member of the ward staff who will be pleased to help.

Fig. 40.1 Information about ECT (from Wilby 1986).

patient refuses to consent to ECT, it may only be given if a second independent doctor, appointed by the Mental Health Act Commission, certifies that the treatment should be given. The second doctor is required by law to consult with at least two other non-medical members of the clinical team, one of whom must be a nurse.

As well as factual information, patients should be encouraged to discuss their concerns about the treatment and to ask questions. Bird (1979) found that the most commonly feared aspects of ECT were the anaesthetic and memory loss and some patients even feared dying. If nurses can find out what beliefs and fears their patients hold, it is possible to correct misconceptions and allay worries. Not surprisingly, patients are influenced by sensational and sometimes inaccurate or outdated accounts of ECT as portrayed in the media.

In order to give consent patients should be informed about the side-effects of ECT which may include headaches, muscle soreness and dizziness (Kreigh & Perko 1983). The more serious side-effects are transient confusion and memory loss, which may persist for hours or days. Several studies have shown that unilateral ECT produces earlier immediate recovery and less confusion and memory impairment (e.g. Fromm-Auch 1982).

If possible nurses may arrange for their patients to meet another person who has benefited from ECT and is willing to discuss it. Prospective patients may be reassured that their fears are not unique and that the treatment is not as frightening as they imagine. A visit to the ECT clinic before treatment may also help, so that it is familiar territory on the day of treatment.

Physical preparation

Physical preparation for ECT begins with a full physical examination by a doctor to ensure fitness for treatment. Pippard & Ellam (1981) found that about half of the psychiatrists in their study also gave their patients chest X-rays and haemoglobin and erythrocyte sedimentation rate estimations. The nurse will assist the patient with these investigations as necessary, drawing any contra-indications to the doctor's attention.

The patient must fast for 6 to 8 hours before ECT, in accordance with the policy of the anaesthetist, because of the risk of aspirating vomit. If possible, ECT should be carried out in the morning, to minimize discomfort and distress to the patient. Medication may be withheld during fasting and sedatives may be withheld for 24 hours as they can prevent a convulsion. On the other hand, a mild sedative may be prescribed the night before treatment to ensure a good sleep and reduce anxiety.

On the day of treatment, hairclips, jewellery, dentures, glasses, contact lenses and other prostheses are removed in order to prevent injury during the convulsion, and are stored in a safe place. Loose clothing should be worn in case resuscitation is required in an emergency. Nail varnish and make-up should be removed so that circulation can be assessed during treatment. The hair should be clean and oil free to prevent it acting as an insulator. Patients should wear an identification bracelet so that identity can be checked when they are unconscious. The patient should be asked to pass urine before treatment to limit the risk of incontinence. A note should be made of temperature, pulse, respiratory rate and blood pressure as baseline measures prior to administration of ECT. A premedication of atropine sulphate may be prescribed to decrease bronchial and tracheal secretions. This may be given by the nurse an hour before treatment, in which case the patient should be warned about its drying effect on the mouth, or it may be given intravenously by the anaesthetist.

Administration of ECT

In their guidelines the Royal College of Nursing (1982) recommended that ECT should be carried out in a specially designated department of a hospital, managed by a nurse whose responsibilities would include 'ensuring that all necessary equipment is available and where relevant has been serviced in accordance with the manufacturer's instructions, that drugs and equipment are re-ordered and that nurses attending ECT sessions are familiar with the procedure'. The Royal College of Nursing (1982) also recommended that waiting, treatment and recovery areas should be separate to ensure adequate privacy for patients.

Equipment required for the administration of ECT includes:

- the ECT machine, electrodes, contact solution and headbands
- oxygen cylinders with masks and ambu bags
- syringes and needles
- tourniquets and elastoplast
- airways and mouthgags
- laryngoscope, endotracheal tubes and connections
- anaesthetic, muscle relaxant and emergency drugs
- emergency equipment including suction machine and intravenous fluids
- patients' charts
- high firm beds or trollies.

In their visits to ECT units, Pippard & Ellam (1981) found that several clinics used obsolete machines which were unsafe because there was little control over the intensity or duration of shocks.

Inpatients should be accompanied to the ECT clinic by a familiar nurse who should stay with the patient throughout the procedure until return to the ward. Outpatients should be accompanied by a relative or friend or a community nurse. Case notes, consent form, drug and observation charts should be taken to the ECT clinic. The waiting area should be comfortable and homely and a nurse should stay with the patients to provide reassurance, support, information and distraction.

When the patient is called into the treatment area, unfamiliar staff should be introduced and the patient should lie supine on the bed with hands and feet exposed. Tight clothing should be loosened and the nurse should ensure that the patient is safe, comfortable and calm. Soothing music may help to relax the patient.

The Royal College of Nursing (1982) emphasized that mixing, drawing up and administering anaesthetics, positioning of electrodes, administering the electrical current and oxygenating the patient are solely medical responsibilities and should not be carried out by a nurse. Pippard & Ellam (1981) found that ECT was usually given by junior doctors who received only minimal training in the procedure. An anaesthetist should be present because of the risk of post-anaesthetic complications.

A light and short-acting general anaesthetic, usually thiopentone sodium or methohexitone sodium is given intravenously. This is immediately followed by a muscle relaxant such as suxamethonium chloride which reduces the muscle spasm caused by the convulsion. The muscle relaxant is always given after the anaesthetic, because the experience of being paralysed while conscious would be frightening.

A mouth gag is inserted to prevent damage to the teeth during the convulsion and the electrodes are positioned. Gregory et al (1985) found that patients receiving bilateral ECT recovered from depression more rapidly than those receiving unilateral ECT, and required significantly fewer treatments. The patient is oxygenated and the controlled electric shock administered. Throughout the treatment the nurse should observe the patient and may immobilize the limbs gently. Bilateral rhythmic jerking of the toes, fingers and face may be the only sign that a convulsion has taken place. The patient continues to be oxygenated until spontaneous breathing resumes and is turned into the three-quarter prone recovery position and a clear airway maintained. The nurse may need to carry out oral suction.

A course of ECT continues as long as it is clinically indicated, and typically consists of between 6 and 12 treatments, usually given twice a week and never more than three times a week.

The recovery period

The nurse responsible for the recovery area should be specially trained in recovery procedures. Until the patient regains consciousness medical assistance should be readily accessible and a nurse should stay with the patient to monitor pulse, respirations, colour and blood pressure. Patients usually regain full consciousness within about 15 minutes, then they should be helped to get up slowly, tidy clothes and hair and replace dentures, spectacles etc. The patient should then be escorted by a nurse to a quiet and comfortable recovery area where a drink and possibly a light meal can be offered. All this time the patient should be reassured and oriented to reality to promote a feeling of security and to minimize confusion. Accompanying relatives or friends will also need support. Patients are then accompanied back to the ward or taken home. It is important that outpatients are reminded not to drive immediately after ECT.

The nurse must listen to the patient and observe for any expression of side-effects so that appropriate interventions may be taken, such as simple analgesics for headaches. All side-effects should be recorded and persistent or serious side-effects should be reported to a doctor.

The nurse should also observe and record changes in mood, so that the effectiveness of the treatment can be assessed and the duration of the course determined. It is particularly important to observe for suicidal intent as suicide may be contemplated as severe psychomotor retardation lifts and the patient has more energy.

As patients begin to respond to ECT they will become more accessible to other treatments, including psychotherapeutic interventions and counselling. Patients will also be able to participate more fully in occupational therapy and other activities. Nurses should, of course, encourage patients to participate in any other activities which form part of their total treatment programme.

In preparing patients for subsequent ECT treatments, nurses should consider whether it is necessary to repeat previously given information about the treatment. Patients may forget what they have been told, either because of anxiety or depression or because of the temporary memory impairment associated with the treatment itself.

Cohen (1971) discussed the use of group therapy for ECT patients. It may be helpful for several patients undergoing courses of ECT to form a group to share their feelings about being depressed and about the treatment. Nurses could establish and lead groups and could offer support, factual information and advice. A group could help patients to regain contact with reality, improve communication, increase feelings of self-worth, motivate patients to examine their behaviour and to learn new methods of coping.

The nurses' dilemma about participating in ECT

ECT in a controversial treatment and mental health professionals have become involved in acrimonious debates about whether or not its use is justified. Some nurses have argued that they are entitled to refuse to participate in ECT in the same way as they are entitled to refuse to participate in abortion. There have been widely publicized cases of psychiatric nurses being dismissed for refusing to assist with ECT and in 1985 the National Board for Nursing, Midwifery and Health Visiting for Scotland (NBS) held that 'no health care worker has an automatic right of objection to legitimately prescribed medical treatment'.

The principal arguments that have been used to oppose ECT are that: it is ineffective; it has dangerous side-effects; its mode of action is uncertain; it is crude and degrading to the patient; it may be given without consent; it may be abused and overused, when other types of intervention would be more appropriate; and it is banned in some places.

In considering these thorny issues, it is essential to put emotional and polemical arguments aside in favour of objective analysis and research findings.

In its notes of guidance for nurses on objecting to participate in ECT, the NBS (1985) attempted to counter some of the objections. They dismissed the comparison with conscientious objection to abortion because this right is based on the principle that people may hold particular religious or moral convictions and should not be restricted in the exercise of their profession. Objection to ECT on the other hand was not principally religious or moral, but is based on a belief that the treatment is harmful to the recipient.

The NBS claimed that uncertainty about the mode of action of ECT was irrelevant, as many effective treatments were used in all areas of medicine before their precise action was known. The description of ECT as crude and degrading was dismissed as emotionally laden and spurious, an objection which could be raised against innumerable surgical and medical procedures. The NBS argued that the only justifiable objection to ECT would be if it were used indiscriminately or inappropriately and this could be demonstrated as a breach of good practice by reference to the Royal College of Psychiatrist's (1977) Guidelines. Many treatments in psychiatry and general medicine can be over-used or used inappropriately, but this is not a justification for rejecting the treatment when it is used appropriately.

One of the most important ethical aspects of ECT is the issue of whether the therapeutic benefits outweigh the risks. Evidence in relation to this question was reviewed by Merskey (1981) who concluded that ECT is an effective treatment for depression with only a minute risk to life and that the benefits outweigh the main complication of possible loss of memory for some events around the time of treatment. Addressing the issue of the curtailment or banning of ECT in some American states, Merskey (1981) argued that this owes little to knowledge of clinical practice and more to vociferous claims by pressure groups that ECT has in the past sometimes been over-used, or used as a punishment or behavioural control. American doctors sometimes avoid controversial treatments because of the risk of expensive litigation. Far from protecting patients' rights, Merskey (1981) claimed that political involvement interfered with patients' rights to free choice to receive effective treatments. It is true that in certain carefully defined circumstances, ECT may be given to detained patients without consent. This is, however, fairly uncommon and although this may be claimed to be paternalistic, patients' rights are well protected under current British legislation. The rights of severely mentally ill people to receive effective treatment are at least as important as their rights to deny it.

It is vital that nurses working in areas where ECT is used should learn as much as possible about the treatment and should keep up to date with current research. Only then can they provide full, accurate and impartial information to patients and their families. Nurses may work closely with patients who are having difficulty in deciding whether or not to agree to ECT. It is important that nurses recognize their personal biases and that these are not allowed to influence patients' decisions. Should a nurse feel unable to offer unbiased information, it is preferable to acknowledge this and refer patients to colleagues who can. Like many treatments, ECT inevitably has a powerful placebo effect. Once patients have given fully informed consent, it is important for nurses to maximize and exploit the placebo effect by encouraging patients to believe that ECT will relieve their depression.

PSYCHOSURGERY

Psychosurgery was defined by the World Health Organization (1976) as 'the selective surgical removal or destruction of neural pathways . . . with the view to influencing behaviour'. However, Bridges & Bartlett (1977) argued that modern psychosurgery is concerned with the treatment of intractable affective illnesses, without any intended effect on behaviour at all. They define it as 'the surgical treatment of certain psychiatric illnesses by means of localized lesions placed in specific cerebral sites' (Bridges & Bartlett 1977). Psychosurgery is sometimes called psychiatric surgery, psychiatric neurosurgery or functional neurosurgery (Kleining 1985).

It is important to look briefly at the history of psychosurgery, since the early operations still tend to influence people's views of these contentious procedures. The frontal leucotomy was introduced in 1935 by Moniz, a Portuguese neurologist. Over the next 10 years the techniques were developed further by Freeman and Watts. About l0 000 standard leucotomies were performed in Britain between 1944 and 1955, two-thirds for schizophrenia (Tooth & Newton 1961). This procedure resulted in 6% mortality, and undesirable side-effects included haemorrhage, convulsions, incontinence, hypersomnia and personality changes, such an disinhibition and gross emotional blunting. Gradually modifications were devised, based on increasing knowledge in the neurosciences, but the use of leucotomies declined because of high morbidity, failure to relieve the symptoms of schizophrenia and the development of ECT and phenothiazine drugs (Drugs and Therapeutics Bulletin 1980).

The popularity of psychosurgery has waxed and waned during its history and the view of it remains highly contentious. Rylander (1973) claimed to see something of a 'renaissance of psychosurgery' 20 years after its decline in the 1950s. The general consensus in the 1980s seems to be that psychosurgery is justified as 'the last hope of escape from crippling and incessant suffering' (Merskey 1981). In a questionnaire survey of the attitudes of British consultant psychiatrists to psychosurgery, Snaith et al (1984) found that most of their 164 respondents considered there is still a place for psychosurgery and most wanted facilities for the referral of patients.

Indications and contraindications

A number of writers (Schurr 1973, Kelly 1976, Rees 1982, Bartlett et al 1981) have commented on the circumstances in which patients should be considered for psychosurgery. They state that suitable candidates for psychosurgery fulfil at least some of the following criteria:

- severe psychiatric illness
- chronic duration of illness of about ten years
- persistent emotional distress, suffering and incapacity severe enough to interfere with well-being
- failure to respond to all other therapies
- high risk of suicide
- poor prognosis
- stable pre-morbid personality, and

- adequate social circumstances with supportive relationships.

The main psychiatric problems for which psychosurgery might be considered are:

- depression
- anxiety states
- obsessional/compulsive neuroses
- aggressiveness, and
- schizophrenia.

Schizophrenia was originally the main indication for psychosurgery, but is now rare. Kelly (1976) argued that surgery was unlikely to abolish delusions and hallucinations, or help apathy and withdrawal, but could be effective in reducing associated anxiety, depression and obsessional symptoms.

A number of personality characteristics and psychiatric and physical disorders are claimed to be important contraindications to psychosurgery (Kelly 1976, Dally & Connolly 1981, Bartlett et al 1981). These include:

- lifelong inadequate personality
- violent urges
- poor impulse control
- pronounced hysterical personality
- antisocial personality and psychopathy
- alcoholism
- primary drug addiction
- paranoid schizophrenia
- dementia and organic brain damage
- bleeding propensity
- severe hypertension, and
- arteriosclerosis.

Major surgical procedures and their effects

Neurosurgical techniques have been refined over the years to permit smaller, less destructive lesions with fewer and milder side-effects than the older 'freehand' operations which have been largely overtaken by stereotactic procedures. As Bartlett et al (1981) wrote 'psychosurgery has evolved with so much fundamental change in indications and surgical techniques that the present clinical situation has little in common with that obtained during the period of widespread enthusiasm for standard prefrontal leucotomy'.

Two major centres for psychosurgery in Britain are at the Geoffrey Knight Unit at Brook Hospital in London and the Atkinson Morley's Hospital in London. Various centres specialize in different surgical techniques, of which three will be discussed.

Stereotactic subcaudate tractotomy

Under general anaesthesia, radioactive yttrium seeds are placed each side of the posterior orbital aspect of the frontal lobes, the radiation destroying surrounding tissue. Larger subcaudate lesions are also used. This procedure has been used in the treatment of chronic endogenous depression, chronic tension, obsessional neurosis and schizo-affective disorders.

Stereotactic limbic leucotomy

A cryogenic probe is used to freeze white matter in the subcaudate area and cingulum bundle of the limbic system. Mitchell-Heggs et al (1976) followed up 66 patients who had this operation and found that three-quarters were improved at 6 weeks and 16 months. The best results were found in patients suffering from obsessional neurosis, anxiety and depression, although 6 out of 7 schizophrenics also responded.

Improvement occurred gradually and continued up to a year postoperatively. Patients with good pre-morbid personalities did better than those with poor pre-morbid adjustment in their social and work life. Adverse effects were few and included confusion, headache, apathy and incontinence immediately after surgery, but cleared up within a few weeks. There was no mortality and little change in patients' personality.

Stereotactic bilateral amygdalotomy

This procedure consists of implanting indwelling electrodes to achieve graded ablation through electrical stimulation. It is used for severe pathological and uncontrollable aggressiveness associated with psychiatric or neurological disorders such as epilepsy. Kiloh (1977) reviewed studies over 12 years and concluded that this procedure

and posterior hypothalamotomy reduced anger and aggression in a significant number of case.

Between 1974 and 1976 431 operations were performed at 31 hospitals in the UK. 63% were for depression, 12% for anxiety and phobic states, 8% for violence, 7% for obsessional disorders and 6% for schizophrenia and schizo-affective disorders (Barraclough & Mitchell-Heggs 1978).

Effectiveness of psychosurgery

Much of the controversy surrounding psycho-surgery is related to uncertainty about its therapeutic effectiveness. Clare (1980) pointed out that there is an unfortunate tendency in psychiatry for treatments to be 'enthusiastically and passionately endorsed by one group of supporters, while vehemently and sharply rejected by another', without either side critically examining available evaluative research. Debate in this area is too often informed (or misinformed) by unsubstantiated accounts of 'almost miraculous effects' (Journal of Medical Ethics 1980), which are then countered by isolated examples of surgical failure (Dickson 1979) and reference to research on outmoded procedures (Robin 1958, Tooth & Newton 1961).

Most research evaluating psychosurgery is based on subjective clinical assessment by a single re-searcher in uncontrolled studies. Valenstein (1977, 1980) reviewed over 150 studies and rated more than 90% of them as extremely low on scientific merit. Research in this area has numerous methodological flaws, some of which were ident-ified by Flor-Henry (1981) and Kleining (1985), and which render findings invalid and unreliable. These flaws include:

- Diagnostic criteria are rarely explicit, so that comparisons between groups of patients are dubious.
- Patients are rarely assessed objectively or fully described prior to surgery.
- No allowance is made for spontaneous changes and remissions and placebo effects.
- Little allowance is made for the heterogeneity of psychosurgical procedures.
- The researcher assessing patients postoperatively is very rarely blind to the treatment condition, and is sometimes a

doctor clinically involved with the case who must have an interest in the success of the treatment.

- Studies vary in the length of follow-up. If follow-up is too short, therapeutic gains may subsequently disappear, but will not be reported in the research.
- Important therapeutic variables, which could account for improvements, are rarely considered. These include extra attention, intensive medical and nursing care before and after surgery and prolonged rehabilitation.
- Descriptions of symptom changes after surgery are often subjective and impressionistic, rather than using objective measures.
- Control groups are rarely used, but when they do exist are not comparable to the surgical group on numerous important variables.

A research committee of the Royal College of Psychiatrists (1977) proposed a controlled trial with random allocation of patients to surgical and non-surgical groups, but the proposal had to be abandoned because of active political lobbying by the opponents of psychosurgery (Clare 1980). In an editorial, the Drugs and Therapeutics Bulletin (1980) argued that a randomized controlled trial was needed, comparing the outcomes of patients who had brain lesions with those who had everything except the lesion. This would involve 'mock surgery' for the control group and would probably be considered unethical.

In their Second Biennial Report, the Mental Health Act (MHA) Commission (HMSO 1987) commented on the possibility of establishing a national follow-up survey of all patients undergoing psychosurgery in Britain. This would be relatively simple as all cases have to be referred to the Commission for consent.

In summary, and bearing in mind the methodological problems of work in this area, it is clear from the research that modern psychosurgical techniques are consistently reported as beneficial to carefully selected patients suffering from chronic intractable anxiety, depression, obsessional states, schizo-affective disorders and uncontrollable aggressiveness.

ROLE OF THE NURSE IN RELATION TO PSYCHOSURGERY

Nursing interventions will be described in chronological order: preparation of the patient for psychosurgery; pre- and postoperative care in the neurosurgical unit; and rehabilitation after surgery.

Preparation of the patient for psychosurgery

Legal aspects of consent

Section 57 of the 1983 Mental Health Act deals with consent to surgical operations for destroying brain tissue or its function and applies to informal as well an detained patients. This treatment requires: the patient's consent, the validity of which must be confirmed by three people appointed by the MHA Commission, only one of whom may be a doctor; and a second independent opinion from a doctor appointed by the MHA Commission, who must consult with at least two other members of the clinical team, one a nurse and the other neither a doctor nor a nurse.

Although the independent doctor must consult with a nurse and one other person — usually a clinical psychologist, occupational therapist or social worker — the nurse and other professional have no formal power to influence the doctor's opinion. The doctor is entitled to reject their recommendations.

In order to contribute fully to decision-making, the nurse should have a full understanding of the procedure and its implications, as well as its role in the patient's overall treatment plan. The nurse must be able to provide the appointed doctor with full information about the patient and the family. The Draft Code of Practice (HMSO 1985) pointed out the importance of all professionals sharing full information with the appointed doctor to enable him or her 'to have the broadest possible understanding and perspective in evaluating the patient's capacity to give consent and the appropriateness of the proposed treatment'.

Guidelines for practice were set out in the Draft Code of Practice (HMSO 1985). When a patient is referred to the MHA Commission under Section 57, the responsible doctor is expected to show that:

the disorder is such that the patient might be relieved of suffering by surgery; that other circumstances, such as pre-morbid personality and family support, are favourable; that all other suitable treatments have been used vigorously, with unsatisfactory results; that there has been a full, recent multi-disciplinary assessment; that the relatives and other family advisers have been fully informed and consulted; and that a consultant psychiatrist with specialist expertise has seen the patient and agrees to psychosurgery.

The referring consultant is expected to hold multi-disciplinary case conferences, which include planning for after-care and rehabilitation. The consultant must be satisfied that the patient is capable of understanding the nature, purpose and likely effects of the treatment and is likely to give valid consent.

The MHA Commissioners visit and interview the patient and relatives at the referring hospital. They also expect to consult with the multi-disciplinary team and to inspect case notes, patient assessment forms and records of case conferences. Permission will usually only be given for surgery to be carried out in specialist centres experienced in psychosurgery, and the Commissioners will require regular follow-up reports on the patient's progress.

In their second Biennial Report (HMSO 1987), the MHA Commission reported that between September 1983 and June 1987, they received applications for second opinions on behalf of 92 patients. Approval was given for 74 patients, of whom 63 had psychosurgery.

Psychological preparation

The nurse has an important role in preparing the patient and family preoperatively. As previously discussed, the responsible doctor has a legal obligation to provide full information about all aspects of the treatment, but this will need to be reinforced, repeated and clarified by the nurse. The nurse should ensure that the patient and relatives understand all aspects of the treatment, recovery and rehabilitation process and can provide more detailed explanations of aspects which are worrying the patient and relatives. Patients may be embarrassed or feel too rushed to admit

their fears to the consultant and the nurse can provide sufficient time to answer all questions and explore their worries.

Patients and relatives need to be warned that surgery in itself is unlikely to produce a sudden 'cure', but that long-term rehabilitation and effort by the patient and family are essential to obtain full benefits (Bridges & Williamson 1977). Relatives will need help to understand their role in rehabilitation and will need to explore the likely effects of the treatment on relationships and roles within the family. The patient may have been seen as a dependent invalid and an object of pity for many years, so that relatives may have difficulty in adjusting to the patient's increased independence and confidence if the treatment is successful. Relatives may have to travel long distances to the few psychosurgical units, so that assistance with travelling expenses and accommodation may be required.

Pre- and postoperative care in the neurosurgical unit*

Pre-anaesthetic care is no different from other neurosurgery. At Atkinson Morley's Hospital in London this includes general physical examination, head and chest X-rays, a pre-anaesthetic consent form signed by the next-of-kin and obtained by the ward doctor or anaesthetist, baseline observations, skull measurements, a bath and hairwash. The patient fasts from midnight before surgery and dentures, jewellery and make-up are removed before going to theatre. The premedication consists of atropine or glycopyralade, but no sedative. A light general anaesthetic is given so that the patient regains consciousness early after surgery. Small areas of hair have to be shaved around the burr hole areas, but this may be done in theatre to avoid distressing the patient.

Immediately postoperatively, patients at Atkinson Morley's Hospital go to the intensive care unit for about 6 hours. Patients are carefully observed for possible complications such as cerebral

---

* Much of this information was kindly provided by Mrs Sheila Bruce, Clinical Teacher to the Post-Basic Neurosurgical Nursing Course at Atkinson Morley's Hospital, London

haemorrhage, epilepsy and infections. Neurological observations are initially half hourly, reducing to hourly, 2 hourly and 4 hourly as the patient recovers. Other observations include temperature, pulse, respiratory rate and blood pressure, and the patient is also observed for changes in the level of consciousness, restlessness, vomiting and pain. The head of the bed is raised 10 degrees for the first 24 hours.

The patient is usually nil by mouth for about 6 hours after surgery, but once the swallow reflex has return, gradually starts taking sips of water, then drinks, then a normal or light diet. The burr holes are covered with dry dressings and the sutures are removed on the second postoperative day.

Codeine phosphate may be given for headache, as this drug only minimally masks neurological signs, but these patients rarely complain of pain. Phenytoin is usually given prophylactically for 2 years after inter-cranial surgery because of the risk of epileptic fits.

At Atkinson Morley's Hospital, pre- and post-operative care is carried out by neurosurgical nurses, and a psychiatric nurse would be involved only if the patient was suicidal or violent. The patient returns to the referring psychiatric hospital for rehabilitation after about 5 days.

Rehabilitation after psychosurgery

Rehabilitation is a complex and long-term process which should be individually planned to meet the needs of the patient. Those who have been in hospital for many years may continue to need the protective hospital environment for some time, gradually progressing to the greater independence of a hostel or day hospital. In the longer term many patients may be able to return home, supported to varying degrees and for varying periods by community psychiatric nurses, social workers and other community resources. It is important to set realistic long-term goals as some severely disabled patients may be left with residual difficulties which make completely independent living in their own homes unlikely.

Irrespective of the patient's disorder and individual needs, rehabilitation after psychosurgery has two broad aims: to help speed the process of symptom resolution and to help overcome the secondary effects of years of illness (Kelly 1976). The whole approach should be positive and forward looking, with nurses conveying optimism for the future and a sense of encouragement. Although morbid patterns of behaviour may be weakened or removed, specific problems may remain which need to be tackled. For example, Kelly (1976) described how anxious patients should be exposed to anxiety-provoking situations in a structured and progressive manner, and how obsessional patients need to be repeatedly encouraged to resist the urge to carry out rituals and to engage in more useful and enjoyable pursuits. Nurses will use a variety of behavioural as well as psychotherapeutic techniques to resolve specific problems after psychosurgery.

Patients who have suffered from severely disbling illnesses over many years are likely to have lost many of the skills necessary to live an independent and fulfilling life and may have become apathetic and institutionalized. Rehabilitation therefore needs to focus on teaching and practising basic self-care, activities of daily living, domestic, social and work skills, with the aims of restoring confidence and resuming work, family and social life.

Relatives need support, advice and practical help to cope with day-to-day problems and to contribute to rehabilitation. It is likely that they will have become physically and emotionally exhausted by the strain of the patient's long-term illness by the time of psychosurgery. Having already seen numerous treatments given without success, they may be sceptical about the likely effects of psychosurgery, but it is important that their pessimism is not communicated to the patient.

ETHICAL ASPECTS OF PSYCHOSURGERY

Ethics and efficacy are inseparable, as it is clearly not ethical to carry out an operation which has not been shown to work. Evaluative research has already been discussed in this chapter, but concepts of therapeutic success themselves raise many ethical problems. It is not always clear whether the desired clinical outcomes are intended to benefit the patient or others. If the results of surgery are to make patients more passive, submissive and compliant to the will of carers, then clearly the primary benefits are not to the patient but to others. This is particularly problematic when the psychiatric disorder is more troubling to carers than to the patient, for example when the patient is extremely aggressive or hyperactive.

These problems are related to concerns about psychosurgery as 'mind control' or 'social control', criticisms levelled at many areas of psychiatry, but particularly relevant to psychosurgery because of the direct and irreversible effects on brain tissue. Fears that psychosurgery could become a socially acceptable instrument of control over deviant behaviour have been frequently expressed (e.g. Whitlock 1977, Mark & Eivin 1970, Schwarz 1972). Whitlock (1977) argued that it is incompatible with humanity to impose this on people judged ill solely on account of antisocial behaviour. The 1983 Mental Health Act provides clear safeguards against this possibility as psychosurgery can only be carried out in Britain under rigorously controlled circumstances with the explicit and informed consent of the patient.

Another ethical concern described by Kleining (1985) relates to 'the sanctity of the brain'. He describes the deep conviction, held by society, that the brain has unique status as the site of selfhood or personality, so that destruction of brain tissue is an invasion of personality and an assault on the repository of one's identity as a unique individual.

Kleining (1985) identifies a further ethical issue relating to the currently crude understanding of brain function. He considers that there is little clear rationale for psychosurgery, which is a largely pragmatic and experimental procedure. This is particularly problematic when the tissue destroyed is only questionably pathological and the results are irreversible as brain tissue is generally non-generable.

Psychosurgery is generally considered only after all conventional treatments have been tried and failed. If conventional treatments such as behavioural psychotherapy are not carried out vigorously and skilfully, then it may be unethical to refer a patient for psychosurgery. With limited health service resources and shortages of skilled and experienced therapists this objection may be valid in some cases or at some referring hospitals.

Furthermore, after surgery it is essential to provide adequate rehabilitation to maximize the likelihood of a successful outcome, and it is questionable whether rehabilitation is always carried out as skillfully as possible. This problem points to the desirability of establishing a single national psychiatric and neurosurgical centre for this treatment.

Finally, a number of writers have argued that it is more unethical to deny a possible treatment to those with severely disabling mental problems than it is to offer it. Pippard (1976) argued, for example, that the reduction in psychosurgery by half since 1962 means that patients 'are being cheated' of 'the excellent chance' of 'great improvement' which can be provided by surgery. Similarly Clare (1980) claimed that severe obsessional disorders are rarely successfully treated by anything but psychosurgery.

OTHER PHYSICAL TREATMENTS
Narco-analysis and abreaction

Intravenous barbiturates and amphetamines are sometimes used to help patients to express repressed conflicts and emotionally charged feelings more readily without inhibition. This differs from other physical treatments in that the drugs themselves are not the therapeutic agent, but are used to facilitate a form of psychotherapy. According to Dally & Connolly (1981) the most commonly used drugs are barbiturates such as sodium amylobarbitone, thiopentone and methohexitone and methyl amphetamine. Inhalants such as ether or nitrous oxide are rarely used today.

Techniques may be used for a variety of problems: for hysterical conversion symptoms, such as paralysis or amnesia; in inhibited obsessional people, to relieve depersonalization; in psychosexual problems to loosen inhibitions, and enable patients to talk freely; for mute or withdrawn psychotics and catatonic stupors; as a diagnostic tool when schizophrenia is suspected, etc.

It is not easy to adjust drug dosages to achieve just the right degree of disinhibition safely, and these procedures are potentially dangerous, e.g. too much intravenous barbiturate will produce anaesthesia. Narco-analysis and abreaction should only be carried out by suitably qualified doctors in safe surroundings and with full resuscitation equipment.

Sleep-related treatments

In some very acute problems it is thought that patients need a period of complete mental and physical rest before beginning other treatments. In modified narcosis the patient is kept asleep or drowsy for much of the time over two or three days, using a combination of sedatives and tranquillizers adjusted in dosage and frequency to achieve the desired effect. The patient is nursed in a quiet single room and is given similar general nursing care to any patient on bed rest or semiconscious. In many ways this treatment parallels the common tendency for people to take to their beds for a day or two as a means of coping with a major crisis, such as a sudden bereavement. Variants of modified narcosis are occasionally used as a preventive measure in coronary prone people with Type A personality, on the assumption that stress is reduced by increased sleep. Patients treated by modified narcosis risk all the well-known complications of bed-rest, such as urinary retention, muscle wasting and chest infections, which emphasize the need for continuous nursing observation and good physical care.

In contrast, sleep deprivation has been described as an effective treatment for patients with severe unipolar or bipolar depression, associated with loss of appetite, early waking, guilt and diurnal variation of symptoms (Bhanji & Roy 1975). Patients are either kept awake all night or selectively deprived of REM sleep. Improvement has been noted the day after deprivation.

Insulin coma therapy

Insulin coma therapy is now only of historical interest, although it may still be used in some parts of the world. This treatment was developed for schizophrenia and other major mental disorders in the 1930s and was described by Sakel (1938). It was a long complex procedure, requiring continuous nursing observation and care, with a danger of life-threatening complications. Insulin was injected to produce hypoglycaemia, the patient was closely observed and before going into a coma was revived with glucose and a high carbohydrate meal. In so far as it had any benefits, it is likely that the therapeutic ingredient was the intensive medical and nursing attention. The good meals may also have improved the nutrition of very debilitated patients. Insulin coma therapy declined from the late 1950s following the introduction of antipsychotic drugs.

REFERENCES

Barraclough B M, Mitchell-Heggs N A 1978 Use of neurosurgery for psychological disorders in the British Isles during 1974–1976. British Medical Journal IV: 1591–1593

Bartlett J, Bridges P, Kelly D 1981 Contemporary indications for psychosurgery. British Journal of Psychiatry 138: 507–511

Bhanji S, Roy G A 1975 The treatment of psychotic depression by sleep deprivation: a replication study. British Journal of Psychiatry 127: 222–226

Bird J M, 1979 Effect of the media on attitudes to ECT. British Medical Journal 2: 26–27

Brandon S, Cowley P, McDonald C, Neville P, Palmer R, Wellstood-Eason S 1984 Electro-convulsive therapy: results in depressive illness from the Leicestershire trial. British Medical Journal 288: 22–25

Bridges P K, Williamson C 1977 Psychosurgery today. Nursing Times, September 1, 1363–1367

Bridges P K, Bartlett J R 1977 Psychosurgery: yesterday and today. British Journal of Psychiatry 131: 249–260

Clare A 1980 Psychiatry in dissent, 2nd ed. Tavistock, London

Cohen R 1971 EST + group therapy = improved care. American Journal of Nursing 71: 6, 1195–1198

Crow T J 1979 The scientific status of ECT. Psychological Medicine 9: 401–408

Dally P, Connolly J 1981 An introduction to physical methods of treatment in psychiatry, 6th ed. Churchill Livingstone, Edinburgh

Dickson D 1979 Psychosurgery supporters sued for malpractice. Nature 277: 5693, 164–165

Drugs and Therapeutics Bulletin 1980 Is leucotomy ever justified? Editorial 18: 15, 57–58

Flor-Henry P 1981 Psychosurgery yesterday and today: a review. In: Dongier M, Wittkower E(eds) Divergent views in psychiatry. Harper & Row, Magerstown Md

Fraser M 1982 ECT: a clinical guide. Wiley, Chichester

Freeman C P L, Basson J V, Creighton A 1978 Double-blind controlled trial of ECT and simulated ECT in depressive illness. Lancet 1: 738–740

Fromm-Auch D 1982 Comparison of unilateral and bilateral ECT: evidence for selective memory impairment. British Journal of Psychiatry 141: 608–613

Gregory S, Shawcross C R, Gill D 1985 The Nottingham ECT study: a double-blind comparison of bilateral, unilateral and simulated ECT in depressive illness. British Journal of Psychiatry 146: 520–524

HMSO 1983 The Mental Health Act 1983. HMSO London, ch 20

HMSO 1985 Mental Health Act 1983 Draft Code of Practice. Mental Health Division, DHSS. HMSO, London

HMSO 1985 Mental Health Act Commission. First Biennial Report 1983–1985. HMSO, London

HMSO 1987 Mental Health Act Commission, Second Biennial Report 1985–1987. HMSO, London

Johnstone E C, Lawler P, Stevens S, Deakin J F W, Frith C D, McPherson K, Crow T J 1980 The Northwick Park ECT trial. Lancet 2: 1317–1320

Journal of Medical Ethics 1980 Surgery for the mind. Editorial 6: 3, 115–116

Kelly D 1976 Neurosurgical treatment of psychiatric disorders. In: Granville Grossman K (ed) Recent advances in clinical psychiatry 2. Churchill Livingstone, Edinburgh

Kiloh L G 1977 The treatment of anger and aggression and modification of sexual deviation. In: Smith J S, Kiloh L G (eds) Psychosurgery and Society. Pergamon, Oxford

Kleining J 1985 Ethical issues in psychosurgery. Allan and Unwin, London

Kreigh H, Perko J E 1983 Psychiatric and mental health nursing: a commitment to care and concern. Prentice-Hall, New York

Lambourn J, Gill D 1978 A controlled comparison of simulated and real ECT. British Journal of Psychiatry 133: 514–519

Mark V H, Eivin F R 1970 Violence and the brain. Harper & Row, New York

Merskey H 1981 Ethical aspects of the physical manipulation of the brain. In: Bloch S, Chodoff P (eds) Psychiatric ethics. Oxford University Press, Oxford

Mitchell-Heggs N, Kelly D, Richardson A 1976 Stereotactic limbic leucotomy: a follow-up at 16 months. British Journal of Psychiatry 128: 226–240

National Board for Nursing, Midwifery and Health Visiting for Scotland 1985 Guidance Paper: Questioning of, or objecting to participation in medical procedures. ECT. NBS, Scotland

Pippard J, Ellam L 1981 Electro-convulsive treatment in Great Britain 1980. A Report to the Royal College of Psychiatrists. Gaskell, London

Rees L 1982 A short textbook of psychiatry. Hodder & Stoughton, London

Robin A A 1958 A controlled study of the effects of leucotomy. Journal of Neurology, Neurosurgery and Psychiatry, 21: 262

Royal College of Nursing 1982 Nursing guidelines for ECT. RCN, London

Royal College of Psychiatrists 1977 Memorandum on the use of ECT. British Journal of Psychiatry 131: 261–272

Rylander G 1973 The renaissance of psychosurgery. In: Laitenen L V, Livingston K E (eds) Surgical approaches to psychiatry. Medical and Technical Publishing Co, Lancaster

Sakel M 1938 The pharmacological shock treatment of schizophrenia. Nervous and Mental Diseases, Monograph Series No 62, New York

Schurr P H 1973 Psychosurgery. British Journal of Hospital Medicine 10: 6, 53–59

Schwarz J P 1972 Stereotactic hypothalamotomy for behavioural disorders. Journal of Neurology, Neurosurgery and Psychiatry 35: 356

Snaith R P, Price D J E, Wright J F 1984 Psychiatrists' attitudes to psychosurgery: proposals for the organization of a psychosurgical service in Yorkshire. British Journal of Psychiatry 144: 293–297

Tooth G C, Newton H P 1961 Leucotomy in England and Wales 1942–1954. Reports on Public Health and Medical Subjects, No 14. HMSO, London

Trimble M R 1981 Neuropsychiatry. Wiley, Chichester

Valenstein E S 1977 The practice of psychosurgery: a review of the literature 1971–1976. Psychosurgery Report. DHEW Publ No (OS) 77 — 0002. Washington, DC

Valenstein E S 1980 (ed) The psychosurgery debate: scientific, legal and ethical perspectives. Freeman, San Francisco

Wilby L 1986 The role of the nurse in psychological preparation of patients for ECT. Dissertation submitted for the BSc (Hons) Nursing Studies, University of London, King's College

World Health Organization 1976 Health aspects of human rights. WHO, Geneva

Whitlock F A 1977 The ethics of psychosurgery. In: Smith J S, Kiloh L G (eds) Psychosurgery and society. Pergamon, Oxford

---

ESSENTIAL GENERAL READING ON PHYSICAL TREATMENT IN PSYCHIATRY

Bloch S, Chodoff P 1981 (eds) Psychiatric ethics. Oxford University Press, Oxford — Clear and thought-provoking discussions of the ethical aspects of several physical treatments.

Clare A 1980 Psychiatry in dissent, 2nd edn. Tavistock, London — Chapters on ECT and psychosurgery critically examine the research evidence for the effectiveness of these treatments.

Dally P, Connolly J 1981 An introduction to physical methods of treatment in psychiatry. Churchill Livingstone, Edinburgh — This is the classic introductory text in this area.

Fraser M 1982 ECT: a clinical guide. Wiley, Chichester — A very clear and well-structured account with an emphasis on clinical aspects.

Johnstone E C et al 1980 The Northwick Park ECT trial. Lancet 2: 1317–1320 — Describes in detail the methodological aspects of a major study to evaluate ECT.

Kleining J 1985 Ethical issues in psychosurgery. Allen & Unwin, London — A careful examination of the many ethical questions surrounding psychosurgery.

Pippard J, Ellam L 1981 Electro-convulsive treatment in Great Britain, 1980. Gaskell, London — The results of a major survey on the use of ECT.

41

Individual psychotherapy and counselling

G. E. Chapman

Most nurses working with troubled people have experienced the pleasure associated with listening to patients in such a way that both they and the patient share a feeling of having understood a personal conflict, problem or painful life event. Listening, understanding and reformulating troubled perceptions are the basis of the psychotherapeutic exercise. Therapeutic listening of this kind and psychotherapy are not, however, the same thing. This is because the setting, the level of formality of the intervention, the theoretical framework and the type of training involved differ. In this chapter I will examine these differences, seeking to make helpful distinctions between therapeutic listening, counselling, psychotherapy and psychoanalysis. Such a discussion, in one chapter, can only provide a flavour of the complexities and richness of the psychotherapeutic approach to psychiatric problems. Readers interested in developing their understanding further should find the further reading list helpful. The structure of the chapter will be as follows: firstly an outline of the theory which underpins most psychotherapeutic approaches; secondly a description of the range of types of psychotherapy available in Great Britain; thirdly, a discussion about the way nurses may use the psychodynamic approach in everyday nursing work; and finally a comment on counselling and psychotherapy as a clinical nurse speciality.

THEORY AND PRACTICE OF PSYCHOTHERAPY

Brown & Pedder (1979) describe psychotherapy as a 'conversation which involves listening to and talking with those in trouble with the aim of helping them understand and resolve their predicament'. What distinguishes psychotherapy and counselling from everyday supportive conversations with patients is:

- the theory which underpins the intervention
- the training in theory and clinical techniques expected of practitioners
- the purpose of the therapeutic intervention.

To a greater or lesser extent most psychotherapies and much counselling work draw on psychoanalytic theory to inform practice. A brief review of the main propositions and concepts will be useful.

Psychoanalytic theory

The work of psychoanalysts suggests that neurotic symptomatology is a result of unresolved childhood experiences long forgotten in adulthood. This basic proposition arises out of the theory of human development formulated by Freud after decades of clinical work with neurotic patients (Sulloway 1980). His model of psychological functioning stressed the importance of the early formative years as a factor in the way we feel and behave as adults. Indeed Freud was to argue that adult personality is determined by childhood experiences. An examination of the ideas behind this proposition will be helpful. Freud suggested that far from being a blank sheet upon which the norms of social conduct are writ, infants and children are actively sensuous beings. They are responsive not only to the external psychosocial stimuli provided by their parents and family, but also to the changing internal physiological and emotional stimuli associated with human biological development. This active, responsive sensuality is termed the libido or libidinal drive. As they develop, infants and children are said to gain sexual or libidinal pleasure from a range of sites on their body (Freud 1905). Internal and external

prohibitions and inhibitions associated with experiencing the pleasure derived from the body cause conflict. The way the child resolves the conflict inherent in the natural process of growing up, together with the way parents respond to the child during periods of growth and change, will determine the formation of adult personality. It is our adult personality which will determine to a greater or lesser extent how we respond to the joys and sorrows of everyday life.

One of Freud's (1915) major contributions to the study of personality was the idea that unconscious wishes and impulses can influence our behaviour as readily as our conscious thoughts and wishes. He suggested that mental life could be separated into several levels: the conscious level, where thoughts, feelings and experiences are readily available to us; the pre-conscious level from which forgotten experiences could be recalled; and the unconscious level which contains repressed and uncomfortable instincts, feelings, memories and experiences. Repressed material is often associated with 'forbidden' instinctual drives associated with sexual or murderous wishes. Repressed unconscious material of this nature, according to Freud, often underlies the neurosis which psychotherapists seek to ameliorate. Evidence to support the notion of an unconscious level of mental operation, of which by definition we cannot be aware, was drawn from two observable phenomenon: dreams and slips of the tongue.

Freud (1900) hypothesized that the hidden content of dreams might include a range of anxiety-provoking desires and fantasies censored from waking thought. These censored thoughts, once revealed to his clients through analysis, evoked distress, then relief and a means of resolving conflicts. He argued, too, that everyday slips of the tongue (Freud 1901) and 'forgetting' of important events and engagements demonstrated the power of the unconscious to affect our behaviour. We 'forget' things and make 'slips of the tongue' because at some level we wish to. It takes little imagination to understand, for example, why we might 'forget' a dentist appointment. Consistently 'forgetting', say, the date of our parents' birthday may conceal a wish that we ourselves will not grow old. Other censored thoughts might be more harmful, however, and it was Freud's contention

Table 41.1   Stages in human development (adapted from Erikson 1974)

Age	Stage	Key elements	Central issues
0–1	Oral	Satisfaction/pleasure derived from mouth via sucking and feeding	Attachment/dependency Trust v mistrust
1–3	Anal	Satisfaction/pleasure derived from gaining control of eliminating faeces	Accommodation of instinctual pleasure to social reality. Separation. Autonomy v shame
3–5	Oedipal	Awareness of genitalia and consequent curiosity/anxiety about sexual differences. Passionate attachment to opposite sex parent, jealous rivalry with same sex parent	Development of gender identity and conscience. Initiative v guilt
6–12	Latency	Sexual quiescence; interest focused on external social world, intellectual and sporting activities	Psychosexual moratorium and development of social identity. Industry v inferiority
12–18	Puberty/adolescence	Hormonal and physical changes rekindle sexual drives; herald in genital sexuality. Reworking of previous stages prior to adulthood	Formation of adult social and sexual identity. Separation from parents. Identity v identity diffusion

that forbidden infantile experiences arising out of the way we grow through certain stages of development, are often the source of neurosis. The stages of psychosexual development suggested by Freud and reformulated by Erikson (1983) are listed in Table 41.1. Certain mental structures arise out of these developmental tasks, and they provide the basic framework of adult personality. These structures are the id, the ego and the super-ego. The id is associated with early, primitive childhood fantasies and feelings; it operates at the unconscious level and is driven by the libido. It is present at birth and is concerned with the life principle, the enjoyment of pleasurable experiences for their own sake. The ego is that aspect of the personality associated with 'common sense', the capacity to modify pleasurable impulses and actions in the light of the perceived consequences of the action.

The ego operates at both conscious and unconscious levels and is formed during the anal period when we learn to control our eliminations in the interests of gaining parental approval and avoiding disapproval. Finally the super-ego, operating at conscious and unconscious levels, is concerned with the conscience. It is the internalized parent whom we seek to please, and against whom we might rebel, who guides our actions and feelings and may prohibit our wishes and desires. The super-ego may be rewarding or punitive; it is never morally neutral. Formed during the oedipal phase, the development of the conscience is associated with the ability to feel guilt and remorse and the impulse to punish self and others for moral wrongdoing. For psychotherapists, behavioural and emotional difficulties may arise from these structures. For example, poor ego strength may result in poor impulse control associated with aggressive or delinquent acts. Similarly, too savage a super-ego may make experiencing sexual pleasure impossible for some people.

According to Freud (1936), there are mental mechanisms which act as the cogs in the machinery of our mental life. The defence mechanisms act as filters and brakes to our feelings, memories and experiences; thus they constitute a vital part of our ability to function in the world. They are listed in Table 41.2. It is paradoxical that the defences which hold us together in order for us to function, may act against us by suppressing unwelcome psychological material. Freud's (1895) classic examples describe how some of his patients experienced a range of symptoms, from neuralgia to paralysis, as a result of suppressed psychic material.

It is important to stress that mental mechanisms are unconscious and may come into play, particularly when feelings or anxieties threaten to overwhelm us. Psychic material which is particularly painful may be suppressed, and when this occurs in the context of a psychotherapy session the term resistance is used. The term refers to an unconscious process of denial rather than a wilful refusal to accept the analyst's ideas.

In summary, psychoanalytic theory suggests that neurotic symptomatology, including depression, hysterical symptoms, phobias, obsessions and 'sexual perversions', are a result of traumatic or unresolved childhood experiences. Psychopathology of this type may occur where early experiences associated with the individual's psychosexual development are such as to prevent resolution of anxiety-provoking conflicts. To some extent all human beings are vulnerable to neurotic symptomatology, but, for those whose experiences have been particularly damaging, a neurotic illness will result which severely inhibits their capacity to function. The psychoanalyst's task is associated with seeking to explore specific experiences by listening to patients' accounts and offering interpretations of them. This activity of untangling the patient's memories and perceptions through talk enables him to find different, less pathological, ways of coping.

Freud's theories were always controversial and his stress on the sexuality of children shocked his 19th century audience. Other clinicians and theorists in the field challenged or revised elements in his theoretical model. Jung (1964), a contemporary of Freud, was to develop ideas stressing the way cultural and social metaphysical beliefs affect individual consciousness.

Klein (Segal 1975) and Anna Freud (1936), working with children, re-examined Freud's

Table 41.2 Mental defence mechanisms

Term	Key elements
Repression	Placing into the unconscious and losing from conscious thought unacceptable feelings, desires, wishes
Projection	Putting or attributing own feelings, thoughts, onto other people, places or objects
Denial	Non-recognition of unacceptable thoughts, feelings, drives, wishes
Reaction formation	Turning unacceptable feelings, actions into their opposite
Rationalization	Using reasoning to accomodate feelings, desires, wishes
Regression	Returning to ealier levels of development as a means of coping with feelings etc.
Displacement	Transferring feelings etc. to a different person, place, objects
Sublimation	Using other activities, people, situations as outlet for suppressed feelings, etc.
Conversion/psychosomatic symptoms	Conversion of internal psychic conflict into physical symptoms
Phobic avoidance	Non-rational avoidance of situations, objects people, imbued with threat arising from own feelings, desires, wishes
Depersonalization	Treating people as objects rather than human subjects as means of coping with own feelings etc. towards them
Confusion	Disintegration of personal intent

assumptions about the timing and nature of child-hood attachments. They were to stress how early the infant's passionate attachment to his mother, or parts of her, occurs. From this, the object relations theory, stressing the need to understand the role of ambivalence, splitting and projective identification in the formation of personality, arose. Later, 'Neo-Freudians' (Brown 1964) were to stress the importance of the ego rather than the unconscious as a means of facilitating the patient to function. Feminists (Strouse 1974, Eichenbaum & Orbach 1982) writing in the late 70s and early 80s began to question Freud's assumptions about femininity and the formation of sexual identity. They pointed out the differing social and cultural expectations and experiences of girls and boys, and took into account the way social norms permeate consciousness. Such values often served to perpetuate oppressive and repressive attitudes towards women and the poor self-image women have of themselves. Most theorists working in this field share, however, a preoccupation with seeking to understand people's troubles in the present in terms of internal conflicts generated by the past. Most share the view that painful feelings and thoughts troubling to adults are often formed during the early years and enacted or reflected in present relationships. Similarly, most psychotherapy writers would agree that to render these experiences visible, discussable and understandable in order that they can be resolved and worked through, is the primary aim of therapy.

Types of psychotherapy

As noted above, there are several types of psychotherapy based on one or other of the theoretical positions. A summary of types of psychotherapy can be found in Table 41.3. Brown & Pedder (1979) argue that there are basic similarities between different types of therapy. These are: a stress on unburdening problems and the ventilation of feelings; a supportive alliance

Table 41.3   Types of psychotherapy

Type	Participants	Duration*	Location	Frequency
Psychoanalysis	Client & trained psychoanalyst	Long term	Consulting room with couch	5 sessions a week (50 mins)
Psychotherapy	Client & trained analyst/therapist	Medium to long term	Consulting room with couch or chair	1–3 sessions weekly (50 mins)
Group psychotherapy	Up to 10 clients and trained group analyst	Medium term	Office or room with chairs	1–2 sessions weekly (50 mins)
Family therapy	Family and therapist	Short to medium term	Office or room with chairs	1–2 sessions weekly (50 mins)
Encounter groups	8 clients or more and therapist	Short term	Varies	1 session a week or 2–3 in series
Counselling	1 client and counsellor	Short to medium term	Varies	Flexible
Self-help groups	Up to 10 people with common interest. Shared leadership	Varies	Varies	Flexible

* Long term: 3 years or more
Medium term: 1 year or more
Short term: 1 session or more
Notes
Many psychotherapies are undertaken on an outpatient basis.
This is only a summary of types of therapy. Interested readers should refer to the reading list.

between therapist and client; and a reliable and consistent time and place for the work to proceed. The differences lie in the psychological depth with which these problems are addressed and explored. Thus, in exploratory therapy, dreams may be analyzed and medication withheld, while with supportive therapy, advice or medication may be offered. They find Cawley's (1977) description helpful. As they summarize it, Cawley suggests that there are three levels of therapy.

1. Outer level

Support and counselling are offered and the client unburdens problems to a sympathetic listener, ventilates his feelings within a supportive relationship, and discusses his difficulties with a non-judgemental helper. A working alliance of this type is often possible in schemes where a nursing process approach is adopted and the patient feels understood and supported by the nurse (Barnes 1968, Chapman 1984, Jones 1980, Green 1983, Smith 1980).

2. Intermediate level

The client discusses his problems with a non-judgemental helper and clarifies their nature and origin within a deepening relationship with the therapist. Some confrontation of defences occurs. There are a range of workers who adopt this approach, from general practitioners and psychiatrists to social workers. Some nurses with special training, such as student counsellors and clinical nurse specialists in drug dependency or family therapy, adopt this approach. The nursing process is, however, probably less useful because of the emergent nature of the discoveries which the client and therapist make.

3. Deeper level

In the context of a therapeutic relationship the client's defences are confronted and interpretation of the unconscious motives and transference phenomena occurs. The term transference refers to the way feelings arising from important relationships in the client's life (usually parental relationships) are transferred to the therapist. Other features of the deeper level include repetition, remembering and reconstruction of the past, and regression to less adult and rational ways of functioning. The aim is to resolve internal conflicts which are thought to be impeding current functioning by re-experiencing them and understanding them. Only those with specific training in psychotherapy or psychoanalysis undertake this type of therapy. A prerequisite of such training is that the therapist herself undergoes therapy. Cawley's levels of psychotherapy have been elaborated further in the unit in which he was a consultant (Ritter 1988).

Evaluation of and criteria for psychotherapy

Stafford-Clarke (1983) asserts that critiques of psychoanalytically-based therapy seem often to be made by writers who have either relied on secondary sources or who have not read Freud in much depth. Thus a critical mythology has arisen around Freud's ideas, while at the same time many concepts have become embedded in our everyday thinking about people. An example is the notion of a 'Freudian slip' to explain embarrassing or revealing slips of the tongue. Other writers have sought to examine whether psychoanalytical concepts can be substantiated empirically. Eysenck & Wilson (1973), for example, have vigorously argued that empirical evidence refutes Freudian theory. On the other hand Kline (1981), in an exhaustive review of the literature, suggests that confirming evidence can be found. Much of this debate rests on the writer's perception of what constitutes a scientific discipline (Bocock 1980). I will not discuss this debate further here but rather concentrate on the problem of whether or not psychotherapy is an effective form of treatment. Here, too, there are difficulties associated with providing conclusive evidence. Kline summarizes these in the following way:

1. Patient variables
   The research studies share a common fallacy of assuming the patients are a homogenous group.

2. Therapist variables
   Studies rarely achieve the aim of including sufficient numbers of therapists to ensure statistical validity.
3. Criteria for success
   There are no fixed, generally agreed criteria for successful therapeutic outcome amongst researchers, psychiatrists and psychotherapists.
4. Control groups
   It is difficult to obtain matched groups of clients to satisfy the criteria for case-controlled studies.
5. Spontaneous remission
   In the field of mental health it is difficult to establish whether the patient might have recovered spontaneously without the help of therapy.

Kline concludes that while writers seeking to refute psychoanalytic theory and practice have not entirely succeeded, neither have the writers seeking to confirm or validate it. For psychotherapists and their clients, subjective assessments continue to be the most effective means of evaluating the therapeutic experience.

There is a consensus of opinion amongst practitioners that psychotherapy is most effective for patients suffering from neurotic illnesses rather than psychoses. This is because a capacity for insight, self-reflexivity and the ability to resolve problems through talk is a prerequisite of this form of treatment. The patient should also be able to distinguish between thoughts which arise from himself and those which originate from others. Furthermore the capacity of the patient to acknowledge his own problems and the motivation to change is essential. Without these the client will find it difficult to sustain a therapeutic alliance with the therapist when painful or threatening issues arise. Finally, the patient requires sufficient ego strength and the capacity to form supportive relationships if he is not to disintegrate during painful moments in therapy. Some critics of the method have argued, mistakenly I would suggest, that the above qualities favour middle class clients who are more articulate and psychologically sophisticated. In practice it is often the ability to pay for treatment rather than the technique itself which favours this group.

Supportive therapy on the other hand, does not make the same demands on patients. It is therefore generally considered suitable for both neurotic and some psychotic patients. Some therapists have put forward the view that psychotic patients can be helped by psychotherapy (Birckhead 1984), and accounts of in-depth programmes have been recorded in biographies of 'Mary Barnes' (Barnes & Berke 1982) and 'Sybil' (Schreiber 1985). Overall, this type of work is highly intensive and requires considerable commitment and skill on the part of the therapists concerned.

PSYCHODYNAMIC APPROACHES TO NURSING

The psychodynamic approach to nursing has proved helpful in a range of orthodox and specialist psychiatric settings. Such input may occur at three main levels. Firstly, the ward, department or hospital may be organized with psychoanalytic principles in mind (Barnes 1968, Kennedy 1986, Kennard & Roberts 1985). Secondly, small groups of patients may be offered group psychotherapy where the nurse acts as therapist or co-therapist (Loomis 1970, Kynaston et al 1981). The third level relates to individual care and it is this area I will concentrate on here.

The individual patient

The emphasis on developing a relationship with a patient and understanding this in terms of what the patient says and feels as well as how he behaves, in conjunction with understanding how the nurse feels about him, has its basis in psycho-analytical thinking. Andrews (1982) describe this in a case study of a patient who is relieved by a nurse's understanding of links between her mother's death and difficulties she had in using her arms. The nursing process approach offers nurses the opportunity, not only of systematic history taking and identification of problems, but also of developing an understanding of the patient during the course of a continuous working relationship with him. Similarly, gaining insight about the patient's day-to-day experiences from a psychodynamic viewpoint may be useful. Julia Segal (1985), now a psychotherapist, describes how, as a nursing assistant, she cared for an elderly demented patient who used constantly to ask: 'When am I going, dear?' or 'Where am I going?' Segal writes: 'There were, of course, many possible interpretations to be put on these questions, but when I once gave a minute to ask her if she was worried where she would go when she died, and when she would die, the response was quite startling. For a while she seemed to become sane and she looked at me with a new expression, as if she really saw me for the first time'. Segal notes how frightened she was at the result of her interpretation in an environment more task- than patient-oriented. It is tempting to suggest that had this ward adopted an individual patient care approach her insights might have been transformed into nursing care plans, for example by arranging for a sympathetic clergyman to visit. The point this example illustrates is that in most areas of nursing work we may use our psychotherapeutic imagination to seek to empathize with, understand and put into words patients' feelings about themselves, their experiences and others. Once put into words and acknowledged, such feelings and thoughts may be rendered safe as the patient gains a different perspective from which to view them. There is more to nursing care and psychotherapy than imaginative empathy however, and the case study described in Boxes 41.1a and b outlines the nursing care of a patient undergoing psychotherapy in a therapeutic community.

Nurses as psychotherapists and counsellors

In some health authorities clinical nurse specialists are employed to provide psychotherapy or counselling sessions. It is usually expected that the nurse has undertaken a formal training in either of these disciplines. Brooking (1985) in her review of training facilities notes how few facilities there are for psychiatric nurses to train in these fields. Dopson (1984) reports a clinic in Wales where nurses practise as psychotherapists. Most nurses may, however, practise as counsellors. A review of

---

Box 41.1a Jane: a case history

Jane was a 15-year-old girl from a working class family in East London. She was admitted because of an escalating history of absence from school, one attempted overdose of Aspro, and two incidents in which she cut her wrists. Her father, towards whom she had a provocative and hostile attitude, was an inarticulate and distant man of 50 years. She had lived alone with him since her mother's death 2 years before. It was felt that working through her hostility towards her father, as the surviving parent, and coming to terms with her grief and anger about her mother's death would be the initial focus of therapy. Two psychotherapy sessions a week were provided as a means of tackling the grief, depression and despair underlying her behaviour. It was acknowledged that psychotherapeutic intervention would not only be painful but might provoke previous acting out behaviours. The nursing task during this early period was to provide a safe, sympathetic but firm environment in which she could express her feelings but not act on them. At the same time opportunities would be provided for her to engage in activities appropriate to her age. It was acknowledged that Jane might feel ambivalent towards her nurse and psychotherapist.

---

the wide range of theories and techniques associated with counselling is provided by Jones (1980) and Patterson (1980). Chalmers & Farrel (1985) describe a model of counselling suited to nursing worth outlining here. They argue that diagnostic clarity is essential prior to the selection of nursing intervention. Pointing out that the association between life-style behaviours and health outcomes is well substantiated, they acknowledge that less is known about which counselling techniques facilitate change. They offer three basic approaches based on a scheme of problem assessment and diagnosis.

1. Health education approach

This is most effective when the client has the ability and motivation to use the educational material provided. Here, accurate sources of information are given and the client himself is responsible for implementing change.

Box 41.1b Nursing care plan: Jane

Problem assessment	Aim of care	Nursing plan of action	Evaluation criteria
Grief re loss of mother & poor relationship with father = 1. Difficulty in sustaining rewarding relationship with others	Establish continuity, reliability of primary nurse rltshp as means of re-establishing rltshp with father	Meet once per shift to discuss day. Inform Jane re own timetable, be reliable. Be honest not evasive, be direct. Arrange regular meeting Jane/Dad. Arrange attendance parent/adolescent gp. Arrange weekends home. Say goodbye when go off-duty. Note next meeting time	Improved rltshp with father in terms of communications, visits home, expressed emotion
2. Hostility, distrust ambivalence towards carers	Provide opportunity for expression of disappointment/ ambivalence within acceptable parameters	Be accepting not judgemental re feelings. Respond firmly if feelings greater than situation warrants, understand but disagree. Point out provocative behaviour, don't be provoked. Set boundaries & expectations. Acknowledge sadness/despair. Meet regularly with staff team & discuss	Open expression of feeling. Reduction in hostile & provocative remarks
3. Despair, depression, withdrawal from peers/activities	Provide opportunity to engage in range of activities with peers & adults	Enrol at school & activity groups. Take on expeditions, shopping, cinema. Provide with opportunity to give. Acknowledge need to withdraw at times. Accept pain, but invite functioning	Decrease in level of withdrawal to normal parameters. Increased participation in social events
4. Potential risks: wrist slashing, overdose of drugs, leaving hospital without permission	Be aware of moments of risk and appropriate actions to take	Be sensitive to levels of distress/communicate with therapist. Share concern with Jane, explain expectations/plans re acting out. Involve other patients in support gp. Arrange patient rota. Ensure no knives, drugs available, Jane to stay in hosp. Arrange special nurse if essential. Keep father, care staff informed, involve as appropriate	Diminished or end to acting out behaviour

2. Behaviour modification approach

This is most effective when the client not only needs the information but lacks the ego strength to change his own behaviour without external help. Thus group or individual behaviour modification programmes are designed.

3. Exploration therapy approach

This is most effective when the problem is situated within the whole context of the patient's life and where multiple psychological and social factors in- fluence the client's behaviour. Here an exploration of the causes of behaviour, as they relate to the client's feelings and perceptions, is offered by a trained therapist.

Chalmers & Farrel conclude that 'while it is inappropriate to apply the more simplistic information-giving techniques to complex client problems, it is equally inappropriate to use in-depth exploratory assessments of clients when simpler, more effective strategies are available'. Glover (1982) provides an example of how similar assessment techniques help nurses undertaking psychosexual counselling.

CONCLUSION

In this chapter I have not attempted to provide a training guide in psychotherapy or counselling. Training in these areas is complex, experientially based and requires supervised clinical practice. Instead I have outlined the theory which underpins most psychotherapeutic work, and noted criticisms and reformulations of this theory. The types of psychotherapy available in Great Britain are described and criteria for treatment noted. I have not examined the wealth of therapies available in the United States. A discussion about the relevance of psychodynamic techniques and ideas to nursing was followed by a case study which illustrated the nursing care of a patient undergoing psychotherapy in a hospital setting. Most psychotherapy and counselling is offered on an outpatient basis, however. Examples of the way nurses have acted as psychotherapists and counsellors in this setting have been noted. Throughout the paper I have stressed the importance of distinguishing between therapeutic listening, counselling and psychotherapy, and the need for training and supervision in each.

REFERENCES

Andrews R 1982 The psychoanalytical mode in psychiatry. Nursing 3

Barton R 1959 Institutional neurosis. Wright, Bristol

Barnes E 1968 Psychosocial nursing. Tavistock Publications, London

Barnes M, Berke J 1982 Mary Barnes. Penguin, Harmondsworth

Birckhead L M 1984 The nurse as leader: group psychotherapy with psychotic patients. Journal of Psychosocial Nursing 22(6): 24–30

Bocock R 1980 Freud and modern society. Nelson, London

Brooking J 1985 Advanced psychiatric nursing education in Britain. Journal of Advanced Nursing 10

Brown D, Pedder J 1979 Introduction to psychotherapy. Tavistock Publications, London

Brown J A C 1964 Freud and the post-freudians. Pelican, Harmondsworth

Cawley R H 1977 The teaching of psychotherapy. Association of University Teachers of Psychiatry Newsletter Jan 77

Chalmers K, Farrel P 1985 Lifestyle counselling: the need for diagnostic clarity. Journal of Advanced Nursing 10

Chapman G E 1984 A therapeutic community, psychosocial nursing and the nursing process. International Journal of Therapeutic Communities 5(2)

Dopson L 1984 Psychotherapy in Powys: down your way. Nursing Times July 4

Eichenbaum L, Orbach S 1982 Outside in, inside out. Pelican, Harmondsworth

Erikson E 1 1974 Childhood and society. Penguin, Harmondsworth

Eysenck H J, Wilson G D 1973 The experimental study of Freudian theories. Methuen, London

Freud S 1895 Studies on hysteria, standard edn, vol 2 Breuer and Freud. Hogarth Press and Institute of Psychoanalysis, London

Freud S 1900 The interpretation of dreams, standard edn, vol 14. Hogarth Press and Institute of Psychoanalysis 1955, London

Freud S 1901 The psychopathology of everyday life. Pelican 1982, Harmondsworth

Freud S 1905 Three essays on the theory of sexuality, standard edn, vol 7. Hogarth Press and Institute of Psychoanalysis 1962, London

Freud S 1915 The unconscious; on metapsychology: the theory of psychoanalysis. Penguin 1984, Harmondsworth

Freud S 1916 The development of the libido and the sexual organizations: introductory lectures on psychoanalysis. Penguin 1975, Harmondsworth

Freud A 1936 The ego and mechanisms of defence. London & Hogarth Press, London

Glover J 1982 Psychosexual counselling. Nursing 35. Medical Education (International) Ltd

Green B 1983 Primary nursing in psychiatry. Nursing Times Jan

Jones M P 1980 The nursing process in psychiatry. Nursing Times 17 July

Jung C 1964 Man and his symbols. W H Allen, London

Kennard D, Roberts J 1983 An introduction to therapeutic communities. Routledge & Kegan Paul, London

Kennedy R 1986 The family of patients. Free Association Press, London

Kline P 1981 Fact and fantasy in Freudian theory. Methuen, London and New York

Kynaston T, Meade H, Jackman K 1981 The Henderson hospital: nursing in a therapeutic community. Nursing 30.

Loomis M E 1970 Group processes for nurses. C V Mosby Co, New York

Nelson Jones R 1982 The theory and practice of counselling psychotherapy. Holt Rinehart & Winston

Patterson C H 1980 Theories of counselling and psychotherapy. Harper & Row, New York

Ritter S 1988 In: Collister B (ed) Person to person. Edward Arnold, London

Schreiber F R 1985 Sybil. Penguin, Harmondsworth

Segal H 1975 Introduction to the work of Melanie Kline. Hogarth Press and The Institute of Psychoanalysis, London

Segal J 1985 Phantasy in everyday life. Penguin, Harmondsworth

Smith L 1980 A nursing history and data sheet. In:

Psychiatry under review. Nursing Times Publication. Macmillan, London, pp. 18–24

Stafford-Clarke D 1983 What Freud really said. Penguin, Harmondsworth

Strouse J 1974 Women and analysis: dialogues on psychoanalysis and feminity. Viking Press, London

Sulloway F J 1980 Freud: biologist of the mind. Fontana Paperbacks, London

Group techniques

M. T. Reed

The practice of group work is important for psychiatric nurses, most of whom are confronted in their working lives by a number of different types of groups. Many nurses are expected to lead or co-lead patient groups. It is vital, therefore, that nurses have a good understanding of theories of group work, as well as guidelines to begin their own group work. This work is challenging, exciting and a rich learning opportunity. To the novice, it is also daunting and, indeed, at times overwhelming. This chapter reviews types of groups, theories of groups, group leadership and gives guidelines for establishing a group. Examples are used to make the information interesting and it is intended that the material will be of practical use.

TYPES OF GROUPS

We all live and work as members of groups, as human beings are inherently social and group-oriented. We belong to and think of ourselves as members of a nation, culture, community, class and family as well as countless other groups, both formal and informal. In trying to classify the various groups that exist, it is useful to consider what a group is. Gordon (1985) defines a group as a collection of people who possess these qualities:

- a definable membership — three or more people

- group consciousness — members who think of themselves as a group and identify with each other
- a sense of shared purpose and common goals
- interaction — members communicate with each other, influence one another, react to each other's ideas and opinions
- interdependence in satisfaction of needs and the need to help each other to accomplish purposes for which they joined the group.

Several types of groups are encountered in psychiatric nursing. The next section identifies three important types of groups and defines their key characteristics. These definitions are discussed more fully by Marram (1978).

Group psychotherapy is a branch of psychiatry and psychotherapy. This type of group is used with patients in psychiatric treatment and is aimed at helping patients to resolve some of their problems in relating to others and to take on more successful patterns of adapting. The emphasis of each group may differ according to the skill and interest of the group therapist and the composition of the group. Psychiatric nurses are involved in different ways in this type of group work.

Therapeutic groups have their emphasis on treating basically healthy individuals who may be in some form of crisis. These groups are concerned with preventing psychological deterioration. They may include groups with medical/surgical patients, AIDs sufferers, the elderly, children, preoperative patients and people experiencing a similar emotional or physical problem. Psychiatric nurses as well as general nurses are involved in such groups.

Self-help groups are, for the most part, organized and operated by the members themselves, without the supervision or leadership of professionally trained group leaders. They aim to solve problems as defined by members, and do not intend to focus on members' insight or on personality reconstruction. Chiefly their focus is on the repression of impulses. Alcoholics Anonymous, one of the best known self-help groups, attempts to stop members from drinking. Although the benefits of these groups are varied, the members get support, empathic understanding and the impetus to change. Nurses should be aware of existing self-help groups, should try to attend a meeting to gain insight into these groups and should not underestimate the value of such groups for clients.

There exist two formats for groups, generally termed 'open' and 'closed'. An open group means that as one group member leaves, another is added; in a closed group, membership remains the same. The duration of sessions also varies in groups. Some groups, such as Alcoholics Anonymous and some therapy groups, continue indefinitely, while others may have a fixed number of sessions.

THEORY OF GROUP WORK
Overview

All major theories of psychotherapy can be applied to group work. This is logical, as the practice of group work focuses on individuals in group settings, as well as on the properties of a group. The nurse will undoubtedly be influenced by the setting in which the group is taking place. If the prevailing theory is psychoanalytic, for example, then those ideas will be used to explain group phenomena. This chapter will not review these theories, as they are covered elsewhere in this text, but will focus on the theory of group psychotherapy as defined by Yalom (1975).

Yalom outlines what he calls the 'curative factors' of group therapy and these are listed below:

1. Installation of hope. Hope is required to keep the patient in the group, and faith in the treatment can be effective in itself. It is hopeful for members to see the improvement of older members.

2. Universality. It is a great relief for people to realize that they are not alone in their fear, misery and pain.

3. Imparting of information. Some groups, such as those in antenatal clinics, are primarily intended for this purpose. Even when education is not explicit, such as in psychotherapy groups, the members learn a great deal about group dynamics, the meaning of symptoms and psychic functioning.

4. Altruism. Psychiatric patients beginning therapy are demoralized and have a deep sense of having nothing to give. It is refreshing and boosts their self-esteem to find that they can be of help to others. They offer support, reassurance, suggestions, insight and share problems with each other.

5. Corrective recapitulation of the primary family group. The group resembles the family and the therapists the parents. Early familial contacts are recapitulated and can be relived correctively. This is working through business of long ago and understanding the past.

6. Development of socializing techniques. Members learn about their maladaptive social behaviour with honest feedback from other members.

7. Imitative behaviour. Members benefit from observing the therapy of other members with similar problems.

8. Interpersonal learning. Members learn about the impression they make on each other: how others see them. They re-create in the group their relationships with others in the outside world and have the chance to examine and change these relationships.

9. Group cohesiveness. This provides a sense of belonging and understanding for members.

10. Catharsis. A chance to express troublesome and affect-laden material is provided.

11. Existential factors. In the group, members face the basic issues of life and death. They learn to take ultimate responsibility for their own lives.

Yalom (1975) explains that the major difference between a therapy group, which is hoping to bring about behavioural and characterological changes, and other groups is that the therapy group takes place in the 'here-and-now'. The immediate events in the meeting are the focus and these will facilitate feedback, catharsis and self-disclosure. The leader first has to steer the group to the 'here-and-now' and then comment on the 'process'.

This idea of process is crucial for the beginner to understand. In all human interactions there are two major ingredients: content and process. The first deals with the subject matter or the task upon which the group is working; in most interactions, the focus of attention of all persons is on the content. Group process deals with such items as morale, feeling, tone and conflict. It deals with the 'how' and the 'why' of what is said, as they illuminate some aspects of the patient's relationship to others with whom he is interacting (Box 42.1).

Learning to tune into and comment on process is not easy. In many ways the nurse needs to be listening at different levels, and always listening carefully to content as well. It is a skill which, like others, must be developed and practised. If there is a golden rule of group work, however, that rule is, 'Attend to Process!'

Box 42.1 An example of process analysis in a group

In a group session for carers of terminally ill patients, David expressed quite movingly his feelings of guilt about putting his wife into long-term care. John, who appeared to be a self-righteous 'know-it-all' who had some years before put his wife into care, responded quickly, 'Well you don't have any choice if you're going to save yourself. You can't feel guilty or you won't be any good to anyone.' This statement broke the sense of sadness and cohesiveness the group had been sharing together and others began speaking about long-term facilities available. Some examples of process to be considered are:

1. Why was John so uncomfortable with the issue of guilt? Is he still overwhelmed with guilt after all these years and has he adopted this self-righteous stance as a defence?
2. How does John's response make David feel? He has exposed a very vulnerable side of himself and has been told he 'can't' feel that way.
3. What is the response of the rest of the group? Is this topic too 'hot' to handle? Are they angry at John for silencing David? Do they need more time to stay with this issue? Can they comfort each other by sharing the pain, at the same time realizing there is no way to take it away, or are they still at the stage where they feel obliged to try and provide answers?

All these thoughts, and others, will be in the nurse's mind as the group is in session. The response of the nurse depends on the nurse's skill, stage of the group, goals of the group, needs of the group and timing.

Stages of development

Groups are never static; they change and develop in a somewhat predictable way. Much has been written about the different stages a group passes through, and these stages, condensed from different authors, will be discussed below. In each stage different themes, issues and behaviours will be prominent and will call for different roles on the part of the leader, so it is important that the nurse is aware of the stage the group is in.

Stage I. Pre-affiliation or orientation stage

Anxiety is high here, both on the part of the group members and the leader. Members tend to be hesitant — they want to avoid conflict. The leader must allow this slow process; the task of the leader is to create an atmosphere of interpersonal safety. Members will speak mostly to the leader rather than to each other. It is in this stage that the group norms are being set. The leader must support members, review the contract and help establish norms by role-modelling.

Stage II. Conflict or power and control stage

Anxiety is again high. Themes are power, position and authority. This stage can be very difficult for novice group leaders. The leader should remember that to have reached this stage is a good sign that the group is developing! She needs to permit the rebellion, protect and support the threatened members and clarify the power struggle.

Stage III. Cohesion

Anxiety decreases here somewhat and this is an enjoyable stage both for the leader and the members. It is the goal of the group to reach this stage. There is free expression, shared concerns, intimacy, fewer problems. The leader has less to do here, as the group is 'running itself'.

Stage IV. Termination or separation

Anxiety increases again and themes are loss, grief and separation. There may be denial, regression and re-enacting of Stage I. The leader needs to give feedback, encourage feelings and help the members to evaluate the group. What impact did it have on them? Were goals met? Why not?

LEADERSHIP

Leadership is a personal, interactional process. It is basic to effective group experience and is probably the aspect of group work the novice finds most daunting. 'What kind of leader am I? What will I need to do in the group? Who will help me?' This section will examine these and other questions about leadership.

Types of leaders

It is a good idea for group leaders to examine their own style of leadership already developed from other settings and experiences. Lewin et al (1939) first defined leadership styles as authoritarian, laissez-faire and democratic.

An authoritarian leader determines all policies and dictates techniques, activities and tasks. This leader may give orders to each member and uses the pronoun 'I'. Members react with hostility and aggression, are dependent on the leader and they may drop out.

A democratic leader encourages and assists the group to make policies and decisions, the division of tasks is left for the group to decide and 'we' is used much more frequently than 'I'. Members react with openness and high interest, and group cohesiveness is apparent.

A laissez-faire leader participates minimally, takes no part in group discussions and does not attempt to appraise or regulate the course of events. Members react with less interest, less satisfaction and feel less stimulated.

In preparing to be group leaders nurses should not only understand their own styles of leadership, but also examine their expectations of themselves and their groups. In the early days it is important to have realistic expectations. Group work and leadership are learning opportunities, and with every experience, both successful and unsuccessful, more will be learned about the group process and about oneself.

Supervision of group leaders

To facilitate the learning process, the use of supervision cannot be overstated. Although the nurse may be 'leading' or 'conducting' or 'facilitating' the group, she is also part of it and it is vital, therefore, to arrange to share with someone the progress of the group. Both Yalom (1975) and Marram (1978) stress the importance of supervision in the case of co-leadership, to enable the co-leaders to assess their relationship and examine the impact it is having on the group. Whether leading or co-leading, supervision is essential and should be built into the time allotted for the group. Supervisors should be chosen with care, as they must be expert in the theory and practice of group work, entirely trustworthy (in order that the nurse can share it *all*) and willing to give honest feedback.

Nurses new to group work will wonder whether they can ever develop the skills necessary to lead groups effectively. Different individuals find particular skills more or less difficult to master and learning will be a life-long process. Practice and the support of good supervision will bring confidence and the pleasure of increased knowledge and understanding.

Leadership functions

The leadership functions outlined by Marram (1978) are general and apply to all groups, regardless of composition.

Firstly, the leader facilitates the benefits of group membership; she starts a process whereby members meet their needs for security, belonging and companionship. The leader can increase the interdependence of members on one another, for example by saying, 'Mary, you've said a lot about your experiences with the district nurse. I wonder what Martin thinks, as he's in a very similar situation'.

Secondly, the leader must maintain a viable group atmosphere. Members must feel safe to talk about what concerns them. In a group of chronic schizophrenic clients, the leader may have to set behavioural limits, i.e. she may need to ask a client who is verbally abusive to leave the session so that the group feels secure.

Thirdly, the leader must oversee group growth. Most groups have goals and the leader may have to redirect the group to the goals. If, for example, the group has been set up for eight sessions to talk about emotional issues involved in caring for chronically ill relatives, the leader may need to interrupt an interesting discussion of different types of illnesses if that is preventing the group from growing and moving towards its goals.

Fourthly, the group leader regulates individual members' growth. At any one stage, the leader may be more focused on one or other individual as the individual members of the group must always be considered, as well as the group itself.

Leadership skills

As stated earlier, the leader must constantly attend to the process of the group. The leader must also observe many aspects of verbal and non-verbal participation of group members. Questions to be answered include:

- Who is a high participator?
- Who is low?
- How are silent people treated?
- Who talks to whom?
- Who keeps the ball rolling?
- Who cuts off others or interrupts?
- Are members listening?
- Who seems to prefer a friendly environment?
- What signs of feelings do you see?
- Do you see any attempt to block expression of certain feelings?
- Are certain areas avoided?
- What is the atmosphere in the group?
- How do you feel?

In addition to making the above observations, Gordon (1986) suggests that the leader needs to keep her eyes moving, be aware of the focus of the group and how it shifts, be able to generate energy, draw members out, cut members off and model to the group self-disclosure and deep listening.

ESTABLISHING A GROUP

This section will give guidelines that the nurse may find useful in establishing a group. There is a great deal of work to be done long before the first group session. The successful completion of pre-group work by the nurse determines, to a large degree, the success or failure of the group. The following outline comes largely from Marram (1978).

Identifying the purpose and objectives of the group

The aims of the group will be determined by the theoretical background and philosophy of the nurse, the nurse's skill and, if the group is set within an institution, that institution's philosophy. The characteristics and needs of the client population also affect the group's purpose.

Marram identifies the following as general aims of any group:

- to enable members to gain greater knowledge of their behaviour and relationships with others
- to provide reassurance and support
- to decrease members' sense of loneliness and isolation and thereby modify feelings of powerlessness and hopelessness
- to facilitate the opportunity for members to try out new communication patterns
- to provide a safe environment where members can share concerns and learn from the experience of others.

There may be other, more specific goals. For a group of newly discharged psychiatric patients, for example, the goals may include sharing of feelings and experiences about leaving the hospital and providing ongoing contact with the hospital. It is extremely important that the nurse is clear about the goals, and writing them down may prove a useful exercise.

Selecting members

The most obvious difference between group members is whether they choose to attend the group or if they are required to go. Often psychiatric nurses in hospitals are working with 'captive' groups, so that selection is not an issue. If this is not the case, then the nurse will meet with prospective group members individually and assess them. During this assessment, the nurse will discuss the goals of the group and ask the client about his own expectations and goals. The nurse will take note of the client's mood, thinking patterns (are there delusions, hallucinations, ideas of reference?), self-esteem and ego strength. The client's communication patterns should be assessed as well as his ability to tolerate feedback. The client should be asked about previous group experiences; were they positive? In this selection process the nurse is striving for some degree of homogeneity and also bearing in mind factors such as age, sex, socio-economic background and degree of physical or mental handicap. Heterogeneity cannot be and should not be avoided completely, as differences in clients' life experiences can be useful learning. Members need to locate a basis of similarity, however, and a member who is strikingly 'different' from the others may not be able to benefit from the group.

Making agreement

In order for the client to be committed to involvement in the group, the client must understand the purpose of the group, how the purpose is to be achieved, what is expected of him and what can be expected from the leader. The goals of the group can be listed.

For the client to understand what is expected, the agreement with him should include the number of sessions, time of each session and provision for what to do if the client is unable to attend. At this pre-group stage, the client's sense of trust in the leader is vital. Yalom (1975) stresses the importance of leaders believing in their own efficacy and in the group. This may not be easy for the first-time group leader, but is important to remember.

The goals will be discussed in the pre-group interview and need to be reviewed in at least the first session and thereafter according to how the group unfolds. As already discussed, it is part of the leader's task to keep the group working towards its goals.

Structuring the group

The size of the group needs to be decided. There should be at least five members, and eight is often considered ideal. The leader may want to consider whether there are likely to be frequent absences and plan accordingly. Leaders should also consider their own anxieties and decide what number of members they are most comfortable with. The setting of the group should be comfortable, private, free from interruption and lend itself to intimacy without causing claustrophobia. Chairs are usually arranged in a circle and the leader will consider the smoking/non-smoking issue. The time of the sessions can be 45–90 minutes and should be strictly adhered to in order to foster trust in the leader. Meetings need to start and finish on time, even if (as is sometimes the case) a client says something especially crucial when there is one minute left in the session. The leader will have already decided whether the group is open or closed.

The first meeting of the group

It is worth discussing briefly the first session as it is inevitably the one that terrifies novices. It is most important to acknowledge one's own anxiety and be aware that the clients' anxiety will also be very high. The room should be prepared and the chairs ready for the group. If a structured exercise is planned it should be ready, with all the materials needed to do it.

The leader should:

- Review mentally the tasks for the first meeting. These probably include reviewing the agreement and covering ground rules.
- Be prepared for what many novices find excruciating — silence
- Remember that the group is establishing norms in the early stage and the leader is most important in setting the scene for future groups.
- Review mentally the worst thing that can happen and be ready for it.
- Keep a sense of humour and use humour to help diffuse tension.
- Take heart from Yalom who assures us that the first group is inevitably a success!

AN EXAMPLE OF PRACTICE

Professor Verona Gordon (1986) has carried out several studies in the USA and Britain, to evaluate the effectiveness of a nurse-facilitated group intervention to reduce depression in women. A discussion of the group work involved in her research will help to illuminate some of the points made in the previous sections.

The group sessions which Gordon and her colleague Canedy have devised are designed to help women gain increased self-esteem through learning to cope appropriately with daily stress and crisis. Another intention is to provide data to document that nurses can lead these groups effectively. To furnish reliable data, research studies are essential. In a study conducted by Gordon (1986) in London, women who met screening criteria were randomly assigned to the experimental (treatment n = 10) or control (no treatment n = 10) condition. The treatment consisted of 14 weekly (2 hour) group sessions, led by two experienced psychiatric nurses with group experience, one of whom was the author of this chapter.

The theoretical underpinnings for the group work were carefully outlined. Nursing theory provided concepts of assessment, intervention and evaluation. Concepts from cognitive-behavioural theory explained why women were depressed and feeling helpless, and offered guidelines to treatment. Concepts from the work of Yalom were applied to explain the role and function of the group facilitators.

This group experience was a closed group of 14 sessions. The goals of the group experience were carefully discussed with each potential group member before beginning the group meetings. The overall goals, which were to provide a supportive place to talk about feelings, to help women learn from each other and to give support for any changes made, were carefully outlined again in the first group meeting. Each woman also wrote down her own personal, individualized goals during the first session, and goal attainment was discussed each week.

The women had been carefully selected. To be eligible they had to be 40 to 60 years of age, they had to speak English and they were not to be seeing a counsellor or psychiatrist at the time. The group members had been tested to ensure that they were not psychotic, psychopathic or suicidal and all were moderately depressed.

This was a highly structured group programme. The first hour each week consisted of a support group session and the second hour of didactic presentations of different topics such as assertion, nutrition, relaxation, feelings and stress. The first meeting was carefully planned by the facilitators, so that the chairs were in place and the room was welcoming. Ground rules about confidentiality, sub-grouping and smoking were reviewed, as well as instructions about what to do if a member could not attend. Opportunity for questions about concerns was provided.

The nurse facilitators were supported and supervised by Dr Gordon, and early group sessions were audio-taped to aid in supervision. The facilitators spent time after each meeting discussing the group process and dynamics observed. The intervention strategy for the next session was planned and the facilitators examined their own relationship and how that was affecting the group. The facilitators kept notes of each session. The date, number of members present and reactions to lateness or absence of peers were recorded. Individual behaviour was described, as well as indications of group stages, themes and cohesiveness.

The unfolding of the stages of the group was a fascinating experience for the facilitators to observe. The group moved from initial stages of mistrust and hostility to a cohesiveness which allowed sharing and support. One member was able, with the group's support, to make major changes in her life, and all of the women, in evaluating the group, described it as insightful and supportive. The sadness at the last session and tearful hugs demonstrated how meaningful the experience had been.

The findings of this study and others done by Gordon and Canedy have been convincing. The women attending the group sessions were found to be less depressed and have higher self-esteem than women in the no-treatment control condition. These results, as well as the personal testimony of the women, support the idea that psychiatric nurses can be very effective in group work.

CONCLUSION

This chapter has provided an overview of the theory of group work and given guidelines for establishing a group. The problems and processes which become apparent after the group is established will be, to a degree, unique to that group. Yalom (1975) reviews 'problem patients' and discusses common problems, and the beginner may find that useful. It is in the supervision setting that the leader's problems, anxieties and learning unfold. It is hoped that this chapter has given a concise review of relevant theory and has conveyed the sense of challenge and fun that group work can have.

REFERENCES

Foukes S H 1964 Therapeutic group analysis. Allen and Unwin, London — An authoritative statement on group analysis by the originator of the Institute of Group Analysis, London.

Gazda G M 1972 Group counselling, a developmental approach. Allyn and Bacon, Boston — Outlines an approach for persons who have early signs of inappropriate coping behaviours.

Glasser W 1965 Reality therapy. Harper & Row, New York — By the originator of reality therapy.

Gordon V C 1985 Group facilitators' manual — Unpublished manuscript available from the author to nurses intending to use Gordon's structured group approach.

Gordon V C 1986 Treatment of depressed woman by nurses in Britain and the USA. In: Brooking J I (ed) 1986 Psychiatric nursing research. Wiley, Chichester — Describes Gordon's evaluative research in Britain and the USA.

Lewin, Lippit, White 1939 Cited in Secord P F, Backman C W 1964 Social psychology. McGraw-Hill, New York

Marram G 1978 The group approach in nursing practice, 2nd edn. C V Mosby, St Louis

Ohlsen M M 1970 Group counselling. Holt, Rinehart & Winston, New York — Problem solving for those who do not have serious emotional problems.

Rogers C 1971 Carl Rogers describes his way of facilitating encounter groups. American Journal of Nursing (71): 275–279 — Describes Rogers' way of working with groups. Appropriate, therapeutic use of self and self-disclosure discussed.

Yalom I D 1975 The theory and practice of group psychotherapy, 2nd edn. Basic Books, New York — Essential reading on the basic principles of group work.

43

Behavioural psychotherapy

K. Gournay

THE NATURE OF BEHAVIOURAL PSYCHOTHERAPY

The development of behavioural approaches has two distinct origins. Firstly, the classical conditioning theories developed by Pavlov and other experimental psychologists arguably formed the original basis of the so-called deconditioning treatments of anxiety, obsessions and sexual problems. Secondly, the operant theories formulated by Skinner and others underpin the behavioural approaches to the maladaptive behaviour of chronic schizophrenic patients, the mentally handicapped and others. These operant approaches are exemplified by token economics and other techniques based on reinforcement. In order to provide a detailed account of method, this chapter focuses on the former group of approaches to neurotic and personality problems. The terms behaviour therapy and behavioural psychotherapy are used interchangeably in this chapter.

Having stated that behaviour therapy for neurotic disorder was originally based on principles of classical conditioning, it should be noted that there are many problems associated with the explanation of behaviour therapy (as practised today) in terms of psychological theories of learning. Marks (1981) asserted that psychologists have transformed these theories into 'Idols of Origin'. Marks further argues that learning theories are inadequate to explain neurotic disorders and their treatment. A review of the competing theories in this area is beyond the scope of this chapter, but, in summary, many behaviour therapists now draw from non-psychological sources such as pharmacology, physiology, general medicine and anthropology for explanations of both problems and treatment. Behaviour therapy has increasingly become an empirical approach used by many non-psychologists, including nurses, with great effectiveness.

Behavioural psychotherapy departs from the psychodynamic psychotherapies in several important ways. Firstly, the approach focuses only on observable behaviour. Most behaviour therapists would now extend the concept of 'behaviour' to include speech and thoughts, in so far as the client may be able to give a self-report of thoughts and thought patterns. Secondly, behavioural psychotherapy does not assume the presence of dynamic processes or unconscious motives. Behaviour therapists of course accept that unconscious thought processes do occur (as the early experiments with dichotic listening demonstrate) (Moray 1969). However, they would argue that these processes are not amenable to reliable observation and therefore the role of unconscious processes in psychological problems is largely a matter of speculation. Finally, behavioural psychotherapy takes into account the influence of biological, genetic and other variables. Behaviour therapists assert that any theories of causation need to be validated by a scientific method of enquiry, that is, one characterized by the components of observation, hypothesis formation and testing and the use of multiple objective evaluations. An exact clarification of cause is not necessary for effective treatment to take place. This is shown by the existence of many highly successful treatments, not only in behaviour therapy but also in general medicine, of conditions with unclear aetiology. Diabetes and some forms of cancer would be obvious examples where treatment provides cure or dramatic symptom relief without causal mechanisms being fully understood.

NURSES AS BEHAVIOUR THERAPISTS

The training of Registered Mental Nurses in behavioural psychotherapy has arguably been the most important advance in psychiatric nursing since the formation of community psychiatric nursing services. Factors which led to this advanced clinical role for nurses were described by Bird et al (1979) as pressures:

- on demand for services
- for more democracy within psychiatry
- to economize
- to expand community psychiatric services
- from nurses dissatisfied with professional limits, and
- to follow (within nursing) the wider trend of confirming therapist status.

There are a number of centres in England and Scotland offering training courses. There are now well over 150 nurses who have completed the intensive training of 18 months and who hold the clinical certificate. Marks et al (1977) described the training as being as much in general clinical management skills as in behavioural psychotherapy. The nurse therapy training is based on an apprenticeship model with emphasis on gradually enabling the nurse therapist to become an independent, expert practitioner.

Bird et al (1979) summarize the general principles of behavioural psychotherapy which are acquired by nurse therapists during training as:

- detailed behavioural analysis
- explicit negotiation and planning
- plentiful real life practice
- multiple concrete evaluations, and
- flexibility based on those evaluations.

The general skills acquired by nurse therapists are:

- interviewing
- problem-oriented record-keeping and correspondence
- case-load planning
- the understanding and application of ethical issues

- liaison, and
- recognition of limits of competence.

Training methods include:

- demonstrations, both live and via videotape
- role rehearsal of interviews and treatment procedures
- closed circuit television monitoring
- feedback and prompting by ear receiver.

These methods are augmented by lectures, seminars and reading lists, with a gradual phasing out of supervision to the 12th month of training. At this point trainees are, in some centres, seconded for a period of practice with minimal supervision before qualifying as certified nurse therapists. The syllabus also ensures that nurse therapist trainees gain considerable experience working with families, with patients in their home environment and within inpatient settings.

Bird et al (1979) discussed the various controversies which attended the development of nurse behaviour therapy in a paper which still holds as an excellent summary of the issues. The major criticisms of nurse therapists are that they are ill equipped by training and intellect for the role and that an extensive knowledge of learning theory is necessary to carry out behavioural psychotherapy. These arguments can be countered by several points.

Firstly, there is little indication that psychological problems or behavioural treatments can be satisfactorily or comprehensively explained by psychological theories. Marks (1981) cites extensive evidence in support of his criticisms of psychological explanations of neurotic behaviour.

Secondly, research evidence clearly shows that nurse therapists are at least as successful as clinical psychologists or psychiatrists with neurotic patients (Marks 1985). Nurse therapy training, with its emphasis on the acquisition of specific skills, seems far more relevant to developing clinical ability than other more academic courses. Nurses gain a wide experience of dealing with psychological problems during student nurse training and this can obviously be a most advantageous precursor to nurse therapy training.

Criticisms that nurse therapists may not be acceptable to the general public have proved groundless, with two studies (Marks et al 1977, Marks 1985) specifically examining this question and demonstrating high levels of consumer satisfaction with nurse therapists. Other criticisms of nurse therapists are that they function as an elite and that the case manager role is contrary to the model of multi-disciplinary care. In practice, nurse therapists function as experts within either primary care or psychiatric teams and, as a recent survey (Lindley & Marks 1985) showed, they seem to work well within a wide variety of settings.

There is now clear evidence that nurse therapists are cost-effective providers of treatment for neurotic patients (Ginsberg et al 1985). Additionally, the most encouraging result of recent research is that nurse therapists work very effectively in primary care settings (Lindley & Marks 1985). Marks (1985) has suggested that an efficient attachment for one nurse therapist would involve working with about 12 general practitioners serving a catchment area of 30 000 people. Marks has therefore stated that 1 800 nurse therapists might meet most needs of primary care patients in the United Kingdom for behavioural psychotherapy.

In summary, this role has provided a most welcome addition to the range of work of the psychiatric nurse, while complementing rather than competing with other professional groups in psychiatry.

INDICATIONS FOR BEHAVIOURAL PSYCHOTHERAPY

There are several problems for which behavioural psychotherapy is the treatment of choice. These categories are covered in the training of nurse therapists and are as follows:

- Agoraphobia
- Specific phobias
- Social phobias and social skills problems
- Sexual dysfunctions
- Sexual deviations
- Obsessive compulsive disorder.

As well as these major diagnostic groups, behavioural treatments are helpful in the management of tics, enuresis and a range of problems subsumed under the heading 'habit disorders'. These also include problems of self-control such as shoplifting and some types of alcohol abuse.

COGNITIVE-BEHAVIOUR THERAPY

Over the past few years behavioural techniques have been extended to disorders such as general anxiety and depressive states. This trend has also been accompanied by an increasing use of so-called cognitive strategies. This has meant the extension of behavioural principles to the area of thinking or cognition. In many circles behaviour therapy is now synonymous with cognitive-behaviour therapy and many cognitive therapists explicitly ally themselves to behaviour therapy by joining the same professional organizations, e.g. the British Association of Behavioural Psychotherapy. This extension of behaviour therapy is welcome in principle; however, it is not entirely supported by experimental evidence. While there is enormous evidence supporting the efficacy of behavioural treatments for many neurotic disorders (e.g. agoraphobia, obsessive rituals), similar evidence is lacking with the cognitive approaches to general anxiety and depression. Treatment of these problems is notoriously difficult to evaluate because depressions and anxiety states remit for many reasons apart from therapeutic endeavour. Thus the current optimism and enthusiasm for the expansion of the scope of behaviour therapy may be premature in relation to general anxiety and depression. The danger is that possibly ineffective treatments are potentially damaging to the credibility of other more effective behavioural approaches.

BEHAVIOURAL MEDICINE

There are several other areas where behavioural methods have been extended with more promise. In these cases there are data to support either superiority to other methods, or their efficacy as adjunctive procedures. In particular, the area known as behavioural medicine has expanded from the early days of treatments for obesity and smoking to many diverse problems. Examples are treatment of essential hypertension, helping to prepare children for surgery, assisting cancer patients to tolerate the nausea of chemotherapy and helping to manage spastic colon. Other areas of promise involve helping people with prolonged or morbid bereavement reactions (Ramsey 1979) and the management of post-traumatic stress disorder in victims of war and urban violence (Keane & Kaloupek 1982).

MEASUREMENT AND EVALUATION

There are a number of problems in attempting to evaluate psychotherapy: these include, for example, how to ensure that the therapist is unbiased; how to ensure that any improvement is directly attributable to treatment; and what criteria to use to define improvement. Rachman & Wilson (1980) have reviewed these and related issues. They argue convincingly that psychoanalytic therapists consistently overestimate the benefits of their therapy, that many problems improve for reasons completely unconnected with 'treatment' and that the improvement criteria used by psychoanalytic therapists are often vague or ill-defined.

Evaluation must always be a comprehensive procedure. It measures not only the presenting problem, but also the effect of the problem on the client's functioning. Furthermore, it is wise to apply several measures to each area in order to ensure that as many perspectives as possible are gained. Each measure must be both valid and reliable in that it should measure the same thing in different people; should measure what it says it measures; and should be able to be used accurately at different times in different situations.

Thus a problem such as agoraphobia can be measured in several ways.

- Firstly, by direct observation of the avoidance behaviour and physiological anxiety of an agoraphobic client could be observed in a busy shop.
- Secondly, the client may rate problems in terms of severity using a simple scale (for an example see Ch. 31).
- Thirdly, the client may rate the problem in terms of its effect on areas of function.

- Fourthly, other aspects of the problem, such as general anxiety and depression, may be measured by the use of established rating scales.

The therapists commonly use a battery of measures, which may involve someone 'blind' to the problem to act as an independent assessor. (This is often used as an extra safeguard in clinical research.) In summary, the battery of measures should include:

- those specific to the problem
- those which measure secondary difficulties or symptoms
- those which measure general life adjustment and social, familial and marital function.

Evaluation in therapy is essential for several reasons. Measurement of the problem and its effects is integral to assessment. The repetition of the various measures during treatment, at the end of treatment and at follow-up intervals gives objective evaluation. Evaluation of groups of patients will aid managers to justify expenditure on various services and prove, for example, the value of a community nurse working in particular settings. Using such evaluations in research leads to the evolution of new treatments and may lead to a greater theoretical understanding. This particular aspect of evaluation is clearly beyond the scope of this book, but an excellent and comprehensive text is provided by Barlow et al (1984).

SOME BEHAVIOURAL TECHNIQUES

A full description of all behavioural techniques is beyond the scope of this chapter. For a clear description of the range of procedures used by nurse therapists the reader is referred to Marks et al (1977).

What follows are descriptions of three techniques. It is hoped that this material together with the account in Chapter 31 will give a flavour of behavioural psychotherapy. It should be emphasized that the use of a behavioural technique in isolation does not constitute a behavioural programme. Behavioural techniques should only be used after a comprehensive assessment, including a systematic analysis of the problem and its context, followed by a definition of treatment targets (goals) and the use of a rigorous evaluative system. It is quite common to see patients who have allegedly had previous behaviour therapy which has apparently been unsuccessful. Closer enquiry often reveals that a behavioural technique, for example relaxation training, has been used out of context, applied haphazardly and naturally has proved ineffective.

Social skills training

This procedure has been increasingly used over the years to help patients who either lack social skills or who are phobic of social situations. Commonly patients present with a mixture of both of these difficulties. Training is most effectively carried out in groups, and many centres use a training package of 10 to 12 weekly sessions of 2 hours each. Ideally the group should consist of 8 to 10 patients of similar age and background, with equal numbers of males and females. One therapist would take overall responsibility for running the group with two or three co-therapists. These co-therapists may include volunteers or former social skills group trainees.

Before the group begins each patient is individually assessed. (Detail of some assessment procedures can be found in Chapter 31.) This will not only involve taking a detailed history and account of the presenting problem, but therapist and patient will also negotiate a list of several behavioural treatment targets. Examples of such targets may be 'to attend social functions at least twice a week', 'to initiate conversation with at least three people each day', 'to converse with an attractive member of the opposite sex and maintain appropriate eye contact'. The therapist will, at this assessment, obtain various measures of anxiety and depression and will also make objective evaluations of current social skills function, using real life behaviour tests. For example, the therapist may use a colleague to act as a stooge, and ask the patient to engage the stooge in conversation. Ideally the role play should be video-taped so that the exercise can be repeated after treatment and a comparison made.

Date	Time	Assignment	Anxiety rating 0 – 8 0 = no anxiety 8 = worst anxiety	Percentage success

Figure 43.1 Diary form used for social skills training homework.

Each group session begins with a review of the previous week's homework which will be recorded on specially designed cards or sheets (see Fig. 43.1). Session work uses situations arising from the patients' homework problems or standard situations (e.g. dating behaviour, receiving criticism, job interviews). Group members are asked to act in a role play based on these situations and ideally this is video-taped. The video-tape is watched by the group, and then the role players, the group and the therapists give feedback. This consists of looking firstly at what was done well and then looking at behavioural deficits. The group members suggest alternatives to these deficits, the emphasis being on constructive criticism. Feedback is based only on observable behaviour, i.e. verbal behaviour such as voice tone and verbal content, and non-verbal behaviours such as posture, eye contact or gestures. The therapist's role in feedback is to guide a brief discussion aimed towards formulating optimum behaviour. Then other group members or therapists repeat the role play, thus 'modelling' appropriate behavioural responses for the original role player. The client is asked to repeat the role play and may be coached or prompted accordingly until performance is satisfactory. Thus, over a number of sessions all members are involved in

similar exercises in rotation. Eventually a spectrum of social behaviours is acquired and trainees become more proficient.

The sessions are often augmented by specific assignments in real life which may be assisted by the presence of a therapist who prompts and encourages. For example, a group member may be asked to go into a pub in order to engage someone in conversation. The group member will also attend to other secondary behaviour which may have been problematic. For example, he may need to make sure that eye contact is maintained and that speed of speech is reduced from its previously high 'nervous' rate. The therapist will keep at a discrete distance and provide instant feedback and encouragement.

Each group meeting usually ends with homework assignments (based on the content of the session) to be carried out before the next meeting.

Social skills training may also be carried out on an individual basis, and for some individuals such programmes may complement other behavioural strategies.

Although this treatment is very popular and used with a wide spectrum of problems, its results are limited. In a review by Marks (1981) it seems clear that socially phobic patients with reasonably circumscribed problems do best, perhaps achieving a 50% reduction in anxiety and avoidance. Schizophrenic patients may show early response to social skills training, but follow-up after treatment is very disappointing (Marks 1981). It is doubtful whether skills training is the main therapeutic ingredient, but rather it facilitates adequate exposure and practice. For a detailed examination of this method in psychiatric nursing, the reader is referred to Hargie & McCartan (1986). For a more theoretical perspective Trower (1984) is recommended.

Stimulus control procedures

Very simply, these approaches involve modifying or developing behaviour by changing the events which prompt behaviour (stimuli) or which are consequent to or reinforcing of a behaviour.

One example of such procedures is currently used in the management of insomnia. This approach has been shown to be the most enduringly effective of all non-drug treatments for insomnia. The method is probably twice as effective as relaxation training (Borkovec 1982). In view of the addiction potential of benzodiazepine tranquillizers, stimulus control programmes will probably become more widely used.

After detailed assessment of the problem the client is asked to use five simple principles, which are tailored to individual circumstances. These are:

1. To retire to bed *only* when sleepy
2. To rise from bed at the same time each morning *regardless* of amount of sleep
3. Absolutely *no* naps during the day
4. To ensure that nothing else other than sleeping is done in the bedroom (e.g. reading, eating, watching television). One exception is engaging in sexual activity!
5. If awake during the night, to get up and engage in dull, not stimulating activity, e.g. jigsaw puzzles, needlework and only return to bed when sleepy.

The patient is instructed to adhere to this programme indefinitely, although great improvement is very often reported within 3–6 weeks. Thereafter the patient should be counselled regarding a maintenance programme, perhaps paying less attention to some of the principles in the long term. Stimulus control procedures for sleeping problems can be used in a wide range of settings and can be adapted successfully to different patient groups. It is easy to see how much programmes might be used within inpatient settings, but unfortunately sleeping pills continue to be widely prescribed.

Self-monitoring

This simple procedure is very useful in several respects.

Assessment

Many problems are difficult for patients to describe. Asking the patient to give an account of the frequency of the problem and its magnitude is a complex request. Considering that the first as-

sessment interview is often anxiety provoking, it is easy to see that an objective problem assessment is made impossible by interview alone. It is true that the therapist can set a behavioural test, e.g. asking the agoraphobic patient to go for a walk away from the clinic, but this will not give information about overall patterns of behaviour. The simplest procedure is to ask the patient to self-monitor by recording when the problem occurs and describe in a few words what happens. A form for doing this is shown in Figure 43.2. Keeping a diary like this may well help to isolate particular cues which prompt a behaviour. For example, one patient described having panic attacks which did not seem to have any particular pattern. After keeping a diary, it became clear that the panic attacks always occurred after events, conversations or situations involving illness or sudden death. Thus it became clear that the panic attacks had consistent cues on the death and dying theme. Subsequently a programme of graduated exposure to 'death and dying themes' led to a dramatic cessation of panic attacks. Likewise, recording the consequences of a behaviour may reveal things which may consistently reinforce a behaviour. For example, a particular symptom such as anxiety may be unwittingly reinforced by a spouse who always gives loving care and attention when anxiety occurs.

Date	Time	Description of behaviour	What happened before	What happened after

Figure 43.2 General purpose diary form.

Keeping diaries will also reveal true patterns of behaviour such as drinking alcohol, smoking or over-eating, and there is ample evidence to suggest that such diaries are very reliable (e.g. Heather & Robertson 1983). The simple act of recording, for example drinking alcohol, is very often revealing for the patient. This information alone may be enough to help the patient to decide to exercise control and reduce consumption.

Self-monitoring procedures are now commonly used for assessment purposes in many non-psychiatric settings. Diaries are widely used in the assessment of pain, pre-menstrual symptoms and other physical disorders.

Evaluation

Self-monitoring provides a very simple but good method for evaluating treatment. It yields a measure of frequency of behaviour, and a spouse's help can be enlisted in order to carry out a similar exercise. Thus, for example, an agoraphobic patient and his spouse can count the number of journeys undertaken from home during a week. This dual rating tends to ensure that the measure is reliable. If the patient is asked to rate anxiety levels during each journey, it can be seen whether a change in behaviour is accompanied by a change in anxiety/discomfort.

Self-monitoring is extremely useful in dealing with 'thinking problems' such as obsessive thoughts (ruminations) or urges to commit deviant acts. Such problems are based on private events and as such external assessment or observation is of little value.

Treatment

Teaching a patient to self-monitor for purposes of assessment and evaluation very often leads to the procedure becoming a treatment in its own right. In essence this procedure helps patients become their own behaviour modifier. Patients who use the process over a period may well see clearly, for the first time, a true pattern to the problem. They are then able to identify the consistent antecedents and consequences of a problem behaviour. If so motivated, the patient can change these to make the behaviour less likely to occur by modifying its cues and reinforcers. This also aids the patient, perhaps with the help of a therapist, to target new, non-problem behaviours. In problems such as drinking or delinquent behaviour, such a definition of alternative behaviour is essential to prevent relapse.

CONCLUSION

Psychiatric nursing has been radically changed by the integration of behavioural psychotherapy into its scope. Furthermore, the rigorous evaluation, essential to behavioural approaches, is slowly leading to the psychiatric nurse becoming more of a scientist-practitioner and less of a servant to other professionals.

REFERENCES

Barlow D H, Hayes S C, Nelson R O 1984 The scientist practitioner. Pergamon, New York

Bird J, Marks I M, Lindley P 1979 Nurse therapists in psychiatry — developments, controversies and implications. British Journal of Psychiatry 135: 321–329

Borkovec T D 1982 Insomnia. Journal of Consulting and Clinical Psychology 50: 880–895

Ginsberg G, Marks I M, Waters H M 1985 A controlled cost benefit analysis. In: Marks I M (ed) Psychiatric nurse therapists in primary care. Royal College of Nursing, London

Hargie O, McCartan P 1986 Social skills training and psychiatric nursing. Croom Helm, London

Heather N, Robertson I 1983 Controlled drinking. Methuen, London

Keane T M, Kaloupek D G 1982 Imaginal flooding in the treatment of a post-traumatic stress disorder. Journal of Consulting and Clinical Psychology 50: 138–140

Lindley P, Marks I M 1985 The work of a nurse therapist in primary care. In: Marks I M (ed) Nurse therapist in primary care. Royal College of Nursing, London

Marks I M 1981 Behavioural concepts and treatments of neurosis. Behavioural Psychotherapy 9(2): 137–154

Marks I M 1985 Psychiatric nurse therapists in primary care: the expansion of advanced clinical roles in nursing. Royal College of Nursing, London

Marks I M, Connolly J, Hallam R S, Philpott R 1977
  Nursing in behavioural psychotherapy, Royal College of
  Nursing, London
Moray N 1969 Attention: selective processes in vision and
  hearing, Hutchinson, London
Rachman S J, Wilson G T 1980 The effects of psychological
  therapy. Pergamon, Oxford

Ramsey R, 1979 Bereavement: a behavioural treatment to
  pathological grief. In: Sjoden O, Bates S, Delkins W Eds
  Trends in behaviour therapy. New York, Academic Press
Trower P 1984 Radical approaches to social skills training.
  Croom Helm, London

44

Social, recreational, creative and occupational activities

J. I. Brooking

The therapeutic activities described in this chapter serve a variety of purposes, but all are intended to help to bring the patient to the maximum possible level of functioning and independence. Most of these activities can be initiated by nurses or occupational therapists, with input from a variety of specialist therapists. The boundaries between nursing and occupational therapy are vague and most often determined by availability of staff with particular interests and skills. What is important is that professional rivalries should not be allowed to obscure the needs of patients for planned programmes of therapeutic activities.

In the past, and even to some extent now, patients were engaged in various forms of simple diversion, intended mainly to fill the time, keep them occupied and to disguise the purposelessness of their time in hospital. Such standardized activity programmes had little meaning or value to individuals as they were not planned as part of the overall treatment programme and only accidentally contributed to overall therapeutic goals. Even worse than standardized programmes is the absence of any activity. Even today it is possible to find both admission and long-stay psychiatric wards where patients have little or no planned activity and where they sit aimlessly waiting for the next meal or drug round, with little more than television to occupy their time.

The social, recreational, creative and occupational activities described in this chapter are just some of the many activities which could be incorporated into individually planned programmes. These should be based on careful assessment, should have clear goals and should be frequently evaluated as part of the overall care plan. Although the actual activities may be useful and enjoyable in themselves, they are not intended to be ends in themselves, but should take place within the context of the overall therapeutic plan.

Box 44.1 The range of social, recreational, creative and occupational activities in psychiatry

Self-care and domestic
Work
Hobbies and craftwork
Creative and artistic
Social
Educational
Relaxation
Exercise

SELF-CARE AND DOMESTIC ACTIVITIES

Psychiatric patients, especially those who are institutionalized, often lose the capacity to care for themselves and to manage their home environment. These skills need to be learned or relearned, constantly maintained and reinforced. Different patients will have deficits and needs in different areas. Some of the skills to assess include:

- personal hygiene, grooming and choice of clothes
- laundry and ironing
- hair styling, nail care and use of cosmetics
- shopping for food and other daily necessities
- managing money
- cleaning
- bedmaking
- cooking and kitchen management
- nutrition and table manners.

Patients will need assistance at various levels. In relation to money, for example, an institutionalized long-stay patient may need to learn the most basic skills of handling money, whereas less disabled patients may require more complex financial counselling to help them sort out debts or poor investments which have contributed to depression. Similarly, in relation to cooking, a chronic patient may need to learn the most basic skills, whereas a neurotic patient may be able to use cooking to facilitate communication with others, to gain a sense of accomplishment, or to channel tensions and aggression through the physical tasks of food preparation (Parrish 1980). In general, self-care and domestic skills are important to increase capacity for independent living and to raise self-esteem through a sense of achievement.

Many psychiatric hospitals take over domestic functions like cooking and cleaning, but some therapeutic communities, such as the Cassel Hospital at Richmond, Surrey, deliberately use the process of everyday domestic activities as an important part of the therapeutic work of the community.

WORK-RELATED ACTIVITIES

Large psychiatric hospitals have traditionally provided many opportunities for patients to work in areas such as carpentry, plumbing, decorating, gardening, laundry, sewing, typing etc. Industrial Therapy Units have provided opportunities for light assembly, packing and other factory-type work. In theory such activities could and should have considerable therapeutic value, but in practice long-stay patients have sometimes been used as cheap labour and the work has lost any real benefit. If an ex-mental patient is to obtain employment after discharge, then rehabilitation should teach work-related skills such as punctuality, concentration, responsibility, coping with stress and getting on with workmates. In practice, few jobs are available on the open market to ex-mental patients, although legislation requires large employers to take a proportion of handicapped people. Despite these problems, work still has a place in psychiatric rehabilitation, as long as it is carefully planned and monitored. Work can be planned to teach useful skills, and work in itself may be important in raising self-esteem, giving a sense of accomplishment and a sense of contributing to society.

For some acute patients, work stress may have contributed to psychiatric breakdown and may precipitate a desire to reconsider work goals. Vocational guidance and counselling may be provided by occupational and clinical psychologist. In the private sector, psychiatric professionals have become increasingly involved in helping people in demanding jobs to cope with the stress of work and to prevent adverse physical and psychiatric reactions to stress. Executive stress management has become big business.

HOBBIES AND CRAFTWORK

Hospital wards tend to have one large day room, typically dominated by the television, and often noisy, overcrowded and unattractive. While it is useful to have a large room in which the whole ward community can meet, it is generally preferable to have several smaller sitting rooms and to separate noisy and quiet areas.

Television and radio should be used selectively, with patients choosing programmes from the newspaper. In a discussion of soap opera therapy Kilguss (1980) describes how television programmes, particularly 'soap operas' deal with critical psychological themes such as incest, suspicion, distrust, dependency, victimization, loneliness, fear, relationships, sexuality and aggression. He argues that soap operas can be used as a therapeutic tool to open up discussion and as a path to the patient's fantasy life. He argues that although mental health professionals typically denigrate popular television shows, they can be comparable to using play therapy in children, and are particularly useful with young, depressed, non-intellectual women. Kilguss (1980) argues that the patient's use and interpretation of media can be a route to the unconscious.

Newspapers should be available on wards to maintain orientation and contact with the outside world. Local newspapers can also be valuable in helping patients to feel part of the local community. A variety of individual, pair and group games should be available, including draughts, chess, popular board games, table tennis, snooker and cards. Nurses need to be competent in these games in order to play with patients, which helps to develop friendly relationships. Letter writing and telephoning are important for patients to keep in contact with family and friends. Writing paper, envelopes and stamps should be made available to patients who lack their own supplies, and there should be a quiet room for reading and writing.

Craft activities can give a great sense of achievement as there is an attractive end-product which the patient can keep. They help to promote concentration and manual dexterity and can be done individually or as collaborative group exercises. Group work encourages social interaction and helps to develop social skills. Relationships among patients and between patients and nurses can be developed. The range of craft activities offered will depend on the expertise of staff. Some possibilities include leatherwork, jewellery-making, toy-making, weaving, basketwork, woodwork, pottery, knitting and sewing.

Gardening has long been advocated for its beneficial effects on physical and mental well-being. Relf (1980) describes the range of horticultural projects, such as vegetable and herb gardens, greenhouses, lawns, indoor plants and flower arranging. He recommends horticulture as therapy for all age groups and types of disorders.

CREATIVE AND ARTISTIC ACTIVITIES

The use of the creative arts in therapy has become more common in recent years and many hospitals employ specialist — art, music and drama — therapists to develop these approaches. These therapies allow leisure time to be used constructively and creatively; they provide an outlet for the expression of painful emotions, which patients might be unable or unlikely to express verbally; and they allow unacceptable emotions and impulses to be channelled into more socially acceptable forms.

The use of literature

Literature may be used in two distinct ways: reading and discussing published work, and writing as a therapeutic activity.

Sclabassi (1980) comments that reading published work can be divided into the use of didactic and imaginative material. Reputable self-help books are now widely available to help lay people to cope with a variety of mental health problems, such as stress, depression, anxiety, phobias, sexual and relationship problems. These books sell in large numbers and are presumably found to be helpful by their readers. Examples are the books produced by the British Holistic Medical Association of which *Overcoming Depression* (Gillett 1987) is particularly relevant to psychiatric care. Another example is Professor Isaac Marks' (1978) *Living with Fear*, which is frequently prescribed by nurse behaviour therapists and which has been found to be highly effective for selected patients. Other books are aimed at the families of sufferers, schizophrenia (e.g. Arieti 1979) and mental illness in the elderly (e.g. Alzheimer's Disease Society 1984) being popular subjects. Nurses should familiarize themselves with popular literature relevant to their patients and should prescribe this material as an adjunct to professional help. Well-motivated people with minor problems may find that self-help material is an adequate alternative to professional help. A good selection of these books should be available in the hospital or ward library, as they can be expensive to buy.

Imaginative literature such as novels, plays and poetry may be used in group and individual work with all age groups. Relevant material is selected by the therapist, read either alone or aloud in a group, and is then used as the basis for discussion. Patients need reasonable cognitive function, orientation to reality and insight into their problems to benefit from this approach. Sclabassi (1980) described four levels of therapeutic intervention:

- *intellectual* in which the material is used to acquire knowledge, to think about and analyse behaviour and attitudes
- *social* in which the material is used to expand experience beyond the patient's own frame of reference, e.g. to illustrate the experience of racism, poverty or violence
- *behavioural* in which the material is used to

contribute to competence by showing how others coped with particular problems, and
- *emotional* in which the material provides vicarious experience which can be discussed and which permits the release of repressed emotion.

Writing poetry, diaries and to a lesser extent fiction, has traditionally been used as a form of self-expression and release. Troubled people have often translated unbearable feelings into the written word, thus purging themselves in a form of catharsis. Patients can be asked to write about specific themes or whatever concerns them, and this work can be discussed individually or in groups according to the patient's mental state, which can be shared with the whole multi-disciplinary team. The use of poetry in therapy is discussed more fully by Leedy & Reiter (1980), and the use of an intensive personal diary is discussed by Morrow (1980).

The use of music

Music has a powerful effect on mind and body and provides a good medium for therapeutic work. Music therapy can fulfil a variety of purposes. Sackett & Fitzgerald (1980) wrote that 'music therapy aims to bring the individual into contact with a world of perceptual and emotional reality; to encourage a more successful adjustment to his environment; to promote his self-knowledge and to develop his awareness'. Duerksen (1980) wrote that music could be used to change mood and feelings, for stimulation and sedation. It is a vehicle for non-verbal communication, which can evoke feelings and encourage the expression of feelings. It frees the imagination and distracts from pain and loneliness. It can promote psychological closeness and can help orientate to reality. Active music-making promotes self-esteem and participation in a group endeavour.

There are several varieties of music therapy which can be employed by nurses as well as by trained music therapists. At the simplest level music can provide entertainment and diversion, but it can also have a profound emotional impact. Music therapy is not specifically intended to improve musical knowledge or performance skills, although these can be valuable outcomes in themselves. Because of its versatility, music therapy can be used with all age groups and all forms of mental disorder, as well as having a place in the treatment of physical and mental handicap.

Three types of music therapy, described by Sackett & Fitzgerald (1980), are creative music, music appreciation and music discussion. In all types the group should meet regularly in a quiet, sound-proofed room, with the same group members and the same therapist. This enables trusting relationships to develop and reduces patients' inhibitions about discussion and music-making.

Creative music-making can range from simple clapping, through using simple instruments, to establishing a band, orchestra or choir. Singing may be a valuable adjunct or alternative to the use of instruments. Music appreciation consists of playing carefully selected pieces of music, followed by discussion of memories and associations evoked. Music discussion focuses on the communication of emotions stimulated by particular passages of music, carefully chosen for their mood content. For example, Sackett & Fitzgerald (1980) describe how a tape might be compiled containing pieces which move from aggression and anguish to sadness and nostalgia to peace and joy.

Blair et al (1973) emphasized that music therapy is an ancillary treatment which, however successful, could not 'be effective in securing a remission of illness by its own unaided efforts'. It must also be remembered that music therapy is not synonymous with 'the ceaseless emissions of the ward radio' (Sackett & Fitzgerald 1980) which are more likely to be irritating and meaningless than therapeutic.

The use of drama

Dramatic techniques can be used in many ways in psychiatric nursing, all of which have in common that patients *enact* their problems or conflicts in a form of role play, instead of simply talking about them. This takes place with the support and participation of a group of patients and a group leader, who may be a qualified drama therapist.

Psychodrama was developed by Dr J. L. Moreno in the 1920s and 1930s and there are now many schools of psychodrama and drama therapy, incorporating the ideas of other theorists, mainly psychoanalysts. Techniques derived from psycho-drama include role play, role reversal, mirroring, drama exercises and experiential games. Yablonsky (1980) describes how Moreno was initially interested in developing a 'theatrical cathedral' for the release of the spontaneity and creativity he believed existed in everyone. Initially this was not seen as a form of psychotherapy, but only later did Moreno observe the positive psychological consequences of the psychodramatic process. Techniques derived from Moreno's work are widely used in education and training, e.g. experiential learning methods, assertion and social skills training (Langley & Langley 1983).

All psychodramatic techniques are designed to construct or reconstruct significant personal events and their associated feelings and to act them out in a safe, structured environment. This provides insight for the patient through actions and verbal feedback and aids the resolution of emotional conflicts and problems.

According to Schützenberger (1983) psychodrama groups usually consist of: a group leader, sometimes called the director, who acts as a catalyst for the session; a main actor, protagonist or subject, who acts out his or her problems on the stage; auxiliary egos or co-actors who take on different roles as required by the action; and a small audience consisting of the remaining group members. A stage or suitable space, with props such as tables and chairs, is required for the action.

Each session begins with a warm-up. Cooperative games can be used for the warm-up or can become ends in themselves, as described by Davison (1986), who gives several examples of games used by nurses. Orlick (1978) claims that these games foster cooperation, enjoyment, acceptance and involvement. After the warm-up the main actor role plays a particular problem he or she has encountered in the past or anticipates in the future. Other group members portray other characters needed for the action. Role play enables the patient to rehearse useful skills, reduce anxiety and understand past and present conflicts. Various techniques such as role reversal, mirroring and empty chair may be suggested by the group leader. In role reversal the patient plays the part of someone with whom he or she has difficulties. This gives insight into how the other person feels and enables the patient to communicate more effectively in future. Finally, the whole group share their feelings about and experiences of the action, with feedback to the actors and discussion of the group dynamics. Role play and its variants may also be used by nurses in one-to-one interactions with patients.

Although these techniques are useful for patients of all ages with many types of problems, Davison (1986) points out that drama therapy is contraindicated in circumstances where an increase in stimulation is likely to bewilder and further confuse the patient, e.g. acutely psychotic patients and others very unsure of their own identities. Davison (1986) also pointed out some of the difficulties he experienced in persuading nurses to participate in drama therapy. Nurses may regard it as childish, as applicable only to those with acting ability, or as a form of amateur dramatics. Nurses may fear that taking an active part in drama therapy exercises will reduce the social and emotional distance between them and their patients, leaving them exposed and vulnerable.

The use of art

Art therapy is a relatively new discipline defined as 'the use of art and other visual media in a therapeutic or treatment setting' (Dalley 1984). Art therapists may work in wards or special art rooms; they may work with groups or individuals; they work with many types of patients; and they bring varying theoretical perspectives to their work, most commonly psychodynamic. Although trained art therapists have special knowledge and skills, nurses should also utilize the principles of art therapy in their work with patients. Dalley (1984) explained that art is traditionally concerned with the end-product, the creative process being secondary or irrelevant. However, in art therapy the process and the person are central as art is

used primarily as a vehicle of communication. Liebmann (1986) considers that art therapy uses art as a means of expressing feelings and is available to everyone, not just the aesthetically gifted.

Following planning, an individual or group art therapy session involves a period of painting or other creative activity, using paint, collage, clay, sand or any other medium. Patients may be invited to work on particular themes or to paint a subject of their choice. There is finally a discussion focusing on the production process, how the picture makes the patient feel and how these feelings relate to the patient's own circumstances.

Waters & Bowden emphasized that art therapy should never be compulsory. Many patients are reluctant to paint because they believe they have no artistic talent, and some may just want to sit in on sessions. Dexter & Walsh (1986) suggest that nurses should join in as a way of breaking the ice. Competition between patients should be avoided. In his art room Bowden tries to encourage spontaneous painting by providing a relaxed safe atmosphere, with readily available art materials and lots of visual stimulus from paintings on the walls. He found that many patients felt safe enough to discuss their pictures, but this should arise from an empathic relationship and should not be forced. The art therapist should, of course, share insights gained with the rest of the therapeutic team.

Patients with different types of problems will derive different benefits from art therapy. For some, painting is a means of expressing emotions; for others, the benefits come from building confidence and self-esteem or the sheer pleasure of producing a picture; some gain most from social interactions in the art group or from the relationship with the therapist; for some painting provides pleasurable stimulation to relieve boredom and apathy; and finally some patients benefits from improved concentration, manual dexterity and visual awareness.

SOCIAL ACTIVITIES

An enormous range of social activities can be organized by nurses and patients, both within and outside hospital. In planning social activities, it is important to consider:

- patients' interests, abilities and disabilities, level of independence and concentration span
- patients' clinical conditions, risks of aggression and self-injury and need for nursing supervision
- legal constraints imposed on patients who are compulsorily detained
- rules about alcohol intake, seniority of nurses accompanying patients outside the hospital and other health authority regulations
- resources available, such as money, transport, equipment and the number of nurses needed to accompany patients.

Some social activities can be organized for small groups or for individuals, and other activities can be organized for larger groups of patients or whole wards. Participation in group activities can be intolerably stressful for some patients, so careful planning is necessary.

Day and weekend trips and longer holidays should be offered with the same frequency as would be expected by people outside hospital. Day trips to local places of interest, seaside resorts and beautiful gardens are usually popular and easy to arrange. Weekend trips with 1 or 2 nights away from the hospital are valuable in rehabilitation, but are more costly. Residents in long-term care should, if possible, be given an annual holiday, either in Britain or abroad. One intensive rehabilitation ward at Springfield Hospital, London, takes almost all its patients for a week abroad each summer. This very successful holiday is demanding for staff, but has great therapeutic value for residents as part of their rehabilitation programme. The associated planning and preparation provide useful and enjoyable activity for many months beforehand.

Parties can be organized to celebrate special personal and public events, such as birthdays and royal weddings. Examples might include a buffet supper prepared by the patients, a wine and cheese tasting, a picnic or barbeque in the garden, a fancy dress party etc. Visits to the local cinema, theatre, disco etc. might be enjoyable for small groups, and some hospitals put on their own concerts, pan-

tomines and plays organized largely by patients. Dances are usually popular and relatively easy to organize.

Social activities give patients something enjoyable to look forward to and provide pleasurable experiences. They encourage relaxed social interaction, helping patients to make new friends. It is commonly observed by nurses that hospital patients' behaviour becomes more 'normal' in relaxed social events, particularly outside the hospital. These activities are also important as markers of significant personal and public events, and thus help to prevent institutionalization.

It is desirable for patients to take as much responsibility as possible for selecting, organizing and hosting their own social activities, as this increases competence, confidence and responsibility and provides opportunities to work with and lead others. In some therapeutic communities, such as the Cassel Hospital, patients are closely involved in the day-to-day running of the community, with various patients' committees managing specific functions and elected patient representatives having particular responsibilities. In some hospitals patients produce their own magazine and contribute to the management of a hospital radio station.

EDUCATIONAL ACTIVITIES

There is a statutory responsibility on local education authorities to provide teaching to all children and adolescents in hospital, so their needs are usually met by qualified teachers. Some adults use a period of crisis or hospitalization to re-evaluate their educational achievements and may decide to take various educational and vocational courses. Nurses should be fully informed about local courses open to adults and should be able to provide up-to-date advice. This is equally important for community and hospital nurses.

In Special Hospitals, where patients are compulsorily detained for periods of years, help is usually available to improve basic literacy as well as to prepare for formal qualifications, such as Open University degrees. Similarly, in therapeutic communities, where young patients with predominantly neurotic and personality disorders stay for about a year, it is quite common for patients to attend local further education colleges part-time, particularly when their psychiatric problems limited their achievements at school.

Even in day hospitals and short-stay wards, it should be possible to provide informal educational activities. These might include language study by linguaphone, discussion groups on current affairs and controversial topics, crossword competitions, quizzes and access to a well-stocked library. Some patients are unaware of the existence of their local library or need help to gain confidence to use it. Computing, typing and word-processing skills are often taught in hospital.

RELAXATION

The importance of deep physical and mental relaxation is now well recognized as an important antidote to stress, with its accompanying physical and psychopathology. Numerous methods of relaxation are being incorporated into health care, particularly in the private sector, some well established scientifically, some associated with holistic or 'alternative' practice and some derived from Eastern mysticism. Despite medical scepticism about some of the more extravagant therapeutic claims made by proponents of particular techniques, there is widespread acknowledgement that these techniques are helpful in combatting stress, even if some of the other claims made for them cannot be substantiated. Numerous books on relaxation have been published in the last few years, of which some of the better general accounts include Pietroni (1986), Kirsta (1986) and Hewitt (1982). Two of these authors recommend a holistic perspective which involves 'stress-proofing' all aspects of life by examining and taking action on relationships, sexuality, work and play, time management, personal space, comfort, nutrition, exercise and the environment, as well as considering specific relaxation methods.

Box 44.2 lists some of the better known methods of relaxation, yet very few are commonly taught to patients in psychiatric wards and few nurses have more than a superficial knowledge of them. Stress reduction through relaxation should be offered to suitable patients and may also be

---

Box 44.2 Summary of relaxation techniques

Methods which can be carried out alone after apprioriate training

Progressive relaxation	see: Jacobson 1962, Hewitt 1982, Pietroni 1986
Self-hypnosis	see: Hewitt 1982
Autogenic training	see: Hewitt 1982
Meditation	see: Burnard 1987, Court 1984
Breathing exercises	see: Kirsta 1986, Pietroni 1986
Alexander technique	see: Barlow 1973
Imagery and visualization	see: Gawain 1982

Methods which involve exercises

Relation exercises	see: Kirsta 1986
Yoga	see: Hittleman 1969
T'ai Chi Chuan	see: Crompton 1986

Methods which require a specialist therapist

Massage and shiatsu	see: Lidell 1984, Kirsta 1986
Reflexology	see: Lidell 1984
Aromatherapy	see: Kirsta 1986
Hypnosis	see: Hewitt 1982

Methods which require technical equipment

Biofeedback	see: Carroll 1984

---

beneficial for nurses in coping with their own stresses and maintaining mental well-being.

EXERCISE

Almost all psychiatric patients can benefit from some form of exercise as a means of promoting physical fitness. Ashton & Davies (1986) reviewed research on the role of exercise in disease prevention and concluded that regular physical activity is important in preventing heart disease and should be regarded 'as the cornerstone of good health policy'. Regular exercise is also associated with the reduction of obesity, improved flexibility, coordination and posture, and healthy physical tiredness leading to better sleep and reduced reliance on sedatives. Exercise has several important psychological benefits: it aids relaxation and reduces stress; it aids the discharge of negative emotions, such as hostility and anxiety; it increases self-esteem through progressive achievement; and it gives a sense of pleasure and well-being. Team sports also encourage the development of friendships and cooperative behaviour.

Many psychiatric patients are extremely unfit because of lack of exercise, cigarette smoking, obesity and an unbalanced diet. Exercise programmes should be offered to everyone and carefully planned according to fitness, age, interests and abilities. Of course unaccustomed exertion does have some risks, so it is important that the patient starts gently and that the intensity, duration and frequency of exercise is planned and monitored. With the increasing involvement of physiotherapists in psychiatry (Hare 1986), it is likely that fitness assessment will become more widespread.

The most important elements of a fitness programme are activities which increase the heart rate and respiration. Examples of aerobic exercises are running, jogging, swimming, cycling, rowing, squash, badminton, disco dancing and volley ball. Brisk walking is also an aerobic exercise and is suitable for even the most unfit people.

An exercise programme should also promote strength and suppleness and some aerobic exercises are also effective in these two areas. Weight training using free weights or machines such as the multigym is beneficial in increasing muscle strength, and is becoming popular with women as well as men. Stretching exercises and yoga increase suppleness. Ashton & Davies (1986) recommend flexibility exercises prior to aerobic exercise as part of the warm-up, to reduce the chances of injury.

Self-defence classes are increasingly popular, especially among women. Quinn (1983) believes that martial arts training also improves women's mental resources to look after themselves by promoting a sense of strength, dignity, power and self-worth and by reducing fear. Frager (1980) claims that Aikido, derived from Japanese martial arts, helps patients to deal with fear and aggressive impulses, develops a more positive self-image and eliminates physical and psychological tension.

Dance therapy

Dance therapy is described by the American Dance Therapy Association as 'the psychotherapeutic use of movement as a process which furthers the emotional and physical integration of the individual' (Payne 1977). It is based on the assumption that there is a relationship between the way a person moves and the way he or she feels.

Dance therapy developed in the USA in the 1930s and 1940s with the recognition that dance classes seemed to have psychotherapeutic benefits. The use of dance and movement as therapy grew out of the modern dance tradition, exemplified by Isadora Duncan, which attempts to express the totality of the human experience through music without the limitations imposed by ballet and folk dancing (Payne 1977). Dance therapy has increased in prominence in the USA where there are now at least eight theoretical approaches, mostly derived from psychoanalysis (Bernstein 1979). The applications are fully described by Espenak (1981). Dance therapy is still in its infancy in Britain, although a number of qualified dance and movement therapists work in psychiatric hospitals.

According to Sarah Holden, Dance Therapist at Springfield Hospital, London, the therapist seeks to extend gradually the patient's vocabulary of movements until it is more balanced and the patient is encouraged to feel 'good feedback' from the body. In this way the therapist improves the patient's body image, self-esteem and feelings of potency. A second area of importance, according to Sarah Holden, is social interaction, either between therapist and patient, or between members of a group. Some patients may be able to give verbal interpretations of the feelings evoked by dance and movement. Others prefer a purely non-verbal approach. Thirdly, dance therapy offers the patient a chance of creative expression. The use of dance and movement therapy is adaptable to almost all patients, even those with minimal movement or who are severely regressed.

Nurses should try to work with dance therapists in order to incorporate at least some of the basic principles into their own work with patients.

PLANNING AN ACTIVITY PROGRAMME

Like any other part of the nursing care plan, an activity programme should be planned on the basis of a careful assessment of the patient; it should be goal directed; and it should be evaluated at regular intervals and modified accordingly. Not all the activities mentioned in this chapter will be available in all treatment settings, so planning must take into account available resources, time and personnel. When occupational therapists, remedial gymnasts, physiotherapists and creative arts therapists are available, the scope of possible activities is considerably widened. As a general principle, the patient should participate fully in planning the programme and should have as much choice as possible. The programme should be varied and balanced, which might be accomplished by selecting one or two activities from each section of this chapter.

Patient assessment

1. Is the proposed activity appropriate to the patient's age, sex, education, social class and cultural background?
2. Is the activity appropriate to the degree and type of handicap resulting from the mental disorder?
3. Does the plan take account of the degree of institutionalization or chronicity?
4. Are there any physical or psychological risks associated with the activities? Are the risks justified and can they be avoided or minimized?
5. What are the likely benefits to the patient from the activity?
6. Is the patient physically, intellectually and emotionally capable of the activity? Is the activity sufficiently stretching to be interesting and rewarding? Is the activity too demanding and likely to cause disappointment and frustration? Are the goals achievable?
7. How much assistance and guidance will the patient need? Who can best provide this?
8. Is the activity meaningful in relation to the patient's normal life outside hospital and previous experience?
9. How long should the activity last?
10. Does the programme include group as well as individual activities? Can the patient cope with group activities? Will the programme provide meaningful social interaction? Are the proposed group members compatible in terms of age, background, interests and level of incapacity?
11. Is the programme interesting and varied? Does it include indoor and outdoor activities, both within and outside the hospital?

REFERENCES

Alzheimer's Disease Society 1984 Caring for the person with dementia: a guide for families and other carers, ADS, London
Ashton D, Davies B 1986 Why exercise? Blackwell, Oxford
Arieti S 1979 Understanding and helping the Schizophrenic. Penguin, Harmondsworth
Barlow W 1973 The Alexander principle. Arrow, London
Bernstein P L (ed) 1979 Eight theoretical approaches in dance-movement therapy. Kendall Hunt, Iowa
Blair D, Werner T A, Brooking M 1973 The value of individual music therapy as an aid to psychotherapy. The British Society for Music Therapy, London
Burnard P 1987 Meditation: uses and methods in psychiatric nursing education. Nurse Education Today 7: 187–191
Carroll D 1984 Biofeedback in practice. Longman, London
Court S 1984 The meditator's manual. Aquarian, Northamptonshire
Crompton P 1986 Chinese soft exercises: a T'ai Chi workbook. Unwin, London

Dalley T 1984 Art as therapy: an introduction to the use of art as a therapeutic technique. Tavistock, London
Davison J 1986 Dramatherapy for psychiatric patients. Nursing Times, June 4: 48–50
Dexter G, Walsh M 1986 Psychiatric nursing skills: a patient-centered approach. Croom Helm, London
Duerksen G L 1980 Music therapy. In: Herink R (ed) The psychotherapy handbook. Meridian, New York
Espanak L 1981 Dance therapy: theory and application. Thomas, Illinois
Frager R 1980 Aikido. In: Herink R (ed) The psychotherapy handbook. Meridian, New York
Gawain S 1982 Creative visualization. Bantam, New York
Gillett R 1987 Overcoming depression: a practical self-help guide to prevention and treatment. British Holistic Medical Association, Dorling Kindersley, London
Hare M 1986 Physiotherapy in psychiatry. Heinnemann, London
Hewitt J 1982 The complete relaxation book: a manual of

Eastern and Western techniques. Rider, London

Hittleman R 1969 Introduction to yoga. Bantam, New York

Jacobson E 1962 You must relax. McGraw-Hill, New York

Kilguss A F 1980 Soap opera therapy. In: Herink R (ed) The psychotherapy handbook. Meridian, New York

Kirsta A 1986 The book of stress survival. Unwin, London

Langley D M, Langley G E 1983 Dramatherapy and psychiatry. Croom Helm, London

Leedy J L, Reiter S 1980 Poetry therapy. In: Herink R (ed) The psychotherapy handbook. Meridian, New York

Lidell L 1984 The book of massage. Ebury, London

Liebmann M 1986 Art therapy for groups: a handbook of themes, games and exercises. Croom Helm, London

Marks I M 1978 Living with fear. McGraw-Hill, New York

Morrow F 1980 The intensive journal. In: Herink R (ed) The psychotherapy handbook. Meridian, New York

Orlick T 1978 The cooperative sports and games book. Writers and Readers Publishing Cooperative, London

Parrish L 1980 Cooking as therapy. In: Herink R (ed) The psychotherapy handbook. Meridian, New York

Payne H 1977 Dance therapy: its origins, present applications and future development. The Association for Dance Movement Therapy, London

Pietroni P 1986 Holistic living. Dent, London

Relf P D 1980 Horticulture therapy. In: Herink R (ed) The psychotherapy handbook. Meridian, New York

Sackett J, Fitzgerald J 1980 Music in hospitals. Nursing Times, October 16: 1845–1848

Schützenberger A A 1983 Psychodrama, creativity and group processes. In: Jennings S (ed) Creative therapy. Kemble, Banbury

Sclabassi S H 1980 Bibliotherapy. In: Herink R (ed) The psychotherapy handbook. Meridian, New York.

Waters M A, Bowden D. Art therapy in psychiatric treatment. Smith, Kline and French services to Psychiatry. Pamphlet, Herefordshire (undated)

Yablonsky L 1980 Psychodrama. In: Herink R (ed) The psychotherapy handbook. Meridian, New York.

45

Rehabilitation

*H. Macdonald**

This chapter presents an appraisal of the recent historical setting of the role of the nurse in psychiatric rehabilitation. Difficulties which are characteristic of patients are described in order to consider the nursing care that they require. Current ideas on the subject of rehabilitation are reviewed at the level of patient assessment and unit organization.

HISTORICAL PERSPECTIVE

In order to understand fully the field of psychiatric rehabilitation and nursing care of institutionalized patients, it is necessary to consider the relevant historical developments both in psychiatry and psychiatric nursing and the way in which these are informed by social policy.

The two world wars provided impetus for change. In the aftermath of World War I, psychiatric casualties needed both work and convalescence in order to readjust to social life and cope with their disability. Treatment was influenced by developments in psychiatry in Europe during the 1920s and in the United States during the 1930s. These related to the idea that institutional care was detrimental to the patients. The consequence of this was a move away from such care. This trend was interrupted by World War II, which created a 'situation of broader social need'

---

* This chapter is based on undergraduate work which was undertaken under the supervision of Julia Brooking.

(Strauss 1966). The most significant feature of this was the need for manpower, so that soldier survivors from World War I who were unfit for active service could be employed in other useful capacities. As well as this need, there was also a sense of moral obligation to these men.

Under the guidance of Maxwell Jones, the implications of the importance of the social environment were recognized in the development of the 'therapeutic community'. Rapaport & Rosow (1960) noted that the staff considered they were giving treatment which was at the same time rehabilitating. Concurrently, other writers were drawing attention to the disabling effects of life in the traditional mental hospital (Goffman 1961). It was demonstrated that much of the behaviour associated with a particular diagnosis, most frequently schizophrenia, could be accounted for by the treatment the patient received in hospital and also by the environment. Features of this 'institutional neurosis' were described by Barton (1966). They include loss of contact with the outside world, enforced idleness, loss of personal friends and possessions, poor ward atmosphere and loss of prospects outside the institution. Wing & Freudenberh (1961) reiterated the importance of the social environment, using a different perspective which documented the increase in relapse rates in schizophrenics in excessively stimulating and stressful environments.

With electroconvulsive therapy (ECT), which began in 1945, and insulin coma therapy (ICT), commencing in 1952, it was thought that many more patients were able to occupy themselves constructively, and opportunities to do so were made available. The development of new drugs, phenothiazines and antidepressants, became a most important variable in rehabilitation programmes, and potentially increased the effectiveness of social therapies. The complex interaction between these various developments led to questioning of the concept of rehabilitation. As the success of resettlement and rehabilitation of patients was evaluated, it prompted the question as to how many more hospital residents could benefit and what features of inpatient life would facilitate successful transfer from hospital to community.

However, the mental hospital was already in decline in the 1950s and this was expected to continue. At the time the Minister of Health, Enoch Powell confidently stated that by 1975 half the mental hospitals, our nineteenth century inheritance, would have been closed down and their function split between psychiatric units in district general hospitals (DGHs) and care in the community. In fact, only two hospitals closed in that time; nonetheless, it cannot be denied that the last 30 years have been a period of significant change in British psychiatry. The trend has been towards a more community-based pattern of services. The 1975 Government White Paper 'Better services for the mentally ill' provides one expression of this trend (DHSS 1975).

In many large mental hospitals firm plans for the complete relocation of current services have already been approved and many others are expected to close in the next decade. Such plans are endorsed by WHO (1976). Concern about such proposals have been voiced through many channels, not least of which is the National Association of Mental Health (MIND). They fear two main problems: firstly, the lack of adequate preparation and unrealistic goals for long-term patients who may be discharged prematurely, and secondly, the inadequate provision for the chronically ill leading to a two-tier system of care and the creation of new 'back' wards in the district general hospital unit.

DEFINITIONS

The concept of rehabilitation has often been confused with resettlement. Many 'definitions' of rehabilitation concentrate on the restoration of the disabled person to his former state. In consequence, there has been a failure to distinguish between the end product of successful rehabilitation and the process itself.

Rehabilitation as a process has two essential features. Firstly, there is identification and minimization of the cause of disability. Secondly, at the same time help must be given if individuals are to develop and use their talents, through which they will acquire confidence and self-esteem from success in social roles. Resettlement, on the other hand, is an event which occurs at some stage in the process of fulfilment and acceptance of social positions such as living in independent accommodation within the community, and being employed. More specifically, resettlement involves discharge of a patient from hospital to live in the outside world once again or the placement of a person in a job following a long period of unemployment (Morgan & Cheadle 1974).

It is important to retain the idea of these two separate concepts of rehabilitation and resettlement in order to ensure that efforts are made not only to rehabilitate those for whom resettlement is a realistic goal but also to ensure that rehabilitation will continue after resettlement. Moreover, the discussion as to whether or not rehabilitation should be attempted with a psychiatric patient should be based on the prospects of eventual resettlement (Bennett & Watts 1983).

The work of the Medical Research Council (MRC) Social Psychiatry Unit in London, under the influence of J. K. Wing, was instrumental in formulating and refining the concept and definition of disablement and rehabilitation. Disablement was broken down into three components:

1. The psychiatric impairments of dysfunction
2. Social disadvantage, both pre-morbid and after onset
3. Personal reaction to impairments or disadvantage or to a combination of both, i.e. secondary handicap.

The acceptance by the handicapped person of limitations that are not actually necessary is the essence of secondary disablement, a typical example being that of institutionalization: when the longer a patient has been in hospital the less favourable his attitude is likely to be towards discharge (Wing & Brown 1970). But it can be difficult to distinguish secondary handicap from those which are part of the disease process (Wing 1963).

PROBLEMS OF LONG-STAY PATIENTS

Since the mid 1950s there has been a continuing decline in the number of inpatients: in 1955 the number was 143 l000; by 1965 it was 120 000; by 1970 it was 111 000; by 1975 it was 87 000 (Cohen 1988). By 1991 the Department of Health hopes to reduce the number of beds to 45 000.

Many of the patients who had been treated in hospital for some years were able to leave and lead more independent lives. The use of behavioural techniques for the acquisition of social skills, recognition of the importance of work and the discovery of new forms of psychotropic drugs, allied to more positive attitudes towards rehabilitation and resettlement, have resulted in many patients being discharged to lead satisfactory lives outside hospital.

Despite all the innovative therapeutic policies, a number of patients continue to need hospital care. They are increasingly frail and aged and now, understandably, their rate of discharge is very low (Goldstone 1977). Goldstone suggests that if this pattern continues it is likely that the workload of psychiatric nurses will increase and alter in character as physical nursing needs increase. The new long-stay patients are defined by the DHSS (1975) as those patients who have been in hospital for not less than 1 year and not more than 5 years. The distinction between these patients and the previous group of long-stay patients (old long-stay) arises from the fact that they are accumulating, despite all available modern methods of treatment and rehabilitation. The previous old long-stay patient population had grown during a different era of predominantly custodial care.

About 5% of those admitted during a year remain in hospital for long periods (i.e. 1 year or more). However, it is estimated that if new long-stay patients represented only 1% of all acute patients they would have filled up half of all beds in psychiatric units in district general hospitals after only 7 years (MIND 1974). At the end of 1976 there were 83 940 inpatients in English psychiatric hospitals. Of this number 48.5% were under 65 years of age and 54% of inpatients of all ages had been in hospital for 5 years or less (DOH 1976).

The disabilities of these patients are 'permanent, severe and crippling' (Bennett 1980), rehabilitation being a process of a lifetime rather than once and for all. The new long-stay patients tend to be much more impaired than in the past and have been shown to adopt institutional attitudes rather more quickly (Mann & Cree 1976). One of the problems that caused considerable discussion in the study undertaken by the author was the patients' motivation (Macdonald 1985). Wing & Brown (1970, Wing 1983) describe lack of motivation as a secondary disablement, whereas Morgan (1980) suggests that the illness contributes more to the disability than institutionalization. Nurses had mixed opinions about this issue. Some thought that low motivation in the patients was the reason for failure to progress. Others have attributed low motivation to the illness, which requires more treatment. Others attributed it to the laziness of patients who need to make more effort (Macdonald 1985).

ASPECTS OF NURSING CARE

Assessment

The way mental illness is identified not only specifies the problem and its origins but also the appropriate modes of intervention (Burgess 1981). The medical model, for example, postulates that an individual who is sick demonstrates signs and symptoms which can be diagnosed, treated and cured (or at least alleviated). The cause of symptomatic behaviour is hence located within the individual, removed from its social context or interpersonal relationships. The function of the hospital becomes that of care and treatment for individual sufferers. For the patient it facilitates the adoption of the sick role and absolves him of responsibility for his behaviour. Expectations change so that exemption from everyday tasks of living is permitted and in return he is expected to accept that he is ill and cooperate with treatment (Parsons 1961). The extent to which psychiatric nurses adopt this model is of concern, as it seems to be contrary to the process of rehabilitation and promotion of independence (Macdonald 1985). Lewis (1980) suggests that sickness and illness must not be the raison d'être for nurses. Consequently, not only does the medical model preclude the identification of pathological aspects of the social environment and the ways to alter and prevent them, but it also fails to provide a framework for interpersonal and psychological care. The provision of general care becomes dissociated from the individual, as the routine manner in which the activities of daily living are undertaken by nurses demonstrates their failure to appreciate that these activities are actually problems faced by the patient (Macdonald 1985). Problems are only determined in the context of possible outcomes, outside of which they are not acknowledged. Twenty-five per cent of nurse subjects in Macdonald's study (n = 19) felt that their patients had no problems since they were all institutionalized. A further 25% stated that the only problem was mental illness. Similarly, the model of care in use makes implicit assumptions about the origin and cause of problems. If it is not acknowledged that patients are responsive to the social environment, for example, then there will be a failure to recognize the signs of institutionalization and an inability to act upon them.

It is clear that the needs of a particular individual are unique and that any programme of care must be uniquely tailored. Shepherd (1983) criticizes the pervading assumption in psychiatry of 'generality' whereby problems are not seen as specific to situations but are identified irrespective of the situational context. It is also a valuable exercise to consider the patients' assets and the way they could be developed. Wing & Brown (1970) categorized the various factors that might hinder the rehabilitation of schizophrenic patients in three large groups:

1. Pre-morbid handicapping factors, such as poor education, difficult personality or low intelligence.
2. Primary disabilities which are part of the illness, such as incoherent thought processes, delusions, hallucinations. Negative symptoms include social withdrawal, poor motivation and flattened affect.
3. Secondary handicaps which are not part of the illness itself but have accumulated with the reaction of the patient and the others around him to the illness. The results of past treatments, insulin courses, psychosurgery,

multiple ECT and drug therapy also contribute to patients' conditions by causing some degree of deterioration of cognitive function, disinhibition, flattening of affect and apathy.

Goals set for each individual must be small, realistic and negotiated with the patient (Shepherd 1983). Hall (1980) suggests that this is not easy, and perhaps the most difficult part of guiding and advising ward staff is to communicate an expectation of change in the patients that is positive and yet at the same time realistic.

In the following section only a brief summary is given of rehabilitation techniques with long-stay psychiatric patients, as many of these areas are dealt with in more detail in other chapters. Rigorous treatment of the underlying disorder by the psychiatrist, and regular drug reviews to prevent iatrogenic damage from the therapeutic regimen are imperative. Reversal of institutional neurosis by modification of the environment and nurse–patient interaction is discussed in a following section. Behavioural techniques are effective in changing behaviour. Ethical objections are raised in all forms of behaviour therapy, and these must be considered. The important questions, though, are therapeutic ones: how quickly will the new behaviours extinguish if reward is withdrawn, and whether this is really a good preparation for discharge. In the outside world the relationship between behaviour and reward is not so simple or constant. Nevertheless, token economies have been found to bring about quite remarkable behaviour changes in regressed chronic schizophrenics. The value of group activities, occupational, recreational and social therapies is covered in Chapter 44.

The nurse may also be usefully engaged in regular, larger scale assessments which provide an overall picture and monitor progress, particularly as long-time spans are involved. An example of such a scale is the Morningside Rehabilitation Status Scale (Affleck & McGuire 1984). Such an assessment of the individual patient, to be repeated at each stage of rehabilitation, was recommended by the Working Party of the Royal College of Psychiatrists (1980).

Physical and psychosocial environment

The attitudes of nurses are particularly relevant in the light of Wing & Brown's (1970) discussion of secondary handicaps. The relationship of these handicaps to the environment can be understood by considering them to be similar to secondary deviance. It is argued that once a patient is admitted to hospital, he is obliged to adjust and to conform to the expectations of the staff. Patients who originally have no intention of staying in hospital gradually change their attitudes and may not wish to leave. As the hospital provides all necessities, so motivation to leave dwindles. For various reasons, relatives and friends gradually stop coming; these reasons include long journeys, unattractive wards, pestering by other patients. Consequently, the gap between the hospital and the outside world widens. Bennett (1980) suggests that the determinants of long hospital stay are a mixture of clinical, social and demographic variables.

Traditional wards provided little privacy and personal territory, with few patients having their own possessions. Patients cannot retain personal information about themselves if it is public property to be shared by all the staff. Some wards remain physically unattractive, unstimulating, dirty and noisy. Communication with fellow patients can be difficult. The effect on patients of a ward environment characterized by poor physical surroundings, under-stimulation and apathy of other patients is to increase what Wing (1970) called 'clinical poverty syndrome'. The patient draws away from other people and environment by reduced communication. Flatness of affect and poverty of speech then emerge. Altschul (1972) identified a lack of interaction on psychiatric wards when she defined interaction as an event where nurse and patient talked together for 5 minutes or more. She found that 40% of patients had no interaction, while some nurses never interacted with some patients; the longer a patient stayed in hospital the less likely they were to interact with nurses, and the more senior a nurse became the less likely she was to interact with patients. The reasons advanced for this included:

1. The original diagnosis: schizophrenia and institutionalization.
2. The social structure of the ward, with the nurses being identified with authority.
3. Nurses are taught not to get involved.
4. Talking with patients is a low priority — a residual activity if there are no other jobs on the ward.

The potential for nurses to act in a stimulating manner and to maintain social interaction is described by Breton & Cockram (1977) in a report on a programme designed to increase sociability and spontaneity among long-term patients.

Traditional staff structures are very hierarchal. This is thought to increase authoritarian attitudes, with the patient being at the bottom of the hierarchy. The social distance created between the nurse and patient is a characteristic of restrictive authoritarian environments. Areas of the ward are specially designated for staff use only. The staff may wear 'protective' and 'identifying' uniforms. Sometimes the forms of address are non-reciprocal, to indicate status differences. In contrast to these records of interaction, staff–patient distance and authoritarianism, Garety & Morris (1984) noted, in a description and evaluation of a new unit for long-stay psychiatric patients, staff optimism, patient oriented practices and perceived involvement in decision-making as being positive attitudes contributing to a therapeutic milieu. Similarly, Wing & Brown (1970) showed that the staff with the most optimistic attitudes were employed in the hospitals with the least restrictive environments. Barton (1966) has suggested that, in order to combat institutionalization, the patient's living environment should encourage:

1. contact with the outside world
2. personal possessions and personal events
3. a homely permissive ward atmosphere
4. patient involvement in planning and decision-making.

Nurses need to believe that long-stay patients can be rehabilitated. Currently, the expectation of success with this group of patients is low and so becomes a self-fulfilling prophecy.

Towell & Harries (1979) describe an example of action research in a psychiatric hospital which was aimed at counteracting such a situation. They describe changes that were brought about at a psychiatric hospital following the appointment of a social research adviser. The adviser responded to invitations from wards or units for help. It was important that the initiative come from ward level and not management. One example of a study on a long-stay ward which identified a need to change is the following. The researcher helped the nurses to devise an interview schedule to use with patients to get to know them better and provide useful information. Each nurse was made responsible for interviewing certain patients and reporting back to a special meeting. At first, the researcher took a leading role in the groups, helping them to understand the material gathered in the interviews. Eventually, that function was taken over by a senior nurse. As a result of the interviews, patient allocation was introduced, care became more individualized and nurse–patient interactions moved in the direction of a counselling approach. From the development of this interview schedule, a number of improvements occurred which culminated in a dramatic increase in discharge rates.

This example illustrates how the introduction of a nursing process approach would bring about changes and certain clear benefits. These include:

- individual identification of need and planning
- patient involvement in planning
- closer nurse–patient relationships.

Nursing organization of psychiatric units

Over two decades ago, Wing et al (1964) described rehabilitation as a series of small steps. The outcomes of such steps are difficult to predict but the result at each stage determines whether it is possible to move on to the next. The practical consequences of this were taken up by Barton (1966) and Early (1968) in advocating the 'ladder system' where the patient is seen as taking steps up the rungs, with the assumption that at the end of the process he would emerge as an individual able to cope with instrumental tasks and adult roles; and, in so doing, the patient with cognitive defects would be able to grasp such notions as progress and the future. Many patients, however, do not recognize these concepts. This is perhaps best demonstrated by the accumulation of patients along the way in day centres (Richards 1971), in hostels (Hewett et al 1975) and on the wards where the toughest problems collect. Implicit in such a system is the process of selection which is widely advocated. Hall (1983) suggests that one of the first steps in rehabilitation, irrespective of the type of regimen, is to carry out at least some selection; although in practice the opportunity to select an entire ward on the basis of level of handicap is unusual. There are, however, serious negative consequences of such a system. When the majority of patients on a ward designated 'rehabilitation' actually have little prospect of leaving and need residential care for the rest of their lives, an anomalous two-tier system may develop in one rehabilitation unit. The medical model encourages such anomalies. There is a danger, too, that nurses' vulnerable morale will be threatened by poor facilities and low multi-disciplinary involvement.

The provision of support and counselling is now being recognized as an essential part of rehabilitation (Ekdawi 1980, Bennett & Morris 1983), and the potential for the nurse working in this area is being acknowledged (Grant 1980, Ramsden 1980, Bennett & Morris 1983).

In a study by Mitchell & Birley (1982) concerning the use of ward support by psychiatric patients in the community, it was found that there were two distinct patterns of uptake. Some patients used the ward support in an 'unengaged' way — a high rate of visits for 'company without intimacy' by those requiring an accepting atmosphere. Other patients found that it provided a more active normal social contact and had a lower rate of visits.

The specific important task of supporting and counselling relatives is only just beginning to be appreciated. Support has now been shown to be a crucial factor in the care of mentally disabled people, and the relatives involved need all the help they can get. Wing (1983) suggests that nurses often prove the most sympathetic helpers, since they themselves take over the responsibility for patients from relatives from time to time and are in a position to understand the problems of management that can arise from day to day.

The concept of support also embraces security and protection, which together are recognized as important functions of nursing. The participants in the author's study reiterated this (Macdonald 1985). It is argued that the most severely disabled patient needs the degree of shelter and support provided by a hospital environment. This, indeed, may be a specific gain for a patient when compared to the loss over the years in accepting such care. The asylum provided both shelter and support but this was irrespective of individual need, so that for some it may have extinguished the patients' resources (Bennett & Morris 1983). Support that focuses upon disability and pathology is more likely to promote dependency than that directed towards the encouragement of skills, autonomy and self-reliance. Thus the provision of shelter or support should not be concentrated in those areas where the patient can already function adequately. Supportive environment must be designed to improve the functioning of the disabled person. It has often been assumed that these aims would be best achieved by moving support and shelter out of the institution. However, in day visits and centres (Shepherd & Richardson 1979) evidence of institutional practice was found. The components which are likely to lead to institutionalization can be present in other settings including hostels, workshops and families. Shepherd & Richardson (1979) concluded that the effectiveness of long-term care is therefore ultimately dependent on the exact nature of the service and not on its location.

The nurse's role

In the author's study, a low proportion of nurses in psychiatric rehabilitation could not identify any specific role in their field apart from giving a description of their work (Macdonald 1985). However, those in the study who did suggest a role for themselves described a role model or parent figure. The parental role is identified by Ramsden (1980), who also points out that it is difficult to know when to adopt and when to relinquish such a role. There are overtones of the nurturing mother figure described by Schilman (1960) and Hessler (1980), who deal with the everday aspects of living in which there is an element of intimacy, tenderness and compassion. But, as Altschul (1980) observes, the role of the mother normally gives her not only obligations towards her dependent offspring, but also rights to make demands for approved behaviour from the child.

Various authors refer to the nurse as a model, a representative of normality and carrier of the important healthy attitudes of expectations for normal living, e.g. hygiene, table manners and dressing. The nurse may be the patient's only contact with a person from outside the institution. Being a model implies that the patients are able to learn from this, which for some will be limited. Ramsden (1980) included these aspects in describing the role of the nurse as teacher imparting practical knowledge and social skills. Participatory teaching is an essential component.

Certain problems have been documented in the literature concerning the role of the nurse in psychiatric rehabilitation. The realization that not all chronic patients will leave the hospital has profound implications for nurses. For some nurses the raison d'être must be that of improving the 'quality of life' of patients. Wing (1980) suggests that preservation of the best level possible is a humane and dignified task, and the morale of staff involved is likely to be sustained if their training and function are clearly identified within the rehabilitation framework. Practically however, this may be problematic. Wing & Brown's (1970) account showed that positive change can be achieved and then reversed. Hicks & Tutt (1982) stated that in their situation the maintenance of 'enthusiastic staff' depended upon an influx of new staff every few years. Staff who remain on the same ward for many years may become set in their ways. Ramsden (1980) advocates that rehabilitation is as much about failure as about success, and the pressures to fall back on institutional and custodial practices are always very great.

Historically, nurses have been trained to care for people, whereas now they are called upon to help people to care for themselves and so the traditional role of the nurse is out of place with its authoritarian and rigid attitudes and concern over routines. Associated with this are the responsibility and accountability of the nurse to protect the patient and the community. Unless these issues are resolved, the possibility of independence for patients remains doubtful (Morgan & Cheadle 1974, Ramsden 1980). A grievance commonly voiced by nurses is lack of adequate numbers of staff but Macdonald (1985) suggests that this is genuine when only two or three staff are on a shift for a ward of up to 30 patients. Low staff levels are characteristic of long-term care. In a parallel situation on geriatric wards, Wells (1980) has suggested that the constant cry for more staff is based on a belief that, should better nurse–patient ratios be available, this would solve all problems and that this is a rationalization to alleviate feelings of failure. Improvements in patient care do not necessarily follow from improved staffing. Harris et al (1974) found that an increase in the number of staff did not necessarily improve the quality of social interaction. Raynes et al (1979) proposed that these circumstances would lead to an increase in staff–staff interaction at the expense of staff–patient communication.

CONCLUSION

Views within the profession concerning the role of the nurse in psychiatric rehabilitation are still evolving and will continue to do so. Historically, great emphasis was placed on institutional care but recent developments have brought about a radical reassessment. Nurses need to develop a body of knowledge regarding the specific nature of their work, in working with the patients individually and in the organization of therapeutic environments where individual assessment of patients should produce specific and flexible care.

REFERENCES

Affleck J W, McGuire R J 1984 The measurement of psychiatric rehabilitation status. A review of the needs and a new scale. British Journal of Psychiatry 145: 517–525

Altschul A T 1972 Patient nurse interaction: a study of interaction in acute psychiatric wards. Churchill Livingstone, Edinburgh

Altschul A T 1980 The role of professionals: psychiatry under review — 3. Nursing Times 76: 555–556

Barton R 1966 Institutional neurosis. Wright, Briston

Bennett D H 1980 The chronic psychiatric patient today. Journal of the Royal Society of Medicine 7: 301–303

Bennett D H, Morris I 1983 Support and rehabilitation. In: Watts F N, Bennett D H (eds) Theory and practice of psychiatric rehabilitation. Wiley, Chichester

Bennett D H, Watts F N 1983 The concept of rehabilitation. In: Watts F N, Bennett D H (eds) Theory and practice of psychiatric rehabilitation. Wiley, Chichester

Breton S, Cockram M 1977 A simple programme designed to counteract some of the effects of institutionalization in long term wards. Journal of Advanced Nursing 2: 495–501

Burgess A W 1981 Psychiatric nursing in the hospital and community, 3rd edn. Prentice-Hall, Englewood Cliffs, NJ

Cohen D 1988 The forgotten millions. Paladin Books, London

Department of Health and Social Security 1975 Better services for the mentally ill. Cmmd 6233. HMSO, London

DOH 1976 Mental Health Enquiry, HMSO, London

Early A F 1968 The industrial therapy organization 1960–1965. British Journal of Psychiatry 2: 1–13

Ekdawi M 1980 The role of day units in rehabilitation. In: Wing J K & Morris B (eds) Handbook of psychiatric rehabilitation practice. Oxford Medical Publications, Oxford, Ch 9

Garety P A, Morris I 1984 A new unit for long stay psychiatric patients: organizations, attitudes and quality of care. Psychological Medicine 14: 183–192

Goffman E 1961 Asylums. Penguin, London

Goldstone L A 1977 Long stay of patient population in a psychiatric hospital. Part 2: Nurses opinions and assessments. Nursing Mirror 73 (12): 71–72

Grant P 1980 The role of the nurse. In: Wing J K, Morris B (eds) Handbook of psychiatric rehabilitation practice. Oxford Medical Publications, Oxford

Hall J 1980 Ward-based rehabilitation programmes. Theory and practice of psychiatric rehabilitation. In: Wing J K, Morris B (eds) Handbook of psychiatric rehabilitation practice. Oxford Medical Publications, Oxford

Harris J, Veint S, Allen G, Chinsky J 1974 Aide resident ratio and ward population density as mediators of social interaction. American Journal of Mental Deficiency 72: 320–326

Hessler I 1980 Roles, status and relationships in psychiatric nursing. Psychiatry under review 2. Nursing Times 76: 508–509

Hewett S, Ryan P, Wing J K 1975 Living with the mental hospitals. Journal of Social Policy 4: 391–404

Hicks J, Tutt M 1982 A progressive approach to rehabilitation. Nursing Times Occasional Paper 29. 78: 81–84

Lewis S 1980 The role of the nurse. In: Wing J K, Morris B (eds) Handbook of psychiatric rehabilitation practice. Oxford Medical Publications, Oxford

National Association of Mental Health (MIND) 1974 Co-ordination or chaos. The run down of psychiatric hospitals. Report No. 13. MIND, London

Macdonald H 1985 A humane and dignified task? An exploratory study of nursing in rehabilitation. BSc thesis, Kings College, London, Unpublished

Mann S A, Cree W 1976 'New' long stay psychiatric patients: a national sample survey of 15 mental hospitals in England and Wales 1972/73. Psychological Medicine 6: 603–616

Mitchell S, Birley J 1982 The use of ward support by psychiatric patients in the community. British Journal of Psychiatry 142: 9–15

Morgan R 1980 A regional rehabilitation unit. In: Wing J K, Morris B (eds) Handbook of psychiatric rehabilitation practice. Oxford Medical Publications, Oxford

Morgan R, Cheadle J 1974 A scale of disability and prognosis in long-term mental illness. British Journal of Psychiatry 125: 475–478

Parsons T 1961 Social structure and dynamic process. The case of modern medical practice. In: Parsons T (ed) The social system. Free Press, New York

Ramsden A 1980 The role of the nurse. In: Wing J K, Morris B (eds) Handbook of psychiatric rehabilitation practice. Oxford Medical Publications, Oxford

Rapaport R N, Rosow I 1960 Community as doctor. Tavistock, London

Raynes N, Pratt M 1979 Organizational structure and care of the mentally retarded. Croom Helm, London

Richards H 1971 Local authority day centre for the mentally ill. Lancet i: 793–795

Royal College of Psychiatrists 1980 Report of the Working Party on Rehabilitation: psychiatric rehabilitation in the 1980s. Royal College of Psychiatrists, London

Schilman S, 1960 Basic functional role of nursing. In: Jacu E G (ed) Patients, physicians and illness. Free Press, New York

Shepherd G, Richardson A 1979 Organization and interaction in psychiatric day centres. Psychological Medicine 8: 573–579

Shepherd G 1985 Planning the rehabilitation of the individual. In: Watts F N, Bennett D H (eds) Theory and practice of psychiatric rehabilitation. Wiley, Chichester

Strauss R 1966 Social change and the rehabilitation concept. In: Sussman M B (ed) Sociology and rehabilitation. American Sociological Association, Washington

Towell D, Harries C 1979 Innovations in patient care. Croom Helm, London

Wells T J 1980 Problems in geriatric nursing care. Churchill Livingstone, Edinburgh

Wing J K 1963 Rehabilitation of psychiatric patients. British Journal of Psychiatry 109: 635–641

Wing J K 1980 Clinical basis of psychiatric rehabilitation. In: Wing J K, Morris B (eds) Handbook of psychiatric rehabilitation practice. Oxford Medical Publications,

Oxford, ch 1

Wing J K 1983 Schizophrenia. In: Watts F N, Bennett D H (eds) Theory and practice of psychiatric rehabilitation. Chichester

Wing J K, Freudenberh R 1961 The response of severely ill chronic schizophrenic patients to social situations. American Journal of Psychiatry 118: 311–322

Wing J K, Bennett D H, Denham J 1964 The industrial rehabilitation of long-stay schizophrenic patients. Medical Research Memo 420. HMSO, London

Wing J K, Brown G W 1970 Institutionalism and schizophrenia — a comparative study of three mental hospitals. Cambridge University Press, London

World Health Organization 1976 Mental Health Services for Europe. HMSO, London

Index